Concepts of Fitness and Wellness

A COMPREHENSIVE LIFESTYLE APPROACH

third edition

Charles B. Corbin

Arizona State University

Ruth Lindsey

California State University—Long Beach

Greg Welk

Cooper Institute for Aerobics Research

Boston   Burr Ridge, IL   Dubuque, IA   Madison, WI   New York   San Francisco   St. Louis
Bangkok   Bogotá   Caracas   Lisbon   London   Madrid
Mexico City   Milan   New Delhi   Seoul   Singapore   Sydney   Taipei   Toronto

McGraw-Hill Higher Education

A Division of The McGraw-Hill Companies

CONCEPTS OF FITNESS AND WELLNESS: A COMPREHENSIVE LIFESTYLE APPROACH, THIRD
EDITION

This book is printed on recycled, acid-free paper containing 10% postconsumer waste.

2 3 4 5 6 7 8 9 0 QPD/QPD 0 9 8 7 6 5 4 3 2 1 0

ISBN 0–697–29566–4

Vice president and editorial director: *Kevin T. Kane*
Publisher: *Edward E. Bartell*
Executive editor: *Vicki Malinee*
Developmental editor: *Tricia R. Musel*
Senior marketing manager: *Pamela S. Cooper*
Project manager: *Renee C. Russian*
Senior production supervisor: *Mary E. Haas*
Coordinator of freelance design: *Michelle D. Whitaker*
Photo research coordinator: *John C. Leland*
Senior supplement coordinator: *Audrey A. Reiter*
Compositor: *Precision Graphics*
Typeface: *10/12 Times Roman*
Printer: *Quebecor Printing Book Group/Dubuque, IA*

Freelance cover/interior designer: *Rebecca Lloyd Lemna*
Cover image: © *Richard Price/FPG International*
Photo research: *Connie Gardner Picture Research*

The credits section for this book begins on page C-1 and is considered
an extension of the copyright page.

Library of Congress Cataloging-in-Publication Data

Corbin, Charles B.
   Concepts of fitness and wellness : a comprehensive lifestyle
approach / Charles B. Corbin, Ruth Lindsey, Greg Welk. — 3rd ed.
     p. cm.
   Includes bibliographical references and index.
   ISBN 0–697–29566–4
    1. Exercise. 2. Physical fitness problems, exercises, etc.
I. Lindsey, Ruth, 1926– . II. Welk, Greg. III. Title.
RA781.C644   2000
613.7—dc21   99–14990
                            CIP

www.mhhe.com

Contents

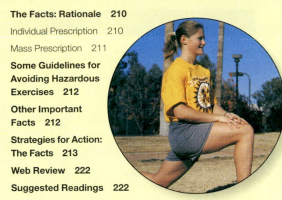

Section IV

Physical Activity: Special Considerations

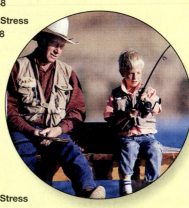

Section VII

Avoiding Destructive Behaviors

Section VIII

Making Informed Choices

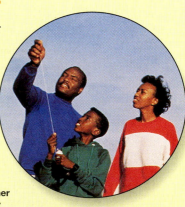

Preface for the Instructor

Meeting the Challenges of the New Millennium

The publication of this third edition, *Concepts of Fitness and Wellness: A Comprehensive Lifestyle Approach,* occurs in the year 2000, the beginning of the new millennium. With the challenges of the new millennium, we feel the addition of a new author, Greg Welk of The Cooper Institute for Aerobics Research, will continue our tradition of excellence in writing and research. As the new subtitle implies, the focus of the third edition is on lifestyle changes that help prevent disease and, more importantly, promote good fitness and wellness. This focus on lifestyle change is consistent with national health goals for the year 2010, which emphasize taking control of personal behaviors as part of permanent lifestyle change. The new focus for the new millennium is a "process" rather than the "product."

As we pioneered the development of fitness and wellness classes over 30 years ago, we focused on trying to get people fit and well. To be sure, fitness is an important product, as is wellness, another product of healthy lifestyle change. But scientific advances have shown that health, fitness, and wellness (all products) are not things you can "do" to people. You have to help them help themselves. Educating them and giving them the self-management skills that help them adopt healthy lifestyles can do this.

The focus of the new millennium is on the *process*. Healthy lifestyles, or what a person does, rather than what a person can do, constitute process. If a person does the process (i.e., adopting a healthy lifestyle), positive changes will occur to the extent that change is possible for that specific person. As noted in the first concept of the book, lifestyles are the most important factors, influencing health, fitness, and wellness. Healthy lifestyles (the processes) are also within a person's individual control. *Any person* can benefit from lifestyle change, and any person can change a lifestyle. These lifestyle changes will make a difference in health, fitness, and wellness for all people.

The emphasis on lifestyle change in the third edition is consistent with the focus of national health objectives for the new millennium. Though the principal national health goals are to increase years and quality of life (products) for all people, the methods of accomplishing these goals focus on changing lifestyles. As we move into the new century, we must adopt a new way of thinking to help all people change their lifestyles to health, fitness, and wellness.

New Features of this Edition

The HELP Philosophy

The "new way of thinking" for the new millennium is based on the HELP philosophy, which is outlined and emphasized in the text. **H** is for *health*. Health and its positive component—wellness—are central to the philosophy. Health, fitness, and wellness are for all people. **E** is for *everyone*. **L** is for *lifetime lifestyle* change, and **P** is for *personal*. The goal is to HELP all people to make personal lifetime lifestyle changes that promote health, fitness, and wellness.

The book adheres to this HELP philosophy. To assure that it is useful to everyone, we include discussions to adapt healthy lifestyles based on personal needs. Separate sections are *not* included for specific groups such as older people, women, ethnic groups, or those with special needs. Rather, we focus on healthy lifestyles *for all people* throughout the book.

Meeting Higher-Order Objectives

The "new way of thinking" based on the HELP philosophy suggests that each person must make decisions about healthy lifetime lifestyles if the goals of longevity and quality of life are to be achieved. What one person chooses may be quite different from what another chooses. Accordingly, our goal in preparing the third edition is to help readers to become good problem solvers and decision makers. Rather than focusing on telling them what to do, we offer information to help readers make informed choices about lifestyles. The stairway to lifetime fitness and wellness that we present helps readers understand the importance of "higher-order objectives" devoted to problem solving and decision making.

Strategies for Action

You will notice a new system of organization as well as many other new features in this edition. These changes are designed to put the HELP philosophy and higher-order objectives into action. The changes are also designed to increase the educational effectiveness of the book. At the end of each concept, *strategies for action* are provided. These are suggestions for putting content into action. Many of these strategies require readers to perform or practice self-assessment or other self-management techniques.

Organization

Consistent with the focus on process or lifestyle change, the table of contents has changed to sequentially study healthy lifestyles. The concepts are rearranged in several ways. First, the focus is on lifestyles rather than fitness. The physical activity concepts are organized sequentially around the physical activity pyramid. Nutrition and stress management are two additional priority healthy lifestyles that follow. A section on time management is added to one of the two stress concepts, which both have expanded coverage. Second, the concepts on planning are moved up to help students begin the planning process early. Third, the concept on body composition has been placed with nutrition after the physical activity concepts. This is done at the request of several reviewers. Finally, a new concept on performance is added. While the focus of the book is on lifestyle changes for health, fitness, and wellness, there are people who are especially interested in high-level performance. The new concept provides information for these people.

Activity Features with Activity Labs

Each of the exercises described in the book is now contained in new activity features using the new magazine format. This format allows students to get immediately involved in activity and to keep activity logs using the newly designed labs. New "Basic 8" tables feature many new and easy to use exercises.

Web Icons

As we begin the new millennium, it is appropriate that students be provided with state-of-the-art technology to promote educational effectiveness. The web icons are unique to this book. It allows learners to locate (at point of use) additional pictures, tables, and figures that illustrate concepts presented in the book. Web addresses to supplemental resource materials such as a self-study guide, sample exam questions, and definitions of terms, as well as other enrichment materials, are also provided on the Online Learning Center.

Redesigned and Expanded Labs

There are many new labs in this third edition. Some of these labs were created based on recommendations of users. They are designed to get users involved in practicing self-management skills that will promote healthy lifestyle change. The labs are in a new attractive and educationally effective format. They are easy to find and easy to use. In many cases, lab resource materials that aid the student in performing lab activities precede them. These resources are retained in the book even when the labs are torn out. This allows future use of such materials as fitness self-assessments. The physical activity labs are designed to get people active early in the course and ultimately to allow each user to plan his or her own personal activity program.

Focus on Self-Management Skills

The educational effectiveness of a book depends on more than just presenting information. If lifestyle changes are to be implemented, there must be opportunities to learn how to make these changes. Research suggests that learning self-management skills is important to lifestyle change. A new expanded section is included early in the book, and additional discussions of how to practice and implement these skills are included throughout the book.

Health Goals for the Year 2010

The health goals are based on the revised health goals for the new millennium (Health Goals for the Year 2010). These goals are provided at the beginning of each concept to help readers relate content to goals.

Magazine Format

The attractive format supports student reading and studying with a more appealing look in a new magazine format. This format has been shown to be educationally effective.

Student User's Guide

This new guide follows the Preface to the Instructor, and it is designed to help students use the book more effectively. Instructors are encouraged to urge students to read this section prior to using the book.

Terms at Point-of-Use

It greatly pleased us that the *Surgeon General's Report on Physical Activity and Health* adopted our physical fitness definitions in their report. Just as we have led the way in defining fitness, we now include state-of-the-art definitions related to wellness and quality of life. These—and all other definitions—are now included at the first point-of-use to make them easier to locate.

Continued Use of Conceptual Format

We use concepts rather than chapters, and each concept contains factual statements that follow concise informational paragraphs. This tried-and-true method has proven to be educationally sound and well received by students and instructors.

Pedagogical Aids

Suggested Readings

Because students want to know more about a particular topic, a list of readings is given at the end of each chapter. Most suggested readings arc readily available at bookstores or public libraries.

Appendixes

Concepts of Fitness and Wellness: A Comprehensive Lifestyle Approach, third edition, includes five appendixes that are valuable resources for the student. The metric conversion chart, metric conversions of selected charts and tables. Caloric guide to common foods, calories of protein, carbohydrates, and fats in food, and the Canadian food guide are included for your use.

Ancillaries

A Note for Instructors

As with past editions, you will see that we have updated this edition with the most recent scientific information. As noted earlier, we have changed the organization, and we have included many new labs that require learners to participate in healthy lifestyles. We have designed experiences to promote higher-order thinking. There is another consideration we think to be important. As usual, we have worked to keep the price of the book low. We have eliminated section pages, reduced the number of concepts, and reduced duplication to achieve this goal.

As always with our *Concepts* books, an extensive list of ancillary materials is available to help you provide the most effective instruction. Brief descriptions of these materials follow.

Instructor's Resource Materials

Instructor's Manual (IM)

The Instructor's Manual contains all new lesson plans, as well as lab plans, suggestions for grading, audiovisual resources, sources of equipment, objectives, and discussion questions.

Microtest III

A completely revised version of our computerized testing software is available with the new editions of *Concepts.* This test bank software provides a unique combination of user-friendly aids that enables the instructor to select, edit, delete, or add questions, as well as construct and print tests and answer keys. The computerized test bank package is available for IBM Windows and Macintosh computers.

Course Organizer

In order to put it all together, we offer this special course-planning binder, which conveniently organizes all the ancillary package items with tabbed dividers.

Visual Resources

PowerPoint Presentation Program. With the publication of the third edition, we continue to provide PowerPoint slide presentations for instructor use. This is also available as a gratis downloadable ancillary on the Concepts book-specific web site. **www.mhhe.com/hper/physed/clw**.

Instructional Videos

Video 1: Introduction to Physical Fitness. This video includes a statement of fitness philosophy, a look at important fitness objectives, including the Stairway to Lifetime Fitness, and a description of the fitness tests included in the *Concepts* books. Test descriptions include estimated 1 RM for strength, the trunk rotation test for flexibility, and the curl-up test for muscular endurance. Other fitness test descriptions are newly described. This video may be viewed by instructors or shown to students to help them understand the various tests. It has been proven popular with both students and instructors. The HELP philosophy is part of the flow of the video presentation of concepts.

Video 2: Introduction to Wellness. This second instructional video defines wellness and puts wellness, health, and fitness in perspective for both students and instructors. The video helps establish common ground for the study of wellness. This proven video has helped provide the basic foundation for the study of wellness that is needed by many students.

The Lifetime Fitness Concepts Course Video Series

This is a series of fifteen 28-minute video programs designed to provide basic conceptual physical fitness information to young adults. When used in conjunction with either of the *Concepts* textbooks on fitness and wellness, the videos help interested students learn how to do self-tests of fitness and wellness, plan effective lifetime fitness and wellness programs, and learn concepts that will make them better fitness and wellness decision makers, problem solvers, and informed consumers.

McGraw-Hill *Fitness and Wellness* Transparencies

Illustrations and graphics are available as transparency acetates. Attractively printed in full color, these useful tools facilitate learning and classroom discussion. They were chosen specifically to help explain complex concepts.

Concepts Transparencies

Fifty four-color acetate transparencies illustrate anatomical and physiological concepts, and help instructors to describe the scientific concepts of physical fitness and health-related fitness.

Student Self-Assessment Materials

Fitness/Wellness *Profile Diskette.*   This proven computer diskette includes several valuable fitness and wellness program applications that will enhance student learning. Included are a fitness evaluation profile as well as the target heart rate, heart disease risk, and nutrition and stress programs, which have proven to be effective in the past. The fitness profile allows students to enter fitness test results and receive ratings on a "learn as you go" basis. Ratings and test results can be displayed on the computer screen or printed on paper. This profile is excellent for use in program planning.

The Fitness Analyst Software.   This software is designed to provide comprehensive support for health and fitness appraisal, prescription, and performance tracking. It is ideally suited to provide student/client appraisal data, generate exercise prescription, track performance data, and create well-designed and informative charts and reports. Five disks for Standard Edition and six disks for the Master Edition runs on IBM and compatibles and in Windows-based platforms.

Fitsolve II Software.   Fitsolve is educational software designed to facilitate the teaching of high-order physical fitness objectives such as self-evaluation, diagnosis, and problem-solving skills, which in turn enable the achievement of fitness independence, and a state of self-sufficiency in which individuals can design and implement their own fitness programs.

Mosby's NutriTrac Software.   Available for Windows and Macintosh computers, this nutrient-analysis software allows you and your students to analyze diets easily, using an icon-based interface and on-screen help features. Foods for breakfast, lunch, dinner, and snacks may be selected from more than 2,250 items in the database. Records may be kept for any number of days. The program can provide intake analyses for individual foods, meals, days, or for an entire intake period. Intake analyses can compare nutrient values to RDA or RNI values and to the USDA food guide pyramid and provide breakdowns of fat and calorie sources.

Testwell *by the National Wellness Institute.*   This is a self-scoring, pencil-and-paper wellness assessment booklet developed by the National Wellness Institute in Stevens Point, Wisconsin, and distributed exclusively by McGraw-Hill Publishers. It adds flexibility to any personal health or wellness course by allowing adopters to offer pre- and postassessments at the beginning, end, or anytime during the course.

Internet Resources

Book-Specific Web Site.   This is a special ancillary that allows instructors and students to get book-specific resources on the Web. Instructors and students can access the Online Learning Center to find online quizzes, interactive key terms, hot-off-the-press articles, and web links. The instructor using the book will have access to these downloadable ancillaries and much more. The web icons in the book indicate the location of web materials related to specific information present at that point of use.

Interactive CD-ROMs

HealthQuest *CD-ROM.*   *HealthQuest* is designed to help students explore the behavioral aspects of personal health and wellness through a state-of-the-art interactive CD-ROM. Your students will be able to assess their current health and wellness status, determine their health risks, and explore options and make decisions to improve the behaviors that impact their health.

Interactive Personal Trainer CD-ROM.   The Interactive Personal Trainer CD-ROM provides users with a variety of features. First, self-assessments for all parts of health-related fitness are provided. Still pictures and QuickTime movies illustrate the assessments, and written statements describe each one. Second, a fitness profile allows users to input assessment results to get a rating profile. In many cases (e.g., skinfolds), calculations are made automatically. Third, physical activities and exercises are provided for each part of fitness and for care of the back and good posture. Users can select exercises for any part of fitness or for different body parts and get descriptions, still pictures and real-time videos of each. Finally, pictures and descriptions of risky exercises are provided followed by descriptions and real-time movies of appropriate alternatives. The CD-ROM is available in either Windows or Mac versions. Instructors may encourage use on a computer accessible to students.

Print Publications

UC Berkeley Wellness Letter. This highly regarded health-related newsletter keeps you informed of the latest developments in the health and wellness field.

The AIDS Booklet, sixth edition, **by Frank Cox.** This booklet provides current and accurate facts about AIDS and HIV: what it is, how the disease is transmitted, its prevalence among various population groups, symptoms of HIV infection, strategies for prevention, etc. Also included are various legal, social, medical, and ethical issues related to HIV and AIDS. Updated semiannually, this short booklet makes HIV and AIDS understandable to your students and insures that they get the most current information possible on HIV and AIDS.

Acknowledgments

It is only fitting as we enter the new millennium that we acknowledge those people who have contributed to the development of this book over its 30+ year history. For this edition an exceptionally large number of people contributed reviews and comments. At the risk of inadvertently failing to mention someone, we want to acknowledge the following people for their role in the development of this book.

First, we would like to acknowledge a few people who have made special contributions over the years. Linus Dowell, Carl Landiss, and Homer Tolson, all of Texas A & M University, were involved in the development of the first *Concepts* book, and their contributions were also important as we helped start the fitness movement in the 1960s. Other pioneers were Jimmy Jones of Henderson State University, who started one of the first *Concepts* classes in 1970 and led the way in teaching fitness in the years that followed; Charles Erickson, who started a quality program at Missouri Western; and Al Lesiter, a leader in the East at Mercer Community College in New Jersey. David Laurie and Barbara Gench (now at Texas Women's University) at Kansas State University, as well as others on that faculty, were instrumental in developing a prototype concepts program, which research has shown to be successful. A special thanks is extended to Andy Herrick and Jim Whitehead, who have contributed to much of the development of most recent editions of the book, including excellent suggestions for change. Mark Ahn, Keri Chesney, Chris MacCrate, Guy Mullin, Stephen Hustedde, Greg Nigh, Doreen Mauro, Marc vanHorne, along with other employees of the Consortium for Instructional Innovation and the Micro Computer Resource Facility at Arizona State University, and Betty Craft and Ken Rudich and other employees at the Distance Learning Technology Program at Arizona State University deserve special recognition.

Second, we wish to extend thanks to the following people who provided comments on the current editions of our *Concepts* books: David Horton, Liberty University; Robert Selvin, Towson University; Lindy S. Pickard, Broward Community College; Laura L. Borsdorf, Ursinus College; Frederick C. Surgent, Frostburg State University; James A. Gemar, Moorhead State University; Vincent Angotti, Towson University; Judi Phillips, Del Mar College; Joseph Donnelly, Montclair State University; Harold L. Rainwater, Asbury College; Candi D. Ashley, University of South Florida; Dennis Docheff, United States Military Academy; Robin Hoppenworth, Wartburg College; Linda Farver, Liberty University; Peter Rehor, Montana State University; Martin W. Johnson, Mayville State University; Keri Lewis, North Carolina State University; J. D. Parsley, University of St. Thomas; Marika Botha, Lewis-Clark State College; and Robert J. Mravetz, University of Akron.

Third, we want to acknowledge the following people who have aided us in the preparation of past editions: Debra A. Beal, Northern Essex Community College; Roger Bishop, Wartburg College; David S. Brewster, Indiana State University; Ronnie Carda, University of Wisconsin—Madison; Curt W. Cattau, Concordia University; Cindy Ekstedt Connelley, Catawaba College; J. Ellen Eason, Towson State University; Bridgit A. Finley, Oklahoma City Community College; Diane Sanders Flickner, Bethel College; Judy Fox, Indiana Wesleyan University; Earlene Hannah, Hendrix College; Carole J. Hanson, University of Northern Iowa; David Horton, Liberty University; John Merriman, Valdosta State College; Beverly F. Mitchell, Kennesaw State College; George Perkins, Northwestern State University; James J. Sheehan, Fitchburg State College; Mary Slaughter, University of Illinois; Paul H. Todd, Polk Community College; Susan M. Todd, Vancouver Community College—Langara Campus; Kenneth E. Weatherman, Floyd College; Newton Wilkes, Bridget Cobb, John Dippel, and Todd Kleinfelter of Northwestern State University of Louisiana and John R. Webster, Central Connecticut State University. A special thanks is extended to Patty Williams, Ann Woodard, Laurel Smith, Bill Carr (Polk Community College), James Angel, Jeanne Ashley, Stanley Brown, Ronnie Carda, Robert Clayton, Melvin Ezell Jr., Brigit Finley, Pay Floyd, Carole Hanson, James Harvey, John Hayes, David Horton, Sister Janice Iverson, Tony Jadin, Richard Krejei, Ron Lawman, James Marett, Pat McSwegin, Betty McVaigh, John Merriman, Beverly Mitchell, Sandra Morgan, Robert Pugh, Larry Reagan, Mary Rice, Roberts Stokes, Paul Tood, Susan Todd, Marjorie Avery Willard, Karen Cookson, Dawn Strout, Earlene Hannah, Ken Weatherman, J. Ellen Eason, William Podoll, John Webster, James Shebban, David Brewster, Kelly Adam, Lisa Hibbard, Roger Bishop, Mary Slaughter, Jack Clayton Stovall, Karen Watkins, Ruth Cohoon, Mark Bailey, Nena Amundson, Bruce Wilson, Sarah Collie, Carl Beal, George Perkins, Stan Rettew, Ragene Gwin, Judy Fox, Diane Flickner, Cindy Connelley, Curt Cattau, Don Torok, and Dennis Wilson.

Finally we want to acknowledge others who have contributed, including Virginia Atkins, Charles Cicciarella, Donna Landers, Susan Miller, Robert Pangrazi, Karen Ward, Darl Waterman, and Weimo Zhu. Among other important contributors are former graduate students who have contributed ideas, made corrections, and contributed in other untold ways to the success of these books. We wish to acknowledge Jeff Boone,

Laura Borsdorf, Lisa Chase, Tom Cuddihy, Darren Dale, Bo Fernhall, Ken Fox, Connie Fye, Louie Garcia, Steve Feyrer-Melk, Kirk Rose, Jack Rutherford, Scott Slava, Dave Thomas, Min Qui Wang, Jim Whitehead, and Ashley Woodcock.

Author Acknowledgments

A very special thanks goes to David E. Corbin of the University of Nebraska at Omaha and Karen Welk of Dallas, Texas. Dr. Corbin is a health educator who made valuable contributions to the stress and destructive habits concepts. Karen is a physical therapist who advised us concerning correct performance of the exercises in the book. Last, but not least, we want to thank Ron Hager and Lynda Ransdell. Dr. Hager was instrumental in assisting Greg Welk with the development of the Web resources and Dr. Ransdell was instrumental in the development of the test bank materials.

Preface for the Student

This book is designed to help you—the reader—adopt behaviors that lead to lifelong fitness, health, and wellness. The focus on lifetime behaviors (lifestyle change) is consistent with national health goals for the new millennium (the year 2010).

First, you are given a brief introduction to lifestyles for health, wellness, and fitness. Information is then presented to advise you about the fundamental principles and health benefits of physical activity. A variety of self-management skills are discussed and opportunities to practice these skills are provided in laboratory activities. You are also provided with information concerning nutrition and body composition, stress management, and other healthy lifestyles. The emphasis is on making informed choices about active healthy living.

Before you begin reading this book, it is important that you become familiar with its special features, each of which is designed to help you use the book more effectively.

Features

Concept Statement. Chapters in the book are referred to as concepts. Each concept begins with a title and a conceptual statement that characterizes the nature of the material. Be sure to read the statement prior to reading the content of the concept.

Health Goals. The health goals that appear on the second page of each concept (green box) are adapted from the national health goals (*Healthy People 2010*). These health goals help the reader understand how the content of each concept relates to meeting national health objectives. They are meant to be realistic goals that can be accomplished by the year 2010. A more complete description of the health goals is included at the beginning of Concept 1.

Concept Introduction. After the health goals, an introduction to each concept is provided. This expands on the concept statement and is designed to set the stage for the materials that follow.

Fact Statements. Each concept includes "fact statements" followed by a discussion that expands on the fact statement. Fact statements are important points that are highlighted as much as you might emphasize material with a highlighter in other books. We have done this for you.

Definitions of Terms. As you read, you will come across terms that are **bold.** All terms in bold are defined in a light-blue definition box on the right page. Look for this box when you see a bold-faced term.

Web Icons. As you read, you will come across icons to indicate that materials are available on the Web to supplement the content described in the book. Look for the icon in the book. To access the information, type the web address, URL). Then select the appropriate concept number, and the column (1 or 2) of the icon.

Exercise Features. In many of the concepts on physical activity, exercise features are included on specially tabbed pages. You can look at the side of the book and easily locate the dark-blue tabs. The featured exercises are ones you can incorporate into your personal plan and record on an activity log.

Strategies for Action. Toward the end of each concept you will find strategies for action, which provide a basis for action. You can find information about self-management skills that enhance adherence to healthy lifestyles. In many cases, the strategies refer you to labs that allow you to perform activities or refer you to informational sources that lend you to lifestyle changes.

Web Review. At the end of each concept, you will find Web Review section. These sites link you to study questions, sample test questions, supplemental pictures and tables, and the definitions of terms. You may get information about access to the Web at **www.mhhe.com/hper/physed/clw/student.**

Suggested Readings. Suggested readings are at the end of each concept. These readings are not original research articles but rather review articles that give easy-to-read, scientifically sound, information on topics covered in the concept. The research articles that document concept content are included in the reference list at the end of the book and in a supplementary list in Web Review.

Lab Resource Materials. Lab resource materials are special materials and information that you will need to complete the various lab activities in the book. They are on the yellow pages with dark red tabs that precede the labs. Unlike labs, lab resource materials are *not* meant to be torn from the book. You can re-use these if you removed the lab report pages from the book. Not all concepts contain lab resource materials.

Tear-Out Labs. The tear-out labs are located at the end of each concept. The page is bright yellow with a blue tab. Read the Purpose and Procedures sections carefully before entering data or answering questions. In many cases, the labs are self-explanatory, though some require lab resource materials. Some labs may require use of information from the appendix.

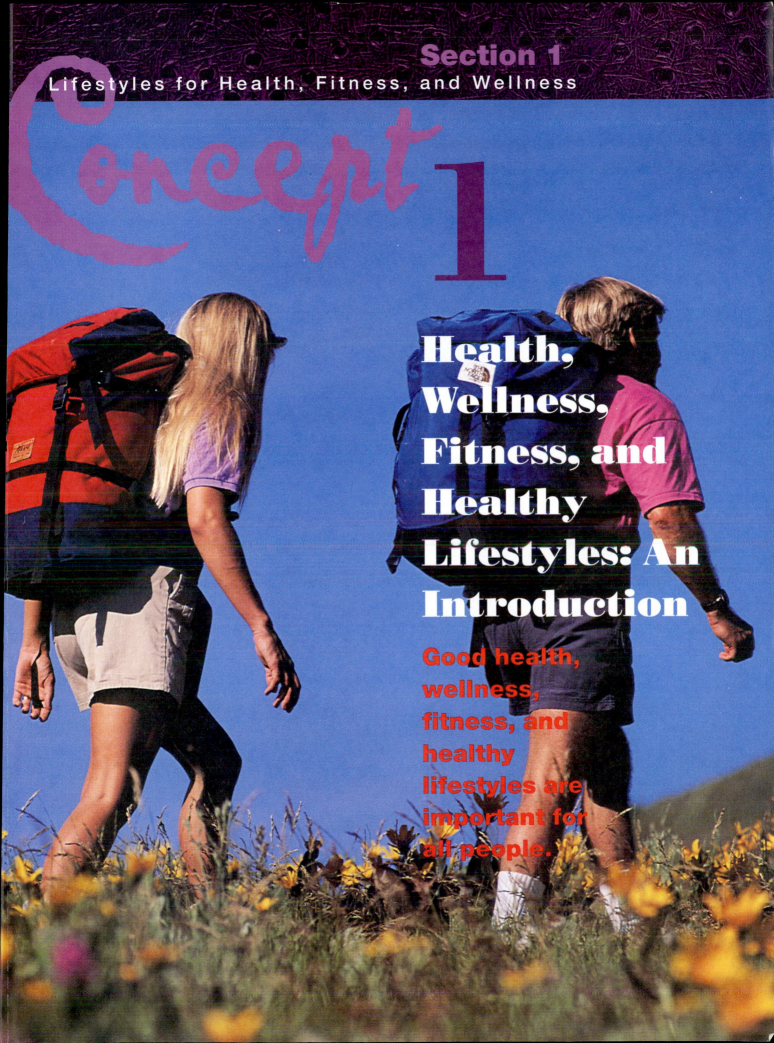

Concept 1

Health, Wellness, Fitness, and Healthy Lifestyles: An Introduction

Good health, wellness, fitness, and healthy lifestyles are important for all people.

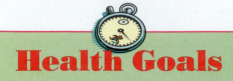

Health Goals
for the year 2010

Increase quality and years of healthy life.

Eliminate health disparities.

Increase incidence of people reporting "healthy days".

Increase incidence of people reporting "active days".

Increase access to health information and services for all people.

A Statement about National Health Goals

At the beginning of each concept in this book is a section containing abbreviated statements of the new national health goals from the document *Healthy People 2010: National Health Promotion and Disease Prevention Objectives.* These statements, established by expert groups representing more than 300 national organizations, are intended as realistic national health goals to be achieved by the year 2010. These objectives for the first decade of the new millennium, are intended to improve the health of those in the United States, but they seem important for all people in North America and in other industrialized cultures throughout the world. The health objectives are designed to contribute to the current World Health Organization strategy of "Health for All." This book is written with the achievement of these important health goals in mind.

Introduction

www.mhhe.com/hper/physed/clw/student/

The first national health goals were developed in 1979 to be accomplished by the year 1990. The focus of those objectives was on reduction in the death rate among infants, children, adolescents, young adults and adults. Except for reducing death rates among adolescents, those goals were met and the average life expectancy was increased by more than 2 years by the 1990s. Those first national health objectives gave way to the Healthy People 2000 objectives designed to be accomplished by the turn of the century. The emphasis in these objectives shifted from reduction in premature death to disease prevention and health promotion. While many of these objectives have been achieved, others have yet to be accomplished.

The goals of the Healthy People 2010 continue to focus on disease prevention and health promotion, but have areas of expanded focus. First, the goals emphasize quality of life, well-being, and functional capacity—all important wellness considerations. This emphasis is based on the World Health Organization statement that "It is counterproductive to evaluate development of programs without considering their impact on the quality of life of the community. We can no longer maintain strict, artificial divisions between physical and mental well-being (World Health Organization, 1995)." Second, the new national health goals take the "bold step" of trying to "eliminate" health disparities as opposed to reducing them as outlined in Healthy People 2000. Consistent with national health goals for the new millennium, this book is designed to aid all people in adopting healthy lifestyles that will allow them to achieve lifetime health, fitness and wellness.

The Facts about Health and Wellness

Good health is of primary importance to adults in our society.

When polled about important social values, 99 percent of adults in the United States identified "being in good **health**" as one of their major concerns. Two other concerns expressed most often were good family life and good self-image. The one percent who did not identify good health as an important concern had no opinion on any social issues. Among those polled, none felt that good health was unimportant. Results of surveys in Canada and other Western nations show similar commitments to good health.

Health varies greatly with income, gender, age, and family origin.

Reducing health disparities among adults over 18 is a major national health goal. We have some distance to go in accomplishing this goal because health varies widely depending on income, gender, age, and family origin. Self-ratings of health have been shown to be good general indicators of health status. When asked to rate health as excellent, good, fair, or poor, more than a few adults indicated that their health was only fair or poor (see Figure 1). It is evident that many more people in poor or near-poor income groups are considered to be fair or poor in health as opposed to good or excellent. African Americans and Hispanics are more often classified as fair or poor in health than white non-Hispanics. Minority women are also likely to be classified as fair or poor in health. Though not indicated in Figure 1, there is good evidence that older adults are especially likely to report poor health and wellness. An important national health goal is to increase the number of **healthy days** people have each month.

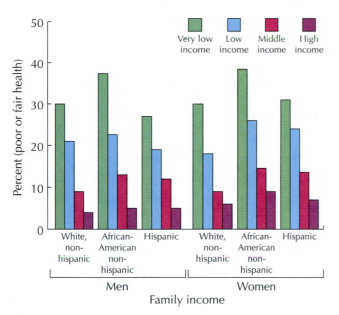

Figure 1

Fair or poor health among adults 18 and over by income, gender, and family origin.

NOTE: Percents are age adjusted.

SOURCE: Centers for Disease Control and Prevention, National Center for Health Statistics, National Health Interview Survey. *Health United States, 1998.*

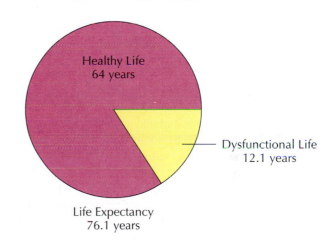

Figure 2

Life expectancy.

SOURCE: National Center for Health Statistics.

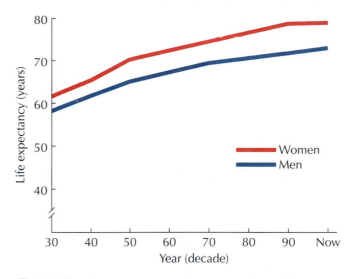

> Increasing the span of healthy life is a principal health goal.

www.mhhe.com/hper/physed/clw/student/
WEB
The principal public health goal of Western nations is to increase the healthy life span of all individuals. During this century, the life expectancy for the average person has increased by 60 percent. A child born in 1900 could expect to live only 47 years. By 1930, the life expectancy increased by more than 10 years; currently, the average life expectancy is slightly more than 76 years. As illustrated in Figure 2, women live longer than men, with the difference between men and women becoming more dramatic with each passing decade. Unfortunately, the average person can expect only about 64 years of healthy life. Approximately 12 years are characterized as dysfunctional or lacking in quality of life (see Figure 3). Disease and illness often associated with poor health limit length of life and contribute to the dysfunctional living.

> Health is more than freedom from illness and disease.

Over 50 years ago, the World Health Organization defined *health* as being more than freedom from illness, disease, and debilitating conditions. In recent years, public health experts

Figure 3

Years of healthy life as a proportion of life expectancy (U.S. population).

SOURCE: Data from *National Vital Statistics System* and *National Health Interview Survey.* Centers for Disease Control and Prevention, Atlanta, GA.

Health   Health is optimal well-being that contributes to quality of life. It is more than freedom from disease and illness, though freedom from disease is important to good health. Optimal health includes high-level mental, social, emotional, spiritual, and physical wellness within the limits of one's heredity and personal abilities.

Healthy days   A self-rating of the number of days (per week or month) a person considers himself or herself to be in good or better than good health.

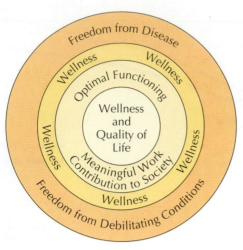

Figure 4
A model of optimal health including wellness.

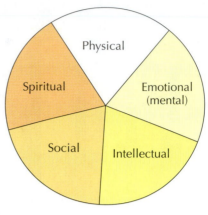

Figure 5
The dimensions of health and wellness.

have identified **wellness** as "a sense of well-being" and **"quality of life."** Healthy People 2010 objectives use the number of **"activity days"** as one indicator of wellness.

Many illnesses are manageable and have only limited effect on total health.

Many **illnesses** are curable and may have only a temporary effect on health. Others, such as diabetes, are not curable but can be managed with proper eating, physical activity, and sound medical supervision. It should be noted that those possessing manageable conditions may be more at risk for other health problems, so proper management is essential. For example, unmanaged diabetes is associated with high risk for heart disease and other health problems.

Wellness is the positive component of optimal health.

Death, disease, illness, and debilitating conditions are negative components that detract from optimal health. Death is the ultimate opposite of optimal health. Disease, illness, and debilitating conditions obviously detract from optimal health. Wellness has been recognized as the positive component of optimal health as evidenced by a sense of well-being reflected in optimal functioning, a good quality of life, meaningful work, and a contribution to society (see Figure 4). Wellness allows the expansion of one's potential to live and work effectively and to make a significant contribution to society.

Health and wellness are multidimensional.

The dimensions of health and wellness include the emotional (mental), intellectual, physical, social, and spiritual.

Figure 5 illustrates the importance of each dimension to total wellness. Throughout this book, references will be made to these wellness dimensions (see Table 1) to help reinforce their importance.

Wellness reflects how one feels about life as well as one's ability to function effectively.

A positive total outlook on life is essential to wellness and each of the wellness dimensions. A "well" person is satisfied in his/her work, is spiritually fulfilled, enjoys leisure time, is physically fit, is socially involved, and has a positive emotional-mental outlook. This person is happy and fulfilled. Many experts believe that a positive total outlook is a key to wellness (see Table 2).

The way one perceives each of the dimensions of wellness affects total outlook. Researchers use the term *self-perceptions* to describe these feelings. Many researchers believe that self-perceptions about wellness are more important than actual ability. For example, a person who has an important job may find less meaning and job satisfaction than another person with a much less important job. Apparently, one of the important factors for a person who has achieved high-level wellness and a positive life's outlook is the ability to reward himself/herself. Some people, however, seem unable to give themselves credit for their life's experiences. The development of a system that allows a person to positively perceive the self is important. Of course, the adoption of positive **lifestyles** that encourage improved self-perceptions is also important. The questionnaire in the Lab 1A will help you assess your self-perceptions of the various wellness dimensions. For optimal wellness, it would be important to find positive feelings about each dimension.

Table 1 Health and Wellness Definitions

Emotional health—A person with emotional health is (1) free from emotional-mental illnesses or debilitating conditions such as clinical depression and (2) possesses emotional wellness. The goals for the nation's health refer to mental rather than emotional health and wellness. In this book, mental health and wellness are considered to be the same as emotional health and wellness.

Emotional wellness—Emotional wellness is a person's ability to cope with daily circumstances and to deal with personal feelings in a positive, optimistic, and constructive manner. A person with emotional wellness is generally characterized as happy, as opposed to depressed.

Intellectual health—A person with intellectual health is free from illnesses that invade the brain and other systems that allow learning. A person with intellectual health also possesses intellectual wellness.

Intellectual wellness—Intellectual wellness is a person's ability to learn and to use information to enhance the quality of daily living and optimal functioning. A person with intellectual wellness is generally characterized as informed, as opposed to ignorant.

Physical health—A person with physical health is free from illnesses that affect the physiological systems of the body such as the heart, the nervous system, etc. A person with physical health possesses an adequate level of physical fitness and physical wellness.

Physical wellness—Physical wellness is a person's ability to function effectively in meeting the demands of the day's work and to use free time effectively. Physical wellness includes good physical fitness and the possession of useful motor skills. A person with physical wellness is generally characterized as fit versus unfit.

Social health—A person with social health is free from illnesses or conditions that severely limit functioning in society, including antisocial pathologies.

Social wellness—Social wellness is a person's ability to successfully interact with others and to establish meaningful relationships that enhance the quality of life for all people involved in the interaction (including self). A person with social wellness is generally characterized as involved as opposed to lonely.

Spiritual health—Spiritual health is the one component of health that is totally comprised of the wellness dimension; for this reason, spiritual health is considered to be synonymous with spiritual wellness.

Spiritual wellness—A person's ability to establish a values system and act on the system of beliefs, as well as to establish and carry out meaningful and constructive lifetime goals. Spiritual wellness is often based on a belief in a force greater than the individual that helps one contribute to an improved quality of life for all people. A person with spiritual wellness is generally characterized as fulfilled as opposed to unfulfilled.

Table 2 The Dimensions of Wellness

–	Wellness Dimensions	+
Depressed	Emotional-mental	Happy
Ignorant	Intellectual	Informed
Unfit	Physical	Fit
Lonely	Social	Involved
Unfulfilled	Spiritual	Fulfilled
Negative	Total outlook	Positive

Health and wellness are integrated states of being.

The segmented pictures of health and wellness shown in Figure 5 and Table 2 are used only to illustrate the multidimensional nature of health and wellness. In reality, health,

Wellness Wellness is the integration of many different components (mental, social, emotional, spiritual, and physical) that expand one's potential to live (quality of life) and work effectively and to make a significant contribution to society. Wellness reflects how one feels (a sense of well-being) about life as well as one's ability to function effectively. Wellness, as opposed to illness (a negative), is sometimes described as the positive component of good health.

Quality of Life A term used to describe wellness. An individual with quality of life can enjoyably do the activities of life with little or no limitation and can function independently. Individual quality of life requires a pleasant and supportive community.

Activity days A self-rating of the number of days (per week or month) a person feels that he/she can perform usual daily activities successfully and in good health.

Illness Illness is the ill feeling and/or symptoms associated with a disease or circumstances that upset homeostasis.

Lifestyles Lifestyles are patterns of behavior or ways an individual typically lives.

P = Physical   I = Intellectual   Sp = Spiritual
S = Social   E = Emotional

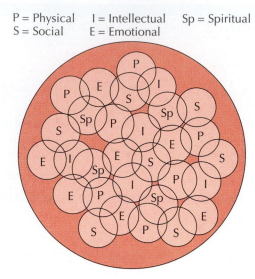

Figure 6
The integration of wellness dimensions.

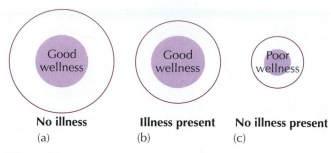

Figure 7
Wellness need not be limited by illness.

and its positive component (wellness), is an integrated state of being that is best depicted as many threads that can be woven together to produce a larger, integrated fabric. Each specific dimension relates to each of the others and overlaps all others. The overlap is so frequent and so great that the specific contribution of each thread is almost indistinguishable when looking at the total (Figure 6). The total is clearly greater than the sum of the parts.

Health and wellness are individual in nature.

Each individual is different from all others. Health and wellness depend on each person's individual characteristics. Making comparisons to other people on specific individual characteristics may produce feelings of inadequacy that detract from one's profile of total health and wellness. Each of us has personal limitations and personal strengths. Focusing on strengths and learning to accommodate weaknesses are essential keys to optimal health and wellness.

It is possible to possess wellness while being ill or possessing a debilitating condition.

All people can benefit from enhanced wellness. Wellness and an improved quality of life are possible for everyone, regardless of disease states. Evidence is accumulating to indicate that people with a positive outlook are better able to resist the progress of disease and illness than those with a negative outlook. Thinking positive thoughts has been associated with enhanced results from various medical treatments and better results from surgical procedures.

Because self-perceptions are important to wellness, positive perceptions of self are especially important to the wellness

of people with disease, illness, and disability. The concepts of wellness and optimal health must be considered in light of one's heredity and personal disabilities and disease states.

Figure 7 illustrates the fact that the most desirable condition is buoyant health (*a*) including freedom from illness and a high level of wellness. However, a person with a physical illness but who possesses a good wellness (*b*) has a better overall health status than a person with no illness but poor wellness (*c*).

Wellness is a useful term that may be used by quacks as well as experts.

Unfortunately, some individuals and groups have tried to identify wellness with products and services that promise benefits that cannot be documented. Because "well-being" is a subjective feeling that is hard to document, it is easy for quacks to make claims of improved wellness for their product or service without facts to back them up.

Holistic health is a term that is similarly abused. Optimal health includes many areas, thus the term *holistic* (total) is appropriate. In fact, the word *health* originates from a root word meaning "wholeness." Unfortunately, many quacks include their questionable health practices under this guise of "holistic health." Care should be used when considering services and products that make claims of wellness and/or holistic health to be sure that they are legitimate.

Facts about Physical Fitness

Physical fitness is a multidimensional state of being.

Physical fitness is the body's ability to function efficiently and effectively. It is a state of being that consists of at least five health-related and six skill-related, physical fitness components, each of which contributes to total quality of life. Physical fitness is associated with a person's ability to work effectively, enjoy leisure time, be healthy, resist **hypokinetic diseases,** and meet emergency situations. It is related to, but

Table 3 Health-Related Physical Fitness Terms

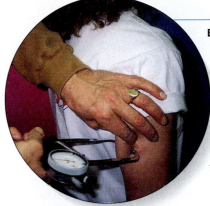

Body composition— The relative percentage of muscle, fat, bone, and other tissues that comprise the body. A fit person has a relatively low, but not too low, percentage of body fat (body fatness).

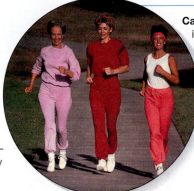

Cardiovascular fitness—The ability of the heart, blood vessels, blood, and respiratory system to supply fuel and oxygen to the muscles and the ability of the muscles to utilize fuel to allow sustained exercise. A fit person can persist in physical activity for relatively long periods without undue stress.

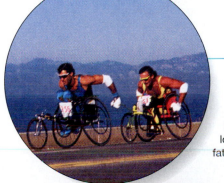

Muscular Endurance— The ability of the muscles to repeatedly exert themselves. A fit person can repeat movements for a long period without undue fatigue.

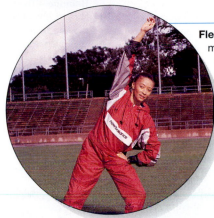

Flexibility—The range of motion available in a joint. It is affected by muscle length, joint structure, and other factors. A fit person can move the body joints through a full range of motion in work and in play.

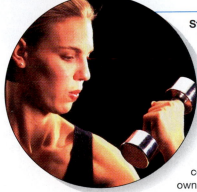

Strength—The ability of the muscles to exert an external force or to lift a heavy weight. A fit person can do work or play that involves exerting force, such as lifting or controlling one's own body weight.

different from, health and wellness. Although the development of physical fitness is the result of many things, optimal physical fitness is not possible without regular physical activity.

The health-related components of physical fitness are directly associated with good health.

The five components of health-related physical fitness are body composition, cardiovascular fitness, flexibility, muscular endurance, and strength (see Table 3). Each health related fitness characteristic has a direct relationship to good health and reduced risk of hypokinetic disease.

Physical Fitness   Physical fitness is the body's ability to function efficiently and effectively. It consists of health-related physical fitness and skill-related physical fitness, which have at least 11 different components, each of which contributes to total quality of life. Physical fitness also includes metabolic fitness (see page 9). Physical fitness is associated with a person's ability to work effectively, enjoy leisure time, be healthy, resist hypokinetic diseases, and meet emergency situations. It is related to, but different from health, wellness, and the psychological, sociological, emotional, and spiritual components of fitness. Although the development of physical fitness is the result of many things, optimal physical fitness is not possible without regular exercise.

Hypokinetic Diseases or Conditions   *Hypo-* means "under" or "too little," and *-kinetic* means "movement" or "activity". Thus, *hypokinetic* means "too little activity." A hypokinetic disease or condition is one associated with lack of physical activity or too little regular exercise. Examples of such conditions include heart disease, low back pain, adult-onset diabetes, and obesity.

Table 4 Skill-Related Physical Fitness Terms

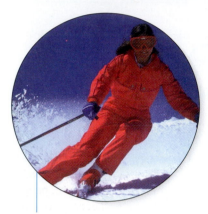

Agility—The ability to rapidly and accurately change the direction of the movement of the entire body in space. Skiing and wrestling are examples of activities that require exceptional agility.

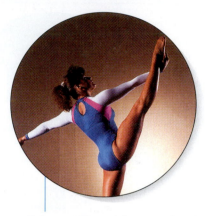

Balance—The maintenance of equilibrium while stationary or while moving. Water skiing, performing on the balance beam, or working as a riveter on a high-rise building are activities that require exceptional balance.

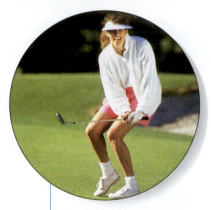

Coordination—The ability to use the senses with the body parts to perform motor tasks smoothly and accurately. Juggling, hitting a golf ball, batting a baseball, or kicking a ball are examples of activities requiring good coordination.

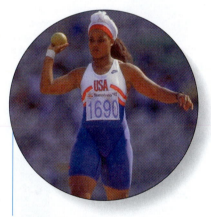

Power—The ability to transfer energy into force at a fast rate. Throwing the discus and putting the shot are activities that require considerable power.

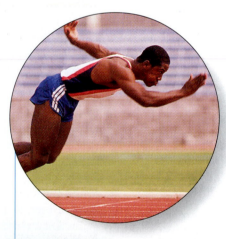

Reaction time—The time elapsed between stimulation and the beginning of reaction to that stimulation. Driving a racing car and starting a sprint race require good reaction time.

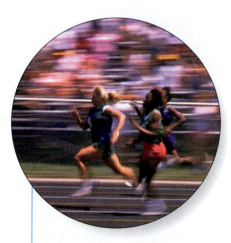

Speed—The ability to perform a movement in a short period of time. A runner on a track team or a wide receiver on a football team needs good foot and leg speed.

Possessing a moderate amount of each component of health-related fitness is essential to disease prevention and health promotion, but it is not essential to have exceptionally high levels of fitness to achieve health benefits. High levels of health-related fitness relate more to performance than health benefits. For example, moderate amounts of strength are necessary to prevent back and posture problems, whereas high levels of strength contribute most to improved performance in activities such as football and jobs involving heavy lifting.

> The skill-related components of physical fitness are more associated with performance than good health.

The components of skill-related physical fitness are agility, balance, coordination, power, reaction time, and speed (see Table 4). They are called skill-related because people who possess them find it easy to achieve high levels of performance in motor skills, such as those required in sports and in specific types of jobs. Skill-related fitness is sometimes called sports fitness or motor fitness.

There is little doubt that there are other abilities that could be classified as skill-related fitness components. Also, each part of skill-related fitness is multidimensional. For example, coordination could be hand-eye coordination such as batting a ball, foot-eye coordination such as kicking a ball, or any of many other possibilities. The six parts of skill-related fitness identified here are those that are commonly associated with successful sports and work performance. It should be noted that each could be measured in ways other than those presented in this book. Measurements are provided to help the reader understand the nature of total physical fitness and to help the reader make important decisions about lifetime physical activity.

Metabolic fitness is a nonperformance component of total fitness.

Research studies show that health benefits often occur even without dramatic improvements in traditional health-related physical fitness measures. Metabolic fitness is a state of being associated with lower risk of many chronic health problems, but not necessarily associated with high performance levels of health-related physical fitness. Examples of nonperformance indicators of reduced risk are lowered blood pressure, lowered fat levels in the blood, and better regulation of blood sugar. Moderate physical activity has been shown to enhance metabolic fitness. Conventional wisdom classifies body composition as a component of health-related physical fitness, but some consider it to be a part of metabolic fitness because it is a nonperformance measure, and it is highly related to nutrition as well as physical activity. You will learn how to assess your metabolic fitness in subsequent concepts.

Bone integrity is often considered to be a nonperformance measure of fitness.

Traditional definitions do not include bone integrity as a part of physical fitness, but some experts feel that it should be. Like metabolic fitness, bone integrity cannot be assessed with performance measures as can most health-related fitness parts. Regardless of whether it is considered as a part of fitness or a component of health, there is little doubt that strong healthy bones are important to optimal health and are associated with regular physical activity and sound diet.

The many components of physical fitness are specific in nature, but are also interrelated.

Physical fitness is a combination of several aspects rather than a single characteristic. A fit person possesses at least adequate levels of each of the health-related, skill-related, and metabolic fitness components. People who possess one aspect of physical fitness do not necessarily possess the other aspects.

Some relationships exist among different fitness characteristics, but each of the components of physical fitness is separate and different from the others. For example, people who possess exceptional strength do not necessarily have good cardiovascular fitness, and those who have good coordination do not necessarily possess good flexibility. Lab 1B is designed to help you distinguish among the different parts of health-related and skill-related physical fitness. A separate questionnaire helps you estimate your current fitness levels.

Good physical fitness is important too, but it is not the same as physical health and wellness.

Good physical fitness contributes directly to the physical component of good health and wellness, and indirectly to the other four components. Good fitness has been shown to be associated with reduced risk of chronic diseases such as coronary heart disease and has been shown to reduce the

Metabolic Fitness Metabolic fitness is a positive state of the physiological systems commonly associated with reduced risk of chronic diseases such as diabetes and heart disease. Metabolic fitness is evidenced by healthy blood fat (lipid) profiles, healthy blood pressure, healthy blood sugar and insulin levels, and other nonperformance measures. This type of fitness shows positive responses to moderate physical activity.

Bone Integrity Soundness of the bones associated with high density and absence of symptoms of deterioration.

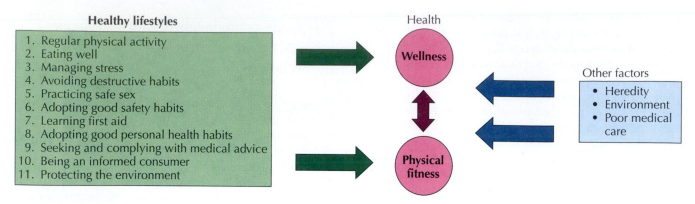

Figure 8

Factors influencing health, wellness, and physical fitness.

consequences of many debilitating conditions. In addition, good fitness contributes to wellness by helping us look our best, feel good, and enjoy life. Other physical factors can also influence health and wellness. For example, having good physical skills enhances quality of life by allowing us to participate in enjoyable activities such as tennis, golf, and bowling. While fitness can assist in performing these activities, regular practice is also necessary. Another example is the ability to fight off viral and bacterial infections. While fitness can promote a strong immune system, other physical factors can influence our susceptibility to these and other conditions.

For optimal health and wellness it is important to have good physical fitness *and* physical wellness. It is also important to strive for good emotional (mental), social, spiritual, and intellectual health and wellness.

The Facts about Healthy Lifestyles

Lifestyle change, more than any other factor, is considered to be the best way of preventing illness and early death in our society.

When people in Western society die before the age of 65, it is considered to be early or premature death. Many factors contribute to early death in Western culture. By far the most important is unhealthy lifestyles that contribute to more than one-half of all early deaths. Eleven healthy lifestyles have been identified that are associated with reduced disease risk

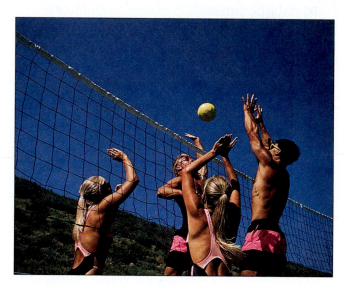

Exercise provides an opportunity for social involvement.

and increased wellness. As shown in Figure 8, these lifestyles affect health, wellness, and physical fitness. The double-headed arrow between health and wellness and physical fitness illustrate the interaction between these factors. Physical fitness is important to health and wellness development, and vice versa. Others factors, some not as much in your control as healthy lifestyles, also affect your health, fitness, and wellness. These factors include environmental factors (e.g., pollution, contaminants in the workplace), human biology (inherited conditions), and inadequacies in the health-care system, to name but a few.

Table 5 Major Causes of Death

1900 Rank	Cause	Current Rank	Cause
1.	Pneumonia	1.	Heart disease
2.	Tuberculosis	2.	Cancer
3.	Diarrhea/enteritis	3.	Stroke
4.	Heart disease	4.	Bronchitis/emphysema
5.	Stroke	5.	Injuries
6.	Liver disease	6.	Pneumonia/influenza
7.	Injuries	7.	Diabetes
8.	Cancer	8.	Suicide
9.	Senility	9.	Chronic Liver Disease
10.	Diphtheria	14.	HIV/AIDS*

*Formerly 8th
SOURCE: National Center for Health Statistics.

The major causes of early death have shifted from infectious diseases to chronic lifestyle-related conditions.

www.mhhe.com/hper/physed/clw/student/

Scientific advances and improvements in medicine and health care have dramatically reduced the incidence of infectious diseases over the past 100 years (see Table 5). For example, new drugs have dramatically reduced deaths from pneumonia and influenza. Small pox, a major cause of death less than a century ago, was globally eradicated in 1977 because of the advent of immunizations. Other examples are the virtual elimination of diphtheria and polio in the United States and Canada.

As infectious diseases have been eliminated, other illnesses have replaced them as the leading causes of early death in Western culture. HIV/AIDS, formerly eighth on the list, has dropped from the top ten, not because of fewer new cases, but because of new treatments that increase length of life among those who are infected. Many among the top ten are referred to as chronic lifestyle related conditions because alteration of lifestyles can result in reduced risk for these conditions.

Healthy lifestyles are critical to wellness.

Just as unhealthy lifestyles are the principal causes of modern-day illnesses such as heart disease, cancer, and diabetes, healthy lifestyles can result in an improved

feeling of wellness that is critical to optimal health. In recognizing the importance of "years of healthy life," the Public Health Service also recognizes what it calls "measures of well-being." This well-being or wellness is associated with social, mental, spiritual, and physical functioning. Being physically active and eating well are two examples of healthy lifestyles that can improve well-being and add years of quality living. Many of the healthy lifestyles associated with good physical fitness and optimal wellness will be discussed in detail later in this book. The Healthy Lifestyle Questionnaire at the end if this concept gives you the opportunity to assess your current lifestyles.

Regular physical activity, sound nutrition, and stress management are considered to be priority healthy lifestyles.

Three of the healthy lifestyles listed in Figure 8 are considered to be priority healthy lifestyles. These are regular **physical activity (exercise)**, eating well, and managing stress. There are several reasons for placing priority on these lifestyles. First, they are behaviors that affect the lives of all people. Second, they are lifestyles in which large numbers of people can make improvement. Finally, modest changes in these behaviors can make dramatic improvements in individual and public health.

To be sure, the other healthy lifestyles listed in Figure 8 are important. For example people who use tobacco, abuse drugs (including alcohol), or practice unsafe sex can have immediate and dramatic health benefits by changing these behaviors. On the other hand, large segments of the population do not have problems in these areas. Obviously, these people cannot benefit from lifestyle changes in these areas. However, the majority of the population can benefit from

Exercise   Exercise is defined as physical activity done for the purpose of getting physically fit.

Physical activity is generally considered to be a broad term used to describe all forms of large muscle movements including sports, dance, games, work, lifestyle activities, and exercise for fitness. In this book, exercise and physical activity will often be used interchangeably to make reading less repetitive and more interesting.

increasing their activity level, eating a better diet, and managing personal stress. For example, statistics suggest that modest changes in physical activity patterns and nutrition can prevent more than 200,000 premature death annually. Similarly, learning to manage stresses that all of us face on a daily basis can result in significant reductions in more than a few health problems. Stress has a major impact on drug, alcohol, and smoking behavior so managing stress can help individuals minimize or avoid these behaviors. Many healthy lifestyles will be discussed in this book, but the focus is on the priority healthy lifestyles because virtually all people can achieve positive wellness benefits if they adopt them.

The change in causes of illness and the new emphasis on fitness, wellness, and healthy lifestyles have resulted in a shift toward prevention and promotion.

Early medicine focused on treatment of disease. Physicians were scarce and were consulted only when illness occurred. A shift toward prevention began with advancements in medical science (e.g., immunizations, antibiotics) and the development of public health efforts (e.g., safe water supplies). Now more than at any other time in history, efforts are being made to promote healthy lifestyles that lead to fitness and wellness. In this text, the emphasis will be on strategies for preventing chronic diseases and promoting fitness and wellness.

The HELP Philosophy: The Facts

The HELP philosophy can provide a basis for making healthy lifestyle change possible.

The four-letter acronym illustrated in Table 6 provides a basis for a philosophy that has helped thousands of people adopt healthy lifestyles. Each letter in the word *HELP* characterizes an important part of the philosophy.

Table 6 The HELP Philosophy

H	=	Health
E	=	Everyone
L	=	Lifetime
P	=	Personal

A personal philosophy that emphasizes Health can lead to behaviors that promote it.

The **H** in HELP stands for "health." One theory that has been extensively tested indicates that people who believe in the benefits of healthy lifestyles are more likely to engage in healthy behaviors. The theory also suggests that people who state intentions to put their beliefs in action are likely to adopt behaviors that lead to health, wellness, and fitness.

Everyone can benefit from healthy lifestyles.

The **E** in HELP stands for "everyone." Accepting the fact that anyone can change a behavior or lifestyle means that *YOU* are included. Nevertheless, many adults feel ineffective in making lifestyle changes. Physical activity is not just for athletes—it is for all people. Eating well is not just for other people—you can do it too. All people can learn stress-management techniques. Healthy lifestyles can be practiced by everyone. As noted earlier in this concept, important health goals include eliminating health disparities and promoting "Health for All."

Healthy behaviors are most effective when practiced for a Lifetime.

The **L** in HELP stands for "lifetime." Young people sometimes feel immortal because the harmful effects of unhealthy lifestyles are often not immediate. As we grow older, we begin to realize that we are not immortal and that unhealthy lifestyles have cumulative negative effects. Starting early in life to emphasize healthy behaviors results in long-term

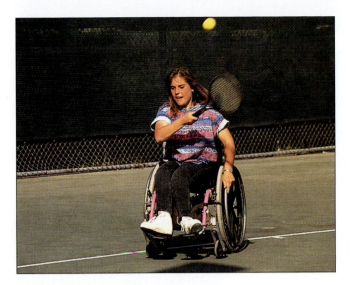

Physical activity is for everyone.

health, wellness, and fitness benefits. One recent study shows that the longer healthy lifestyles are practiced, the greater the beneficial effects. This study also demonstrated that long-term healthy lifestyles can even overcome hereditary predisposition to illness and disease.

Healthy lifestyles should be based on **P**ersonal needs.

The **P** in HELP stands for "personal." No two people are exactly alike. Just as there is no single pill that will cure all illnesses, there is no single lifestyle prescription for good health, wellness, and fitness. It is important for each person to assess personal needs and make lifestyle changes based on those needs.

Strategies for Action: The Facts

Self-assessments of lifestyles will help you determine areas in which you may need changes to promote optimal health, wellness, and fitness.

As you begin your study of health, wellness, fitness, and healthy lifestyles, it is wise to make a self-assessment of

your current behaviors. The Healthy Lifestyle Questionnaire in the lab resource materials will allow you to assess your current lifestyle behaviors to determine if they are contributing positively to your health, wellness, and fitness. Because this questionnaire contains some very personal information, answering all questions honestly will help you get an accurate assessment. As you continue your study, you may want to refer back to this questionnaire to see if your lifestyles have changed.

Initial self-assessments of wellness and fitness will provide information for self-comparison.

www.mhhe.com/hper/physed/clw/student/

The Healthy Lifestyle Questionnaire allows you to assess your lifestyles or behaviors. It is also important to assess your wellness and fitness at an early stage. These early assessments will only be estimates. As you continue your study, you will have the opportunity to do more comprehensive self-assessments that will allow you to see how accurate your early estimates were.

In Lab 1A you will estimate your wellness using a Wellness Self-Perceptions Questionnaire, which assesses five wellness dimensions. Remember, wellness is a state of being that is influenced by healthy lifestyles. Because other factors such as heredity, environment, and health care affect wellness, it is possible to have good wellness scores even if you do not do well on the lifestyle questionnaire. However, over a lifetime, unhealthy lifestyles will catch up with you and have an influence on your wellness and fitness.

Lab 1B allows you to get a better understanding of the different components of health-related and skill-related physical fitness. You will perform some simple stunts to help you distinguish among the different fitness parts. You can use these as a basis for estimating your current fitness levels. Later, you will use more accurate tests to get a good assessment of your fitness. Like wellness, fitness is a state of being that is influenced by healthy lifestyles, especially regular physical activity. Young people sometimes have relatively good fitness—especially skill-related fitness—even if they have not been doing regular activity. Over a lifetime, inactivity greatly influences your fitness.

Web Review

Web review materials for Concept 1 are available are at *www.mhhe.com/hper/physed/clw/student/*.

AMA Health Insight

www.ama-assn.org/consumer.htm

Mayo Health Oasis

www.mayohealth.org/mayo

Healthfinder

www.healthfinder.org

Health Information

www.planethealth.com

Wellness Interactive Network

www.stayhealthy.com

Healthy People 2010

www.health.gov/healthypeople

Centers for Disease Prevention and Control (CDC)

www.cdc.gov

Suggested Readings

Clement, M. and Hales, D. How Healthy Are We? *Parade Magazine.* September 7, 1998, 4.

Corbin, C. B. and Pangrazi, R. P. (Editors), *Towards a Better Understanding of Physical Fitness and Activity.* Scottsdale, AZ: Holcomb-Hathaway, 1998.

National Center for Health Statistics. *Health, United States, 1998: With Socioeconomic Statistics and Health Chartbook.* Hyattsville, MD: National Center for Health Statistics, 1998.

Payne, W. A. & Hahn, D. B. *Understanding Your Health.* (5th ed.) St. Louis: WCB/McGraw-Hill, 1998.

U.S. Department of Health and Human Services. *Physical Activity and Health: A Report of the Surgeon General.* Atlanta, GA: U.S. Department of Health and Human Services, 1996.

U.S. Department of Health and Human Services. *Healthy People 2010 Objectives: Draft for Comments.* Washington, DC:U.S. Department of Health and Human Services, 1998.

Lab Resource Materials:
The Healthy Lifestyle Questionnaire

The purpose of this questionnaire is to help you analyze your lifestyle behaviors and to help you in making decisions concerning good health and wellness for the future. Information on this Healthy Lifestyle Questionnaire is of a very personal nature. For this reason, this questionnaire is not designed to be submitted to your instructor. It is for your information only. Answer each question as honestly as possible and use the scoring information to help you assess your lifestyle.

Directions: Place an X over the "yes" circle to answer yes. If you answer "no," make no mark. Score the questionnaire using the procedures that follow.

(yes) 1. I accumulate 30 minutes of moderate physical activity most days of the week (brisk walking, climbing the stairs, yard work, or home chores).	17. I abstain from sex or limit sexual activity to a safe partner. **(yes)**
(yes) 2. I do vigorous activity that elevates my heart rate for 20 minutes at least three days a week.	18. I practice safe procedures for avoiding STDs. **(yes)**
(yes) 3. I do exercises for flexibility at least three days a week.	19. I use seat belts and adhere to the speed limit when I drive. **(yes)**
(yes) 4. I do exercises for muscle fitness at least two days a week.	20. I have a smoke detector in my home and check it regularly to see that it is working. **(yes)**
(yes) 5. I eat three regular meals each day.	21. I have had training to perform CPR if called on in an emergency. **(yes)**
(yes) 6. I select appropriate servings from the food guide pyramid each day.	22. I can perform the Heimlich maneuver effectively if called on in an emergency. **(yes)**
(yes) 7. I restrict the amount of fat in my diet.	23. I brush my teeth at least two times a day and floss at least once a day. **(yes)**
(yes) 8. I consume only as many calories as I expend each day.	24. I get an adequate amount of sleep each night. **(yes)**
✓ **(yes)** 9. I am able to identify situations in daily life that cause stress.	25. I do regular self-exams, have regular medical check-ups, and seek medical advice when symptoms are present. **(yes)**
✓ **(yes)** 10. I take time out during the day to relax and recover from daily stress.	26. When I receive advice and/or medication from a physician, I follow the advice and take the medication as prescribed. **(yes)**
✓ **(yes)** 11. I find time for family, friends and things I especially enjoy doing.	27. I read product labels and investigate their effectiveness before I buy them. **(yes)**
(yes) 12. I regularly perform exercises designed to relieve tension.	28. I avoid using products that have not been shown by research to be effective. **(yes)**
✓ **(yes)** 13. I do not smoke or use other tobacco products.	29. I recycle paper, glass or aluminum. **(yes)**
✓ **(yes)** 14. I do not abuse alcohol.	30. I practice environmental protection such as car pooling and conserving energy. **(yes)**
✓ **(yes)** 15. I do not abuse drugs (prescription or illegal).	
✓ **(yes)** 16. I take over-the-counter drugs sparingly and use them only according to directions.	**Overall Score—Total Yes Answers** 14

Scoring: Give yourself one point for each yes answer. Add your scores for each of the lifestyle behaviors. To calculate your overall score, sum the totals for all lifestyles.

Physical Activity	Nutrition	Managing Stress	Avoiding Destructive Habits	Practicing Safe Sex	Adopting Safety Habits
— — — 1	— — — 5	— ¦ — 9	— ¦ — 13	— — — 17	— ¦ — 19
— — — 2	— — — 6	— ¦ — 10	— ¦ — 14	— — — 18	— ¦ — 20
— — — 3	— — — 7	— ¦ — 11	— ¦ — 15		
— — — 4	— — — 8	— — — 12	— ¦ — 16		
— 0 — Total +	— 0 — Total +	— 3 — Total +	— 4 — Total +	— — — Total +	— 2 — Total +

Knowing First Aid	Personal Health Habits	Using Medical Advice	Being an Informed Consumer	Protecting the Environment	Sum All Totals for Overall Score
— — — 21	— ¦ — 23	— ¦ — 25	— ¦ — 27	— — — 29	
— — — 22	— ¦ — 24	— ¦ — 26	— — — 28	— — — 30	
— 0 — Total +	— 2 — Total +	— 2 — Total +	— ¦ — Total +	— 0 — Total =	14

Interpreting Scores: Scores of 3 or 4 on the four-item scales are indicative of generally positive lifestyles. For the two-item scales, a score of 2 would indicate the presence of positive lifestyles. An overall score of 26 or more would be a good indicator of healthy lifestyle behaviors. It is important to consider the following special note when interpreting scores.

Special Note: Your scores on the Healthy Lifestyle Questionnaire should be interpreted with caution. There are several reasons for this. First, all lifestyle behaviors do not pose the same risks. For example, using tobacco or abusing drugs has immediate negative affects on health and wellness, while others, such as knowing first aid, may have only occasional use. Second, you may score well on one item in a scale, but not on another. If one item indicates an unhealthy lifestyle in an area that poses a serious health risk, your lifestyle may appear to be healthier than it really is. For example, you could get a score of 3 on the destructive habits scale and be a regular smoker. For this reason, the overall score can be particularly deceiving.

Strategies for Change: In the space below, you may want to make some notes concerning the healthy lifestyle areas in which you could make some changes. You can refer to these notes later to see if you have made progress.

Concept 2

Using Self-Management Skills to Adhere to Healthy Lifestyle Behaviors

Learning and regularly using self-management skills can help you to adopt and maintain healthy lifestyles throughout life.

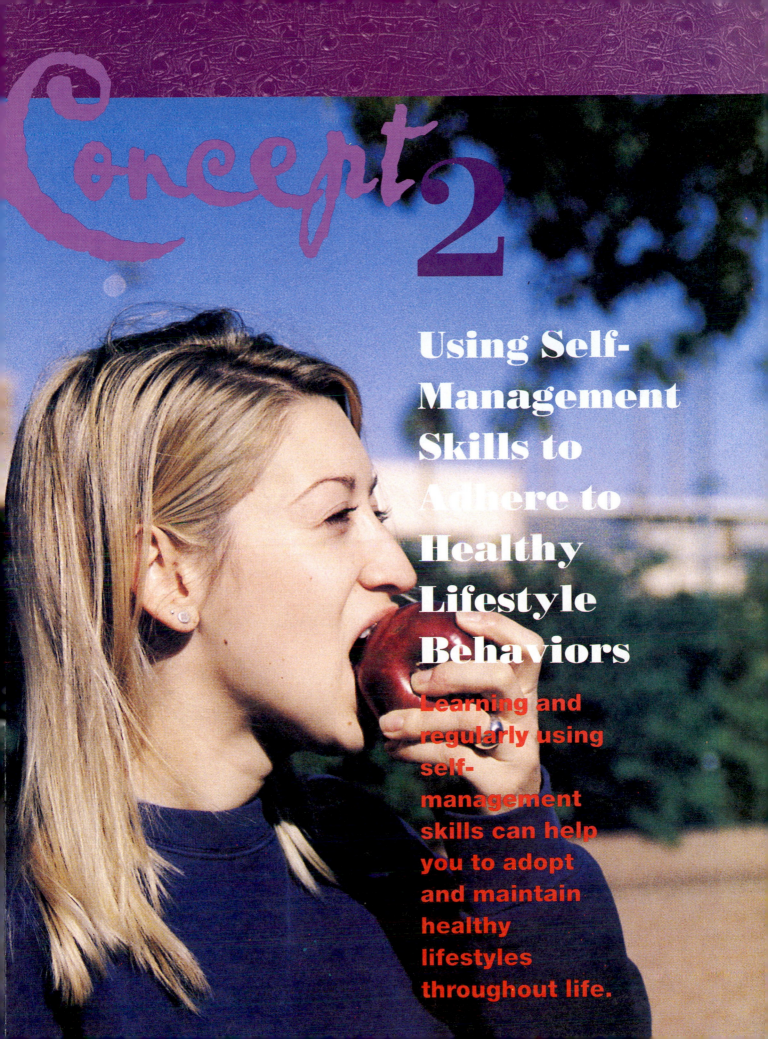

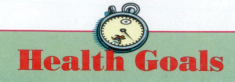

Health Goals

for the year 2010

Increase quality and years of healthy life.

Increase incidence of people reporting "healthy days".

Increase incidence of people reporting "active days".

Increase the adoption and maintenance of daily physical activity.

Increase the proportion of all people who eat well.

Decrease personal stress levels and mental health problems.

Reduce accidents, destructive habits, and environmental pollution.

Introduction

Reducing illness and debilitating conditions and promoting wellness and fitness are important goals for all of us. Practicing lifelong healthy lifestyles is the key to health, wellness, and fitness. Yet, there is considerable evidence that many people are not effective in making lifestyle changes, even when they want to do so. Experts have determined that people who practice healthy lifestyles possess certain characteristics. These characteristics can be modified to improve health behaviors of all people. Researchers have also identified several special skills, referred to as self-management skills, that can be useful in helping you alter factors related to adherence and ultimately help you to make lifestyle changes. Like any skill, self-management skills must be practiced if they are to be useful. In this concept, factors relating to healthy lifestyle adherence and self-management skills will be described.

The Facts about Lifestyle Change

Many adults want to make lifestyle changes but are unable to do so.

The majority of adults (66 percent) would prefer to alter their diet to improve health rather than take medicine. Nine

of 10 people indicate that regular physical activity is important to their health. Approximately two-thirds of adults feel "great stress" at least one day a week and would like to reduce their stress levels. In spite of these statistics, those who profess interest in dietary change often are unsuccessful in making lasting changes. Those who say they value physical activity often fail to adhere to even modest activity schedules. Though stress reduction is important, nearly half of all adults still feel that there is a stigma associated with seeking help for an emotional problem, yet they frequently lack the skills to help themselves. Changes in other lifestyles are frequently desired, but often not accomplished.

Practicing one healthy lifestyle does not mean you will practice another, though adopting one healthy behavior often leads to adoption of another.

College students are more likely to participate in regular physical activity than older adults. However, they are also much more likely to eat poorly and abuse alcohol. Many young women adopt low-fat diets to avoid weight gain and also smoke because they have the mistaken belief that smoking will contribute to long-term weight maintenance. These examples illustrate the fact that practicing one healthy lifestyle does not insure **adherence** to another. However, there is evidence that making one lifestyle change often makes it easier to make other changes. For example, smokers who have started regular physical activity programs often see improvements in fitness and general well-being and decide to stop smoking.

People do not make lifestyle changes overnight. Rather, people progress forward and backward through several stages of change.

www.mhhe.com/hper/physed/clw/student/
When asked about a specific healthy lifestyle, it is not unusual for people to respond with "yes" or "no" answers. If asked, "Do you exercise regularly?", the answer would be "yes" or "no." When asked, "Do you eat well?", the answer would be "yes" or "no." We now know that there are many different stages of lifestyle behavior.

Prochaska and colleagues have developed a model for lifestyle change that suggests at least five different dynamic stages of healthy behaviors (see Figure 1). The stages were originally developed to help understand negative lifestyles.

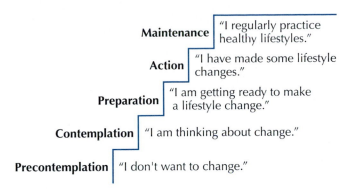

Figure 1
Stages of lifestyle change.

Smokers were among the first studied. Smokers who are not considering stopping are at the stage of precontemplation. Those who are thinking about stopping are classified in the contemplation stage. Those who have bought a nicotine patch or a book about smoking cessation are classified in the preparation stage. They have moved beyond contemplation and are preparing to take action. The action stage occurs when the smoker makes some change in behavior, even a small one. Cutting back on the number of cigarettes smoked is an example. The fifth stage is the stage of maintenance. When a person finally stops smoking for a relatively long period of time (6 months) this stage has been reached.

The **stages of change** model (as illustrated in Figure 1), has now been applied to positive lifestyles as well as negative ones. Those who are totally sedentary are considered to be in the precontemplation stage. Contemplators are thinking about becoming active. A person at the preparation stage may have bought a pair of walking shoes and appropriate clothing for activity. Those who have started some activity, even if infrequent, are considered to be at the stage of action. Those who have been exercising regularly for at least 6 months are said to be at the stage of maintenance.

Whether the lifestyle is positive or negative, people move from one stage to another in an upward or downward direction. Individuals in action may move on to maintenance or revert back to contemplation depending on their attitudes and personal experiences. Smokers who succeed in quitting permanently report having stopped and started dozens of times before reaching lifetime maintenance. Similarly, those attempting to adopt positive lifestyles such as eating well often move back and forth from one stage to another depending on their life circumstances.

> Once maintenance is attained, relapse is less likely to occur.

While it is possible to **relapse** completely, it is generally less likely after the maintenance stage is reached. At this point, the behavior has been integrated into a personal lifestyle and

it becomes easier to sustain. For example, a person who has been physically active for years does not have to undergo the same thought processes as a beginning exerciser—the behavior becomes automatic and habitual. Similarly, a non-smoker is not tempted to smoke in the same way as a person who is currently trying to quit. Some people have termed the end of this behavior change process as "termination."

Factors That Promote Lifestyle Change: The Facts

> There are many factors associated with achieving advanced stages of healthy behavior.

The ultimate goal for any health behavior is to reach the stage of maintenance (see Figure 1). The Surgeon General's Report on Physical Activity and Health outlines some of the factors that relate to reaching and staying at the maintenance level for physical activity. These factors relate equally well to stages of change for other healthy lifestyles. For ease of understanding, they are classified as **personal, predisposing, enabling,** and **reinforcing factors.** Predisposing factors help precontemplators get going—to move them toward

Adherence Adopting a healthy behavior such as regular physical activity or sound nutrition as part of your lifestyle.

Stage of Change A stage of change refers to the level of lifestyle behavior a given individual has for a specific health behavior.

Relapse Reverting back to old lifestyle habits after attempting a change in behavior.

Personal Factor Factors such as age or gender that are related to healthy lifestyle adherence but that are typically not under your personal control.

Predisposing Factor Anything that makes you more likely to decide that you should make a healthy lifestyle such as regular physical activity a part of your normal routine.

Enabling Factor Anything that helps you to carry out your healthy lifestyle plan.

Reinforcing Factor Anything that provides encouragement to maintain healthy lifestyles such as physical activity for a lifetime.

contemplation or even preparation. Enabling factors help those in contemplation or preparation take the step toward action. Reinforcing factors move people from action to maintenance and to help those in maintenance stay there.

Personal factors affect health behaviors but are often out of your personal control.

Your age, gender, and heredity are examples of personal factors. While these factors do not cause differences in behavior, differences in behavior are evident across these factors. For example, there are significant differences in health behaviors among those of various age groups. According to one survey, young adults between the ages of 18 and 34 are more likely to smoke (30 percent) than those 65 and older (13 percent). On the other hand, young adults are much more likely to be physically active than older adults.

Gender differences are illustrated by the fact that women use health services more often than men. Women are more likely than men to have identified a primary care doctor and are more likely to participate in regular health screenings. As you will discover in more detail later in this book, heredity plays a role in health behaviors. For example, some people have a hereditary predisposition to gain weight, and this may affect their eating behaviors.

While personal factors should be considered in making lifestyle changes, there is little you can do about your age, gender, or heredity. However, self-management skills can be effective for all people regardless of personal factors. Your personal characteristics may affect the way you use self-management skills but they do not prevent you from using them effectively.

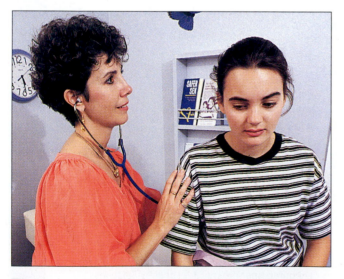

Women are more likely to use health care services than men.

Predisposing factors are important in getting you started with the process of change.

Predisposing factors are factors that are likely to help you move from precontemplation to contemplation or a higher state of healthy behavior. As illustrated in Figure 2, predisposing factors are associated with two basic questions: "Am I able?" and "Is it worth it?"

Am I able to do regular activity? Am I able to change my diet or to stop smoking? People who have "feelings that they are able" are said to have good perceptions of competence. They have the **self-confidence** and **self-efficacy** to embark on behavior changes for health improvement. Perceptions of competence, as evidenced by self-confidence and self-efficacy, are considered to be predisposing factors. If you feel competent, you are more likely to try something than if you feel incompetent. Later in this concept, you will learn several self-management skills that can help you improve perceptions of competence (if you do not already possess them).

Is it worth it? Making a change in behavior takes effort. You are more likely to make a change in behavior if you think your effort is worthwhile. Some factors that make a behavior change worthwhile are having the belief that the change will have benefits. Part of changing your beliefs is becoming knowledgeable about the behavior and its benefits. Enjoyment is another factor that makes a behavior change worthwhile. If you enjoy doing something, the enjoyment is its own benefit. Finally, attitudes make a difference. Research shows that people who have more positive feelings (attitudes) than negative attitudes are likely to adopt healthy behaviors.

Enabling factors are important in moving you from the beginning stages of change to action and maintenance.

Enabling factors help people follow through with decisions to make changes in behavior (see Figure 2). Having **self-management** skills is one type of enabling factor. Examples of self-management skills are self-assessment, self-monitoring, and goal-setting skills. You will learn more about these later in this concept.

Having access to the things you need to make changes in lifestyle is another type of enabling factor. For instance, having access to fitness facilities or cooking facilities would enable you to do regular exercise or cook healthy meals.

Reinforcing factors are important in adhering to lifestyle changes.

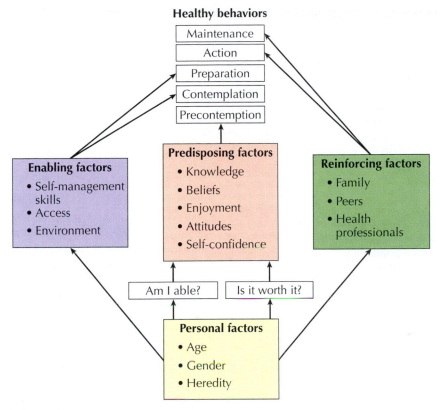

Figure 2
Factors that influence change in healthy behaviors.

Once a person has reached the action stage, it is important to move on to maintenance. Once a person has reached the maintenance stage, it is important to stay at that stage. Reinforcing factors help people stick with a behavior change (see Figure 2). Family, peer, and health professional influence are all reinforcing factors. If your family and friends or a doctor encourage you, it may help you adhere. It is important, however, that support from others does not create unnecessary pressure. Though support from others can be reinforcing, perhaps the most important reinforcing factor is success. If you change a behavior and have success, it makes you want to keep doing the behavior. If you fail, you may conclude that the behavior does not work and give up on it. Planning for success is very important in adhering to healthy lifestyle change.

Being aware of factors that influence lifestyles can lead to lifestyle change.

The factors described in the previous paragraphs and illustrated in Figure 2, are susceptible to change. Learning about these factors and studying how they affect you personally can help you in moving through the stages of lifestyle change.

Self-Management Skills: The Facts

Learning self-management skills can help you alter factors that lead to healthy lifestyle change.

Self-Confidence The belief that you can be successful at something (for example, the belief that you can be successful in sports and physical activities, and can improve your physical fitness).

Self-Efficacy Confidence that you can perform a specific task. (A type of very specific self-confidence.)

Self-Management Skills Skills that you can learn to help you adhere to healthy lifestyles such as regular physical activity. Examples include goal setting, time management, and program-planning skills.

Table 1 Self-Management Skills

Self-Management Skill	Lifestyle Examples	How Is It Useful?
Self-Assessment Skills This involves how to assess your own fitness, health, and wellness. In addition it requires you to learn to interpret your own self-assessment results. It takes practice to become good at doing self-assessments.	A person wants to know his/her health strengths and weaknesses. The best procedure is to select good tests and self-administer them. Practicing the assessments at the end of many concepts in this book will help you become good at self-assessment.	• Helps in setting goals • Provides basis for planning • Helps make success possible • Basis for new way of thinking • Basis for learning skills
Self-Monitoring Skills This involves monitoring behavior and record keeping. Many people think that they adhere to healthy lifestyles, but they do not. They have a distorted view of what they actually do. Self-monitoring helps give you a true picture of your own behavior. Monitoring progress in meeting goals is also important.	A person can't understand why he/she is not losing weight even though restricting calories. Keeping records may show that the person was eating more than he/she thought. Learning to keep records of progress is also important to adherence.	• Provides information • Helps in setting goals • Provides basis for planning • Provides feedback • Increases chance of success • Provides information • Helps alter beliefs
Goal-Setting Skills This involves learning how to establish things that you want to achieve in the future. It is important that goals be realistic and achievable. Learning to set goals for behavior change is especially important for beginners.	A person wants to lose body fat. If he/she sets a goal of losing 50 pounds, success is unlikely. Setting a process goal of restricting 200 Calories a day or expending 200 more a day for several weeks makes success more likely.	• Provides basis for planning • Increases chance of success • Basis for feedback • May enhance enjoyment • May influence attitudes • May alter beliefs • May help build confidence
Planning Skills This involves learning how to plan for yourself rather than having others do all the planning for you. Knowledge and practice in planning can help you develop these skills.	A person wants to be more active, to eat better, and to manage stress. Self-planning skills will help him/her plan a personal activity, nutrition, or stress-management program.	• Provides basis for success • Basis for reinforcement • May help self-confidence • Improves enjoyment
Performance Skills This involves learning skills necessary for performance of specific tasks, such as sport or relaxation. These skills can help you feel confident and enjoy activities.	A person is stressed and anxious in many life situations. Learning stress-management skills, such as relaxation, can help a person cope. Like all skills, stress-management skills must be practiced to be effective.	• Enhances enjoyment • Provides for success • Enhances self-confidence • Influences attitudes
Balancing Attitudes This involves learning to balance positive and negative attitudes. To adhere to a healthy lifestyle, it is important to develop positive attitudes and reduce the negative attitudes.	A person does not do activity because he or she lacks support from friends, has no equipment, and does not like to get sweaty. These are negatives. Shifting the balance to positive things such as fun, good health, and looking good can help promote activity.	• Enhances enjoyment • Basis for planning • Helps in setting goals • Influences beliefs

Personal, predisposing, enabling, and reinforcing factors influence the way you live. These factors are of little practical significance, however, unless they can be altered to promote lifestyle change. Self-management skills influence many of the factors that are associated with healthy lifestyle change. It takes effort to learn self-management skills, but, with practice and effort, they are skills all people can learn. Descriptions of various self-management skills that are especially useful in promoting lifestyles that enhance health, wellness, and fitness are included in Table 1.

It takes time to develop unhealthy lifestyles and time to change them.

People in Western culture are used to seeing things happen quickly. We flip a switch, and the lights come on. We want

Table 1 *(continued)*

Self-Management Skill	Lifestyle Examples	How Is It Useful?
Overcoming Barriers This involves developing skills that allow you to overcome problems such as lack of facilities, lack of equipment, and inconvenience. People who develop skills to overcome barriers can learn to rearrange schedules and acquire personal equipment and other skills to overcome these barriers.	People at work are often exposed to snack foods high in empty calories. For this reason his/her nutrition is not what it could be. Skills in overcoming barriers include planning and preparing your own food and selecting good foods.	• Improves access • Provides good environment • Makes time available • Contributes to enjoyment • Improves self-confidence
Learning Consumer Skills This involves gaining knowledge about products and services. It also may require rethinking untrue beliefs that may lead to poor consumer decisions.	A person avoids seeking medical help when symptoms of illness are present. Instead, the person takes an unproven remedy. Learning consumer skills provides knowledge for making sound medical decisions.	• Builds knowledge • Promotes founded beliefs • Influences attitudes • Improves self-confidence
Finding Social Support This involves learning how to get the support of others for healthy lifestyles you want to adopt. You learn how to get this support from family and friends. Support of an outside authority such as a doctor can help.	A person abuses alcohol. If friends and family also abuse alcohol, the abuse will probably continue. In some cases, it is best to find support elsewhere and then seek support of friends and family.	• Reinforces healthy behavior • Doctor's advice motivates • Supports idea that you are able • Supports idea that it is worth it • Improves self-confidence
Preventing Relapse This involves staying with a healthy behavior once you have adopted it. It is sometimes hard not to relapse to an unhealthy lifestyle. There are skills such as avoiding high risk situations and learning how to say no that can help avoid relapse.	A person stops smoking. To stay at maintenance, the person can learn to avoid situations where there is pressure to smoke. The person can learn methods of saying "no" to those who offer tobacco.	• Builds self-confidence • Alters environment • Promotes success • Builds knowledge
Adopting Coping Skills This involves developing a new way of thinking about things. People with this skill can see situations in more than one way and learn to think more positively about life situations.	A person avoids physical activity because he/she does not have the physical skills equal to peers. Coping skills allows this person to tell him or herself that self-comparisons are not important and then choose to be active anyway.	• Improves enjoyment • Enhances attitudes • Improves self-confidence • Promotes success
Managing Time This involves keeping records similar to self-monitoring. It relates to total time use rather than monitoring specific behaviors. Skillful monitoring of time can help you in planning and adhering to healthy lifestyles.	A person wants more quality time with family and friends. Monitoring time can help a person reallocate time to spend it in ways that are more consistent with personal priorities.	• Provides options • Helps overcome barriers • Provides for skill learning • Aids planning

food quickly, and thousands of fast-food restaurants provide it. The expectation that we should have what we want when we want it has led us to expect instantaneous changes in health, wellness, and fitness. Unfortunately, there is no quick way to health. There is no pill that can reverse the affects of a lifetime of sedentary living, poor eating, or abuse of tobacco. Changing your lifestyle is the key. But lifestyles that have been practiced for years are not easy to change. As you progress through this book, you will have the opportunity to learn how to implement self-management skills. Learning these skills is the surest way to make permanent lifestyle changes.

Strategies for Action: The Facts

Many people feel that factors influencing health and wellness are out of their control.

www.mhhe.com/hper/physed/clw/student/

 A recent poll indicates that 91 percent of adults would like to change their lifestyles to make their lives more enjoyable and to change factors associated with wellness, such as reducing stress and tension. Unfortunately, many people feel that they do not have personal control over good health and wellness. For example, one survey suggests that most of the lifestyle changes deemed important by millions in our society will remain in the realm of fantasies, just beyond realization. Experts have shown that people who feel that health is beyond personal control express such ideas as "Bad things [illness] can't happen to me and good things [wellness] are beyond my reach."

Many people can benefit from a new way of thinking about health, wellness, and fitness.

Many people have unrealistic expectations about health and fitness. They compare their fitness to athletes and their appearance to models and movie stars, often setting standards for themselves that are impossible to achieve. Some say "I could never do that" when considering becoming physically active, altering eating patterns, or learning to manage stress. Many lack information about what is really possible concerning healthy lifestyles. Those who feel a lack of control, set unrealistic standards for themselves, and lack confidence in their own abilities to change.

Adopting a new way of thinking can have dramatic implications. A major purpose of this text is to help you adopt a new way of thinking toward health behaviors. This new way of thinking acknowledges that many of the factors that influence health, fitness, and wellness are largely within your control. Learning and practicing self-management skills can help you develop this new way of thinking.

Assessing factors that influence healthy lifestyles provides a basis for changing those factors that can contribute to health, wellness, or fitness.

Lab 2A allows you to assess predisposing, enabling, and reinforcing factors associated with one healthy lifestyle—regular physical activity. Similar assessments are possible for other healthy lifestyles. Self-assessments allow you to determine the factors that you can alter to make changes in any or all healthy lifestyles.

Assessing your current self-management skills provides a basis for future skill development.

Lab 2B provides you with an opportunity to assess your current self-management skills for one healthy lifestyle—regular

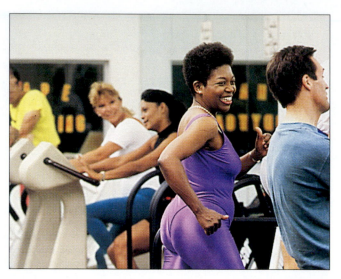

A new way of thinking can help you adopt healthy lifestyles.

physical activity. In subsequent concepts, you will practice the self-management skills relating to a variety of different healthy lifestyles. As you learn more about self-management skills, especially those that relate to physical activity, you can refer to Lab 2B to see if your assessments of your self-management skills were accurate.

You can benefit from a critical analysis of the theories and models that help us understand the factors that lead to healthy living.

www.mhhe.com/hper/physed/clw/student/

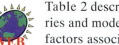

Table 2 describes some of the best-known theories and models used by researchers to study the factors associated with healthy living. Much of the information presented in this concept was derived from research using these theories and models. The suggested readings provide more information about the theories and models for those interested for studying them further.

   Web Review

Web Review materials for Concept 2 are available at *www.mhhe.com/hper/physed/clw/student/*.

American Journal of Health Promotion
   www.ajhp.com
ACSM's Health and Fitness Journal
   www.wwilkins.com/FIT

Table 2 Theorics and Models Associated with Healthy Lifestyle Adoption

Theory	Brief Description
Transtheoretical model	This model is also referred to as the stages of change model. As described earlier in this concept, this model suggests five stages of change that characterize various health behaviors. The model suggests that doing the correct things (processes) at the right time (stage of change) is important to self-change in health behaviors.
Health beliefs model	This model suggests that a person's health behavior is related to the following five factors: the belief that a health problem will have harmful effects, the belief that a person is susceptible to the problem, the perceived benefits of changing a lifestyle to prevent the problem, the perceived barriers to overcoming the problem, and the confidence that he/she can do what is necessary to prevent it.
Social cognitive theory	Social cognitive theory is also referred to as social learning theory. Central to this theory are self-efficacy and positive expectations about behavior change. Also, the theory suggests that a person must value the outcomes of a behavior if he or she is likely to do that behavior.
Theory of reasoned action	This theory suggests that a person's behavior is most associated with the person's intention to do the behavior. The two factors most likely to influence a person's intentions are attitudes (beliefs) and the social environment (opinions of others).
Theory of planned behavior	This theory is often combined with the theory for reasoned action. It has the same basic tenets but adds the concept of "perceived control" over the environment. The person must believe that he or she has some control over the factors that allow performance of that behavior. Perceived control is in many ways similar to self-efficacy in social cognitive theory.
Self-determination theory	Central to self-determination theory is the importance of choice in a person's life (autonomy). Perceptions of competence at mastering life's tasks are also critical to the theory. Making personal choices in attempt to master the tasks of daily living are emphasized rather than making choices based on external pressures to comply. Self-determination theory, and its subtheory cognitive evaluation theory, emphasize intrinsic motivation. The intrinsic motivation inherent in behaviors that are exciting and/or fulfilling to do, is very important in making activity choices.

Journal of Sport and Exercise Psychology

www.humankinetics.com/infok/ journal/jsep/intor.html

Medicine and Science in Sports and Exercise

www.wwilkins.com/FIT

Suggested Readings

Bandura, A. *Social Foundations of Thought and Action: A Social-Cognitive Theory.* Englewood Cliffs, NJ: Prentice-Hall, 1986.

Duda, J. L. (ed.) *Advances in Sport and Exercise Psychology Measurement.* Morgantown, WV:Fitness Information Technology Inc., 1998.

Haussenblas, H. A. et al. "Applications of the Theories of Reasoned Action and Planned Behaviors: A Meta Analysis." *The Journal of Sport and Exercise Psychology,* 19 (1997):36.

Prochaska, J. O. "Strong and Weak Principles for Progressing From Precontemplation to Action on the Basis of Twelve Problem Behaviors." *Health Psychology,* 13 (1994):47–51.

Prochaska, J. O. and Markus, B. H. "The transtheoretical model: Applications to exercise." In Advances in Exercise Adherence, Dishman, R. K. (ed.). Champaign, IL: Human Kinetics.

Marcus, B. H. et al. Longitudinal shifts in employee's stages and processes of exercise behavior change. *American Journal of Health Promotion,* 10 (1997):1105.

Reibe, R., and Nigg, C. "Setting the Stage for Healthy Living." *ACSM's Health and Fitness Journal,* 2(3) (1998):11–15.

Rosenstock, I. M. *The Health Belief Model: Explaining Health Behavior Through Expectancies.* In Glantz, K., Lewis, F. M. and Riner, B. K. *Health Behavior and Education.* San Francisco: Jossey–Bass, 1990.

Sallis, J. F. "Influences of Physical Activity on Children, Adolescents, and Adults or Determinants of Physical Activity." In Corbin, C. B. & Pangrazi, R. P. (eds.), *Towards a Better Understanding of Physical Fitness and Activity.* Scottsdale, AZ: Holcomb-Hathaway, 1999, Chapter 4.

Surgeon General's Office. *Surgeon General's Report on Physical Activity and Health.* Washington D.C.: U.S. Government Printing Office, 1996; Chapter 6.

Welk, G. J. "The Youth Physical Activity Promotion Model: A Conceptual Bridge Between Theory and Practice." *Quest* 51 (1999):5–23.

Whitehead, J. R. "Physical Activity and Intrinsic Motivation." In Corbin, C. B. & Pangrazi, R. P. (eds.), *Towards a Better Understanding of Physical Fitness and Activity.* Scottsdale, AZ: Holcomb-Hathaway, 1999, Chapter 5.

Lab 2A: The Physical Activity Adherence Questionnaire

Name	Section	Date

Purpose: To help you understand the factors that influence physical activity adherence and to see which factors you might change to improve your chances of achieving the action or maintenance level for physical activity.

Procedures:

1. The factors that predispose, enable, and reinforce adherence to physically active living are listed below. Read each statement. Place an X in the circle under the most appropriate response for you: very true, somewhat true, or not true.
2. When you have answered all of the items, determine a score by summing the four numbers for each type of factor. Then sum the three scores (predisposing, enabling, reinforcing) to get your total score.
3. Record your scores in the Results section and answer the questions in the Conclusions and Implications section.

	Very True	Somewhat True	Not True	
Predisposing Factors				
1. I am very knowledgeable about physical activity.	3	2	1	
2. I have a strong belief that physical activity is good for me.	3	2	1	
3. I enjoy doing regular exercise and physical activity.	3	2	1	
4. I am confident of my abilities in sports, exercise, and other physical activities.	3	2	1	
Predisposing Score			=	
Enabling Factors				
5. I possess good sport skills.	3	2	1	
6. I know how to plan my own physical activity program.	3	2	1	
7. I have a place to do physical activity near my home or work.	3	2	1	
8. I have the equipment I need to do physical activities I enjoy.	3	2	1	
Enabling Score			=	
Reinforcing Factors				
9. I have the support of my family for doing my regular physical activity.	3	2	1	
10. I have many friends who enjoy the same kinds of physical activities that I do.	3	2	1	
11. I have the support of my boss and my colleagues for participation in activity.	3	2	1	
12. I have a doctor and/or employer who encourages me to exercise.	3	2	1	
Reinforcing Score			=	
Total Score (Sum 3 Scores)			=	

Classification	Predisposing Score	Enabling Score	Reinforcing Score	Total Score
Adherence likely	11–12	11–12	11–12	33–36
Good	9–10	9–10	9–10	25–32
Adherence unlikely	<8	<8	<8	<24

Results: Record your scores and ratings in the spaces below.

Adherence Category	Score	Rating
Predisposing		
Enabling		
Reinforcing		
Total		

Conclusions and Implications:

In several sentences, discuss your ratings from this questionnaire. Also discuss the predisposing, enabling, and reinforcing factors that you may need to alter to increase your prospects for lifetime activity.

In several sentences, speculate about adherence factors for other healthy lifestyles such as eating well and managing stress. Do you think you need more or less work in these areas as compared to physically active living?

Lab 2B: The Self-Management Skills Questionnaire

Lab 2B The Self-Management Skills Questionnaire

Name _____   **Section** _____   **Date** _____

Purpose: To help you assess your self-management skills that are important to adhering to physically active lifestyles.

Procedures:
1. Each question reflects one of the self-management skills described earlier. Read each statement. After each statement, place an X over the circle indicating whether you think the item is very true, somewhat true, or not true.
2. When you have answered all of the items, score the questionnaire using the information in the Results section. Determine your ratings and answer the questions in the Conclusions and Implications section.

	Very True	Somewhat True	Not True	Score
1. I regularly assess my health-related fitness and rate my fitness test results using health-fitness standards.	3	2	1	
2. I keep regular physical activity logs to monitor current physical activity levels.	3	2	1	
3. I set realistic and attainable fitness and activity goals and monitor progress in meeting these goals.	3	2	1	
4. I have planned a personal program that includes activities for all parts of fitness and for optimal health benefits.	3	2	1	
5. I have the motor skills necessary to perform several physical activities on a regular basis.	3	2	1	
6. I have more positive than negative attitudes about physical activity.	3	2	1	
7. I find a way to do my activity even when the weather is bad or my time is limited.	3	2	1	
8. I know how to identify fitness misinformation and quackery.	3	2	1	
9. I know how to get others to do exercise with me and to get the support of others for doing my own activity program.	3	2	1	
10. I know and use strategies to stick with it especially when I have not been active for a while.	3	2	1	
11. I participate in activities that I am not very good at because I am able to enjoy them even if I don't excel.	3	2	1	
12. I manage my time to allow regular performance of my physical activity program.	3	2	1	
Total Score (Sum 12 Scores)				

Rating	Individual Scores	Total Score
Good	3	30–36
Marginal	2	24–29
May need improvement	1	less than 24

Results: Record your score for each skill as well as the rating in the chart below. There is one question for each self-management skill. Your score for each self-management skill is the number inside the circle for that question. The number of the question for each skill is noted in the chart below. To get your total score, sum the scores for all of the self-management skills.

Self-Management Skill	Item	Score	Rating
Self-assessment	1		
Self-monitoring	2		
Goal setting	3		
Self-planning	4		
Performance skills	5		
Balancing attitudes	6		
Overcoming barriers	7		
Learning consumer skills	8		
Finding social support	9		
Preventing relapse	10		
Adopting coping strategies	11		
Managing time	12		
Total			

Conclusions and Implications:

In several sentences, discuss your ratings regarding self-management skills. In which areas do you think you need to learn more to be able to be a better self-manager?

In several sentences, speculate about your self-management skills for other healthy lifestyles such as eating well and managing stress. Do you think you need more or less work in these areas as compared to managing for physically active living?

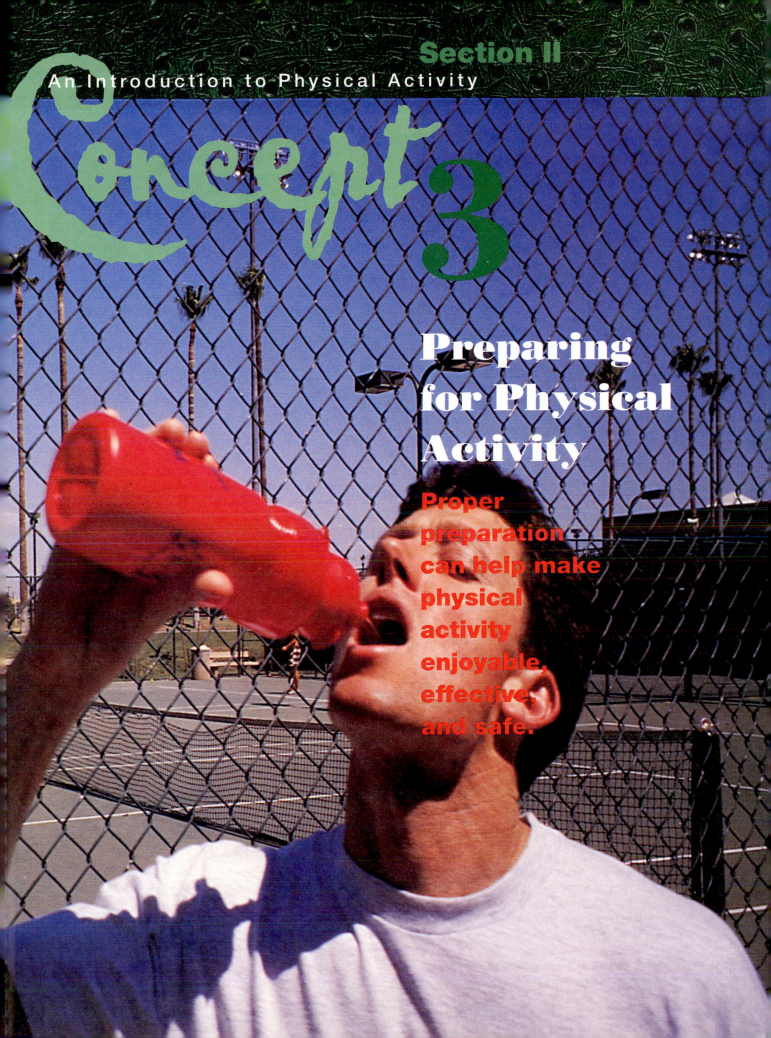

Concept 3

Preparing for Physical Activity

Proper preparation can help make physical activity enjoyable, effective, and safe.

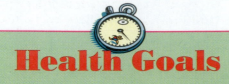

Health Goals

for Year 2010

Improve the health, fitness and quality of life of all people through the adoption and maintenance of regular, daily physical activity.

Increase leisure time physical activity.

Introduction

For people just beginning a physical activity program, adequate preparation may be the key to persistence. For those who have been regularly active for some time, sound preparation can help reduce risk of injury and make activity more enjoyable. It is hoped that a person armed with good information about preparation will become involved and stay involved in physical activity for a lifetime. For long-term maintenance, physical activity must be something that is a part of a person's normal lifestyle. Some facts that will help you prepare for and make physical activity a part of your normal routine are presented in this concept.

The Facts to Consider before Beginning Physical Activity

Before beginning a regular physical activity program, it is important to establish your medical readiness to participate.

Physical activity requires the cardiovascular system to work harder. While this level of stress can promote positive adaptations, the stress on the heart can be unsafe and dangerous for certain individuals. The British Columbia (Canada) Ministry of Health conducted extensive research to devise a procedure that would help people know when it was advisable to seek medical consultation prior to beginning or altering an exercise program. The goal was to prevent unnecessary medical examinations, while at the same time helping people to be reasonably assured that regular exercise was appropriate. The research resulted in the development of the Physical Activity Readiness Questionnaire (**PAR Q**) questionnaire. The most recent revision of the PAR Q consists of seven simple questions you can ask yourself to determine if medical consultation is necessary prior to exercise involvement.

Table 1 American College of Sports Medicine Risk Classification Categories	
Classification	**Description**
Apparently Healthy	Individuals who have no symptoms and are apparently healthy with no more than one of the following major coronary risk factors: age above 45 for men and 55 for women, history of heart attack in a parent, current tobacco use, high blood pressure, high cholesterol, diabetes mellitus, or sedentary lifestyle.
Increased Risk	Individuals with two or more of the risk factors identified above and/or signs or symptoms of possible cardiopulmonary or metabolic diseases such as chest pain, pain down the arm, shortness of breath with mild exertion, dizziness or fainting, ankle swelling, irregular heart beat, or heart murmur.
Known Disease	Individuals with known cardiac, pulmonary, or metabolic diseases.

Source: Adapted from ACSM's Guidelines for Exercise Testing and Prescription (see suggested readings).

The American College of Sports Medicine (ACSM) has developed additional guidelines to help determine if medical consultation or if a **clinical exercise test** is necessary prior to participation in physical activity programs. The ACSM divides people into three general categories (see Table 1). "Apparently healthy" adults (men under 40 and women under age 50) who have no known health problems and answer no to all seven PAR Q questions are generally cleared for participation in both **moderate** and **vigorous physical activity.** For older men and women (men over 40 and women over 50) and those with increased risk, but no symptoms of disease, moderate exercise programs do not necessarily need to be preceded by an exam and clinical exercise test. The ACSM does recommend a medical exam and a clinical exercise test for older adults and those with "increased risk" who plan to begin vigorous exercise programs, for those with symptoms of disease regardless of age, and for those with "known disease." When resuming physical activity after an injury or illness, consultation with a physician is always wise no matter what your age or medical condition.

There is no way to be absolutely sure that you are medically sound to begin a physical activity program. Even a thorough exam by a physician cannot guarantee that a person does not have some limitations that may cause a problem during exercise. The ACSM guidelines are designed to minimize the risk while preventing unnecessary medical cost. However, if there is any doubt about your readiness for activity, a medical exam is the surest way to make certain that you are ready to participate.

Those who plan to do intensive training (particularly for sports) may want to answer some additional questions concerning whether a medical exam is necessary before beginning (see Lab 3A).

It is important to dress properly for physical activity.

The clothing you wear for exercise should be specifically for that exercise. It should be comfortable and not too tight or binding at the joints. Though appearance is important to everyone, comfort in exercise is more important than looks. Clothing should not restrict movement in any way. Preferably, the clothing that comes in direct contact with the body should be porous to allow for sweat evaporation. Some fabrics (e.g., Gortex) allow heat loss and sweat evaporation while protecting against wind and rain. Some women, especially those who need extra support, should consider using an exercise bra, and men may benefit from an athletic supporter. A warm-up suit over other exercise apparel is recommended because it can be removed during exercise if desired. Some exercise apparel marketed to promote weight loss resulting from increased sweating can be dangerous. Suits that are nonporous and trap sweat inside preventing the cooling effect that results from the normal evaporation of sweat should not be worn.

Absorbent socks that fit properly should be worn during exercise. Socks that are too short can cause ingrown toenails, and loose-fitting socks can cause blisters. Not wearing socks can result in blisters, abrasions, odor, and excess wear on shoes.

Some activities require special protective apparel. For example, helmets are recommended for bikers and inline skaters. Statistics indicate a 75 percent decrease in risk of injury when wearing a bike helmet. Special gloves, pads and padded clothing can also help reduce risk of injury. These may be especially important for beginning rollerbladers since there is a high rate of falling for novices. Bikers, joggers, and walkers should consider reflective clothing and shoes, especially if activity takes place when light is restricted. Some experts now recommend water shoes to protect the feet for those who do extensive water aerobic exercise. It would be wise to investigate proper apparel and equipment needs for new activities in your activity program.

Proper footwear is important for safe and effective physical activity.

www.mhhe.com/hper/physed/clw/student/

Most manufacturers now produce athletic shoes in six categories: running/jogging, walking, tennis, court, aerobic/fitness, and **cross-training.** Many produce even more specialized shoes within each category. For example, many manufacturers have separate court shoes for basketball and volleyball. For people who are highly dedicated to a specific activity, a specialized pair of shoes should be purchased. For those who do not specialize in one activity, the cross trainer is a good choice.

The essential characteristics of all athletic shoes are described below (see Figure 1):

- **Support.** The heel counter and the heel stabilizer provide stability and control foot movement. The heel tab protects the Achilles tendon from trauma. The heel in running shoes should not be too narrow. Adequate width in the heel provides stability and protects against ankle turns. For court games such as basketball, a high-top shoe is recommended for additional ankle support.

- **Cushioning.** It is generally agreed that good cushioning is important, especially in the heel and midsole. However, excessive cushioning is not recommended. Too much cushioning may increase risk of injury by inhibiting the reflexes that help the body protect itself against the impact of the foot with the ground.

- **Performance.** A lightweight shoe requires less energy output over lengthy exercise periods. Good traction for a given sport is also important. For lengthy performances, a shoe that is at least partially made from a material that can breathe, such as nylon mesh, helps sweat evaporation and inhibits shoe weight gain.

PAR Q An acronym for Physical Activity Readiness Questionnaire; designed to help you determine if you are medically suited to begin an exercise program.

Clinical Exercise Test A test typically administered on a treadmill in which exercise is gradually increased in intensity while the heart is monitored by an EKG. Symptoms not present at rest, such as an abnormal EKG, may be present in an exercise test.

Moderate Physical Activity Physical activity that is equal in intensity to brisk walking.

Vigorous Physical Activity Physical activity that is more intense than brisk walking; usually associated with elevated heart rate, increased breathing rates, and increased sweating.

Cross-Training A term commonly used to indicate participation in a variety of activities (e.g., running, tennis, resistance training).

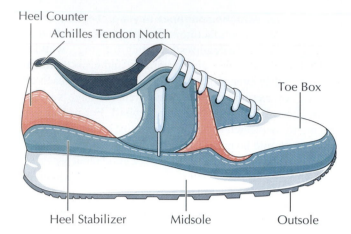

Heel Counter

Achilles Tendon Notch

Toe Box

Heel Stabilizer   Midsole   Outsole

Figure 1

Characteristics of a good activity shoe.

- **Fit.** The toe box should be roomy enough so that you can wiggle your toes. Regardless of the type of shoe, exercise shoes should generally be one-half size larger than your regular shoes. If you wear two pairs of socks while exercising, you should wear two pairs when trying on the shoes. It is important to try on the shoes and move around in them before making a purchase. Make sure they feel good to you.

Probably the biggest mistake made regarding footwear is not replacing them when they wear out. The important cushioning areas of the shoe (heel and midsole) typically wear out before the sole or the fabric. Thus, it may be necessary to replace shoes before they appear worn out.

The Facts to Consider during Daily Physical Activity

There are three key components of the daily activity program: the warm-up exercise, the workout, and the cool-down exercise.

The key component of a fitness program is the daily workout. Experts agree, however, that the workout should be preceded by a **warm-up** and followed by a **cool-down.** The warm-up prepares the body for physical activity, and the cool-down returns the body to rest and promotes effective recovery.

The cardiovascular warm-up prior to the workout is recommended to prepare the muscles and heart for the workout.

www.mhhe.com/hper/physed/clw/student/

There are two good reasons for warming up prior to activity. The first is to prepare the heart muscle and circulatory system. When you start physical activity, blood flow is not immediately available to the heart and muscles. A proper warm-up decreases the risk of irregular heart beats associated with poor coronary circulation. A proper warm-up can also improve performance since it minimizes the premature formation of **lactic acid** at the start of physical activity. Research suggests that two minutes of walking, jogging, or mild exercise is adequate for moderate activities; however, some experts recommend five minutes or more of moderate activity as a warm-up for vigorous activity.

The second reason for a warm-up is to stretch the skeletal muscles. When you begin exercise, muscles and joints are usually cold and stiff. By gradually warming up the body, the muscles become more elastic and extensible. The skeletal muscle warm-up should include static stretching of the major muscle groups involved in the exercise that is to follow. It should be emphasized that even though warming up prior to an activity may help reduce the chance of muscle injury, it is not a substitute for a regular program of exercise designed to improve flexibility.

A warm-up that is suitable for walking, jogging, running, cycling, and even basketball is illustrated in Figure 2. This warm-up can be used for other activities provided stretching exercises for the major muscle groups involved in the activities are added. Additional exercises that are appropriate for inclusion in a stretching warm-up are illustrated in the flexibility concept. The cardiovascular warm-up is suitable for most activities, but other mild exercise (such as a slow swim for swimmers or a slow ride for cyclists) can be substituted.

Many experts recommend that the stretching portion of the warm-up be done after the cardiovascular portion.

Some experts believe that the cardiovascular portion of the warm-up should precede the stretching portion because warm muscles are less likely to be injured by the stretch. Warm muscles also stretch farther. Some experts are concerned that the stretch warm-up may be abandoned by people who feel that they do not have time to do both the cardiovascular and stretching warm-up before doing their activity program. In this case, it is better to do stretching without the cardiovascular warm-up than do nothing at all. If you choose to stretch before the warm-up, make certain it is a gentle, static stretch. This is not the time for a flexibility workout in which you try to increase your normal range of motion. Rather, it should be for the purpose of limbering up or loosening.

A cool-down after the workout is important to promote an effective recovery from physical activity.

Figure 2
Sample warm-up and cool-down exercises.

The exercises shown here can be used before a moderate workout as a warm-up, or after a workout as a cool-down. Perform these exercises slowly, preferably after completing a cardiovascular warm-up. Do not bounce or jerk against the muscle. Hold each stretch for at least 15 seconds. Perform each exercise at least once and up to three times. Other stretching exercises are presented in the concept on flexibility that can be used in a warm-up or cool-down.

Cardiovascular Exercise
Before you perform a vigorous workout, walk or jog slowly for 2 minutes or more. After exercise, do the same. If possible do this portion of the warm-up prior to muscle stretching.

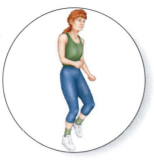

Calf Stretcher
This exercise stretches the calf muscles (gastrocnemius and soleus). Face a wall with your feet 2 or 3 feet away. Step forward on left foot to allow both hands to touch the wall. Keep the heel of your right foot on the ground, toe turned in slightly, knee straight, and buttocks tucked in. Lean forward by bending your front knee and arms and allowing your head to move nearer the wall. Hold. Repeat with the other leg.

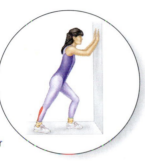

Hamstring Stretcher
This exercise stretches the muscles of the back of the upper leg (hamstrings) as well as those of the hip, knee, and ankle. Lie on your back. Bring the right knee to your chest and grasp the toes with the right hand. Place the left hand on the back of the right thigh. Pull the knee toward the chest, push the heel toward the ceiling, and pull the toes toward the shin. Attempt to straighten the knee. Stretch and hold. Repeat with the other leg.

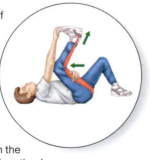

Leg Hug
This exercise stretches the hip and back extensor muscles. Lie on your back. Bend one leg and grasp your thigh under the knee. Hug it to your chest. Keep the other leg straight and on the floor. Hold. Repeat with the opposite leg.

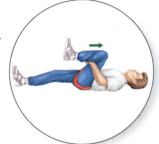

Seated Side Stretch
This exercise stretches the muscles of the trunk. Begin in a seated position with the legs crossed. Stretch the left arm over the head to the right. Bend at the waist (to right), reaching as far as possible to the left with the right arm. Hold. Do not let the trunk rotate. Repeat to the opposite side. For less stretch the overhead arm may be bent. This exercise can be done in the standing position but is less effective.

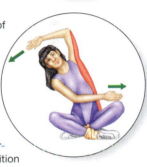

Zipper
This exercise stretches the muscle on the back of the arm (triceps) and the lower chest muscles (pecs). Lift right arm and reach behind head and down the spine (as if pulling up a zipper). With the left hand, push down on right elbow and hold. Reverse arm position and repeat.

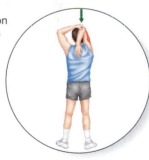

The cool-down is done immediately after the workout. Like the warm-up, there are two principal components of a cool-down: static muscle stretching and an activity for the cardiovascular system. Although not all experts agree, some believe that static muscle stretching *after* the workout is more important than stretching before because it may help relieve spasms in fatigued muscles. Stretching as part of the cool-down may be more effective for lengthening the muscles than stretching at other times because the muscle temperature is elevated and therefore the stretching is more likely to produce optimal flexibility improvements.

A cardiovascular portion of the cool-down is also important. During physical activity, the heart pumps a large amount of blood to supply the working muscles with the oxygen necessary to keep moving. The muscles squeeze the

Warm-Up Light to moderate activity done prior to the workout. Its purpose is to reduce the risk of injury and soreness and possibly to improve performance in a physical activity.

Cool-Down Light to moderate activity done after a workout to help the body recover; often consisting of the same exercises used in the warm-up.

Lactic Acid A byproduct of the metabolic processes that occurs during vigorous physical activity; a cause of muscle fatigue.

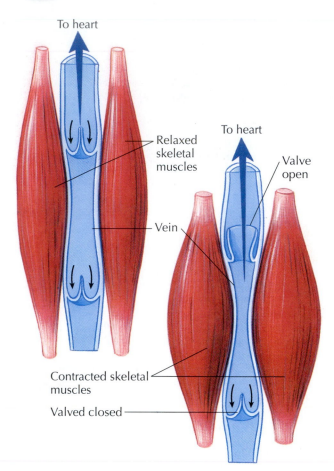

Figure 3
The pumping action of the muscles.

veins (see Figure 3), which forces the blood back to the heart. Valves in the veins prevent the blood from flowing backward. As long as exercise continues, the blood is moved by the muscles back to the heart, where it is once again pumped to the body. If exercise is stopped abruptly, the blood is left in the area of the working muscles and has no way to get back to the heart. In the case of the runner, the blood pools in the legs. Because the heart has less blood to pump, blood pressure may drop. This can result in dizziness, and can even cause a person to pass out. The best way to prevent this problem is to taper off or slow down gradually after exercise. A cardiovascular cool-down should include approximately 2 minutes of walking, slow jogging, or any nonvigorous activity that uses the muscles involved in the workout.

The Facts about Physical Activity in the Heat

Physical activity in hot and humid environments challenges the body's heat loss mechanisms.

www.mhhe.com/hper/physed/clw/student/
The normal human body temperature is 98.6°F. During vigorous activity, the body produces large amounts of heat, which must be dissipated to keep the body temperature regulated. The body has several ways to dissipate heat. Conduction is the transfer of heat from a hot body to a cold body. Convection is the transfer of heat through the air or other medium. Fans and wind can facilitate heat loss by convection and help regulate temperature. The primary method of cooling is through evaporation of sweat. The chemical process involved in evaporation transfers heat from the body and reduces the body temperature. When conditions are humid, the effectiveness of evaporation is reduced since the air is already saturated with moisture. This is why it is difficult to regulate body temperature when conditions are both hot and humid.

Heat-related illness can occur if proper hydration is not maintained.

Maximum sweat rates during physical activity in the heat can approach 1–2 liters per hour. If this fluid is not replaced, **dehydration** can occur. If dehydration is not corrected with water or other fluid-replacement drinks, it becomes increasingly more difficult for the body to maintain normal body temperatures. At some point, the rate of sweating decreases as the body begins to try to conserve its remaining water. It attempts to shunt blood to the skin to transfer excess heat directly to the environment, but this is less effective than evaporation, and various heat-related problems including heat stroke and **hyperthermia** can result (see Table 3).

One way to monitor the amount of fluid loss is to monitor the color of your urine. The American College of Sports Medicine indicates that clear (almost colorless) urine produced in large volumes indicates that you are hydrated and ready for activity. Dark yellow urine produced in small volume is a good indicator of dehydration and need for fluid replacement.

Acclimatization improves the body's tolerance in the heat.

Individuals with good fitness will respond better to activity in the heat than individuals with poor fitness. This is because the ability to sweat improves with training. With regular exposure to the heat, the body becomes conditioned to sweat earlier, to sweat more profusely, and to distribute sweat more effectively around the body. This process of acclimatization makes it easier for the body to maintain a safe body temperature.

When doing physical activity in hot and humid environments, special precautions should be taken to prevent heat-related problems.

Table 2 Exercise in the Heat (Apparent Temperatures)

To read the table, find air temperature on the top, then find the humidity on the left. Find the apparent temperature where the columns meet.

Relative Humidity (%)	Air Temperature (Degrees F)										
	70	75	80	85	90	95	100	105	110	115	120
100	72	80	91	108	132						
95	71	79	89	105	128						
90	71	79	88	102	122						
85	71	78	87	99	117	141					
80	71	78	86	97	113	136					
75	70	77	86	95	109	130					
70	70	77	85	93	106	124	144				
65	70	76	83	91	102	119	138				
60	70	76	82	90	100	114	132	149			
55	69	75	81	89	98	110	126	142			
50	69	75	81	88	96	107	120	135	150		
45	68	74	80	87	95	104	115	129	143		
40	68	74	79	86	93	101	110	123	137	151	
35	67	73	79	85	91	98	107	118	130	143	
30	67	73	78	84	90	96	104	113	123	135	148
25	66	72	77	83	88	94	101	109	117	127	139
20	66	72	77	82	87	93	99	105	112	120	130
15	65	71	76	81	86	91	97	102	108	115	123
10	65	70	75	80	85	90	95	100	105	111	116
5	64	69	74	79	84	88	93	97	102	107	111
0	64	69	73	78	83	87	91	95	99	103	107

■ = Safe Zone
■ = Caution Zone
■ = Danger Zone

"Apparent Temperatures"

Source: Data from National Oceanic and Atmospheric Administration.

www.mhhe.com/hper/physed/clw/student/

WEB

- Limit or avoid physical activity in hot or humid environments. The **apparent temperature** is a combined value determined by both temperature and humidity. When the apparent temperature is below 90°F (32.2°C), exercise is safe for most people. Caution should be used when exercising at apparent temperatures ranging from 90° to 100°F (37.7°C). Above 100°F, apparent temperature is the danger zone, and physical activity should be done with extreme care, be limited, or be canceled (see Table 2). Experienced exercisers who have become acclimatized to the heat may be able to perform at higher apparent temperatures than those who are less experienced. However, care should be used by all people who perform physical activity in hot and humid environments.

- Replace fluids regularly. Drink water before (2 cups or 16 ounces) and during activity (1 cup or 5–10 ounces every 15 to 20 minutes). After activity, replacing 16 ounces of fluid for each pound of weight lost is a good rule. For exercise lasting more than 1 hour, fluid-replacement drinks containing simple carbohydrates (glucose, fructose, or sucrose) and electrolytes are considered beneficial to performance and body cooling. If the concentration of sugars is no more than 4–8 percent, they can replace fluids as quickly as water.

- Gradually expose yourself to physical activity in hot and humid environments. Too much at once is especially dangerous.

Table 3 Types of Heat-Related Problems

Problem	Symptoms	Severity
Heat cramps	Muscle cramps, especially in muscles most used in exercise	Least severe
Heat exhaustion	Muscle cramps, weakness, dizziness; headache, nausea, clammy skin, paleness	Moderate severity
Heat stroke	Hot, flushed skin; dry skin (lack of sweating); dizziness fast pulse; unconsciousness; high temperature	Extremely severe

Dehydration Excessive loss of water from the body, usually through perspiration, urination, or evaporation.

Hyperthermia Excessively high body temperature caused by excessive heat production or impaired heat loss capacity. Heat stroke is an example of a hyperthermic condition.

Apparent Temperature A combination of temperature and humidity used to determine if it is dangerous to perform physical activity.

- When possible, do your activity in the morning or evening.
- Dress properly for exercise in the heat and humidity. Wear white or light colors that reflect rather than absorb heat. Porous clothing allows the passage of air to cool the body. Rubber, plastic, or other nonporous clothing is especially dangerous. A porous hat or cap can help when exercising in direct sunlight.
- Do not change your wet shirt for a dry one. A wet shirt cools the body better.
- Rest at regular intervals, preferably in the shade.
- Watch for signs of heat stress. If signs are present, stop immediately.

If overheating occurs, take immediate steps to cool the body.

Take these steps: stop physical activity; get out of the heat and into the shade; remove excess clothing; drink cool water; immerse the body in cool water; if symptoms of heat stroke are present, seek immediate medical attention; and statically stretch cramped muscles.

Facts about Physical Activity in Other Environments

Physical activity in exceptionally cold and windy weather can be dangerous.

Physical activity in the cold presents the opposite problem as exercise in the heat. In the cold, the primary goal is to retain the body's heat and avoid **hypothermia** or frostbite. Because wind promotes heat loss through convection, the combination of wind and cold temperatures (**windchill factor**) poses the greatest danger. When performing physical activity in cold and windy environments, special considerations should be taken.

- Limit or cancel activity if the windchill factor reaches the danger zone (see Table 4).
- Dress properly in the wind and cold. Wear light clothing in several layers rather than one heavy garment. The layer of clothing closest to the body should ideally help to transfer (wick) moisture away from the skin and transfer it to a second more absorbent layer. Fabric such as polypropylene and capilene are examples of wickable fabrics. A porous windbreaker will keep wind from cooling the body and will allow the release of body heat. Since the hands, feet, nose, and ears are most susceptible to frostbite, these body parts should be covered. Wear a hat or cap, mask, and mittens. Mittens are warmer than gloves. If you do not wear mittens or gloves, a light coating of petroleum jelly on the back of the hands is helpful. A similar treatment of the nose and ears has been shown to be effective.

- Try to keep from getting wet in cold weather.

High altitude and/or air pollution may limit performance and require adaptation of normal physical activity.

www.mhhe.com/hper/physed/clw/student/
The ability to do vigorous physical tasks is diminished as altitude increases. Breathing rate and heart rates are more elevated at high altitude. With proper acclimation (gradual exposure), the body adjusts to the lower oxygen pressure found at high altitude, and performance improves. Nevertheless, performance ability at high altitudes, especially for activities requiring cardiovascular fitness, is usually less than would be expected at sea level. At extremely high altitudes, the ability to perform vigorous physical activity may be impossible without an extra oxygen supply. When moving to a high altitude from sea level, vigorous exercise should be done with caution. Acclimation to high altitudes requires a minimum of two weeks and may not be complete for several months. Care should be taken to drink adequate water at altitude.

www.mhhe.com/hper/physed/clw/student/
Various pollutants such as ozone, carbon monoxide, pollens, and particulates can also cause poor physical performance, and in some cases, health problems. Ozone, a pollutant produced primarily by the sun's reaction to car exhaust, can cause symptoms including headache, coughing, and eye irritation. Similar symptoms result from exposure to carbon monoxide, a tasteless and odorless gas, caused by combustion of oil, gasoline, and cigarette smoke. Most news media in metropolitan areas now provide updates on ozone and carbon monoxide levels in their weather reports. When levels of these pollutants reach moderate levels, exercise may need to be modified for some people. When levels are high, exercise may need to be postponed. Exercisers wishing to avoid ozone and carbon monoxide may want to exercise indoors early in the morning, or later in the evening. It is wise to avoid areas with a high concentration of motor vehicles.

Pollens from certain plants may cause allergic reactions for certain people. Some people are allergic to dust or other particulates in the air. Weather reports of pollens and particulates may help exercisers determine the best times for their activities and when to avoid vigorous activities.

The Facts about Soreness and Injury

Understanding soreness can help you persist in physical activity and avoid problems.

www.mhhe.com/hper/physed/clw/student/
Some people avoid physical activity because they remember earlier experiences such as team practices or training for special events that led to sore-

Table 4 Windchill Factor Chart

Actual Temperature Reading (Degrees F)	Estimated Wind Speed (mph)									Zones
	Calm	5	10	15	20	25	30	35	40	
50	50	48	40	36	32	30	28	27	26	Relatively safe with proper clothing
40	40	37	28	22	18	16	13	11	10	
30	30	27	16	9	4	0	-2	-4	-6	
20	20	16	4	-5	-10	-15	-18	-20	-21	
10	10	6	-9	-18	-25	-29	-33	-35	-37	Danger to exposed skin
0	0	-5	-24	-32	-39	-44	-48	-51	-53	
-10	-10	-15	-33	-45	-40	-59	-63	-67	-69	
-20	-20	-26	-46	-58	-67	-74	-79	-82	-85	Unsafe— postpone exercise
-30	-30	-36	-58	-72	-82	-88	-94	-98	-100	
-40	-40	-47	-70	-85	-96	-104	-109	-113	-116	

*NOTE: Wind speeds above 40 mph do not seem to add to danger of cold.

Based on data from Taylor, K. *Runner's World,* 8 (1973):28.

ness 24 to 48 hours after the intense exercise. They feel that all activity will make them sore, and they want to avoid this unpleasant experience. It is true that intense exercise, especially to muscle groups that are not normally exercised, can cause what is called delayed-onset muscle soreness (**DOMS**). Some people mistakenly believe that lactic acid is the cause of muscle soreness. Lactic acid, however, returns to normal levels 30 minutes after exercise, whereas DOMS occurs at least 24 hours following exercise. We now know that DOMS results from microscopic muscle tears, not a build up of lactic acid. In some cases, DOMS is accompanied by swelling and pain, but in general the condition has no long-term consequences.

There are several steps that can be taken to avoid DOMS and to make activity more enjoyable. Starting gradually (not doing too much after being inactive) is perhaps the most important thing you can do. It is known that lengthening contractions (eccentric) are more likely to cause DOMS than shortening muscle contractions (concentric contractions). For this reason, walking or running downhill or downstairs should be gradually phased into your program. Of course, a regular warm-up is also advised. Fortunately, DOMS lasts only a day or so. Doing moderate exercise when you have soreness does not seem to put you at risk of muscle injury. DOMS is only temporary and not a common occurrence for those who exercise regularly and consistently. Understanding this will keep it from being a deterrent to regular physical activity.

Being able to treat minor injuries will help reduce their negative effects.

Minor injuries such as muscle sprains and strains are not uncommon to those who are persistent in their exercise. If a serious injury should occur, it is important to get immediate medical attention. However, for minor injuries, following the "RICE" formula will help you reduce the pain or the injury and will speed recovery. In this acronym, **R** stands for "rest." Muscle sprains and strains heal best if rested, and rest also helps you avoid further damage to the muscle. **I** stands for "ice." The quick application of cold (ice or ice water) to a minor injury minimizes swelling and speeds recovery. Cold should be applied to as large a surface area as possible (soaking is best). If ice is used, it should be wrapped to avoid direct contact with the skin. Apply cold for 20–30 minutes, three times a day for several days. **C** stands for "compression." Wrapping or compressing the injured area also helps minimize swelling and speeds recovery. Elastic bandages are good for applying compression. For a sprained ankle, wearing a tied high-top shoe

Hypothermia Excessively low body temperature (less than 95°F) characterized by uncontrollable shivering, loss of coordination, and mental confusion.

Windchill Factor An index that uses air temperature and wind speed to determine the chilling effect of the environment on humans.

DOMS An acronym for delayed onset muscle soreness; a common malady that follows relatively vigorous activity especially among beginners.

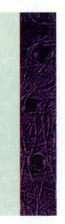

until a bandage can be located provides good compression. Elastic socks may also be useful. Care should be taken to avoid wrapping an injury too tightly because this can result in loss of circulation to the area. **E** stands for "elevation." Keeping the injured area elevated (above the level of the heart) is effective in minimizing swelling. If pain or swelling persists, or if there is any doubt about the seriousness of an injury, seek medical help.

Taking over-the-counter pain remedies can help reduce the pain of muscle strains and sprains. Aspirin and ibuprofen (e.g., Motrin, Excedrin) have anti-inflammatory properties. However, acetaminophen (e.g., Tylenol) does not have anti-inflammatory properties, so it may reduce the pain but it will not reduce the inflammation. Any over-the-counter remedy should be taken only as directed unless otherwise indicated by a physician.

> **The most common injuries incurred in physical activity are sprains and strains.**

www.mhhe.com/hper/physed/clw/student/

A strain occurs when the fibers in a muscle are injured. A sprain is an injury to a ligament—the connective tissue that connects bones to bones. Common activity-related injuries are hamstring strains that occur after a vigorous sprint. A good example would be the occasional athlete who sprints to first base without warming up and after not playing in a long time. Other commonly strained muscles include the muscles in the front of the thigh, the low back, and the calf muscles. The most common sprain is to the ankle. It frequently occurs when the ankle is rolled to the outside when jumping or running. Evidence suggests that lace-up ankle braces made of non-elastic material are effective in reducing ankle sprains. Other common sprains are to the knee, the shoulder, and the wrist. Sprains and strains respond well to RICE.

Tendonitis is an inflammation of the tendon and is most often a result of overuse rather than trauma. Tendonitis can be painful but often does not swell to the extent that sprains do. For this reason, elevation and compression are not especially effective, but ice, and especially rest, are useful.

> **Muscle cramps can be relieved by statically stretching a muscle.**

Muscle cramps are pains in the large muscles of the body that result when the muscle contracts vigorously for a continued period of time. A muscle cramp is usually not considered to be an injury, but they are painful and may seem like an injury. They are usually short in duration and can often be relieved with proper treatment. Cramps can result from lack of fluid replacement (dehydration), from fatigue,

and from a blow directly to a muscle. A true cramp is not the same as a muscle tear, sprain, or strain. A cramp can be relieved by statically stretching the cramped muscle. For example, the calf muscle, which often cramps among runners, football players, and other sports participants, can be relieved using the calf stretcher exercise, which is part of the warm-up in this concept. Other stretching exercises from the concept on flexibility can be used to relieve cramps to other muscles or muscle groups. If stretching causes persistent pain, stop the stretching—you may have a muscle injury rather than a cramp. Of course, replacing fluids regularly during exercise helps avoid cramps, as does the development of flexibility.

Web Review

Web Review materials for Concept 3 are available at *www.mhhe.com/hper/physed/clw/student/*.

ACSM's Health and Fitness Journal
   www.wwilkins.com/FIT

American Alliance for Health, Physical Education, Recreation
   www.ahper.org

American College of Sports Medicine
   www.acsm.org

National Athletic Trainers Association
   www.nata.org

The Physician and Sportsmedicine
   www.physsportsmed.com

Suggested Readings

Agostini, R. Reduce Risks of Activity-Induced Injury. *ACSM's Health and Fitness Journal* 2(2), S29, 1998.

American College of Sports Medicine. *ACSM's Guidelines for Exercise Testing and Prescription*, 5th ed. Baltimore, MD: Williams and Wilkins, 1995.

American College of Sports Medicine. Position Stand on Exercise and Fluid Replacement. *Medicine and Science in Sports and Exercise*, 28 (1)(1996): i .

American College of Sports Medicine. Position Stand on Heat and Cold Illness During Distance Running. *Medicine and Science in Sports and Exercise.* 28(12)(1996):i.

Garrick, J. G. and Schelkun, P. H. "Managing Ankle Sprains: Keys to Preserving Motion and Strains." *The Physician and Sports Medicine,* 25(3)(1997):56.

Martin, D. R. "Athletic Shoes: Finding a Good Match." *The Physician and Sports Medicine,* 25(9)(1997):138.

Peterson, J. "10 ways to avoid heat-related conditions while exercising." *ACSM's Health and Fitness Journal,* 2(3)(1998):48.

Powers, S. K., and Howley, E. T. *Exercise Physiology* (3d ed.) Dubuque, IA: WCB/McGraw-Hill Publishers, 1997.

Sandor, R. P. "Heat Illness." *Physician and Sportsmedicine,* 25(6)(1997):35.

Shephard, R. J. "Preparing for Physical Activity." In Corbin, C. B. & Pangrazi, R. P. (ed.), *Towards a Better Understanding of Physical Fitness and Activity.* Scottsdale, AZ: Holcomb-Hathaway, 1999, Chapter 1.

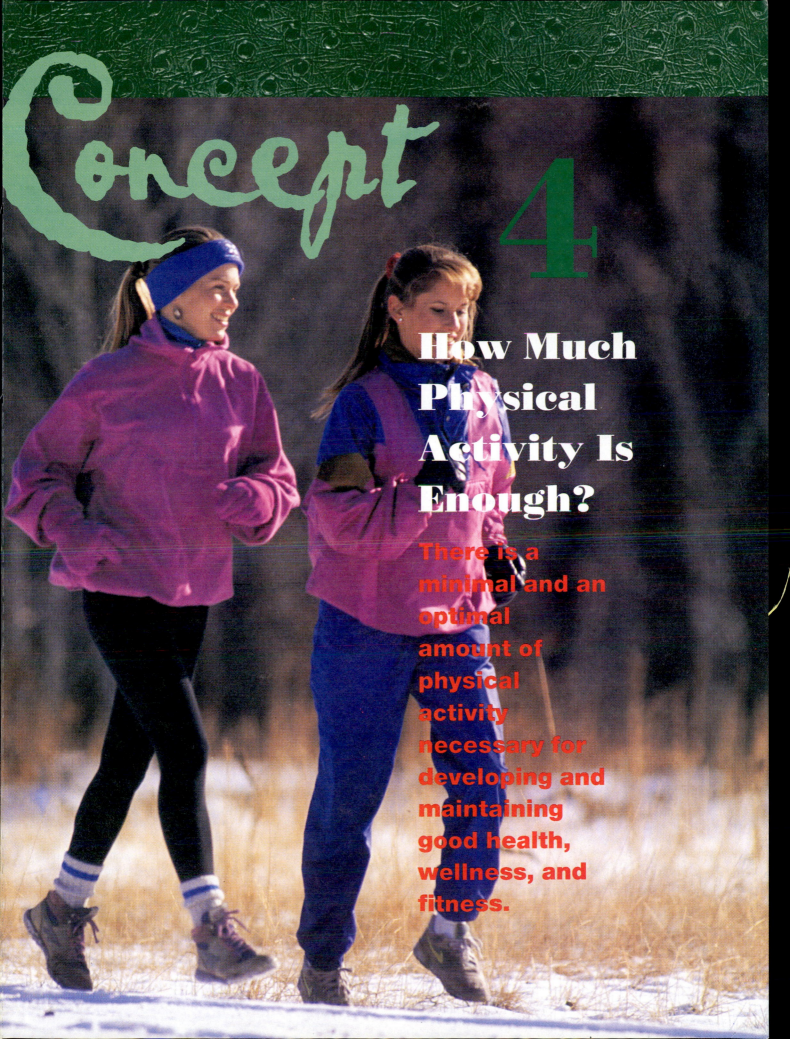

Concept 4

How Much Physical Activity Is Enough?

There is a minimal and an optimal amount of physical activity necessary for developing and maintaining good health, wellness, and fitness.

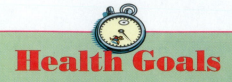

Health Goals

for the year 2010

Improve the health, fitness and quality of life of all people through the adoption and maintenance of regular, daily physical activity.

Increase the proportion of people who do moderate daily activity for 30 minutes.

Increase the proportion of people who do vigorous physical activity three days a week.

Increase the proportion of people who do regular exercises for muscle fitness.

Increase the proportion of people who do regular exercise for flexibility.

Introduction

Just as there is a correct dosage of medicine for treating an illness, there is a correct dosage of physical activity for promoting health benefits and developing physical fitness. Several important principles of physical activity provide the basis for determining the correct dose or amount of physical activity. In this concept, a formula for implementing the important physical activity principles will be presented. This formula and the concepts of "threshold of training" and "target zones" will be described to help you determine how much physical activity is enough. New evidence indicates that the amount of physical activity necessary for developing metabolic fitness, and its associated health benefits, is different from the amount of physical activity necessary for developing health-related fitness and other performance benefits. Research also shows that the amount of activity or exercise necessary for maintaining fitness may differ from the amount needed to develop it.

The Principles of Physical Activity: The Facts

Overload is necessary to achieve health, wellness, and fitness benefits of physical activity.

The **overload principle** is the most basic of all physical activity principles. This principle indicates that doing "more than normal" is necessary if benefits are to occur. In order

for a muscle (including the heart muscle) to get stronger, it must be overloaded, or worked against a load greater than normal. To increase flexibility, a muscle must be stretched longer than is normal. To increase muscular endurance, muscles must be exposed to sustained exercise for a longer than normal period. The health benefits associated with metabolic fitness seems to require less overload than for health-related fitness improvement, but overload is required just the same.

Physical activity should be increased progressively for safe and effective results.

The **principle of progression** indicates that overload should not be increased too slowly or too rapidly if benefits are to result. A simple example relates to working with your hands. If you have not done anything for a while and you do too much work with your hands, you develop blisters. You are less able to work the next day. A day or more of recovery may be necessary before you are back to normal. If, however, you begin gradually and increase the work you do each day, you develop calluses. The calluses make your hands tougher, and you are able to work long or longer without injury or soreness. The benefits of all forms of physical activity are best when you gradually increase overload. Doing too much too soon is counterproductive.

The benefits of physical activity are specific to the form of activity performed.

The **principle of specificity** states that to benefit from physical activity, you must overload specifically for that benefit. For example, strength-building exercises may do little for developing cardiovascular fitness, and stretching exercises may do little for altering body composition or metabolic fitness.

Overload is specific to each component of fitness and each health or wellness benefit desired. Overload is also specific to each body part. If you exercise the legs, you build fitness of the legs. If you exercise the arms, you build fitness of the arms. For this reason, it is not unusual to see some people with disproportionate fitness development. Some gymnasts, for example, have good upper body development but poor leg development, whereas some soccer players have well-developed legs but lack upper body development.

Specificity is important in designing your warm-up, workout, and cool-down programs for specific activities. Training is most effective when it closely resembles the activity for which you are preparing. For example, if your goal is to improve your skill in putting the shot, it is not enough to strenghten the arm muscles. You should perform a training activity requiring overload that closely resembles the motion you use in the actual sport.

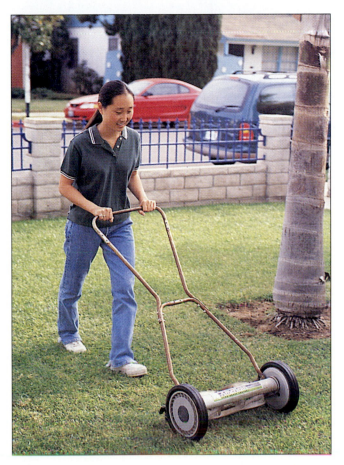

Doing lifestyle activities can benefit your health.

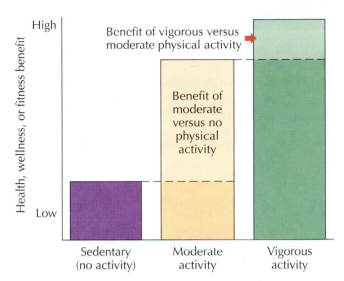

Figure 1

Diminishing returns from increased physical activity.

tive person. This person's fitness is low. The second bar in the figure indicates the same person who did moderately activity and achieved a substantial improvement in fitness. When the person increased activity again by the same amount, fitness increases were not as dramatic. Improvement occurred but not as much as when the person moved from inactivity to moderate activity.

The benefits achieved from overload last only as long as overload continues.

The **principle of reversibility** is basically the overload principle in reverse. To put is simply, if you don't use it, you will lose it. It is an important principle because some people have the mistaken impression that if they achieve a health or fitness benefit, it will last forever. This, of course, is not true. There is evidence that you can maintain health benefits with less physical activity than it took to achieve them. Still, if you do not adhere to regular physical activity, any benefits attained will gradually erode away.

Beginners may find that improvements in health, wellness, and fitness come more quickly than for those who already possess good health, wellness, and fitness.

The **principle of diminishing returns** is illustrated in Figure 1. The bar on the left of the figure characterizes an inac-

Overload Principle A basic principle that specifies that you must perform physical activity in greater than normal amounts (overload) to get an improvement in physical fitness or health benefits.

Principle of Progression A corollary of the overload principle that indicates the need to gradually increase overload to achieve optimal benefits.

Principle of Specificity A corollary of the overload principle that indicates a need for a specific type of exercise to improve each fitness component or fitness of a specific part of the body.

Principle of Reversibility A corollary of the overload principle that indicates that disuse or inactivity results in loss of benefits achieved as a result of overload

Principle of Diminishing Returns A corollary of the overload principle indicating that the more benefits you gain as a result of activity, the harder additional benefits are to achieve.

Health, wellness, and fitness benefits increase your amount of physical activity. But it is important to understand that if you keep increasing physical activity by equal increments, each additional amount of activity will yield less benefit. At some point, improvements will plateau and if activity is overdone, may actually decrease.

The Facts about the FIT Formula

The acronym FIT can help you remember the three important variables for applying the overload principle and its corollaries.

www.mhhe.com/hper/physed/clw/student/
For physical activity to be effective, it must be done with enough frequency and intensity and for a long enough time. The first letter from these three words spells **FIT** and can be considered as the formula for achieving health, wellness, and fitness benefits.

Frequency (how often)—Physical activity must be performed regularly to be effective. The number of days a person does activity in a week is used to determine frequency. Most benefits require at least three days and up to six days of activity per week but frequency ultimately depends on the specific benefit desired.

Intensity (how hard)—Physical activity must be intense enough to require more exertion (overload) than normal to produce benefits. The method for determining appropriate intensity varies with the desired benefit. For example, metabolic fitness and associated health benefits require only moderate intensity; cardiovascular fitness for high-level performance requires vigorous activity that elevates the heart rate well above normal.

Time (how long)—Physical activity must be done for an adequate length of time to be effective. Generally, an exercise period must be at least 15 minutes in length to be effective, while longer times are recommended for optimal benefits. As the length of time increases, intensities of exercise may be decreased. Time of physical activity involvement is also referred to as duration.

The FIT formula provides a practical means of applying the overload principle progressively for each specific benefit expected.

The type of physical activity you do is often considered to be part of the FITT formula.

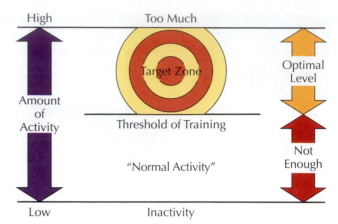

Figure 2
Physical activity target zone.

Sometimes a second *T* is added to the FIT formula to create the FITT formula, which indicates that the **T**ype of physical activity you perform is important. As the specificity principle indicates, different types of activity build different components of fitness and promote different health and wellness benefits. There is a FIT formula for each different benefit and each different type of physical activity. When the formula is applied to one specific type of activity, it is properly referred to as the FIT rather than the FITT formula.

The threshold of training and target zone concepts help you use the FIT formula.

The **threshold of training** is the minimum amount of activity (frequency, intensity, and time) necessary to produce benefits. Depending on the benefit expected, slightly more than normal activity may not be enough to promote health, wellness, or fitness benefits. The **target zone** begins at the threshold of training and stops at the point where the activity becomes counterproductive. Figure 2 illustrates the threshold of training and target zone concepts.

www.mhhe.com/hper/physed/clw/student/
Some people incorrectly associate the concepts of threshold of training and target zones with only cardiovascular fitness. As the principle of specificity suggests, each component of fitness, including metabolic fitness, has its own FIT formula and its own threshold and target zone. The target and threshold levels for **health benefits** are different from those for achieving **performance benefits** associated with high levels of physical fitness. Details of the different FIT formulae, threshold levels, and targets zones for the various benefits of activity are presented later in this book.

It takes time for physical activity to produce health, wellness, and fitness benefits even when the FIT formula is properly applied.

www.mhhe.com/hper/physed/clw/student/

Sometimes people just beginning a physical activity program expect to see immediate results. They expect to see large losses in body fat, or great increases in muscle strength in just a few days. Evidence shows, however, that improvements in health-related physical fitness and the associated health benefits take several weeks to become apparent. Though some people report psychological benefits, such as "feeling better" and a "sense of personal accomplishment" almost immediately after beginning regular exercise, the physiological changes will take considerably longer to be realized. Proper preparation for physical activity includes learning not to expect too much too soon, and not to do too much too soon. Attempts to overdo it and to try to get fit fast will probably be counterproductive, resulting in soreness and even injury. The key is to start slowly, stay with it, and enjoy yourself. Benefits will come to those who persist.

The Physical Activity Pyramid: The Facts

The physical activity pyramid classifies activities by type and associated benefits.

www.mhhe.com/hper/physed/clw/student/

The **physical activity pyramid** (see Figure 3) is a good way to illustrate different types of activities and how each contributes to the development of health, wellness and physical fitness. The pyramid evolved from a pyramid of activity emphasis developed more than 20 years ago and from the food guide pyramid developed by the U.S. Department of Agriculture to help people understand appropriate servings of foods. Like the food guide pyramid, the physical activity pyramid has four different levels. Each level includes one or two types of activity and characterizes the "portions" of physical activity necessary to produce different health, wellness, and fitness benefits.

The four levels of the pyramid are based on the beneficial health outcomes associated with regular physical activity. Activities having broad general health and wellness benefits for the largest number of people are placed at the base of the pyramid. The *Surgeon General's Report on Physical Activity and Health* points out that significant national health and economic benefits will occur if we can

get inactive people, especially those who are totally sedentary, to do some type of activity. The activities at the lower levels can provide these benefits, and because they are relatively low in intensity, they may appeal to the large number of people who can most benefit from beginning an activity program. The activities at the lower levels of the pyramid typically require greater frequency than those at higher levels.

Lifestyle activities are at the base of the physical activity pyramid.

Lifestyle physical activity is encouraged as a part of everyday living and can contribute significantly to good health, fitness, and wellness. Lifestyle activities include walking to or from work, climbing the stairs rather than taking an elevator, working in the yard, or doing any other type of exercise as part of your normal daily activities. The *Surgeon General's Report on Physical Activity and Health* suggests the accumulation of 30 minutes of physical activity equal to brisk walking on most, if not all, days of the week (see pyramid level 1).

Studies that track active versus inactive adults over long periods of time show that lifestyle activities provide many

FIT A formula used to describe the frequency, intensity, and length of time for physical activity to produce benefits. (When "FITT" is used, the second *T* refers to the type of physical activity you perform.)

Threshold of Training The minimum amount of physical activity that will produce benefits.

Target Zone Amounts of physical activity that produce optimal benefits.

Health Benefit A result of physical activity that provides protection from hypokinetic disease or early death.

Performance Benefit A result of physical activity that improves physical fitness and physical performance capabilities.

Physical Activity Pyramid This pyramid illustrates how different types of activities contribute to the development of health and physical fitness. Activities lower in the pyramid require more frequent participation, whereas activities higher in the pyramid require less frequency.

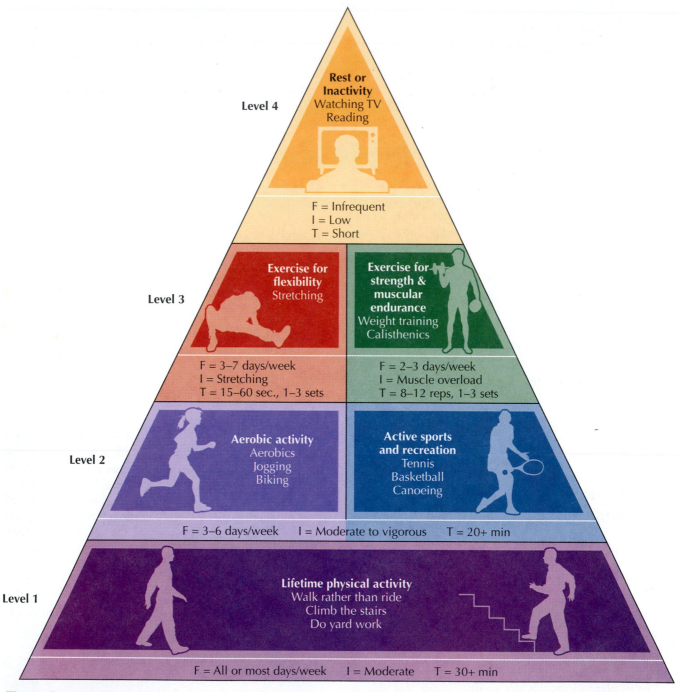

Figure 3

The physical activity pyramid.

health and wellness benefits. Metabolic fitness and modest gains in some parts of health-related physical fitness are associated with lifestyle activities. However, health-related fitness improvement as evidenced by high scores on performance tests are not generally considered to be a major benefit of this type of activity. The fact that lifestyles activities are moderate in intensity may encourage sedentary people to be more active. A summary of the FIT formula for this type of activity is illustrated in level one of Figure 3. If you do no activity at all, lifestyle activity is encouraged, even if it is all you do.

Active aerobics and sports and recreation are at the second level of the pyramid.

Aerobic activities (level 2) include those that are of such an intensity that they can be performed for relatively long periods of time without stopping but that also elevate the heart rate significantly. Lifestyle activities (level 1), also known as **moderate activity,** are technically aerobic in nature but are not especially vigorous and are therefore not considered to be "active aerobics." More **vigorous activities** such as jogging, biking, and aerobic dance are commonly classified as "active aerobic" activities. This type of activity is included in the second level of the pyramid because benefits can be accomplished in as few as three days a week and is especially good for building cardiovascular fitness and helping to control body fatness. This type of activity can provide metabolic fitness and health benefits similar to lifestyle activities.

Active sports and recreation are also included at level 2 of the pyramid. Examples of active sports include basketball, tennis, and racquetball, and active recreation includes hiking, backpacking, skiing, and rock climbing. Some active sports and recreational activities involve short bursts of physical activity followed by rests and therefore may not be considered to be aerobic in nature. If done for relatively long periods of time without stopping, active sports and recreation activities can have the same benefits of active aerobic activities. Sports such as golf and bowling may be classified as lifestyle activities rather than active sports since they are done at more moderate intensities. Activities at level 2 of the pyramid may substitute for activities at level 1 if done according to the FIT formula, but many experts encourage activities from both levels. They reason that people who develop active lifestyles from level 1 will be more likely to stay active later in life when they are less likely to participate in activities from level 2. Others argue that if you are active at level 2 you will be fit enough to continue active aerobics and sports as you grow older. A summary of the FIT formula for level 2 activities is included in Figure 3.

Flexibility and muscle fitness exercises are at level 3 of the pyramid.

Flexibility (stretching) exercises are a type of physical activity that is planned specifically to develop flexibility. This type of exercise is necessary because activities lower in the pyramid often do not contribute to flexibility development. The muscle fitness category includes exercises that are planned specifically to build strength and muscular endurance. This type of exercise is necessary because activities lower in the pyramid often do not contribute to these parts of fitness. A general description of the FIT formula for level 3 exercises is included in Figure 3.

Some rest is necessary, but with the exception of sleep, long periods of inactivity are discouraged.

Rest or inactivity can be important to good health. Some time off just to relax is important to us all, and of course proper amounts of rest and 8 hours of uninterrupted sleep help us recuperate. But, sedentary living (too much inactivity) results in low fitness as well as poor health and wellness. Rest and inactivity are placed at the top of the pyramid (see Figure 3) because they should be done sparingly compared to other types of activity in the pyramid.

There are some important guidelines that should be considered when using the physical activity pyramid.

The physical activity pyramid is a useful model for describing different types of activity and their benefits. The pyramid is also useful in summarizing the FIT formula for each of the different benefits of activity. But as the American College of Sports Medicine (1995) pointed out, physical activity guidelines ". . . cannot be applied in an overly rigid or precise fashion . . . and . . . should be used with flexibility and with careful attention paid to the goals of the individual." This important point should be considered when using the pyramid. The following guidelines for using the pyramid should also be considered.

- *No single activity provides all of the benefits.* More than a few people have asked the question, "What is the perfect form of physical activity?" It is now evident that there is no single activity that can provide all of the health, wellness, and fitness benefits. For optimal benefits to occur, it is desirable to perform activities from all levels of the pyramid because each type of activity has quite different benefits. As other guidelines will indicate, care should be used not to overgeneralize this recommendation.

- *In some cases, one type of activity can substitute for another.* If a person does appropriate activity of either type at level 2 of the pyramid, similar benefit can result.

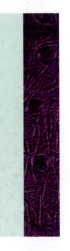

Moderate activity For the purposes of this book, moderate activity refers to activity equal in intensity to a brisk walk. Level 1 activities from the activity pyramid are included in this category and are sometimes referred to as sustained physical activity.

Vigorous Activity For the purposes of this book, vigorous activity refers to activities that elevate the heart rate and are greater in intensity than brisk walking. It is also referred to as moderate to vigorous activity. Those activities from level 2 of the pyramid are included in this category.

Both types are not required. Also, if a person does adequate activity of either type at level 2, it can provide similar benefits to those at level 1 of the pyramid. Selecting activities from more than one category does provide variety and may aid in adherence for some people.

- *Something is better than nothing.* Some people may look at the pyramid and say, "I just don't have time to do all of these activities." This could lead some to throw up their hands in despair, resulting in the conclusion "I just won't do anything at all." The best evidence indicates that something is better than nothing. If you do nothing or feel that you can't do it all, performing a lifestyle physical activity is a good start. Additional activities from different levels of the pyramid can be added as time allows.

- *Activities from Level 3 are useful even if you are limited in performing activities at other levels.* Though flexibility and muscle fitness exercises do not produce all of the benefits associated with regular physical activity, they will produce benefits even if you are unable to perform as much activity from other levels as you like.

- *Good planning will allow you to schedule activities from all levels in a reasonable amount of time.* In subsequent concepts, you will learn more about each level of the pyramid as well as more information about planning a total physical activity program.

The Facts about Physical Activity Patterns

The proportion of adults meeting national health goals varies with activity type and gender.

www.mhhe.com/hper/physed/clw/student/
National goals have been established for each of the different types of activity from the physical activity pyramid. The proportion of adults 18 years of age and older meeting these goals are illustrated in Figure 4. While lifestyle activities are recommended for 30+ minutes on most, if not all, days of the week, an adult is considered to be moderately active if he or she is active 5 days a week. Twenty to 24 percent of adults meet this goal, with more men than women meeting the goal.

Adults are less likely to meet the goal of performing vigorous activities (level 2) at least 3 times a week for 20+ minutes. Interestingly, males and females do not differ much for this type of activity. The type of activity most practiced by adults is flexibility exercise (stretching), performed by 26 percent of all adults with men and women performing similarly. Males are much more likely than females to do muscle

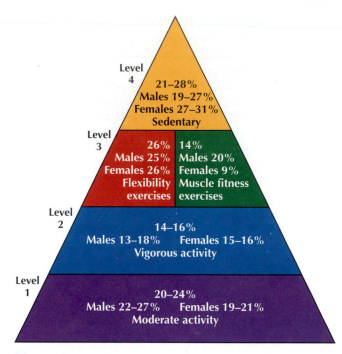

Figure 4
Proportion of adults meeting activity goals.
Based on data from the *Surgeon General's Report on Physical Activity and Health.*

fitness exercises, with 14 percent of all adults doing them regularly. About one-quarter of all adults (21 to 28 percent) do no leisure time physical activity at all. Women are more likely than men to be sedentary.

The proportion of adults meeting national health goals varies based on a variety of characteristics.

Older groups, Hispanics, and African Americans are more likely than younger and white non-Hispanic groups to be inactive. Younger nonminority groups are also more likely to participate in moderate, vigorous, flexibility, and muscle fitness activities.

Physical activity is most common in high-income groups who have had more education. People in the west and north-central parts of the country are least likely to be sedentary, and people in the northeast and south are most likely to be sedentary. In general, people from the west are most active, and those from the south least active. Sedentary living is most common in the winter months, and least frequent in the summer months. January and December are the months in which greater numbers of people are likely to report no leisure time physical activity.

Strategies for Action: The Facts

A self-assessment of your current activity at each level of the pyramid can help you determine future activity goals.

Lab 4A provides you with the opportunity to assess your physical activity at each level of the pyramid. Later you will be developing a program of activity, and these assessments will provide a basis for program planning.

Web Review

Web Review materials for Concept 4 are available at *www.mhhe.com/hper/physed/clw/student/*.

American College of Sports Medicine

www.acsm.org

Morbidity and Mortality Weekly Reports

www.cdc.gov/epo/mmwr/mmwr.html

Medicine and Science in Sports and Exercise

www.wwilkins.com/FIT

National Sports Medicine Institute

www.nsmi.org.uk

Surgeon General's Report on Physical Activity and Health

www.cdc.gov/nccdphp/sgr/sgr.htm

Suggested Readings

American College of Sports Medicine. *ACSM's Guidelines for Exercise Testing and Exercise Prescription,* 5th ed. Baltimore, MD: Williams and Wilkins, 1995.

American College of Sports Medicine. "The Recommended Quantity and Quality of Exercise for Developing and Maintaining Cardiorespiratory and Muscular Fitness, and Flexibility in Healthy Adults." *Medicine and Science in Sports & Exercise* 30(6)(1998):975–990.

Corbin, C. B., and Pangrazi, R. P. "Physical Activity Pyramid Rebuffs Peak Experience." *ACSM's Health and Fitness* 2(1)(1998):12–17.

Franks, B. D. "Personalizing Physical Activity Prescription." *President's Council on Physical Fitness and Sports Research Digest* 2(9)(1997):1–8.

Howley, E. T. and Franks, B. D. *Health Fitness Instructor's Handbook* (3rd ed.). Champaign, IL: Human Kinetics, 1997.

National Center for Health Statistics. *Health, United States, 1998: With Socioeconomic Statistics and Health Chartbook.* Hyattsville, MD: National Center for Health Statistics, 1998.

Roitman, J. L. (ed.) *ACSM's Resource Manual for Guidelines for Exercise Testing and Prescription* 3rd ed. Baltimore, MD; Williams & Wilkins, 1998.

U.S. Department of Health and Human Services. *Physical Activity and Health: A Report of the Surgeon General.* Atlanta, GA: U.S. Department of Health and Human Services, 1996.

Lab 4A: Self-Assessment of Physical Activity

Purpose: To estimate your current levels of physical activity from each category of the physical activity pyramid.

Name	**Section**	**Date**

Procedures:

1. Place an X over the circle that characterizes your participation in each category in the pyramid.
2. Determine if you met the national goal for each type of activity. Place an X over the "yes" circle if you met the goal in each area. (See Results.)

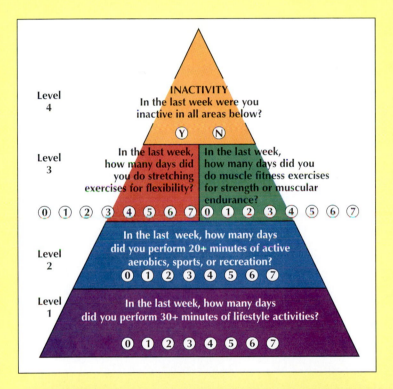

Results

Activity Type	Level	National Goal	Did You Meet the National Health Goal?	
Lifestyle activity	1	5 days or more	Yes	No
Active aerobics/sports	2	3 days or more	Yes	No
Flexibility exercises	3	3 days or more	Yes	No
Muscle fitness	3	2 days or more	Yes	No
Inactivity	4	Avoid total inactivity	Yes	No

Conclusions and Implications: In the space below, write a brief paper describing your current physical activity patterns. Do you meet the national health goals in all areas? If not, in what types of activity from the pyramid do you need to improve? Are the answers you gave for the past week typical of your regular activity patterns? If you meet all national health goals, explain why you think this is so. Do you think that meeting the goals in the table above indicate good activity patterns for you?

Write your physical activity assessment paper in the space below.

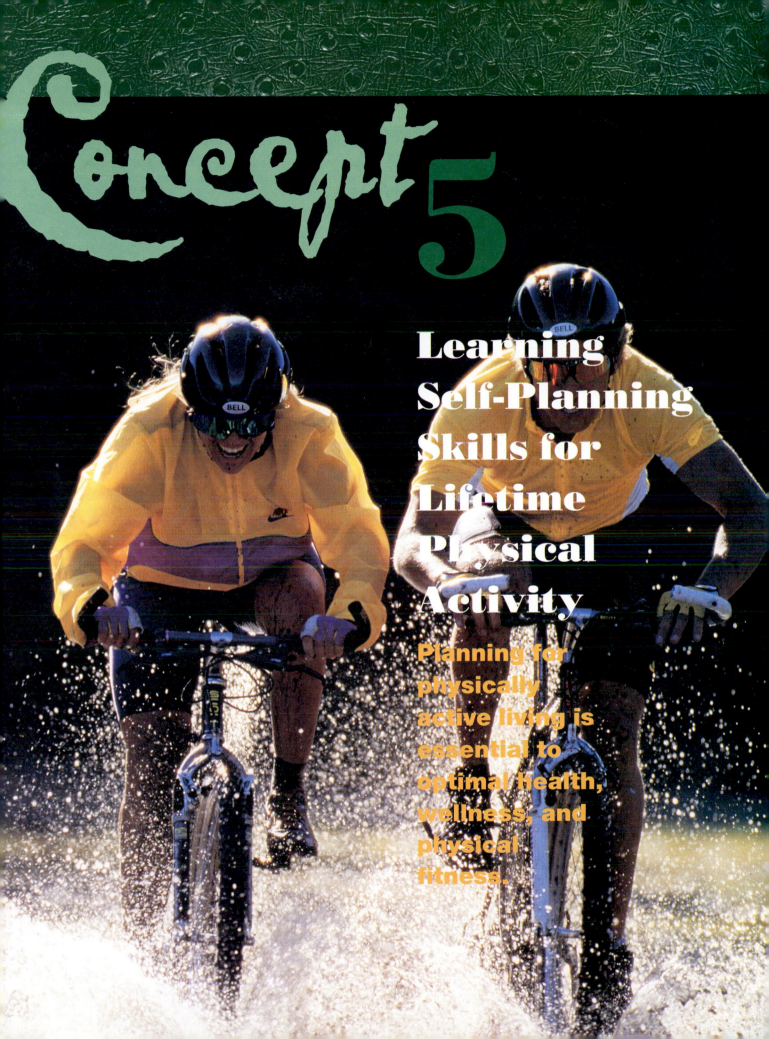

Concept 5

Learning Self-Planning Skills for Lifetime Physical Activity

Planning for physically active living is essential to optimal health, wellness, and physical fitness.

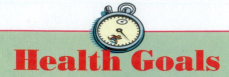

Health Goals

for Year 2010

Improve the health, fitness and quality of life of all people through the adoption and maintenance of regular, daily physical activity.

Increase leisure time physical activity.

Increase proportion of people who do moderate daily activity for 30 minutes.

Increase proportion of people who do vigorous physical activity three days a week.

Increase proportion of people who do regular muscle fitness exercise.

Increase proportion of people who do regular exercise for flexibility.

Increase prevalence of a healthy weight.

Introduction

There is no single exercise program best suited for all people, nor is there one best lifestyle for health, wellness, and fitness. When planning a program, it is important to consider your own unique needs and interests and to self-plan a program that is personal. In concept 2, you learned about self-management skills. In this concept, you will have the opportunity to practice and apply self-management skills that are especially useful in helping you plan for a lifetime of physical activity. Later you will learn self-management skills for use in developing other healthy lifestyles.

Clarifying Reasons for Participation: The Facts

Clarifying your reasons for participating, or not participating, in physical activity is an important step in self-planning.

As you continue your study in this book, you will be presented with a wide variety of physical activity choices. Your personal reasons for choosing to participate or not to participate should be clarified prior to planning your program.

Over time, attitudes change, so periodic reassessment is recommended.

Knowing the most common reasons for inactivity can help you avoid sedentary living.

Some of the common reasons given by those who do not do regular physical activity are outlined in Table 1. Many of the reasons for not being active are considered by experts to be barriers that can be overcome. Overcoming barriers is a self-management skill. Using the solutions in Table 1 helps inactive people to become more active.

Knowing the reasons people give for being active can help you adopt positive attitudes.

www.mhhe.com/hper/physed/clw/student/

Table 2 describes some of the major reasons why people choose to be active. It also offers strategies for changing behavior if you have more than one or two negative attitudes. Active people have more positive than negative attitudes. This is referred to by experts as a positive "balance of attitudes." The questionnaire in Lab 5A gives you the opportunity to assess your balance of attitudes. If you have a negative balance score, you can analyze your attitudes and determine how you can change them to view activity more favorably.

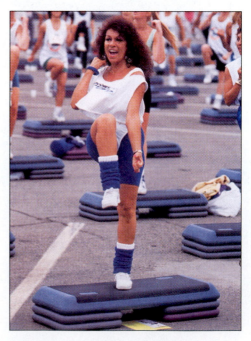

Active people have more positive than negative feelings about physical activity.

Table 1   Common Reasons People Give for Not Being Active

Reason	Description	Strategy for Change
"I don't have the time."	This is the number one reason people give for not exercising. Invariably, those who feel they don't have time indicate that they know they should do more exercise and that they plan to in the future when "things are less hectic." Young people say that they will soon be established in a career and then they will have the time to exercise. Older people say that they wish they had taken the time to be active when they were younger.	Planning a daily schedule can help you find the time for activity and avoid wasting time on things that are less important. Learning the facts in the concepts that follow will help you see the importance of activity and how you can include it in your schedule with a minimum of effort and with time efficiency.
"It's too inconvenient."	Many who avoid physical activity do so because it is inconvenient. They are procrastinators. Specific reasons for procrastinating include: "It makes me sweaty" and "It messes up my hair."	Research shows that if you have to travel more than 10 minutes to do activity or if you do not have easy access to equipment, you will avoid activity. Locating facilities and finding a time when you can shower is important.
"I just don't enjoy it."	Many do not find physical activity to be enjoyable or invigorating. These people may assume that all forms of activity have to be strenuous and fatiguing to count as exercise.	There are many activities to choose from. If you don't enjoy vigorous activity, try more moderate forms of activity such as walking.
"I'm no good at physical activity."	"People might laugh at me"; "Sports make me nervous"; and "I am not good at physical activities" are reasons some people give for not being active. These people often lack confidence in their own abilities. In some cases, this is because of their past experiences in physical education or athletics (sports).	With properly selected activities, even those who have never enjoyed exercise can get hooked. Building performance skills can help, as can changing your way of thinking. Avoiding comparisons to others can help you feel successful.
"I am not fit so I avoid activity."	Some people avoid exercise because of health reasons. Some who are unfit lack energy. Starting slowly can build fitness gradually and help you realize that you can do it.	There are good medical reasons for not doing physical activity, but many people with problems can benefit from exercise if it is properly designed. If necessary, get help adapting activity to meet your needs.
"I have no place to be active, especially in bad weather."	Regular activity is much more convenient if facilities are easy to reach and the weather is good. Still, recreational opportunities have increased considerably in recent years. Some of the most popular activities require very little equipment, can be done in or near the home, and are inexpensive.	If you cannot find a place, if it is not safe, or if it is too expensive, consider using low-cost equipment at home such as rubber bands or calisthenics. Lifestyle activity can be done by anyone at almost any time.
"I am too old."	As people grow older, many begin to feel that physical activity is something they cannot do. For most people, this is simply not true! Studies indicate that properly planned exercise for older adults is not only safe but also has many health benefits, including longer life, fewer illnesses, increased working capacity, an improved sense of well-being, and optimal functioning.	Older people who are just beginning activity should start slowly. Lifestyle activities are a good alternative. Setting realistic goals can help, as can learning new activity skills, such as resistance training and appropriate flexibility exercises.

Table 2 Common Reasons for Doing Regular Physical Activity

Reason	Description	Strategy for Change
"I do activity for my health, wellness, and fitness."	Surveys show this is the number one reason for doing regular physical activity. Unfortunately, many adults say that a "doctor's order to exercise" would be the most likely reason to get them to begin a regular program. For some, however, waiting for a doctor's order may be too late.	Gaining information contained in this book will help you see the value of regular physical activity. Performing the self-assessments in the various concepts will help you determine the areas in which you need personal improvement.
"I do activity to improve my appearance."	In our society, looking good is highly valued, thus physical attractiveness is a major reason why people participate in regular exercise. Regular physical activity can contribute to looking your best.	Some people have failed in past attempts to change their appearance through activity. Setting realistic goals and avoiding comparisons to others can help future attempts to be more successful.
"I do activity because I enjoy it."	A majority of adults say that enjoyment is of paramount importance in deciding to be active. This is not surprising, given statements from participants such as experiencing the "peak experience," the "runner's high," or "spinning free." The sense of fun, the feeling of well-being, and the general enjoyment associated with physical activity are well-documented.	Those people who do not enjoy activity often lack performance skills or feel that they are not competent in activity situations. Improving skills with practice, setting realistic goals, and adopting a new way of thinking about performance can help a person to be successful and to enjoy activities.
"I do activity because it relaxes me."	Relaxation and release from tension rank high as reasons why people do regular physical activity. For years, it has been recognized that activity in the form of sports and games provides a catharsis, or outlet, for the frustrations of normal daily activities. Evidence indicates that regular exercise can help reduce depression and anxiety, both common symptoms in Western culture.	Activities, such as walking, jogging, or cycling, are ways of getting some quiet time away from the job or the stresses of daily living. In a later concept, you will learn about some special exercises that you can do to reduce stress.
"I like the challenge and sense of personal accomplishment I get from physical activity."	A sense of personal accomplishment associated with performing various physical activities is frequently a reason for people doing activity. In some cases, it is merely learning a new skill, such as racquetball or tennis; in other cases, it is running a mile or doing a certain number of crunches that provides this feeling of accomplishment. The challenge of doing something you have never done before is apparently a very powerful experience. Physical activities provide opportunities not readily available in other aspects of life.	Some people get little sense of accomplishment from activity. Taking lessons to learn new skills or attempting activities new to you can provide the challenge that makes activity interesting. Also, adopting a new way of thinking that allows you to avoid comparisons to others with a focus on the task rather than competition with others can help.

Identifying Needs: The Facts

Learning to assess your current levels of health, wellness, and fitness is useful in establishing personal needs, planning your program, and evaluating your progress.

You have already done some self-assessments of wellness, current activity levels, and current lifestyles. In the lab for this concept and others that follow, you will make additional assessments. The results of these assessments help you build a personal profile that can be used as the basis for program planning. With practice, self-assessments become more accurate. It is for this reason that it is important to repeat self-assessments more than one time and to pay careful attention to the procedures for performing them. If ques-

Table 2 *(continued)*

Reason	Description	Strategy for Change
"I like the social involvement I get from physical activities."	Frequent answers to the question, "Why am I physically active?" include: "It is a good way to spend time with other members of the family"; "It is a good way to spend time with close friends"; and "Being part of the team is a satisfying feeling." Physical activity settings can also provide an opportunity for making new friends.	If you find physical activity to be socially unrewarding you may have to find activities that both you and friends or family enjoy. Taking lessons together can help. Also finding a friend with similar skills can aid in sports performance. Focus on the activity rather than the outcome.
"Competition is the main reason I enjoy physical activity."	"The thrill of victory" and "sports competition" are two reasons often given by people who participate in physical activities. For many, the competitive experience can be very satisfying.	Some people simply do not enjoy competing. If this is the case for you can participate without competing or select noncompetitive individual activities.
"Physical activity helps me feel good about myself."	For many people, participation in physical activity is an important part of their identity. They feel better about themselves when they are regularly participating in physical activity.	Physical activity is something that is self-determined and within your control. Participation in a regular program can help you feel good about yourself and build your confidence and self-esteem.
"Physical activity provides opportunities to get fresh air.	"Being outside and experiencing nature are reasons that some people give for being physically active.	Many activities provide opportunities to be outside more frequently. If this is an important reason for you, try to seek out parks and enjoyable settings for your activities.

tions arise, rather than making an error, get a professional opinion.

Periodic physical fitness self-assessments can aid in determining if a person is meeting health-fitness standards and is making progress toward personal goals.

www.mhhe.com/hper/physed/clw/student/

WEB At some point, it is wise to have an expert test your fitness. This helps you get an accurate assessment of your current fitness level and helps you determine if your self-assessment results are accurate. Expert tests are often expensive and require time and effort on your part. When possible, you should learn to perform self-assessments so that you can continue to assess your fitness for a lifetime without dependence on someone else. Tests such as skinfold measures are hard to administer to yourself, but you can learn to teach a friend or relative to assist you with the measurement.

For many components of physical fitness, multiple assessments are provided in this book. For example, four different cardiovascular fitness assessments are included for your selection. You are encouraged to try several assessments and then decide which one best meets your personal needs.

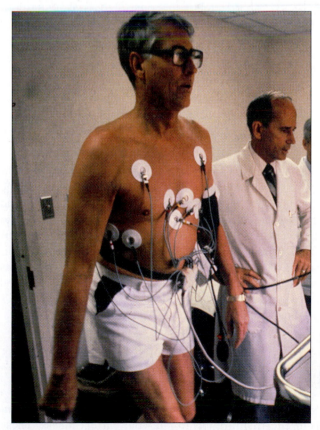

A fitness assessment by an expert can be useful.

Self-assessment of metabolic fitness and all components of health-related fitness is important.

Because fitness has many different components, you will need to do many self-tests if you are going to get an accurate picture of your total fitness. It is recommended that each person do several tests of fitness for each component of health-related fitness. Multiple tests will give you a more complete and accurate picture.

It is more important to compare physical fitness test results to health standards or personal fitness improvement than to compare yourself to other people.

In Western culture, we have a tendency to compare ourselves to others in almost all things we do. Rather than comparing your fitness scores to those of other people, you would be wise to concentrate on meeting good fitness standards and improving your personal fitness. Exceptionally high scores on fitness tests may improve performances in sports but are not necessary for good health. For example, a male having 10 to 15 percent body fat is considered to be more healthy than one having 25 to 30 percent body fat. However, having less than 10 percent of the body as fat is not necessarily more healthy than having 10 to 15 percent fat. Having too little body fat can be harmful to your health.

Results of fitness assessments are influenced by heredity.

Heredity plays an important role in the amount of physical fitness a person can attain. More than a few people have become discouraged after completing an exercise program only to find that they have scored lower on fitness tests than friends who are less active. Though it is clear that regular exercise is critical to optimal physical fitness, each person also has a hereditary predisposition to fitness. Although achieving good scores on fitness tests is a desirable goal, it is important to understand that a person's hereditary predisposition to fitness limits one's potential for achieving exceptionally high scores.

Health-based criterion-referenced standards are recommended for rating your fitness.

Most experts now recommend **health based criterion-referenced standards** to rate your current fitness. These

Table 3 The Four Fitness Zones

High Performance Zone

The high performance zone is a good indicator of adequate fitness, but it is not necessary to reach this level to experience good health benefits. Achievement of high performance scores has more to do with performance than it does with good health. In some cases, extreme fitness scores can increase health risk (eg, very low body fatness).

Good Fitness Zone

If you reach the good fitness zone, you probably have enough of a specific fitness component to help reduce the risk of a specific health condition, assuming that you maintain an active lifestyle. Even achievement in the good fitness zone may not result in optimal health benefits for inactive people.

Marginal Zone

Marginal scores indicate that some improvement is in order, but you are nearing minimal health standards set by experts.

Low Fit Zone

If you score low in fitness, you are probably less fit than you should be for your own good health and wellness.

standards help you determine "how much fitness is enough" for health and wellness. In the past, norms or percentiles have been used to rate physical fitness. These types of ratings compare an individual to a group. Knowing how you compare to someone else is not particularly important. In fact, such comparisons have been shown to be discouraging to many people. Determining if your fitness is adequate to enhance your health and wellness is much more relevant.

In this book, four categories are provided for you to rate each part of fitness. These are illustrated and described in Table 3. Your first goal should be to be sure that you do not rate low on any health-related fitness part. Ultimately, you should achieve the good fitness zone for all parts of fitness. You may, for personal reasons, wish to achieve the high performance zone for some fitness components, but this choice has more to do with personal preference than health and wellness. The fitness ratings used in this book help you determine "how much fitness is enough" for your good health and wellness. They do not require you to compare yourself to others or set unrealistic standards.

Self-assessments have the advantage of consistent error rather than variable error.

As noted previously, the best type of assessments are done by highly qualified experts using precise instruments. Eliminating error is always desirable. Following directions and practicing sound assessment technique reduces error significantly. Still, errors will occur. One advantage of a self-assessment is that the person doing the assessment is always the same—you. Even if you make an error in a self-assessment, it is likely to be consistent over time, especially if you use the same equipment each time you make the assessment. For example, if you measure your own weight using a home scale and your measurement shows your weight to be 2 pounds higher than it really is, you have made a consistent error. You can determine if you are making improvement because you know the error exists, but it is a consistent error. When different people using different instruments assess your fitness, the errors they make may be quite variable.

The Facts about Goal Setting

> Learning to set realistic goals is useful as a basis for physical activity self-planning.

If any lifestyle change is to be of value, it is important to determine—ahead of time—what you hope to accomplish. Goals are specific objectives you hope to accomplish as a result of a lifestyle change. To be effective, goals must be realistic—neither too hard nor too easy. If the goal is too hard, failure is likely. Failure is discouraging. By setting realistic and attainable goals, you will have a greater chance of being successful.

> Beginners are encouraged to focus on short-term goals.

Focus on **short-term goals** first. Short-term goals are easier to accomplish than **long-term goals.** Realistic short-term goals make you successful because one success leads to another. When you meet short-term goals, establish new ones. Long-term goals take a long time to accomplish and may be discouraging to beginners. After a series of short-term goals have been successfully accomplished, set long-term goals. In fact, setting and achieving a series of short-term goals is the best way to achieve long-term goals.

> Short-term goals should be specific.

Many individuals make the mistake of setting vague or nebulous goals such as "be more active" or "eat less." While these may be your long-term objectives, goals should be more specific. Setting specific goals helps you commit to what you want to accomplish. It is also easier to assess whether you are making progress.

> Short-term goals should be behavioral goals rather than outcome goals.

A **behavioral goal** is associated with something you do. Performing physical activity for a specific period of time is something you do, so a **physical activity goal** is a type of behavioral goal. An example of a specific short-term behavioral goal would be "to perform 30 minutes of brisk walking six days a week for the next two weeks." It is specific because you specify how long and how often you expect to do the exercise. It is short-term because you can accomplish it in a few weeks or less. The principal factor associated with success is your willingness to give effort. No matter who you are, you can accomplish this behavioral goal if you give a daily effort. In addition, behavioral goals are easy to self-monitor. Keeping an activity log of your weekly participation in brisk walking will reveal your compliance with the goal.

An **outcome goal** is associated with something you "can do". For example, **fitness goals** such as being able to do 10 push-ups or to run a mile in 7 minutes are examples of outcome goals. Outcome or fitness goals are not recommended for beginners. Three reasons for this are listed below:

- *Typically, it takes time (more than a week or two) to reach fitness and other outcome goals.* For this reason, short-term or fitness goals are often not achieved in the designated time, resulting in a perception of failure.
- *Outcome goals depend on many things other than your lifestyle behavior.* For example, your heredity affects your body fatness and muscle development. Setting a goal of achieving a certain percent body fatness or lifting a

Behavioral Goal A statement of intent to perform a specific behavior (changing a lifestyle) for a specific period of time. An example would be, "I will walk for 15 minutes each morning before work."

Fitness Goal A fitness goal is an outcome goal with a specific fitness score as the intended outcome.

Health Based Criterion-Referenced Standards The amount of a specific type of fitness necessary to gain a health or wellness benefit.

Long Term Goal A statement of intent to change behavior or achieve a specific outcome in a period of months or years.

Outcome Goal A statement of intent to achieve a specific test score (attainment of a specific standard) associated with good health, wellness or fitness. An example would be, "I will lower my body fat level by 3 percent."

Physical Activity Goal An exercise or physical activity goal is a behavioral goal with exercise as the intended behavior.

Short-Term Goal A statement of intent to change a behavior or outcome in a period of days or weeks.

certain weight is influenced by heredity as well as your physical activity program. This makes it hard for beginners to set realistic fitness goals. Too often the tendency is to set the goal based on a comparative standard rather than on a standard that is possible for the individual to achieve in a short period of time. Those more experienced in physical activity learn to set more realistic outcome goals and learn that these goals often take time to achieve.

- *Different people progress at different rates.* People not only inherit a predisposition to fitness and body composition, they inherit a predisposition to benefit from training. In other words, if 10 people do the exact same physical activities, there will be 10 different results. One may improve performance by 60 percent while another improves only 10 percent. Until you gain enough experience to see how you respond to physical activity, it is not wise to set fitness or outcome goals. You need experience to determine the areas of fitness in which you respond quickly and those areas in which your response to activity is slower. It is at this time that fitness or outcome goals become more appropriate.

Long-term goals can be either behavioral or outcome goals.

Long-term goals can be of a behavioral nature similar to short-term goals. If you set as a goal participation in regular physical activity and meet the goal over a long period of time, fitness and other health benefits will occur to the extent that they are possible given your genetics and body type. For this reason, behavioral or physical activity goals are very appropriate. This type of goal is easy to monitor, and self-assessments of fitness will provide feedback of program success.

Outcome or fitness goals can also be useful to the person experienced in physical activity. If realistic, these goals will be met with appropriate physical activity and provide evidence of success. When establishing long-term fitness goals, be careful not to base them on what other people can do. You may be setting yourself up for failure. Be sure that the fitness outcomes you expect are based on health standards or scores slightly above what you can currently perform, rather than on performance scores of other people.

It is appropriate to consider maintenance goals.

There is a limit to the amount of fitness any person can achieve. You cannot improve forever. Limits on physical activity goals are appropriate. At some point, it is reasonable to set maintenance goals to help you to stay active and fit when improvement goals have already been met.

Set goals that that you can maintain for a lifetime. Physical activity and fitness for a lifetime mean maintaining your program forever. If you set exercise or fitness goals that are excessive, you may burn out and quit exercising entirely. Consider the long term in setting your goals.

Putting your goals in writing helps formalize them.

Put your goals in writing. Otherwise, your goals will be easy to forget. Writing them helps establish a commitment to yourself and clearly establishes your goals. You can revise them if necessary. Written goals are not cast in concrete.

Selecting Personally Appropriate Activities: The Facts

The most popular forms of exercise among adults require very little skill or equipment and are easily accessible.

www.mhhe.com/hper/physed/clw/student/
The *Surgeon General's Report on Physical Activity and Health* indicates that the most popular participation activities among adults are walking, gardening or yard work, stretching exercises, bicycling, strength exercises, stair climbing, jogging, aerobic dancing, and swimming. Other national surveys consistently show similar results. All of these can be done in or near the home for little or no cost. None requires a high degree of physical skill in order for a person to be successful or to enjoy the benefits associated with regular involvement. These activities are not often those that people value for their children, nor those in which they themselves were involved in as children. And although football, baseball, basketball, gymnastics, and boxing are the activities adults most enjoy watching, they usually are not the ones in which they participate.

Learning performance skills will expand the choices of appropriate activities.

If you should choose an activity that requires considerable skill (e.g., basketball, tennis, golf), it would be wise to take lessons to improve your performance skills. Even for those activities that require less skill (walking, jogging, and biking), learning the appropriate techniques can enhance the enjoyment from participation. In subsequent concepts, you will learn more about enhancing your performance skills for various activities.

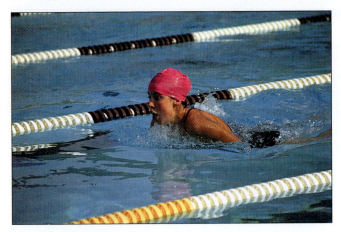

Select activities that help you meet personal goals.

Select activities that match your abilities.

The self-assessments that you perform as you do the activities in this book will help you match your abilities to specific activities. No matter what your abilities, you should choose the activities you think you will enjoy. But finding activities that require the types of fitness in which you excel will increase your prospects for success.

Select activities that provide all of the health, wellness, and fitness benefits.

Each of the activities in the physical activity pyramid provides different benefits. It is important to select activities from each category if optimal benefits are to be achieved. In subsequent concepts, you will learn more about the FIT formula for each of these activities.

The Facts about Keeping Records

Keeping a physical activity log is one important method of record keeping.

www.mhhe.com/hper/physed/clw/student/

Record keeping can help you stick with your physical activity program and can help you attain your goals. Record keeping is a type of self-management skill commonly referred to as self-monitoring. You can monitor your physical activity goals by keeping daily records of the activities you perform. Keeping records in the form of physical activity logs is the preferred method of self-monitoring for beginners. Activity logs help you comply with physical activity goals. In the concepts that follow, you will prepare a plan for different types of physical activity from the pyramid and keep activity logs to chart progress.

Keeping records of fitness improvement should be reserved for those with experience.

By the time you complete your studies associated with this book, you should have the experience necessary to establish and self-monitor fitness goals. Many of you may already have the experience necessary but you are encouraged to focus on physical activity record keeping as you perform the lab experiences presented early in this book.

Periodic self-assessments allow you to monitor progress toward fitness and other outcome goals. If fitness has improved the results can be motivational. If done too frequently, monitoring improvements can be discouraging, since it takes time for fitness to improve. Also, changes that occur from day to day may not be representative of true changes in fitness. Fatigue, time of testing, and nutritional status are but a few of the factors that account for fitness differences from day to day. For example, strength test results may be low if done after a hard day's work, and your weight can vary from day to day or even hour to hour based on nutritional factors such as water loss from physical activity.

Fitness record keeping is important. Periodic self-assessment of each of the different fitness dimensions is encouraged as long as it is not too often. Doing self-assessments under the same conditions including the same time of the day is important if self-monitoring is to be meaningful.

Writing Your Plan: The Facts

Preparing a written plan can improve your adherence to the plan.

A written plan is a pledge or a promise to be active. Research shows that intentions to be active are more likely to be acted on when put in writing. In the concepts that follow, you will be given the opportunity to prepare written plans for all of the activities in the physical activity pyramid. This will be done one activity at a time. When you have developed a plan for each type of activity, you can then develop a comprehensive physical activity plan.

The self-management skills presented in this concept should be used in planning programs for the different types of physical activity.

The self-management skills described in this concept should be used as you develop plans for each of the types of activity in the physical activity pyramid. To use these skills effectively, it is important to practice them and use them regularly. Over time, you will improve in the use of these skills.

Table 4 Self-Planning Skills

Self-Planning	Description	Self-Management Skill
Clarifying reasons	Knowing the general reasons why you might benefit helps you select activities that you will enjoy and adhere to for a lifetime.	Balancing Attitudes: Sections of this concept and Lab 5A help you determine if you have more positive than negative attitudes and help clarify your reasons for doing physical activity.
Identifying needs	If you know your strengths and weaknesses, you can plan to build on your strengths and overcome weaknesses.	Self-Assessment: In the concepts that follow, you will learn how to assess different health, wellness and fitness characteristics. Learning these self-assessments will help you identify needs.
Establishing goals	Goals are more specific than reasons (see above). Establishing specific things that you want to accomplish can provide a basis for feedback that your program is working.	Goal Setting: Guidelines in this concept will help you set goals. In subsequent concepts, you will establish goals for different types of activity from the pyramid.
Selecting activities	A personal plan should include activities that meet your needs and goals (see steps above) and provide fun and enjoyment. Having skill improves enjoyment.	Performance Skills: In subsequent concepts, you will learn how to enhance your performance skills. Self-assessments will also help you match your abilities to specific activities.
Keeping records	Keeping records provides feedback and helps you adhere to your program.	Self-Monitoring: These skills are necessary for accurate record keeping.

Table 4 summarizes the self-planning and associated self-management skills presented in this concept.

Strategies for Action: The Facts

A self-assessment of your attitudes about physical activity is a good first step in planning for lifelong physical activity.

The physical activity attitudes questionnaire included in Lab 5A allows you the opportunity to consider your reasons for participating in physical activity. You will calculate a score for each of the nine attitudes described in Table 2. You will also calculate a balance of attitudes score that will indicate whether you have more positive than negative attitudes about physical activity. If you have low scores for certain attitudes, you should consider the strategies for action outlined in Table 2. Efforts to change attitudes are especially important for people with a negative balance of attitudes (poor or very poor ratings).

Self-planning skills can be used for each of the different types of activity in the physical activity pyramid.

In subsequent concepts, you develop self-plans for each of the types of activity in the physical activity pyramid. As you develop those plans, it will be useful to refer to the self-planning skills outlined in this concept.

Web Review

Web review materials for Concept 5 are available are at *www.mhhe.com/hper/physed/clw/student/*.

American College of Sports Medicine
> *www.acsm.org*

Phys-In Fitness & in Health
> *www.phys.com*

FitLife
> *www.fitlife.com*

Planning Workouts
> *www.thriveonline.com*

Suggested Readings

American College of Sports Medicine. *ACSM's Guidelines for Exercise Testing and Exercise Prescription* 5th ed. Baltimore, MD: Williams and Wilkins, 1995.

Corbin, C. B. & Pangrazi, R. P. (Editors), *Towards a Better Understanding of Physical Fitness and Activity.* Scottsdale, AZ: Holcomb-Hathaway, 1999, Chapters 2 and 3.

Franks, B. D. (1997). "Individualized Recommendations for Physical Activity." *President's Council on Physical Fitness and Sports Research Digest,* 3(1)(1997):1.

Roitman, J. L. (ed.) *ACSM's Resource Manual for Guidelines for Exercise Testing and Prescription* 3rd Ed. Baltimore, MD: Williams & Wilkins, 1998.

Shangold, M. M. (1998). "Beyond the Exercise Prescription: Making Exercise a Way of LIfe." *Physician and Sports Medicine.* 26(11)(1998):35.

Stuhr, R. M. "Strategies for Beating the Barriers to Exercise for Women." *ACSM's Health and Fitness Journal,* 2(5)(1998):20.

U.S. Department of Health and Human Services. *Physical Activity and Health: A Report of the Surgeon General.* Atlanta, GA: U.S. Department of Health and Human Services, 1996.

Lab 5A: Physical Activity Attitude Questionnaire

Name **Section** **Date**

Purpose: To evaluate your feelings concerning physical activity and to determine the specific reasons why you do or do not participate in regular physical activity.

Procedures:
1. Read and answer each question in the questionnaire.
2. Make an X over the circle that best represents whether you strongly agree, agree, disagree, or strongly disagree. If you are unsure place an X on undecided.
3. Write the number in the circle of your answer in the box labeled "score" provided.
4. After you have answered all questions, add the two questions for each score and record the sum of the two items in the box provided on the questionnaire.
5. Record your scores in the chart provided in the results section.
6. Determine your rating for each score and record it in the chart in the results section.
7. Count the number of ratings that were good or excellent and record this number in the box as indicated.
8. Count the number of ratings that were fair, poor, or very poor and record this number in the box as indicated.
9. Subtract the number in the second box from the one in the first box to determine your balance of feelings score.
10. Determine your balance of feelings rating and record it in the appropriate space.

The Physical Activity Attitude Questionnaire

Directions: The term *physical activity* in the following statements refers to all kinds of activities, including sports, formal exercises, and informal activities, such as jogging and cycling. Make an X over the circle that best represents your answer to each question.

	Strongly Agree	Agree	Undecided	Disagree	Strongly Disagree	Score
1. I should do physical activity regularly for my health.	5	4	3	2	1	
2. Doing regular physical activity is good for my fitness and wellness.	5	4	3	2	1	
Health and Fitness Score (1 + 2)						
3. Regular exercise helps me look my best.	5	4	3	2	1	
4. I feel more physically attractive when I do regular physical activity.	5	4	3	2	1	
Appearance Score (3 + 4)						
5. One of the main reasons I do regular physical activity is because it is fun.	5	4	3	2	1	
6. The most enjoyable part of my day is when I am exercising or doing a sport.	5	4	3	2	1	
Enjoyment Score (5 + 6)						

	Strongly Agree	Agree	Undecided	Disagree	Strongly Disagree	Score

7. Taking part in physical activity helps me to relax. — 5 · 4 · 3 · 2 · 1 · ▯

8. Physical activity helps me get away from the pressures of daily living. — 5 · 4 · 3 · 2 · 1 · ▯

Relaxation Score (7 + 8) ▯

9. The challenge of physical training is one reason why I do physical activity. — 5 · 4 · 3 · 2 · 1 · ▯

10. I like to see if I can master sports and activities that are new to me. — 5 · 4 · 3 · 2 · 1 · ▯

Challenge Score (9 + 10) ▯

11. I like to do physical activity that involves other people. — 5 · 4 · 3 · 2 · 1 · ▯

12. Exercise offers me the opportunity to meet other people. — 5 · 4 · 3 · 2 · 1 · ▯

Social Score (11 + 12) ▯

13. Competition is a good way to make physical activity fun. — 5 · 4 · 3 · 2 · 1 · ▯

14. I like to see how my physical abilities compare to others. — 5 · 4 · 3 · 2 · 1 · ▯

Competition Score (13 + 14) ▯

15. When I do regular exercise, I feel better than when I don't. — 5 · 4 · 3 · 2 · 1 · ▯

16. My ability to do physical activity is something that makes me proud. — 5 · 4 · 3 · 2 · 1 · ▯

Feeling Good Score (15 + 16) ▯

17. I like to do outdoor activities. — 5 · 4 · 3 · 2 · 1 · ▯

18. Experiencing nature is something I look forward to when exercising. — 5 · 4 · 3 · 2 · 1 · ▯

Outdoor Nature Score (17 + 18) ▯

Results: Using the chart below record your scores as indicated in the procedures above.

Physical Activity Attitude Questionnaire Results

Attitude	Score	Rating
Health and Fitness		
Appearance		
Enjoyment		
Relaxation		
Challenge		
Social		
Competition		
Feeling Good		
Outdoor		

Rating Chart

Rating Category	Individual Scores	Balance of Feeling Score
Excellent	9–10	+5 to +9
Good	7–8	+2 to +4
Fair	5–6	0 to +1
Poor	3–4	−1 to −2
Very Poor	2	more than −2

Record the number of good and excellent ratings.

Record the number of fair, poor or very poor ratings.

Subtract the number from box 2 from the number in box 1.
This is your balance of feelings score.

Balance of Feelings Rating

Conclusions and Implications:

1. In a few sentences, discuss your results on the Physical Activity Attitudes Questionnaire (ratings for the nine attitude scores). Include comments on whether you think your ratings suggest that you will be active or inactive and whether your ratings are really indicative of your feelings.

2. In a few sentences, discuss your "balance of feelings" rating. Having more positive than negative scores (positive balance of feelings) increases the probability of being active. Include comments on whether you think your ratings suggest that you will be active or inactive and whether your ratings are really indicative of your feelings. Do you think that the scores on which you were rated poor or very poor might be reasons why you would avoid physical activity? Explain.

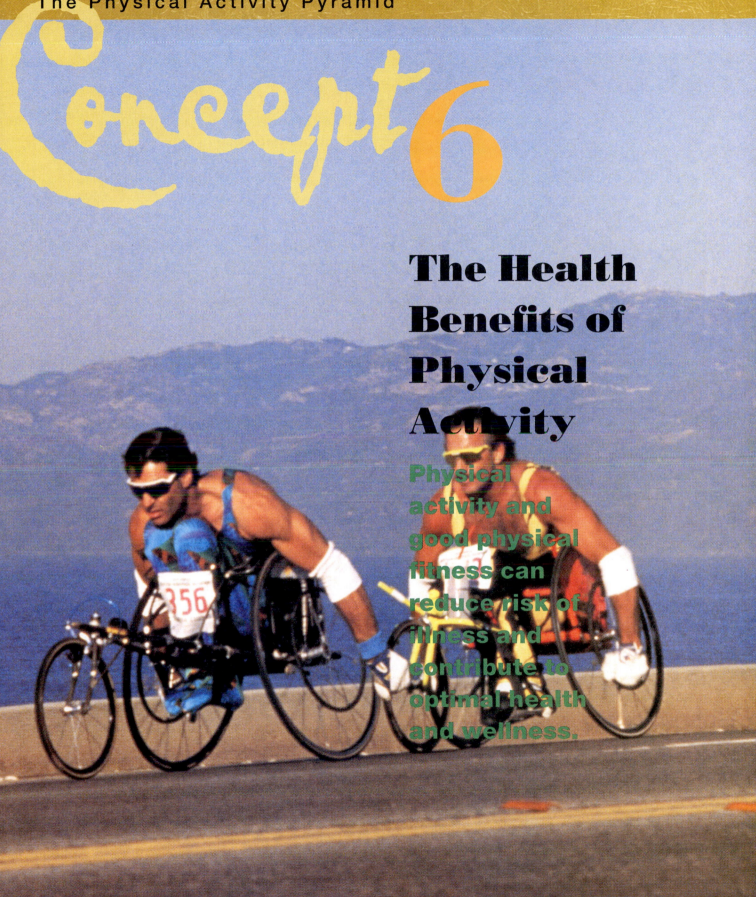

Concept **6**

The Health Benefits of Physical Activity

Physical activity and good physical fitness can reduce risk of illness and contribute to optimal health and wellness.

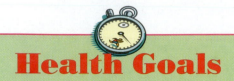

Health Goals

f o r   Y e a r   2 0 1 0

Increase quality and years of healthy life.

Increase incidence of people reporting "healthy days."

Increase incidence of people reporting "active days."

Increase the adoption and maintenance of daily physical activity.

Increase prevalence of a healthy weight and reduce prevalence of overweight.

Reduce days with pain for those with arthritis, osteoporosis and chronic back problems.

Reduce activity limitations, especially among older adults.

Reduce incidence of and deaths from cancer.

Increase diagnosis of and reduce incidence of Type II diabetes.

Decrease incidence of depression.

Decrease incidence of heart diseases including stroke and high blood pressure.

Decrease incidence of high cholesterol levels among adults.

Introduction

At no time in our history has so much evidence been accumulated to demonstrate the health and wellness benefits of physical activity and fitness. The American Heart Association has elevated sedentary living to the status of a "primary risk factor" for heart disease, indicating that activity is of primary rather than secondary importance in preventing heart disease. The recent *Surgeon General's Report on Physical Activity and Health* is an especially powerful document summarizing the benefits of regular physical activity and good fitness. It provides definitive evidence of the value of physical activity and fitness to sound health and wellness. *Healthy People 2010,* the national health goals that take us into the twenty-first century, emphasize physical activity as one of the key healthy lifestyles contributing to optimal health, wellness, and fitness. Each of these documents is cited to support the facts in this concept.

The Facts about Physical Activity, Fitness, and Disease Prevention/Treatment

There are three major ways in which regular physical activity and good fitness contribute to optimal health and wellness.

The methods by which physical activity and fitness contribute to optimal health and wellness are illustrated in Figure 1. First, they can aid in disease/illness prevention. There is considerable evidence that the risk of **hypokinetic conditions** can be greatly reduced among people who do regular physical activity and achieve good physical fitness. Virtually all **chronic diseases** that plague society are considered to be hypokinetic, though some relate more to inactivity than others. Nearly three-quarters of all deaths among those 18 and older are a result of chronic diseases.

Leading public health officials have suggested that physical activity is related to the health of all Americans. It directly reduces the risk for several major chronic diseases. Physical activity also stimulates positive changes with respect to other risk factors for these diseases. Physical activity may produce the shortcut for the control of chronic diseases, much like immunization controlled infectious diseases.

Second, physical activity and fitness can be a significant contributor to disease/illness treatment. Even with the best disease-prevention practices, some people will become ill. Regular exercise and good fitness have been shown to be effective in alleviating symptoms and aiding rehabilitation after illness for such hypokinetic conditions as diabetes, heart attack, back pain, and others.

Finally, physical activity and fitness are methods of health and wellness promotion. They contribute to quality living associated with wellness, the positive component of good health. In the process they aid in meeting many of the nation's health goals for the year 2010.

Too many adults suffer from hypokinetic diseases.

In 1961, Kraus and Raab coined the term "hypokinetic disease." They pointed out that recent advances in medicine had been quite effective in eliminating infectious diseases but that degenerative diseases, characterized by sedentary or "take-it-easy" living, had increased in recent decades. In fact, heart disease is the leading cause of death in North America. High blood pressure, stroke, and coronary artery disease (including heart attack) afflict millions each year. The second leading medical complaint (headache is number one) is low back

Optimal Health

Wellness	Health Promotion
	Disease Prevention
Disease/Illness	Disease Treatment

Death

Figure 1
Contributors to optimal health and wellness.

pain, and as many as one-half of all adults are considered to be obese. Studies show that the symptoms of hypokinetic conditions begin in youth. This suggests that the incidence of hypokinetic disease in our culture will not be reduced without considerable lifestyle change in people of all ages.

The link between regular physical activity and good health is now well documented.

www.mhhe.com/hper/physed/clw/student/
People who do regular physical activity can reduce their risk of death, regardless of the cause. Active people increase their life expectancy by two years compared to those who are inactive. Sedentary people experience a 20 percent to two-fold increase in early death compared to active people. One leading public health official indicates that increasing physical activity among the adult population would do wonders for the health of the nation because there are so many sedentary people who could benefit from active lifestyles. He notes that physical inactivity, in combination with the poor eating patterns, ranks with tobacco use among the leading preventable contributors to death for adults. If adults who lead sedentary lives would adopt a more active lifestyle, there would be enormous benefit to the public's health and to individual well-being. The major health benefits of physical activity as outlined in the *Surgeon General's Report* and other important recent reports are summarized later in this concept.

Regular physical activity over a lifetime may overcome the effects of inherited risk.

Some people with a family history of disease may conclude that there is nothing they can do because their heredity works against them. There is no doubt that heredity significantly affects risk of early death from hypokinetic diseases. New studies of twins, however, suggest that active people are less likely to die early than inactive people with similar genes. This suggests that long-term adherence to physical activity can overcome other risk factors such as heredity—at least for some people.

Hypokinetic diseases and conditions have many causes.

Regular physical activity and good physical fitness are only two of the preventative factors associated with the conditions described in this concept as hypokinetic diseases. Other healthy lifestyle factors cannot be overlooked in the prevention of these diseases.

The Facts about Physical Activity and Cardiovascular Diseases

There are many types of cardiovascular diseases.

There are many forms of **cardiovascular diseases** (CVD). Some are classified as **coronary heart disease** (CHD) because they affect the heart muscle and the blood vessels

Hypokinetic Conditions *Hypo-* means "under" or "too little," and *-kinetic* means "movement" or "activity." Thus, *hypokinetic* means "too little activity." A hypokinetic disease or condition is associated with lack of physical activity or too little regular exercise. Examples of such conditions include heart disease, low back pain, adult-onset diabetes, and obesity.

Chronic Disease A disease or illness that is associated with lifestyle or environmental factors as opposed to infectious diseases (hypokinetic diseases are considered to be chronic diseases).

Cardiovascular Disease (CVD) A broad classification of diseases of the heart and blood vessels that include CHD, as well has high blood pressure, stroke, and peripheral vascular disease.

Coronary Heart Disease (CHD) Diseases of the heart muscle and the blood vessels that supply it with oxygen, including heart attack.

inside the heart. **Coronary occlusion** (heart attack) is a type of CHD. **Atherosclerosis** and **arteriosclerosis** are two conditions that increase risk of heart attack and are also considered to be types of CHD. **Angina pectoris** (chest or arm pain), which occurs when the oxygen supply to the heart muscle is diminished, is sometimes considered to be a type of CHD though it is really a symptom of poor circulation.

Hypertension (high blood pressure), **stroke** (brain attack), **peripheral vascular disease,** and **congestive heart failure** are other forms of CVD. Inactivity relates in some way to each of these types of disease.

The various forms of cardiovascular disease are the leading killers in automated societies.

In the United States, coronary heart disease accounts for approximately 32 percent of all premature deaths. Stroke accounts for an additional 8.6 percent. Men are more likely to suffer from heart disease than women. African American, Hispanic, and Native American populations are at higher-than-normal risk. Heart disease and stroke death rates are similar in the United States, Canada, Great Britain, Australia, and other automated societies.

There is a wealth of statistical evidence that physical inactivity is a primary risk factor for CHD.

Much of the research relating inactivity to heart disease has come from occupational studies that show a high incidence of heart disease in people involved only in sedentary work. Even with the limitations inherent in these types of studies, the findings of more and more occupational studies present convincing evidence that the inactive individual has an increased risk of coronary heart disease. A study summarizing all of the important occupational studies shows a 90 percent reduced risk of coronary heart disease for those in active versus inactive occupations.

Studies also indicate that adults who expend a significant number of calories per week in strenuous sports and other activities have reduced risk of coronary heart disease. In fact, improving activity levels is among the best ways to reduce the risk of heart disease among adults.

The American Heart Association, after carefully examining the research literature, concluded that a sedentary lifestyle is a risk factor comparable to high blood pressure, high blood cholesterol, obesity, and cigarette smoke. After reviewing hundreds of studies on exercise and heart disease, the *Surgeon General's Report on Physical Activity*

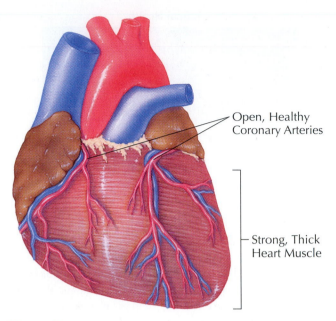

Open, Healthy Coronary Arteries

Strong, Thick Heart Muscle

Figure 2
The fit heart muscle.

and Health concluded that "physical inactivity is causally linked to atherosclerosis and coronary heart disease."

The Facts about Physical Activity and the Healthy Heart

There is evidence that regular physical activity will increase the ability of the heart muscle to pump blood as well as oxygen.

A fit heart muscle can handle extra demands placed on it. Through regular exercise, the heart muscle gets stronger, contracts more forcefully, and therefore pumps more blood with each beat. This results in a slower heart rate (especially during physical activity), and greater heart efficiency. The heart is just like any other muscle—it must be exercised regularly to stay fit. The fit heart has open, clear arteries free of atherosclerosis. (See Figure 2.)

The hypothetical "normal" resting heart rate is said to be 72 beats per minute (bpm). However, resting rates of 50 to 85 bpm are not uncommon. People who regularly do physical activity will typically have lower resting heart rates than people who do no regular activity. Some endurance athletes have heart rates in the 30 and 40 bpm range. This is not considered unhealthy or abnormal. While resting heart rate is *not* considered to be a good measure of health or fitness, decreases in individual heart rate following training reflect positive adaptations. Low heart rates in response to a standard amount of physical activity *are* a good indicator of fitness. The bicycle and step tests presented later in this book use your heart rate response to a standard amount of exercise to estimate your cardiovascular fitness.

The Facts about Physical Activity and Atherosclerosis

Atherosclerosis is implicated in many cardiovascular diseases.

Atherosclerosis is a condition that contributes to heart attack, stroke, hypertension, angina pectoris, and peripheral vascular diseases. Deposits on the walls of arteries restrict blood flow and oxygen supply to the tissues. Atherosclerosis of the coronary arteries, the vessels that supply the heart muscle with oxygen, is particularly harmful. If these arteries become narrowed, the blood supply to the heart muscle is diminished, and angina pectoris may occur. Atherosclerosis increases the risk of heart attack because a fibrous clot is more likely to obstruct a narrowed artery than a healthy, open one.

Atherosclerosis, which begins early in life, is the result of a systematic buildup of deposits in an arterial wall.

Current theory suggests that atherosclerosis begins when damage occurs to the cells of the inner wall or intima of the artery (see Figure 3). Substances associated with blood clotting are attracted to the damaged area. These substances seem to cause the migration of smooth muscle cells, commonly found only in the middle wall of the artery (media), to the intima. In the later stages, fats (including cholesterol) and other substances are thought to be deposited, forming plaques or protrusions that diminish the internal diameter of the artery. Research indicates that the first signs of atherosclerosis begin in early childhood.

There is evidence that regular physical activity can help prevent atherosclerosis.

All of the ways in which regular exercise help prevent atherosclerosis are not yet known. However, three of the most plausible theories are discussed on the next page.

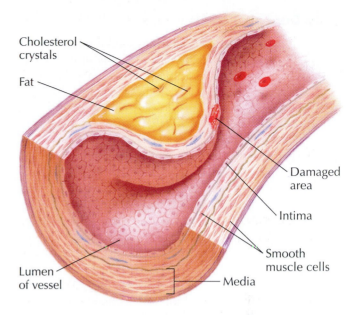

Figure 3
Atherosclerosis.

Coronary Occlusion The blocking of the coronary blood vessels.

Atherosclerosis The deposition of materials along the arterial walls; a type of arteriosclerosis.

Arteriosclerosis Hardening of the arteries due to conditions that cause the arterial walls to become thick, hard, and nonelastic.

Angina Pectoris Chest or arm pain resulting from reduced oxygen supply to the heart muscle.

Hypertension High blood pressure.

Stroke (Cerebrovascular Accident or CVA) A condition in which the brain, or part of the brain, receives insufficient oxygen as a result of diminished blood supply; sometimes called apoplexy.

Peripheral Vascular Disease Lack of oxygen supply to the working muscles and tissues of the arms and legs resulting from decreased blood flow.

Congestive Heart Failure The inability of the heart muscle to pump the blood at a life-sustaining rate.

Lipid Deposit Theory

www.mhhe.com/hper/physed/clw/student/

There are several kinds of **lipids** in the bloodstream, including **lipoproteins,** phospholipids, triglycerides, and cholesterol. Cholesterol is the most well-known, but it is not the only culprit. Many blood fats are manufactured by the body itself, while others are ingested in high-fat foods, particularly saturated fats. Saturated fats are fats that are solid at room temperature.

As noted earlier, blood lipids are thought to contribute to the development of atherosclerotic deposits on the inner walls of the artery. One substance, called low-density lipoprotein (LDL), is considered to be a major culprit in the development of atherosclerosis. LDL is basically a core of cholesterol surrounded by protein and another substance that makes it water soluble. The theory is that regular exercise can reduce blood lipid levels, including LDL-C (the cholesterol core of LDL). People with high total cholesterol and LDL-C levels have been shown to have a higher-than-normal risk of heart disease (see Table 1). New evidence indicates that there are subtypes of LDL cholesterol (characterized by their small size and high density) that pose even greater risks. These subtypes are hard to measure and not included in most current blood tests, but future research will no doubt help us better understand and measure them.

Triglycerides are another type of blood lipid. Elevated levels of triglycerides are positively related to heart disease. Triglycerides lose some of their ability to predict heart disease with the presence of other risk factors, so high levels are more difficult to interpret than other blood lipids. Normal levels are considered to be 200 mg/dL or less. Values of 200 to 400 mg/dL are considered to be borderline and above 400 mg/dL is considered to be high. It would be wise to include triglycerides in a blood lipid profile. Physical activity is often prescribed as part of a treatment for high triglyceride levels.

Protective Protein Theory

www.mhhe.com/hper/physed/clw/student/

Whereas LDLs carry a core of cholesterol that is involved in the development of atherosclerosis, high-density lipoprotein (HDL) picks up cholesterol (HDL-C) and carries it to the liver, where it is eliminated from the body. For this reason, it is often called the "protective protein." High levels of HDL are considered to be desirable. When you have a blood test, it is wise to determine the amount of HDL-C compared to the total amount of cholesterol (TC) in your blood. A low TC/HDL-C ratio is a good indicator of the protection you are receiving from HDL (see Table 1). Individuals who do regular

Table 1 Cholesterol Classifications (mg/dL)

	Total Cholesterol	LDL-C	HDL-C	TC/HDL-C
Goal	200 or less	130 or less	55+	3.5 or less
Borderline	201–239	130–159	36–55	3.6–5.0
High risk	240+	160+	35 or less	5.0+

Source: Data from B. Liebman, "Rating Your Risk" in *Nutrition Action,* 19:8, 1992 and Fifth Committee on Detection, Evaluation, and Treatment of High Blood Pressure in *Archives of Internal Medicine,* 153, 1993.

physical activity have higher HDL levels, lower TC/HDL-C ratios, and therefore less risk of heart disease.

Blood Coagulant (Fibrin and Platelet) Theory

Fibrin is a sticky, threadlike substance in the blood that is important to the clotting process. Platelets are another type of cell involved in blood coagulation. The blood coagulant theory suggests that fibrin and platelets may be involved in the development of atherosclerosis. Specifically, blood coagulants may deposit at the site of an injury on the wall of an artery, contributing to the process of plaque buildup or atherosclerosis. Exercise has been shown to reduce fibrin levels in the blood. The breakdown of fibrin resulting from regular physical activity seems to reduce platelet adhesiveness and the concentration of platelets in the blood. This, in turn, is thought to reduce the risk of atherosclerosis development.

The Facts about Physical Activity and Heart Attack

Heart attack is the most prevalent and serious of all cardiovascular diseases.

A heart attack occurs when a coronary artery is blocked (see Figure 4). A clot or thrombus is the most common cause, reducing or cutting off blood flow and oxygen to the heart muscle. If the coronary artery that is blocked supplies a major portion of the heart muscle, death will occur within minutes. Occlusions of lesser arteries may result in angina pectoris or a nonfatal heart attack.

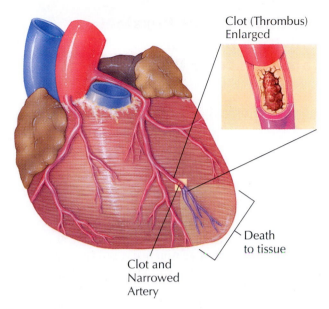

Figure 4
Heart attack.

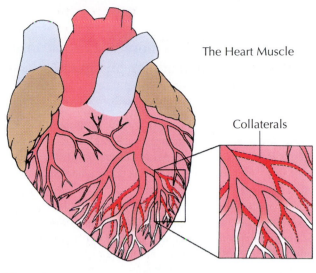

Figure 5
Coronary collateral circulation.

Regular physical activity reduces the risk of heart attack (coronary occlusion).

People who perform regular sports and physical activity have half the risk of a first heart attack compared to those who are sedentary. Possible reasons are less atherosclerosis, greater diameter of arteries, and less chance of a clot forming.

There is evidence that regular exercise can improve coronary circulation and thus reduce the chances of a heart attack or dying from one.

Within the heart, there are many tiny branches extending from the major coronary arteries. All of these vessels supply blood to the heart muscle. Healthy arteries can supply blood to any region of the heart as it is needed. Active people are likely to have greater blood-carrying capacity in these vessels, probably because the vessels are larger and more elastic. Also, the active person may have a more profuse distribution of arteries within the heart muscle (see Figure 5), which results in greater blood flow. A few studies show that physical activity may promote the growth of "extra" blood vessels, which are thought to open up to provide the heart muscle with the necessary blood and oxygen when the oxygen supply is diminished, as in a heart attack. Blood flow from extra blood vessels is referred to as **coronary collateral circulation.**

Improved coronary circulation may provide protection against a heart attack because a larger artery would require more atherosclerosis to occlude it. In addition, the development of collateral blood vessels supplying the heart may diminish the effects of a heart attack if one does occur. These extra (or collateral) blood vessels may take over the function of regular blood vessels during a heart attack.

Lipids All fats and fatty substances.

Lipoprotein Fat-carrying protein in the blood.

Low-Density Lipoprotein (LDL) A core of cholesterol surrounded by protein; the core is often called "bad cholesterol."

Triglyceride A type of blood fat associated with increased risk of heart disease.

High-Density Lipoprotein (HDL) A blood substance that picks up cholesterol and helps remove it from the body; often called "good cholesterol."

Fibrin The substance that in combination with blood cells forms a blood clot.

Coronary Collateral Circulation Circulation of blood to the heart muscle associated with the blood-carrying capacity of a specific vessel or development of collateral vessels (extra blood vessels).

The heart of the inactive person is less able to resist stress and is more susceptible to an emotional storm that may precipitate a heart attack.

The heart is rendered inefficient by one or more of the following circumstances: high heart rate, high blood pressure, and excessive stimulation. All of these conditions require the heart to use more oxygen than is normal and decrease its ability to adapt to stressful situations.

The inefficient heart is one that beats rapidly because it is dominated by the **sympathetic nervous system,** which speeds up the heart rate. Thus, the heart continuously beats rapidly, even at rest, and never has a true rest period. A study of one college basketball coach who was under considerable stress indicated that his lowest resting heart rate during the day was 88 bpm. High blood pressure also makes the heart work harder and contributes to its inefficiency.

Research indicates five things concerning physical activity and the inefficient heart.

1. Regular activity leads to dominance of the **parasympathetic nervous system** rather than to sympathetic dominance; thus the heart rate is reduced and the heart works efficiently.
2. Regular activity helps the heart rate return to normal faster after emotional stress.
3. Regular activity strengthens the heart muscle, making it better able to weather an **emotional storm.**
4. Regular activity decreases sympathetic dominance and its associated hormonal effects on the heart, thus lessening the chances of altered heart contractility and the likelihood of the circulatory problems that accompany this state.
5. Regular activity reduces the risk of sudden death from ventricular fibrillation (arrhythmic heartbeat).

Regular physical activity is one effective means of rehabilitation for a person who has coronary heart disease or who has had a heart attack.

Not only does regular physical activity seem to reduce the risk of developing coronary heart disease, there is also evidence that those who already have the condition may reduce the symptoms of the disease through regular exercise. For people who have had heart attacks, regular and progressive exercise can be an effective prescription when carried out under the supervision of a physician. Remember, however, that exercise is not the treatment of preference for all heart attack victims. In some cases, it may be contraindicated.

The Facts about Physical Activity and Other Cardiovascular Diseases

Regular physical activity is associated with a reduced risk of high blood pressure (hypertension).

www.mhhe.com/hper/physed/clw/student/

Approximately 30 percent of adults have borderline or high-risk hypertension. More men than women are likely to be hypertensive, as are more blacks than whites. Native Americans and Hispanics have a higher-than-normal incidence of hypertension, and the incidence for all groups increases as people grow older. A recent research summary indicates that the effects of physical activity on blood pressure are more dramatic than previously thought and are independent of age, body fatness, and other factors. Inactive, less-fit individuals have a 30 to 50 percent greater chance of being hypertensive than active, fit people. Regular physical activity can also be one effective method of reducing blood pressure for those with hypertension. Physical inactivity in middle age is associated with risk of high blood pressure later in life. The most plausible reason is a reduction in resistance to blood flow in the blood vessels, probably resulting from dilation of the vessels.

The hypothetical "goal" blood pressure is 120 mm Hg (**systolic blood pressure**) over 80 mm Hg (**diastolic blood pressure**). However, systolic pressures as low as 100 mm Hg and up to 130 mm Hg are considered in the normal range. Diastolic pressures of 60 to 85 mm Hg are also considered to be in the normal range. Exceptionally low blood pressures (below 100 systolic and 60 diastolic) do not pose the same risks to health as high blood pressure but can cause dizziness, fainting, and lack of tolerance to change in body positions. Classifications for blood pressure are shown in Table 2. Stage 1 hypertension is sometimes called "mild," Stage 2 "moderate," and Stage 3 "severe." Some experts do not like these terms because people with "mild" or "moderate" hypertension may not feel the need to seek medical help. All stages of hypertension should be taken seriously.

Regular physical activity can help reduce the risk of stroke.

Stroke is a major killer of adults. People with high blood pressure and atherosclerosis are susceptible to stroke. Since regular exercise and good fitness are important to the prevention of both high blood pressure and atherosclerosis, exercise and fitness are considered helpful in the prevention of stroke.

Table 2 Blood Pressure Classifications for Adults*

Category	Systolic Blood Pressure (mm Hg)	Diastolic Blood Pressure (mm Hg)
Goal	<120	<80
Normal	<130	<85
High Normal	130–139	85–89
Stage 1 Hypertension	140–159	90–99
Stage 2 Hypertension	160–179	100–109
Stage 3 Hypertension	≥180	≥110

*Not taking antihypertensive drugs and not acutely ill. When the systolic and diastolic blood pressure categories vary, the higher reading determines the blood pressure classification.

SOURCE: National Institutes for Health, 1997. See Suggested Readings.

Regular physical activity is helpful in the prevention of peripheral vascular diseases.

www.mhhe.com/hper/physed/clw/student/
There is evidence that people who exercise regularly have better blood flow to the working muscles and other tissues than inactive, unfit people. Since peripheral vascular disease is associated with poor circulation to the extremities, regular exercise can be considered one method of preventing this condition.

The Facts about Physical Activity and Other Hypokinetic Conditions

Physical activity reduces the risk of some forms of cancer.

www.mhhe.com/hper/physed/clw/student/
Cancer is the second leading cause of death in the United States. According to the American Cancer Society, cancer is a group of diseases characterized by uncontrollable growth and spread of abnormal cells. Several cancers are considered hypokinetic. Adequate data are now available to document the relationship of inactivity to colon cancer. Inactive people have a 50 to 250 percent greater risk of getting colon cancer than active people. Consistent findings also suggest that rectal cancer is also associated with inactivity. The relationship between fitness, exercise, and other forms of cancer is not yet fully understood. One possible reason why regular exercisers have a reduced risk of colon/rectal cancer (the second most common cause of cancer deaths among males) is the faster intestinal transit time.

Several studies have suggested that fit people who regularly perform physical activity have increased protection against reproductive system and breast cancers. One study indicates a one-third reduction in risk of breast cancer among those who do at least four hours of leisure physical activity each week as compared to those who are less active. (People who do heavy manual labor have an even greater reduction in risk.) In fact, nonathletes have been found to have a greater risk of breast cancer than athletes. On the other hand, a recent study of Harvard graduates failed to find a strong link between activity and breast cancer. Researchers who have shown a relationship between activity and breast cancer hypothesize that regular physical activity in youth may delay the onset of menstruation and reduce the lifelong exposure to estrogen. This suggests a hormonal link between physical activity and breast cancer. A causal link between activity and breast cancer has yet to be established—more research is necessary. For those who have cancer, there is evidence that physical activity can help them lead more fulfilling and productive lives.

Physical activity plays an important role in the management and treatment of Type II diabetes.

www.mhhe.com/hper/physed/clw/student/
Diabetes is a group of disorders that results when there is too much sugar in the blood. It occurs when the body does not make enough

Sympathetic Nervous System Branch of the autonomic nervous system that prepares the body for activity by speeding up the heart rate.

Parasympathetic Nervous System Branch of the autonomic nervous system that slows the heart rate.

Emotional Storm A traumatic emotional experience that is likely to affect the human organism physiologically.

Systolic Blood Pressure The upper blood pressure number often called working blood pressure. It represents the pressure in the arteries at its highest level just after the heart beats.

Diastolic Blood Pressure The lower blood pressure number often called "resting pressure." It is the pressure in the arteries at its lowest level occurring just before the next beat of the heart.

insulin or when the body is not able to use insulin effectively. Diabetes is the seventh leading cause of death among people over 40. It accounts for at least 10 percent of all short-term hospital stays and has a major impact on health-care costs in Western society. By itself, exercise is not an effective treatment for Type I (insulin-dependent) diabetes. However, with proper medical supervision, exercise is encouraged for maintaining physical fitness for most diabetics.

People who perform regular physical activity are less likely to suffer from Type II (noninsulin-dependent, adult-onset) diabetes than sedentary people. For people with Type II diabetes, regular physical activity can help reduce body fatness, decrease **insulin resistance,** improve **insulin sensitivity,** and improve the body's ability to clear sugar from the blood in a reasonable time. All of these factors contribute to controlling the disease. With sound nutritional habits and proper medication, physical activity can be useful in the management of both types of diabetes.

> **Regular physical activity is important to maintaining bone density and decreasing risk of osteoporosis.**

www.mhhe.com/hper/physed/clw/student/
Studies indicate that excessive bed rest can result in deterioration of the bones. When the long bones in our body do not bear weight, they lose calcium and become porous and fragile. When this occurs in the extreme, it is called **osteoporosis.** Even excessive sitting can result in bone deterioration, regardless of age. Bones are strengthened not only by bearing weight, but by the pull of active muscles. Regular physical activity is as necessary for healthy bone development as it is for healthy muscle development.

Physical activity helps prevent osteoporosis in several ways. First, activity increases your peak bone mass, which is the maximum amount of bone you will ever develop. This is usually achieved early in life. Lack of weight-bearing exercise and poor nutrition during this time can result in a low peak bone mass. People who develop greater peak bone mass when young can lose bone density without becoming osteoporotic later in life.

The second way in which physical activity helps prevent osteoporosis is to maintain bone density over the lifespan. The people who are particularly susceptible to osteoporosis are postmenopausal women not taking an estrogen supplement, people who do not consume adequate calcium, and those who do no regular weight-bearing exercise and/or lack a nutritious diet. Weight training has been shown to be valuable for older people because

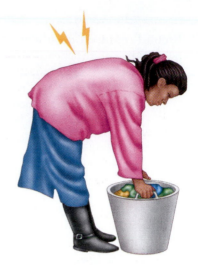

Back pain is a hypokinetic condition, but it may also be caused by incorrect lifting techniques.

bone loss is potentially greater, and this type of exercise can help reduce the rate of loss.

> **Active people who possess good muscle fitness are less likely to have back and other musculoskeletal problems than inactive, unfit people.**

Because few people die from it, back pain does not receive the attention given to such medical problems as heart disease and cancer. But back pain is considered to be the second leading medical complaint in the United States, second only to headaches. Only common colds and flu cause more days lost from work. At some point in our lives, approximately 80 percent of all adults will experience back pain that limits their ability to function normally. Recent National Safety Council data indicated that the back was the most frequently injured of all body parts, and the injury rate was double that of any other part of the body.

Many years ago, medical doctors began to associate back problems with the lack of physical fitness. It is now known that the great majority of back ailments are the result of poor muscle strength and endurance, and poor flexibility. Tests on patients with back problems show weakness and lack of flexibility in key muscle groups.

Though lack of fitness is probably the leading reason for back pain in Western society, there are many other factors that increase the risk of back ailments, including poor posture, improper lifting and work habits, heredity, and disease states, such as scoliosis and arthritis.

> **Physical activity is important in maintaining a healthy body weight and avoiding the numerous health conditions associated with obesity.**

Obesity, as well as lesser degrees of fatness, is not a disease state in itself but is a hypokinetic condition associated with a multitude of far-reaching complications. Obesity is associated with serious organic impairments, shortened life span, psychological maladjustments, poor relationships with peers (especially among children), awkward physical movement, and lack of achievement in athletic activities. Obesity can be both a cause and an effect of physical inactivity. People who are overfat have a higher risk of respiratory infections; are prone to developing high blood pressure, atherosclerosis, and disorders of the circulatory and respiratory systems; and have a greater-than-normal risk of some forms of cancer. The symptoms of adult-onset diabetes are associated with excessive fatness. (Fortunately, fat loss to normal levels is usually followed by remission of adult-onset diabetic symptoms.) Because physical activity, together with sound nutritional management, is an effective means of lowering body fat, it can be helpful in reducing the risk of those conditions associated with fatness and obesity.

> **Physical activity reduces the risk and severity of a variety of common mental (emotional) health disorders. Such disorders can be considered hypokinetic conditions.**

Some mental (emotional) health conditions are prevalent in modern society. According to the *Surgeon General's Report on Physical Activity and Health,* nearly one of every two adult Americans will report having a mental health disorder at some point in life. A recent summary of studies revealed that there are several mental/emotional disorders that are associated with inactive lifestyles.

Depression is a stress-related condition experienced by many adults. Thirty-three percent of inactive adults report that they often feel depressed. For some, depression is a serious disorder that physical activity alone will not cure; however, recent research does indicate that activity, combined with other forms of therapy, can be effective.

Anxiety is an emotional condition characterized by worry, self-doubt, and apprehension. More than a few studies have shown that symptoms of anxiety can be reduced by regular activity. Low-fit people who do regular aerobic activity seem to benefit the most. In one study, one-third of very active people felt that regular activity helped them to better cope with life's pressures.

Physical activity is also associated with better and more restful sleep. People with insomnia (the inability to sleep) seem to benefit from regular activity if it is not done too vigorously right before going to bed. A recent study indicates that 52 percent of the population feel that physical activity helps them sleep better. Regular aerobic activity is associated with reduced brain activation that can result in greater ability to relax or fall asleep.

Even more common than depression and insomnia is the condition called Type A behavior. Type A personalities are stress-prone individuals with a greater than normal incidence of diseases. A Type A person is tense, overcompetitive, and worried about meeting time schedules. Apparently all Type A personalities are not equally stressed. It has been suggested that aggressive Type A personalities are most likely to be prone to negative consequences of stress. Regular physical activity can benefit the Type A person—especially the aggressive Type A. Noncompetitive activities would probably be best for this stress-prone personality type.

A final benefit of regular physical activity is increased self-esteem. Improvements in fitness and appearance can improve self-confidence and self-esteem. The ability to regulate behavior and perform new tasks can also promote higher self-esteem.

> **Regular physical activity can have positive effects on some non-hypokinetic conditions.**

Some non-hypokinetic conditions that can benefit from physical activity are:

- Arthritis. Many, if not most, arthritics are in a deconditioned state resulting from a lack of activity. The traditional advice that arthritics should avoid physical activity is now being modified in view of the findings that carefully prescribed exercise can improve general fitness and, in some cases, reduce the symptoms of the disease.
- Asthma. Asthmatics often have physical activity limitations. New evidence suggests that, with proper management, activity can be part of their daily life. In fact, when done properly, activity can reduce airway reactivity and medication use. Because exercise can trigger bronchial constriction, it is important to choose appropriate types of activity and to use inhaled medications

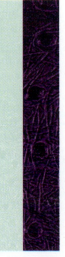

Insulin A hormone secreted by the pancreas that regulates levels of sugar in the blood.

Insulin Resistance A condition that occurs when insulin becomes ineffective or less effective than is necessary to regulate sugar levels in the blood.

Insulin Sensitivity A person with insulin resistance (see above) is said to have decreased insulin sensitivity. The body's cells are not sensitive to insulin so they resist it and sugar levels are not regulated effectively.

Osteoporosis A condition associated with low bone density and subsequent bone fragility leading to high risk of fracture.

to prevent bronchial constriction caused by exercise or other triggers such as cold weather. Cold weather exercise should typically be avoided.

- Chronic pain. There are many sources of pain that persist for long periods of time without relief; some are difficult to understand. Nevertheless, large numbers of adults are victims of chronic pain. Both aerobic exercise and resistance training are currently being prescribed to treat this problem.

- Infections. Infectious diseases are not generally considered to be hypokinetic conditions. However, regular physical activity that fosters physical fitness and good health may help you resist diseases that result from lowered general resistance. On the other hand, when the body is fighting an infection, too much exercise can cause a lowered state of resistance.

- Premenstrual syndrome (PMS). PMS, a mixture of physical and emotional symptoms that occurs prior to menstruation, has many causes. However, current evidence suggests that changes in lifestyle, including regular exercise, may be effective in relieving PMS symptoms.

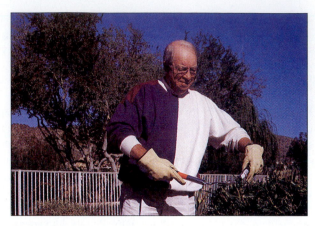

Fitness improves work efficiency.

The Facts about Physical Activity and Aging

Regular physical activity can improve fitness and improve functioning among older adults.

www.mhhe.com/hper/physed/clw/student/
Approximately 30 percent of adults age 70 and over have difficulty with one or more activities of daily living. Women have more limitations than men, and low-income groups have more limitations than higher-income groups. Nearly half get no assistance with the activity in which they are limited.

The inability to function effectively as you grow older is associated with lack of fitness and inactive lifestyles. This loss of function is sometimes referred to as "acquired aging" as opposed to "time-dependent" aging. Because so many people experience limitations in daily activities and often find it difficult to get assistance, it is especially important for older people to stay active and fit. In Africa, Asia, and South America, where older adults maintain an active lifestyle, individuals do not acquire many of the characteristics commonly associated with aging in North America.

The *Surgeon General's Report* indicates that, in general, older adults become much less active than younger adults. Losses in muscle fitness are associated with loss of balance, greater risk of falling, and less ability to function independently. Though the amount of activity performed must be adapted as people grow older, fitness benefits dis-

cussed in the next section and throughout this book apply to people of all ages.

Regular physical activity can compress illness into a shorter period of our life.

www.mhhe.com/hper/physed/clw/student/
An important national health goal is to increase the years of healthy life. Living longer is important, but being able to function effectively during all years of life is equally—if not more—important. "Compression" refers to shortening the total number of years that illnesses and disabilities occur. The average person lives to the national average of 76.1 years and has nearly 12 years of illness. Compressing the illness means dramatically decreasing the years of illness. Healthy lifestyles, including regular physical activity, have been shown to compress illness and increase years of effective functioning.

Facts about Health, Fitness, and Wellness Promotion

Physical activity enhances metabolic fitness that can reduce risk of a variety of health problems.

Metabolism refers to the chemical and physiological processes of the body that lead to the production of energy. When the metabolic systems of the body do not work effectively, it can lead to risk of chronic diseases such as diabetes and heart disease. Metabolic fitness is the positive

Table 3 Health and Wellness Benefits of Physical Activity and Fitness

Major Benefit	Related Benefits	Major Benefit	Related Benefits
Improved cardiovascular fitness and health	• Stronger heart muscle • Lower heart rate • Better electric stability of heart • Decreased sympathetic control of heart • Increased O_2 to brain • Reduced blood fat, including low-density lipids (LDLs) • Increased protective high-density lipids (HDLs) • Delayed development of atherosclerosis • Increased work capacity • Improved peripheral circulation • Improved coronary circulation • Resistance to "emotional storm" • Reduced risk of heart attack • Reduced risk of stroke • Reduced risk of hypertension • Greater chance of surviving a heart attack • Increased oxygen-carrying capacity of the blood	Reduced diabetes risk	• Decreased chance of adult-onset diabetes • Improved quality of life for Type I diabetics
		Reduction in mental tension	• Relief of depression • Improved sleep habits • Fewer stress symptoms • Ability to enjoy leisure • Possible work improvement
		Opportunity for social interactions	• Improved quality of life
		Resistance to fatigue	• Ability to enjoy leisure • Improved quality of life • Improved ability to meet some stressors
		Opportunity for successful experience	• Improved self-concept • Opportunity to recognize and accept personal limitations • Improved sense of well-being • Enjoy life—fun
		Improved appearance	• Better figure/physique • Better posture • Fat control
Greater lean body mass and less body fat	• Greater work efficiency • Less susceptibility to disease • Improved appearance • Less incidence of self-concept problems related to obesity	Reduced effect of acquired aging	• Improved ability to function in daily life • Better short-term memory • Fewer illnesses • Greater mobility • Greater independence • Greater ability to operate an automobile
Improved strength and muscular endurance	• Greater work efficiency • Less chance of muscle injury • Reduced risk of low back problems • Improved performance in sports • Quicker recovery after hard work • Improved ability to meet emergencies	Improved flexibility	• Greater work efficiency • Less chance of muscle injury • Less chance of joint injury • Decreased chance of low back problems • Improved sports performance
Bone development	• Greater peak bone density • Less chance of osteoporosis	Other health benefits	• Extended life • Decrease in dysfunctional years • Aids some people who have arthritis, PMS, asthma, and chronic pain
Reduced cancer risk	• Reduced risk of colon cancer • Possible reduced risk of rectal, reproductive, and breast cancers		

states of these systems, evidenced by healthy blood fat (lipid) profiles, healthy blood pressure, healthy blood sugar and insulin levels, and other nonperformance measures including a healthy body fatness level. It is apparent that many of the factors that constitute metabolic fitness are common to more than a few of the hypokinetic conditions described in this concept. For this reason, good metabolic fitness is important to an overall reduced risk of disease. Concepts presented later in this book will outline the types of physical activity that produce metabolic fitness benefits.

Good health-related physical fitness and regular physical activity are important to health promotion and feeling well.

Optimal health is more than freedom from disease. Regular physical activity and good fitness not only help prevent illness and disease but also promote quality of life and feeling well. Good health-related fitness can help you feel good, look good, and enjoy life. Table 3 presents a summary of some of the more specific benefits associated with physical activity.

Good physical fitness can help an individual enjoy his or her leisure time.

A person who is lean, has no back problems, does not have high blood pressure, and has reasonable skills in a lifetime of sports is more likely to get involved and stay regularly involved in leisure-time activities than one who does not have these characteristics. It is said that enjoying your leisure time may not add years to your life, but can add life to your years.

Good physical fitness can help an individual work effectively and efficiently.

A person who can resist fatigue, muscle soreness, back problems, and other symptoms associated with poor health-related fitness is capable of working productively and having energy left over at the end of the day. Surveys of employees who are involved with employee fitness programs indicate that 75 percent have an improved sense of well-being. Employers indicate that absenteeism decreased by up to 50 percent among program participants. People with good skill-related fitness may be more effective and efficient in performing specific motor skills required for certain jobs.

Good physical fitness is essential to effective living.

Although the need for each component of physical fitness is specific to each individual, every person requires enough fitness to perform normal daily activities without undue fatigue. Whether it be walking, performing household chores, or merely feeling good and enjoying the simple things in life without pain or fear of injury, good fitness is important to all people.

Good physical fitness may help you function safely and assist you in meeting unexpected emergencies.

Emergencies are never expected, but when they do arise, they often demand performance that requires good fitness. For example, flood victims may need to fill sandbags for hours without rest, and accident victims may be required to walk or run long distances for help. Also, good fitness is required for such simple tasks as safely changing a spare tire or loading a moving van without injury.

Physical fitness is the basis for dynamic and creative activity.

Though the following quotation by former President John F. Kennedy is more than 30 years old, it clearly points out the importance of physical fitness.

The relationship between the soundness of the body and the activity of the mind is subtle and complex. Much is not yet understood, but we know what the Greeks knew: that intelligence and skill can only function at the peak of their capacity when the body is healthy and strong, and that hardy spirits and tough minds usually inhabit sound bodies. Physical fitness is the basis of all activities in our society; if our bodies grow soft and inactive, if we fail to encourage physical development and prowess, we will undermine our capacity for thought, for work, and for the use of those skills vital to an expanding and complex America.

President Kennedy's belief that physical activity and fitness are associated with intellectual functioning has now been backed up with research. Recent summaries of the research in this area suggest that, though modest, the effect of activity and fitness on intellectual functioning is positive. Time taken to be active during the day has been shown to help children learn more, even though less time is spent in intellectual pursuits.

There are many economic benefits associated with employee physical activity.

A comprehensive review of the literature indicates that worksite physical activity programs can improve health, wellness, and fitness of employees, reduce health care costs, and decrease absenteeism. The costs associated with providing physical activity for employees more than offsets the cost of medical care and lost days of work associated with inactivity. Active employees are up to three times less likely to be absent or have medical complaints than inactive employees.

The Facts about Risk Factors

There are many different positive lifestyles that can reduce the risk of disease.

Many of the factors that contribute to optimal health and quality of life are also considered risk factors. Changing these risk factors can dramatically reduce the risk of hypokinetic diseases such as heart disease, back pain, diabetes, and cancer. Lack of physical activity, poor nutrition, smoking, and inability to cope with stress are all risk factors associated with various diseases (see Table 4).

Not all risk factors are under your personal control.

Some factors that can contribute to the increased risk of disease are not under your personal control. Three uncontrollable

Table 4 Hypokinetic Disease Risk Factors

Factors That Cannot Be Altered

1. **Age**—As you grow older, your risk of contracting hypokinetic diseases increases. For example, the risk of heart disease is approximately three times as great after 60 as before. The risk of back pain is considerably greater after 40.

2. **Heredity**—People who have a family history of hypokinetic disease are more likely to develop a hypokinetic condition, such as heart disease, hypertension, back problems, obesity, high blood lipid levels, and other problems. African Americans are 45 percent more likely to have high blood pressure than Caucasians; therefore, they suffer strokes at an earlier age with more severe consequences.

3. **Gender**—Men have a higher incidence of many hypokinetic conditions than women. However, differences between men and women have decreased recently. This is especially true for heart disease, the leading cause of death for both men and women. Postmenopausal women have a higher heart disease risk than pre-menopausal women.

Factors That Can Be Altered

4. **Body fatness**—Having too much body fat is now a primary risk factor for heart disease and is a risk factor for other hypokinetics conditions as well. For example, loss of fat can result in relief from symptoms of adult-onset diabetes, can reduce problems associated with certain types of back pain, and can reduce the risks of surgery.

5. **Diet**—There is a clear association between hypokinetic disease and certain types of diets. The excessive intake of saturated fats, such as animal fats, is linked to atherosclerosis and other forms of heart disease. Excessive salt in the diet is associated with high blood pressure.

6. **Diseases**—People who have one hypokinetic disease are more likely to develop a second or even a third condition. For example, if you have diabetes,* atherosclerosis, or high blood pressure, your risk of having a heart attack or stroke increases dramatically. People with poor posture have a high risk of experiencing back pain, and those with too much body fat have a greater-than-normal risk of diabetes. Although you may not be entirely able to alter the extent to which you develop certain diseases and conditions, reducing your risk and following your doctor's advice can improve your odds significantly.

7. **Regular physical activity**—As noted throughout this book, regular exercise can help reduce the risk of hypokinetic disease.

8. **Tobacco Use**—Smokers have a much higher risk of developing and dying from heart disease than nonsmokers. The risk of heart attack is twice as great among young smokers as among young nonsmokers. (Most striking is the difference in risk between older women smokers and nonsmokers.) Smokers have five times the risk of heart attack as nonsmokers. Tobacco use is also associated with the increased risk of high blood pressure, cancer, and several other medical conditions. Apparently, the more you use, the greater the risk. Stopping tobacco use even after many years can significantly reduce the hypokinetic disease risk.

9. **Stress**—There is evidence that people who are subject to excessive stress are predisposed to various hypokinetic diseases including heart disease and back pain. Statistics indicate that hypokinetic conditions are common among those in certain high-stress jobs and those having type A personality profiles.

*Some types of diabetes cannot be altered.

---

risk factors are age, heredity, and gender. These factors that cannot be altered by lifestyle changes are presented in Table 4.

Altering risk factors can help reduce the risk of more than one adverse condition at the same time.

By altering the risk factors that are controllable, you can reduce the risk of several hypokinetic conditions. For example, controlling body fatness reduces the risk of diabetes, hypertension, and back problems. Altering your diet can reduce the chances of developing high levels of blood lipids, and thus reduce the risk of atherosclerosis.

Risk reduction does not guarantee freedom from disease.

Reducing risk alters the probability of disease, but does not assure disease immunity.

Too much physical activity can lead to hyperkinetic diseases or conditions.

www.mhhe.com/hper/physed/clw/student/
The information presented in this concept points out the health benefits of physical activity performed in appropriate amounts. When done in excess or incorrectly, physical activity can result in **hyperkinetic conditions.** The most common hyperkinetic condition is overuse injury to muscles, connective tissue, and bones. Recently, anorexia nervosa and body neurosis have been identified as conditions associated with inappropriate amounts of physical activity. These conditions will be discussed in the concept on performance.

Hyperkinetic Condition A disease/illness or health condition caused by or contributed to by too much physical activity.

Strategies for Action: The Facts

> A self-assessment of risk factors can help you modify your lifestyle to reduce risk of heart disease.

The Heart Disease Risk Factor Questionnaire in Lab 6A will help you assess your personal risk. You can use your self-assessment to determine your alterable, unalterable, and total risk scores. These scores should be useful in preparing a plan for lifestyle change to reduce risk.

 ## Web Review

Web review materials for Concept 6 are available are at *www.mhhe.com/hper/physed/clw/student/*.

American Cancer Society
   www.cancer.org

American Diabetes Association
   www.diabetes.org

American College of Sports Medicine
   www.acsm.org

American Heart Association
   www.amhrt.org

Centers for Disease Control and Prevention
   www.cdc.gov

National Stroke Association
   www.stroke.org

Osteoporosis Online HotLink
   www.nof.org

Suggested Readings

ACSM's Health and Fitness Journal. 2(2)(1998): entire issue. This issue contains 11 articles dealing with the health benefits of physical activity.

Campaigne, B. N. "Exercise and Type I Diabetes." *ACSM's Health and Fitness Journal.* 2(4)(1998):35.

Corbin, C. B., and Pangrazi, R. P. *Towards a Better Understanding of Physical Fitness and Activity.* Scottsdale, AZ: Holcomb-Hathaway, 1999, Sections II, III, and IV.

Corbin, C. B., and Pangrazi, R. P. "What You Need to Know About the Surgeon General's Report on Physical Activity and Health." *Physical Activity and Fitness Research Digest* 2(1996):1.

Etnier, J. L. et al. "The Influences of Physical Fitness and Exercise Upon Cognitive Functioning: A Meta Analysis." *The Journal of Sport and Exercise Psychology* 19(3)(1997):249.

Haskell, W.L. "Physical Activity in the Prevention and Management of Coronary Heart Disease." *Physical Activity and Fitness Research Digest* 2(1995):1.

Leutholtz, B. C. "Exercise Can Reduce Incidence and Severity of Hypertension." *ACSM's Health and Fitness.* 2(5)(1998):36.

McGinnis, J.M., and Lee, P.R. "Healthy People 2000 at Mid Decade." *Journal of the American Medical Association* 273(1995):1123.

National Institutes of Health. The Sixth Report of the Joint National Committee on Detection, Evaluation, and Treatment of High Blood Pressure, NIH Publication Number 98-4080, 1997.

Nieman, D. C. "Moderate Exercise Boosts the Immune System." *ACSM's Health and Fitness Journal.* 1(5)(1997):19.

Ortal, M. & Sherman, C. "Exercise Against Depression." *The Physician and Sports Medicine.* 26(10)(1998):55–60.

Osness, W. H. *Exercise and the Older Adult.* Reston, VA: AAHPERD, 1998.

Plowman, S.A. "Physical Fitness and Healthy Low Back Function." *Physical Activity and Fitness Research Digest* 1(1993):1.

Shaw, J.M., and Snow-Harter, C. "Osteoporosis and Physical Activity." *President's Council on Physical Fitness and Sports Research Digest.* Washington, D.C.: President's Council on Physical Fitness and Sports, 1995.

U.S. Department of Health and Human Services. (1996). *Physical Activity and Health: A Report of the Surgeon General.* Atlanta, GA: U.S. Department of Health and Human Services, Chapter 6.

Van Loan, M. D. "What Makes Good Bones: Factors Affecting bone Health." *ACSM's Health and Fitness Journal.* 2(4)(1998):27.

Youngstedt, S. D. "Does Exercise Truly Enhance Sleep?" *Physician and Sportsmedicine.* 25(10)(1997):72.

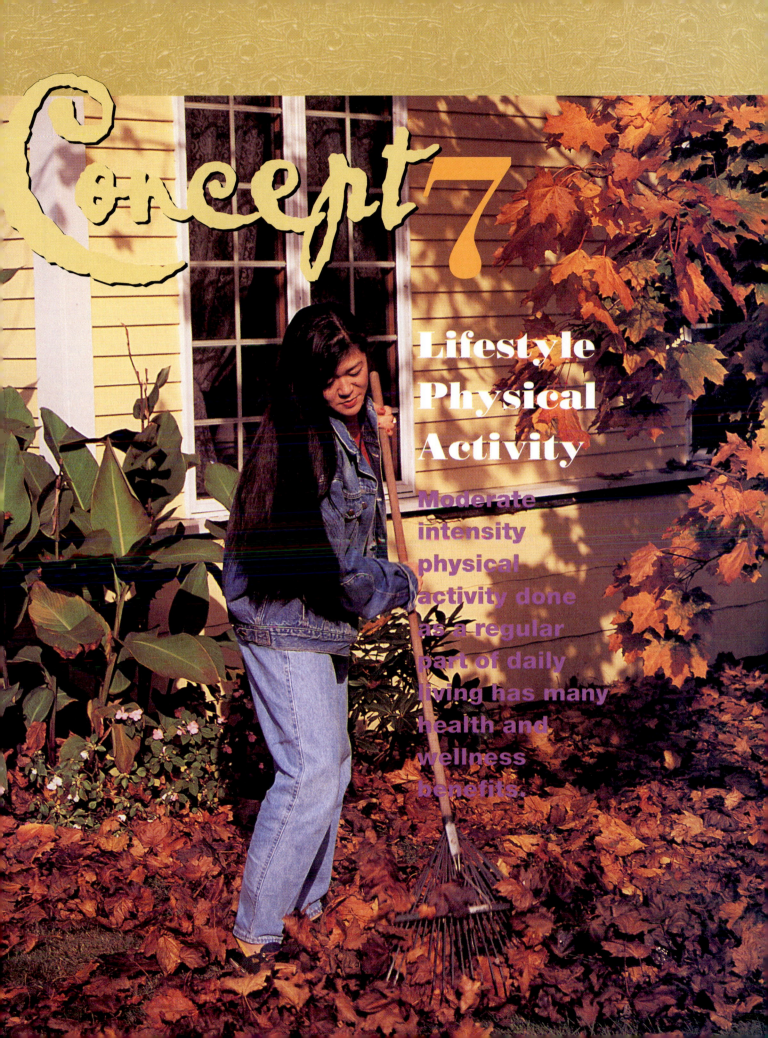

Concept 7

Lifestyle Physical Activity

Moderate intensity physical activity done as a regular part of daily living has many health and wellness benefits.

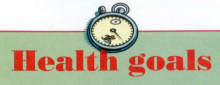

Introduction

The *Surgeon General's Report on Physical Activity and Health* and a recommendation on *Physical Activity and Public Health* from the Centers for Disease Control and Prevention and the American College of Sports Medicine emphasize the value of **moderate physical activity** to good health. These reports refer to moderate intensity physical activity as lifestyle physical activity, which is located at the base of the physical activity pyramid. In this concept, lifestyle physical activity will be explained in detail.

The Facts about Lifestyle Activity

Lifestyle physical activities can easily be integrated into daily living.

During rest, the body is able to meet all of its energy needs. This is done by the aerobic system that allows the body to produce energy by breaking down a food in the presence of oxygen. Thus, sedentary activities like sitting, playing a musical instrument, or even watching television can technically be considered "aerobic" in nature. To improve our health and fitness, activities must challenge the body to work above this resting level on a regular basis. One of the best ways to do this is to perform physi-

cal activity as part of your daily routine. Moderate intensity lifestyle physical activities that involve the larger muscle groups of the body are **aerobic physical activities** that are often referred to as lifestyle activities. Lifestyle activities include daily living activities such as walking to work or to the store, housework, gardening or yard work, and climbing the stairs.

Lifestyle physical activities should expend much more energy than normally expended at rest.

www.mhhe.com/hper/physed/clw/student/
Scientists have devised a method to classify levels of activity by intensity. With this system, all activities are compared against the amount of activity needed at rest. The amount of energy expended at rest is referred to as one metabolic equivalent (1 **MET**). Activities listed as 2 METs require twice the energy of rest, and activities listed as 4 METs require four times the energy required for rest. Table 1 defines different intensity levels so that the reader can distinguish among the various terms used later in this book. You can see that moderate-intensity activities typically require 4.7–7.0 METs. The table also indicates that nearly all people can perform moderate activity aerobically. This means that the aerobic system can meet the energy demands for this activity, and the activity can be performed for relatively long periods of time without stopping.

www.mhhe.com/hper/physed/clw/student/
Anaerobic physical activities are those that are so vigorous that your body cannot supply adequate oxygen to meet the energy demand using the aerobic system. In these instances, the body must rely on short-term energy provided by the anaerobic metabolic system. As indicated in Table 1, those activities classified as hard, very hard, or maximum may be anaerobic in nature (or at least partially anaerobic). Because these activities cannot be sustained, they are not considered lifestyle physical activities.

Activities considered to be "light" when you are young may be considered moderate at older ages.

As noted in Table 1, brisk walking for a young person (20s and 30s) typically requires a 4.7 to 7 MET energy expenditure. The activity is 4.7 to 7 times more intense than lying down doing nothing. As a person grows older, the MET equivalent of the activity can decrease and still result in benefits. This is because fitness levels tend to decrease and less activity is needed to challenge the body. From the 40s to age

Table 1 Classification of Different Intensities of Aerobic and Anaerobic Physical Activity[*]

Classification	Description	Type	Examples
Very light	Activity that is about 2 to 2 1/2 times as intense as lying or sitting at rest (2 to 2.5 METs)	Aerobic	Washing your face, dressing yourself, typing, driving a car
Light	Activity that is 2 1/2 to 4 2/3 times as intense as rest (2.5 to 4.7 METs).	Aerobic	Normal walking, walking downstairs, bowling, mopping
Moderate	Activity about 4 2/3 to 7 times as intense as rest (4.7 to 7 METs).	Aerobic	Brisk walking, lawn mowing, shoveling, social dancing
Hard	Activities more than 7 and up to 10 times as intense as rest (7 to 10 METs).	Anaerobic for some, aerobic for others	Digging, level jogging (5 mph, 12 min. mile), cycling (13 mph), skiing, fencing
Very hard	Activities more than 10 and up to 12 times as intense as rest (10 to 12 METs).	Anaerobic for most, partly aerobic for some	Running (8.5 mph, 7 min. mile), handball, full-court competitive basketball
Maximum	Activities more than 12 times as intense as rest (12+ METs).	Anaerobic for virtually all	Running (10 mph, 6 min. mile)

[*]This table is based on values for healthy adults 20–39 years of age. As you grow older, it takes less intensity to achieve higher level classifications. Based on the ACSM suggested reading, 1998.

65, expending 4–6 METs provides benefits similar to those of 5–7 METs for people in their 20s and 30s. From 65 to 80, an expenditure of 3–5 METs is considered moderate activity. For the older old adults (80+), moderate activity is equal to 2–3 METs. Because the multiples of resting expenditure need not be as great as you grow older, it is easy to see that the speed of walking need not be the same among older people as among the young. The intensity of all activities should be adjusted as you grow older.

> Because they are relatively easy to perform, lifestyle activities are very popular among adults.

www.mhhe.com/hper/physed/clw/student/

According to the *Surgeon General's* report, walking is the most popular of all leisure-time activities among adults 18 years of age and over. Approximately 39 percent of all men and 48 percent of all women walked for exercise in the past two weeks. Also, among the 10 most popular activities among adults is gardening (including yard work), which is done by 34 percent of all male and 25 percent of all female adults. Approximately 10 percent of men and 12 percent of women report that they regularly use the stairs to increase their activity levels.

One very interesting fact about lifestyle physical activities is that the number of people participating in them increases with age. For example, only 33 percent of men 18 to 29 walk regularly, but 50 percent of men over 65 walk for exercise. Among young women, 47 percent walk, while 50 percent over 65 are walkers. Nearly twice as many older men than young men do gardening, and the difference

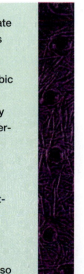

Moderate Activity Physical activity of moderate intensity; referred to as moderate activity in this concept.

Aerobic Physical Activity or Exercise Aerobic means "in the presence of oxygen." Aerobic activity is activity or exercise for which the body is able to supply adequate oxygen to sustain performance for long periods of time.

MET One MET equals the amount of energy a person expends at rest. METs are multiples of resting activity (two METS equals twice the resting energy expenditure).

Anaerobic Physical Activity or Exercise Anaerobic means "in the absence of oxygen." Anaerobic exercise is performed at an intensity so great that the body's demand for oxygen exceeds its ability to supply it.

among women is almost as dramatic. As lifetime physical activity participation increases with age, involvement in sports dramatically decreases.

> **Some sports and recreational activities may be considered to be lifestyle physical activities if classified as light or moderate in intensity.**

Some sports that are of light or moderate intensity can be classified as lifestyle physical activities. Golf, shuffleboard, bocci ball, table tennis, and bowling are examples. Recreational activities of light and moderate intensity can also be classified as lifestyle physical activities. Examples are fishing, canoeing, horseback riding, and gardening.

For children, play is considered to be a lifestyle physical activity because play is a normal activity for this age group. For retired adults, light- to moderate-intensity sports and recreational activities are truly lifestyle activities because they are a part of normal daily living.

Light- to moderate-intensity sports and recreational activities are very popular among adults, especially older adults. A recent Gallup poll indicated that fishing was the second most popular lifetime activity, bowling the fourth, and camping fifth. Though golf is not one of the top 10 participation activities, it is a very popular activity among older adults. More people over 65 play golf than those in the 18–30 group, perhaps because older people have more time for activities that take several hours and because its intensity is more appropriate for older adults.

> **Lifestyle physical activities can easily be performed by most people regardless of fitness level.**

www.mhhe.com/hper/physed/clw/student/

Prior to the last two decades, the conventional wisdom concerning physical activity was that it had to be vigorous to provide health and fitness benefits. Long-term studies of large populations were conducted with a variety of groups showing that moderate activity produced many benefits. For example, postal carriers who delivered mail showed benefits not present in the postal workers who sorted the mail, and bus drivers in England did not get the benefits found for conductors who climbed the stairs in double-deck busses many times during the day. More recently, a study in Finland showed that people who do gardening are much less likely to have health problems than sedentary people, and people who hunt and hike in the forest have even more dramatic reductions in health conditions. Studies of walkers show that brisk walking also produces dramatically less risk health problems and early death. These are

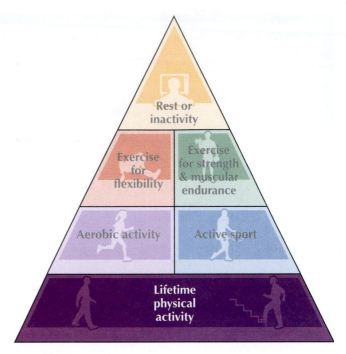

Figure 1
The physical activity pyramid: Level 1.

only a few of the studies now available to show the benefits of lifestyle physical activity.

Because lifestyle activities are moderate, most people can easily perform them. This is one reason lifestyle physical activities are placed at the bottom of the pyramid (see Figure 1). They are basic and provide a foundation for other activities.

> **Moderate activity is more attractive than vigorous activity to many people.**

As the intensity of physical activity increases, it becomes less enjoyable to many people. Studies show that vigorous physical activity is a deterrent for more than a few people. This is another reason why lifestyle physical activities are placed at the base of the physical activity pyramid. Not only does this type of activity provide many health benefits, its intensity level makes it especially attractive to the people who most need to be active.

About one-quarter of all adult Americans do no physical activity at all. They are totally sedentary. Statistics indicate that hundreds of thousands of premature deaths could be prevented if sedentary people would become active. Moderate physical activity is an alternative to vigorous activity that may be especially attractive to sedentary and/or less-fit adults.

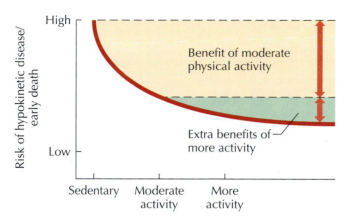

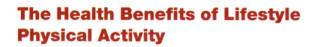

Figure 2
The benefits of moderate lifestyle physical activity.

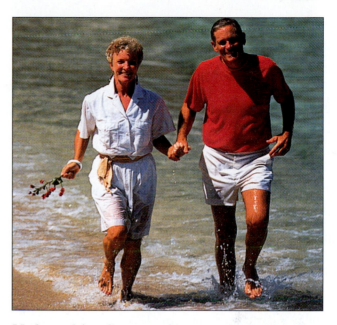

Moderate lifestyle activity has many health benefits.

The Health Benefits of Lifestyle Physical Activity

Many health benefits can be achieved as a result of participation in lifestyle physical activities.

Figure 2 illustrates the fact that disease risk and early death are greatly reduced by moderate lifestyle physical activity. This figure, based on several large studies done worldwide, shows that a great proportion of the **health benefits** of physical activity described in this book result from participation in moderate lifestyle physical activities. Though additional benefits occur with more vigorous activity, they do not produce the proportional gain resulting from moderate activity.

The benefits of moderate or lifestyle physical activities are illustrated by the long arrow in Figure 2. The shorter arrow shows the additional benefits that result from more vigorous activity. The principle of diminishing returns applies. Even modest increases in physical activity are better than doing no activity at all. Clearly, the adage that "something is better than nothing" applies to physical activity.

Lifestyle physical activity promotes metabolic fitness.

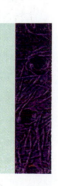 **www.mhhe.com/hper/physed/clw/student/**
Metabolic fitness has been previously defined as fitness of the systems that provide the energy for effective daily living. Indicators of good metabolic fitness include normal blood lipid levels, normal blood pres-

sure, normal blood sugar levels, and healthy body fat levels. While lifestyle physical activity does not promote high-level cardiovascular fitness, commonly referred to as a **performance benefit,** it is effective in promoting metabolic fitness associated with health and wellness benefits. This type of activity can produce enough cardiovascular fitness to help unfit people escape from the low-fit category.

Lifestyle physical activity has wellness benefits.

Reduction in disease risk and early death are important. But equally important is quality of life. Many of the wellness benefits previously described result from moderate lifestyle physical activity. For example, people who do very moderate exercise have been shown to take less time to go to sleep and sleep nearly an hour longer. A very recent study shows that functional limitations are much lower in moderately active people than those who are sedentary. Lifestyle activity and its accompanying metabolic fitness benefits are also associated with enhanced self-esteem and less incidence of depression and anxiety.

Health Benefits Health benefits refer to reduction in hypokinetic disease risk, decreased risk of early death, and improved quality of life.

Performance Benefits Performance benefits refer to improved ability to score well on physical fitness tests or to perform well in athletic or work activities requiring high-level performance.

How Much Lifestyle Physical Activity Is Enough? The Facts

The Surgeon General and the American College of Sports Medicine have outlined a basic recommendation for lifestyle physical activity.

The recommendation for lifestyle physical activity is that adults accumulate 30 minutes or more of moderate-intensity physical activity on most, preferably all, days of the week. Brisk walking is an example of activity that typifies moderate activity. Table 2 provides some other examples of activities that meet the activity recommendation.

Near-daily activity is recommended because each activity session actually has short-term benefits that do not occur if activity is not relatively frequent. This is sometimes referred to as the **last bout effect.** Activity is beneficial only if you do the next bout before the effect of the last bout wears off.

Calories can be counted to determine if a person is doing enough to receive the health benefits of physical activity.

The threshold of training (minimum amount of activity) for producing many of the health benefits can be determined using a weekly calorie count. As few as 500 to 1,000 calories expended in physical activity per week can reduce death rate, but most experts suggest that to insure a health benefit from exercise, a person should expend no less than 1.35 calories per pound of body weight each day. This amounts to 1,000 to 2,000 calories per week for most people if activity is done daily.

As illustrated in Figure 3, additional benefits occur with the expenditure of calories in excess of 2,000. People who expend 2,000 to 3,500 calories from physical activity can reduce risk of early death by 10 to 20 percent in addition to the reduction provided by 2,000 calories per week.

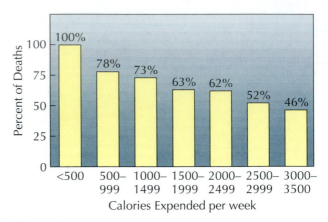

Figure 3

Deaths decrease as caloric expenditure increases.

While it is possible to expend more than 2,000 calories in moderate activity each week, most people with this level of caloric expenditure are performing some sort of more vigorous physical activity. It is for this reason that the 2,000-calorie ceiling is used for the target zone for lifestyle physical activity. Expending more than 2,000 calories is encouraged for those who choose to be that active. However, as pointed out earlier, doing something is better than nothing. Beginners should start with the threshold level of 150 calories expended per day and gradually increase. If doing more activity becomes a deterrent to adherence, additional activity may be more harmful than helpful.

You can "accumulate" lifestyle physical activity to meet the recommendation.

Previous recommendations suggested that physical activity had to be continuous to be effective. The evidence now indicates that all of the activity need not be done in one session to be effective. To achieve the health benefits you can "accumulate activity" throughout the day. While the bulk of the energy or calories expended should be in moderate activities, some light-calorie expenditure can also be beneficial.

Table 2   Examples of Lifestyle Physical Activities

Activity	Length of time	
Washing and waxing a car	45–60 minutes	Less vigorous, more time
Washing windows or floors	45–60 minutes	
Gardening	30–45 minutes	
Wheeling self in wheelchair	30–40 minutes	
Social dancing	30 minutes	
Pushing a stroller (1 1/2 miles)	30 minutes	
Raking leaves	30 minutes	
Walking (2 miles)	30 minutes	More vigorous, less time

Adapted from the *Surgeon General's Report on Physical Activity and Health.*

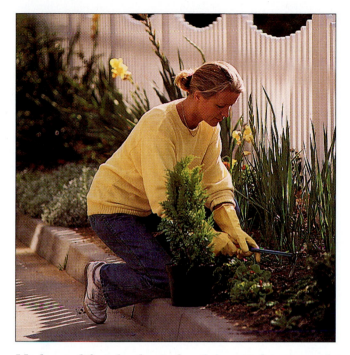 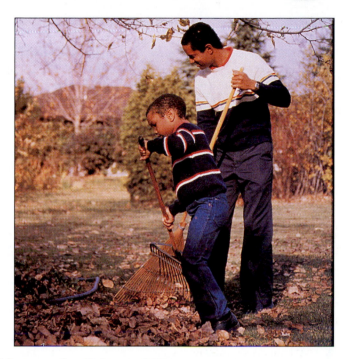

Moderate lifestyle physical activity can be accumulated in several activity sessions.

When some of the accumulated activity is in light activity, the duration of the activity must be increased (e.g., washing windows and floors as seen in Table 2). Some lifestyle physical activities, such as shoveling snow and climbing the stairs, are actually considered to be vigorous in nature. These activities can be counted in the accumulation of daily activities. Performing some of these activities can offset the performance of light activity and make it possible to expend adequate calories in a 30-minute period.

If the goal is to build cardiovascular fitness activity, sessions need to be at least moderate in nature, and activity sessions should probably be at least 10 minutes in length. You will learn more about this in the concept on cardiovascular fitness.

There is a FIT formula for lifestyle physical activity.

Table 3 summarizes the FIT formula for lifestyle physical activity. Both threshold of training (minimum amounts to get a benefit) and target zones (optimal activity levels) are presented.

Last Bout Effect Some of the benefits of physical activity are short-term in nature. If the benefit of a bout of exercise lasts 24 hours, it is beneficial only if the last bout of activity was done before 24 hours elapsed.

Table 3 The FIT Formula for Lifestyle Physical Activity

	Threshold of Training	Target Zone
Frequency	Most days of the week	All, or most, days of the week
Intensity	• Equal to normal walking	• Normal to brisk walking
	• Approximately 150 calories accumulated	• 150 to 300 calories accumulated
	• 500 to 1,000 calories expended per week	• 500 to 2,000* calories expended per week
Time (duration)	30 minutes or three 10 minute sessions.	Approximately 30 to 60 minutes (length of time depends on activity intensity)

*Additional health benefits can result from additional calorie expenditure, but typically expenditure of greater than 2,000 calories per week indicates activity in excess of moderate activity.

Table 4 Calories Expended in Lifestyle Physical Activities.

Activity Classification / Description	METs	Calories used per hour for different body weights				
		100 lb. (45 kg)	120 lb. (55 kg)	150 lb. (70 kg)	180 lb. (82 kg)	200 lb. (91 kg)
Gardening Activities						
Gardening (general)	5.0	227	273	341	409	455
Mowing lawn (hand mower)	6.0	273	327	409	491	545
Mowing lawn (power mower)	4.5	205	245	307	368	409
Raking leaves	4.0	182	218	273	327	364
Shoveling snow	6.0	273	327	409	491	545
Home Activities						
Child care	3.5	159	191	239	286	318
Cleaning, washing dishes	2.5	114	136	170	205	227
Cooking / food preparation	2.5	114	136	170	205	227
Home/auto repair	3.0	136	164	205	245	273
Painting	4.5	205	245	307	368	409
Strolling with child	2.5	114	136	170	205	227
Sweeping / vacuuming)	2.5	114	136	170	205	227
Washing / waxing car	4.5	205	245	307	368	409
Leisure Activities						
Bocci ball / croquet	2.5	114	136	170	205	227
Bowling	3.0	136	164	205	245	273
Canoeing	5.0	227	273	341	409	455
Cross-country skiing (leisure)	7.0	318	382	477	573	636
Cycling (<10 mph)	4.0	182	218	273	327	364
Cycling (12-14 mph)	8.0	364	436	545	655	727
Dancing (social)	4.5	205	245	307	368	409
Fishing	4.0	182	218	273	327	364
Golf (riding)	3.5	159	191	239	286	318
Golf (walking)	5.5	250	300	375	450	500
Horseback riding	4.0	182	218	273	327	364
Swimming (leisure)	6.0	273	327	409	491	545
Table tennis	4.0	182	218	273	327	364
Walking (4 mph)	4.0	182	218	273	327	364
Walking (3 mph)	3.5	159	191	239	286	318
Occupational Activities						
Bricklaying / masonry	7.0	318	382	477	573	636
Carpentry	3.5	159	191	239	286	318
Construction	5.5	250	300	375	450	500
Electrical work / plumbing	3.5	159	191	239	286	318
Digging	7.0	318	382	477	573	636
Farming	5.5	250	300	375	450	500
Store clerk	3.5	159	191	239	286	318
Waiter / waitress	4.0	182	218	273	327	364

Note: MET values and caloric estimates are based on values listed in the Compendium of Physical Activities (see Suggested Readings).

Table 5 Walking Time for Expending 1,000 Calories per Week

Days per Week	Pace	Minutes per Day		
		100 lb.* (45 kg)	150 lb.* (68 kg)	200 lb.* (90 kg)
5	2 mph (3.2 kph)	96	62	46
	3 mph (4.8 kph)	44	48	38
	4 mph (6.4 kph)	48	36	24
6	2 mph	80	52	40
	3 mph	62	40	32
	4 mph	40	26	20
7	2 mph	68	44	34
	3 mph	54	36	26
	4 mph	34	24	18

*Body weight

A combination of several different activities can be used to accumulate lifestyle physical activity.

www.mhhe.com/hper/physed/clw/student/

A variety of different activities can be performed to expend the calories necessary to meet the guidelines for lifestyle physical activity. You may decide to walk to work, do some gardening after work, and do some social dancing in the evening to accumulate the activity for the day. Table 4 provides a general idea of the number of calories expended in a variety of lifestyle physical activities (including moderate-intensity sports and leisure activities). The table helps you account for your body weight when estimating calories expended in activity. This is necessary because bigger people expend more calories than smaller people doing the same activity.

It is also important to account for the intensity of the activity you perform. For example, walking at different speeds results in less time needed to expend the same number of calories. Table 5 illustrates this point for walking. Just as there are a variety of speeds of walking, each of the activities in Table 4 can be performed at different intensities. This walking example shows you how important body weight and intensity level are to expending 1,000 calories in one week. It is impossible to include all activities and their different intensities. You can use the calories in Table 4 as a basis for making decisions about lifestyle physical activity.

You may need to adjust them up or down based on the speed or intensity of the activities you perform.

Strategies for Action: The Facts

A regular plan of lifestyle physical activity is a good place to start.

Lifestyle physical activity is something that virtually anyone can do. In Lab 7A you can set lifestyle physical activity goals and plan a one-week lifestyle physical activity program. In the plan, you can indicate the lifestyle activities you plan to do on all, or most days, of the week. For some, this plan may be the main component of a lifetime plan. For others, it may be only a beginning that leads to the selection of activities from other levels of the physical activity pyramid. Even the most active people should consider regular lifestyle physical activity because it is a type of activity that can be done throughout life.

Self-monitoring lifestyle physical activity can help you stick with it.

Self-monitoring is a self-management skill that can be valuable in encouraging long-term activity adherence. A self-monitoring chart is provided in Lab 7A to help you keep a log of the lifestyle activities you perform during a one-week time period. This is a short-term record sheet. However, charts such as this can be copied to make a log book to allow long-term activity self-monitoring.

> Because lifestyle physical activity is moderate in nature, a specific warm-up may not be necessary.

Lifestyle activities are very similar to the cardiovascular portion of the warm-up described in the concept on preparing for physical activity. For this reason, it may not be necessary to perform a special warm-up prior to doing activities such as walking. It would be wise to perform the stretching activities after the walk as a cool-down.

 ## Web Review

Web review materials for Concept 7 are available are at *www.mhhe.com/hper/physed/clw/student/*.

American College of Sports Medicine
   www.acsm.org

ACSM's Health and Fitness Journal
   www.wwilkins.com/FIT

Centers for Disease Control and Prevention
   www.cdc.gov

Surgeon General's Report on Physical Activity and Health
   www.cdc.gov/nccdphp/sgr/sgr.htm

The Fitness Partner Connection
   www.primusweb.com/fitnesspartner/

Suggested Readings

Ainsworth, B. E., Haskell, W. L., Leon, A. S., Jacobs, D. R., Montoye, H. J., Sallis, J. F., & Paffenberger, R. S. (1993). "Compendium of Physical Activities: Classification of Energy Costs of Human Activities." *Medicine and Science in Sports and Exercise,* 25, 71–80.

American College of Sports Medicine. "Exercise and Physical Activity for Older Adults." *Medicine and Science in Sports and Exercise,* 30(6)(1998):992.

American College of Sports Medicine. "The Recommended Quantity and Quality of Exercise for Developing and Maintaining Cardiorespiratory and Muscular Fitness, and Flexibility in Healthy Adults." *Medicine and Science in Sports and Exercise,* 30(6)(1998), 975.

Blair, S. N. & Connelly, J. C. "How Much Physical Activity Should We Do? The Case for Moderate Amounts and Intensities of Physical Activity." *Research Quarterly for Exercise and Sport,* 67(2)(1996):193.

Corbin, C. B., and Pangrazi, R. P. "Physical Activity Pyramid Rebuffs Peak Experience." *ACSM's Health and Fitness Journal,* 2(1)(1998):12–17.

Pate, R. R., et al. "Physical Activity and Public Health: A Recommendation from the Centers for Disease Control and Prevention and the American College of Sports Medicine." *Journal of the American Medical Association* 273(5)(1995):402–407.

Public Health Service. *Surgeon General's Report on Physical Activity and Health.* Washington, D.C.: U.S. Government Printing Office, 1996.

Lab 7A: Planning and Logging Your Lifestyle Physical Activity

Name	**Section**	**Date**

Purpose: To establish goals for one week of lifestyle physical activity, to prepare a lifestyle physical activity plan, to self-monitor progress in your one-week plan.

Procedures:
1. On chart 1, check the lifestyle activities you plan to perform during the week. Try to plan for at least 30 minutes each day.
2. Keep a one-week log of your actual participation using chart 2. If possible, keep the log with you during the day. List all lifestyle activities you perform for each day, including ones that you didn't originally plan to do. For each activity, record the number of minutes you were active using combinations of 5- or 10-minute blocks. For example, if you perform 15 minutes, you would select one 10-minute block and one 5-minute block. If you perform an activity for a total of 20 minutes, you could check two 10-minute blocks. If you cannot keep the log with you, fill in the log at the end of the day. If you choose to keep a log for more than one week, make extra copies of the log before you begin.
3. Sum the total number of minutes for each day by tallying the number of activity blocks.
4. Answer the questions in the Results section.

Chart 1 Lifestyle Physical Activity Plan

Write the number of minutes you plan to do each activity each day. You may mix activities each day.	Day 1	Day 2	Day 3	Day 4	Day 5	Day 6	Day 7
Brisk walking							
Yard work							
Active house work							
Gardening							
Social dancing							
Occupational activity							
Wheeling self in wheelchair							
Bicycling							
Walking							
Walking up and down stairs							
Other							
Daily Totals							

Results:
Did you do 30 minutes of activity each day?   Did you do 30 minutes of activity on most days?

Conclusions and Interpretations:
1. Do you feel that you will use lifestyle physical activity as a regular part of your lifetime physical activity plan, either now or in the future? Use several sentences to explain your answer.
2. Did the logging of your activity make you more aware of your daily activity patterns? Explain why or why not.

Directions: Record the number of 5- or 10-minute blocks of lifestyle activity you did each day.

Chart 2 Lifestyle Activity Log

		5-Minute Blocks										10-Minute Blocks						Total Minutes
Day 1	Date:	1	2	3	4	5	6	7	8	9	10	1	2	3	4	5	6	
Activity:																		
Activity:																		
Activity:																		
Activity:																		
Activity:																		
																Daily Total:		
Day 2	Date:	1	2	3	4	5	6	7	8	9	10	1	2	3	4	5	6	
Activity:																		
Activity:																		
Activity:																		
Activity:																		
Activity:																		
																Daily Total:		
Day 3	Date:	1	2	3	4	5	6	7	8	9	10	1	2	3	4	5	6	
Activity:																		
Activity:																		
Activity:																		
Activity:																		
Activity:																		
																Daily Total		
Day 4	Date:	1	2	3	4	5	6	7	8	9	10	1	2	3	4	5	6	
Activity:																		
Activity:																		
Activity:																		
Activity:																		
Activity:																		
																Daily Total:		
Day 5	Date:	1	2	3	4	5	6	7	8	9	10	1	2	3	4	5	6	
Activity:																		
Activity:																		
Activity:																		
Activity:																		
Activity:																		
																Daily Total:		
Day 6	Date:	1	2	3	4	5	6	7	8	9	10	1	2	3	4	5	6	
Activity:																		
Activity:																		
Activity:																		
Activity:																		
Activity:																		
																Daily Total:		
Day 7	Date:	1	2	3	4	5	6	7	8	9	10	1	2	3	4	5	6	
Activity:																		
Activity:																		
Activity:																		
Activity:																		
Activity:																		
																Daily Total:		

Weekly Total

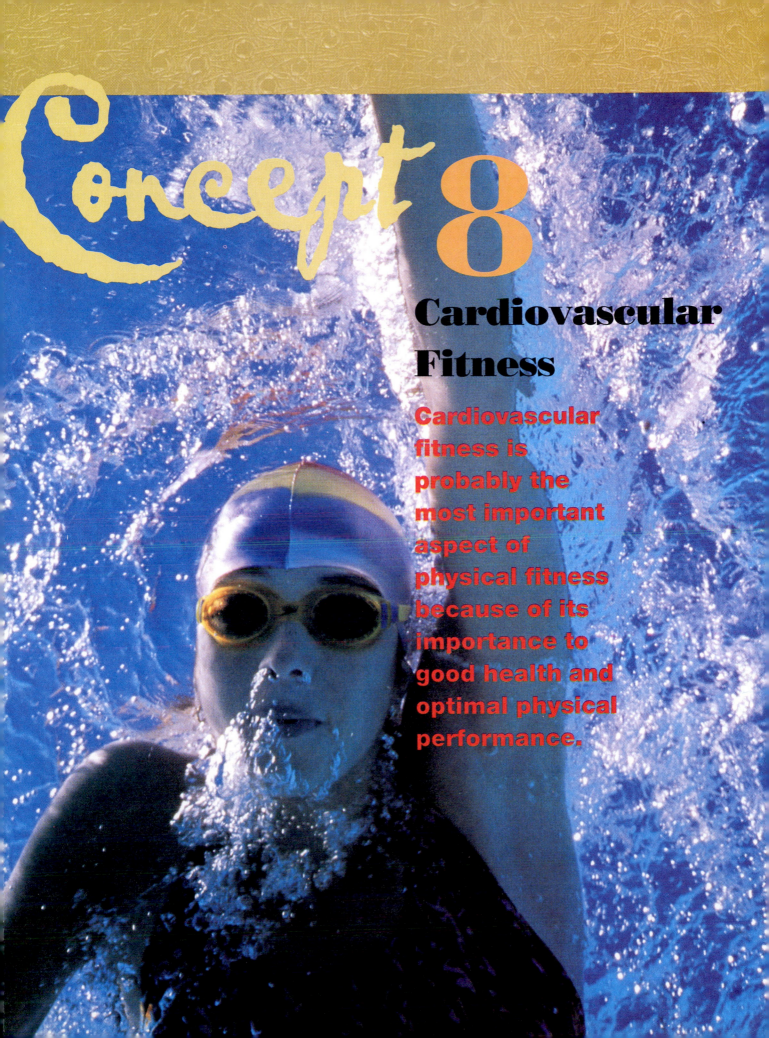

Concept 8

Cardiovascular Fitness

Cardiovascular fitness is probably the most important aspect of physical fitness because of its importance to good health and optimal physical performance.

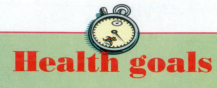

Health goals

for Year 2010

Increase proportion of people who do vigorous physical activity that promotes cardiovascular fitness 3 or more days a week for 20 minutes per occasion.

Decrease deaths from heart attack and stroke.

Decrease incidence of heart attack, high blood pressure, stroke and high blood lipids.

Decrease heart disease among females.

Increase public awareness of symptoms of heart diseases.

Introduction

Cardiovascular fitness is frequently considered the most important aspect of physical fitness because those who possess it have a decreased risk of heart disease—the number-one killer in our society. This is supported by statements of the American Heart Association and the *Surgeon General's Report on Physical Activity and Health,* which indicate sedentary living is a primary risk factor for heart disease. Physical activity that leads to improved cardiovascular fitness has dramatic health and wellness benefits that extend well beyond heart disease risk reduction. Cardiovascular fitness is important to the effective performance of virtually all types of work and play activities.

The Facts about Cardiovascular Fitness

Cardiovascular fitness is a term that has several synonyms.

Cardiovascular fitness is sometimes referred to as "cardiovascular endurance" because a person who possesses this type of fitness can persist in physical activity for long periods of time without undue fatigue. It has been referred to as "cardiorespiratory fitness" because it requires delivery and utilization of oxygen, which is only possible if the circulatory and respiratory systems are capable of these functions.

The term "aerobic fitness" has also been used as a synonym for cardiovascular fitness because aerobic capacity is considered to be the best indicator of cardiovascular fitness, and aerobic physical activity is the preferred method for achieving it. Regardless of the words used to describe it, cardiovascular fitness is complex because it requires fitness of several body systems (see Figure 1).

Good cardiovascular fitness requires a fit heart muscle.

www.mhhe.com/hper/physed/clw/student/

The heart is a muscle; to become stronger, it must be exercised like any other muscle in the body. If the heart is exercised regularly, its strength increases; if not, it becomes weaker. Contrary to the belief that strenuous work harms the heart, research has found no evidence that regular, progressive exercise is bad for the normal heart. In fact, the heart muscle will increase in size and power when called upon to extend itself. The increase in size and power allows the heart to pump a greater volume of blood with fewer strokes per minute. For example, the average individual has a resting heart rate between 70 and 80 beats per minute (bpm), whereas it is not uncommon for a trained athlete's pulse to be in the low 50s or even in the 40s.

The healthy heart is efficient in the work that it does. It can convert about half of its fuel into energy. An automobile engine in good running condition converts only one-fourth of its fuel into energy. By comparison, the heart is a more efficient engine. The heart of a normal individual beats reflexively about 40 million times a year. During this time, over 4,000 gallons, or 10 tons, of blood are circulated each day, and every night the heart's workload is equivalent to a person carrying a 30-pound pack to the top of the 102-story Empire State building.

Good cardiovascular fitness requires a fit vascular system.

As illustrated in Figure 1, blood containing a high concentration of oxygen is pumped by the left ventricle through the aorta (a major artery), where it is carried to the tissues. Blood flows through a sequence of arteries to capillaries and to veins. Veins carry the blood containing lesser amounts of oxygen back to the right side of the heart, first to the atrium and then to the ventricle. The right ventricle pumps the blood to the lungs. In the lungs, the blood picks up oxygen

"Enjoy what we have"

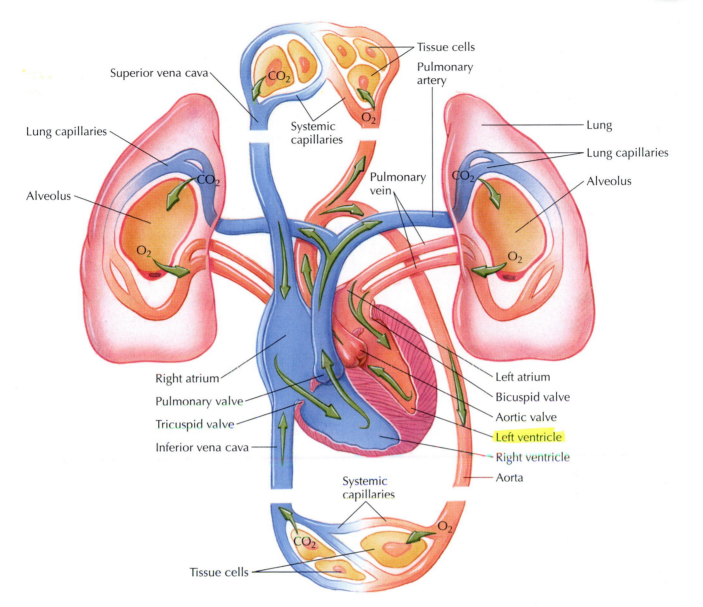

Figure 1
The cardiovascular system.

(O_2), and carbon dioxide (CO_2) is removed. From the lungs, the oxygenated blood travels back to the heart, first to the left atrium and then to the left ventricle. The process then repeats itself.

Healthy arteries are elastic, free of obstruction, and expand to permit the flow of blood (see Figure 2). Muscle layers line the arteries and control the size of the arterial opening upon the impulse from nerve fibers. Unfit arteries (see Figure 3) may have a reduced internal diameter (atherosclerosis) because of deposits on the interior of their walls, or they may have hardened, nonelastic walls (arteriosclerosis).

Fit coronary arteries are especially important to good health. The blood in the four chambers of the heart does not directly nourish the heart. Rather, numerous small arteries within the heart muscle provide for coronary circulation. Poor coronary circulation precipitated by unhealthy arteries can be the cause of a heart attack.

Aerobic Capacity A measure of aerobic or cardiovascular fitness; another term used for maximum oxygen uptake ($\dot{V}O_2$ max).

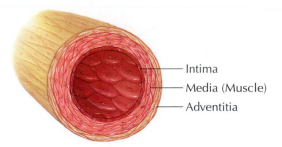

Figure 2
Healthy, elastic artery.

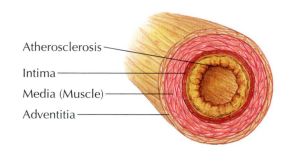

Figure 3
Unhealthy artery.

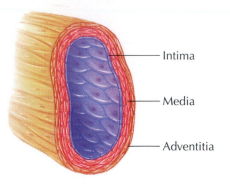

Figure 4
Healthy, nonelastic vein.

Veins have thinner, less-elastic walls than arteries, as shown in Figure 4. Also, veins contain small valves to prevent the backward flow of blood. Skeletal muscles assist the return of blood to the heart. The veins are intertwined in the muscle; therefore, when the muscle is contracted, the vein is squeezed, pushing the blood back to the heart. A malfunction of the valves results in a failure to remove used blood at the proper rate. As a result, venous blood pools, especially in the legs, causing a condition known as varicose veins. Regular physical activity helps reduce pooling of blood in the veins and helps keep the valves of the veins healthy.

Capillaries are the transfer stations where oxygen and fuel are released, and waste products, such as carbon dioxide, are removed from the tissues. The veins receive the blood from the capillaries for the return trip to the heart.

Good cardiovascular fitness requires a fit respiratory system and fit blood.

The process of taking in oxygen (through the mouth and nose) and delivering it to the lungs, where it is picked up by the blood, is called external respiration. External respiration requires fit lungs as well as blood with adequate **hemoglobin** in the red blood cells (erythrocytes). Insufficient oxygen-carrying capacity of the blood is called anemia, a condition caused by lack of hemoglobin.

Delivering oxygen to the tissues from the blood is called internal respiration. Internal respiration requires an adequate number of healthy capillaries. In addition to delivering oxygen to the tissues, these systems remove carbon dioxide. Good cardiovascular fitness requires fitness of both the external and internal respiratory systems.

Cardiovascular fitness requires fit muscle tissue capable of using oxygen.

Once the oxygen is delivered, the muscle tissues must be able to use oxygen to sustain physical performance. Physical activity that promotes cardiovascular fitness stimulates changes in muscle fibers that make them more effective in using oxygen. Outstanding distance runners have high numbers of well-conditioned muscle fibers that can readily use oxygen to produce energy for sustained running. Training in other activities would elicit similar adaptations in the specific muscles used in those activities.

The Facts about Cardiovascular Fitness and Health Benefits

Good cardiovascular fitness reduces risk of heart disease, other hypokinetic conditions, and early death.

The best evidence indicates that cardiovascular fitness is associated with reduced risk for heart disease. A classic research study at The Cooper Institute for Aerobics Research showed that low-fit people are especially at risk. In addition, it has now been demonstrated that improving your fitness (moving from low-fitness to the good-fitness zone) can reduce risk of early death and produce the other health benefits described earlier in this text. Among those who are not low in fitness, further fitness increases bring additional health benefits. However, it is generally acknowledged that the principle of diminished returns applies. Figure 5, illustrates that additional fitness

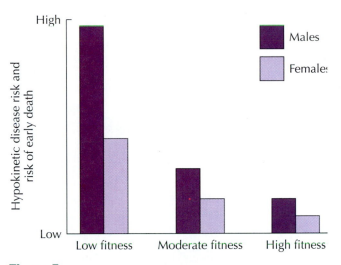

Figure 5

Risk reduction associated with cardiovascular fitness.

Adapted from Blair et al., 1996 (see Suggested Readings).

Table 1	Relative Risk of Major Risk Factors on Heart Disease and Early Death[*]	
Risk Factor	Relative Risk of Heart Disease	Relative Risk of Early Death (All Causes)
Low Cardiovascular Fitness	2.69	2.03
Smoking	2.01	1.89
High Systolic Blood Pressure	2.07	1.67
High Cholesterol	1.86	1.45
Obesity (BMI)	1.70	1.33

[*]Statistically adjusted to assure independence of risk factors.

Based on Blair, S. N. et al. 1996 (see suggested readings)

yields additional benefits but not equal in magnitude to the benefits received from getting out of the low-fitness category.

Low cardiovascular fitness is associated with greater disease risk, and is independent of other risk factors.

Good cardiovascular fitness has been shown to be independent of other risk factors in reducing heart disease risk and of reduction in early death from all causes. Table 1 shows the relative risk of cardiovascular disease in the first column and the relative risk of early death from all causes in the second column. People with virtually no risk factors have a relative risk of 1.0. A person with a relative risk of 2.0 would have two times the risk of a risk-free person. The highest relative risk for heart disease is among people low in cardiovascular fitness (2.69). Those with low cardiovascular fitness also have the highest relative risk of early death (2.03). All of the values in the table were adjusted statistically to exclude the influence of other risk factors. This illustrates that the benefits of good cardiovascular fitness are independent of other primary risk factors for heart disease and early death from all causes.

Good cardiovascular fitness can reduce risk for most people, including those who are overweight.

www.mhhe.com/hper/physed/clw/student/

Some people think that they cannot be fit if they are overweight or overfat. It is now known that appropriate physical activity can build cardio-

vascular fitness in all types of people, including those with excess body fatness. In fact, having good cardiovascular fitness greatly reduces risk for those who are overweight. Poor cardiovascular fitness on the other hand, increases risk for both lean and overfat people. The greatest risk is among people who are both unfit and overfat.

Good cardiovascular fitness enhances the ability to perform various tasks, improves the ability to function, and is associated with a feeling of well-being.

Moving out of the low-fitness zone is of obvious importance to disease risk reduction. Achieving the good zone on tests further reduces disease and early death risk and promotes optimal wellness benefits and a recent position statement by the American College of Sports Medicine also shows an improved ability to function among older adults. Other wellness benefits include the ability to enjoy leisure activities and meet emergency situations, as well as the health and wellness benefits described earlier in this book. Cardiovascular fitness in the high-performance zone enhances the ability to perform in certain athletic events

Hemoglobin Oxygen-carrying pigment of the red blood cells.

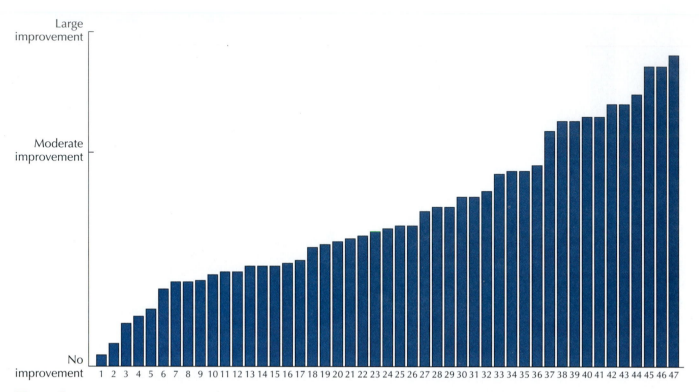

Figure 6

Difference in cardiovascular fitness improvement in 47 different people doing the same activity program for 15 to 20 weeks.

Source: Adapted from Bouchard, 1999 (see Suggested Readings).

and in occupations that require high-level performance (e.g., firefighters). These benefits are commonly referred to as **performance benefits.**

Heredity influences your cardiovascular fitness.

It would be nice if all people who did appropriate physical activity achieved high levels of cardiovascular fitness. Genetic researchers have shown that the type of cardiovascular system you inherit has a good deal to do with your cardiovascular fitness. Further, we do not all respond similarly to physical activity because of our heredity. Figure 6 shows that after 15 to 20 weeks of training, different people who performed the exact same amount of physical activity varied greatly in their cardiovascular fitness improvement. This research led the researchers to draw the following conclusion: "Not only is it important to recognize that there are individual differences in the response to regular physical activity, but research indicates that there are non-responders in the population. Heredity may

account for fitness differences as large as 3 to 10 fold when comparing low and high responders who have performed the same physical activity program" (Bouchard 1999).

As illustrated in Figure 6 one person showed virtually no gain, while one showed dramatic improvements in cardiovascular fitness even though the activity levels were the same. Those with low fitness in the beginning made more improvements than those who were already fit, but the researchers indicated that heredity was more of a factor than beginning fitness level.

You should not conclude from this information that achieving good cardiovascular fitness is impossible for some people. Rather, you should understand that it is harder for some people to get fit than others. No matter who you are, you can improve your cardiovascular fitness, but it takes longer for some than others. This study also points out the futility of comparing your own performance to others. Comparing yourself to fitness standards associated with good health is more reasonable. The research cited above suggests that achieving high-performance levels of cardiovascular fitness will be very difficult for some people.

Threshold and Target Zones for Improving Cardiovascular Fitness

Aerobic physical activity that is more vigorous than lifestyle physical activities is necessary to produce optimal gains in cardiovascular fitness.

Lifestyle physical activity at the base of the pyramid promotes many health benefits and has positive effects on metabolic fitness. Activities at the second level of the physical activity pyramid—including active aerobics and active sports and recreation—are recommended for promoting good cardiovascular fitness (Figure 7). The word *active* implies that these activities must be relatively vigorous in nature.

Cardiovascular fitness can be developed in three to six days per week.

Unlike less-intense lifestyle physical activities, the types of activities that promote cardiovascular fitness may be done as few as three days a week. Additional benefits occur with added days of activity. However, because more vigorous physical activity has been shown to increase risk of orthopedic injury if done too frequently, most experts recommend at least one day a week off.

There are several methods for assessing the intensity of physical activity for building cardiovascular fitness.

www.mhhe.com/hper/physed/clw/student/

The best measure of cardiovascular fitness is **maximum oxygen uptake** ($\dot{V}O_2$ max). This test **WEB** is usually done on a treadmill. Oxygen use is monitored minute by minute as exercise becomes harder and harder. When the exercise becomes very hard, oxygen use reaches its maximum. The highest amount of oxygen used in one minute of maximum intensity physical activity is your maximum oxygen uptake. Your **resting oxygen uptake** subtracted from your maximum oxygen uptake is your **oxygen uptake reserve** ($\dot{V}O_2$R). Calculating a percentage of your $\dot{V}O_2$R is the most accurate way to determine if your exercise is intense enough to promote improvements in cardiovascular fitness.

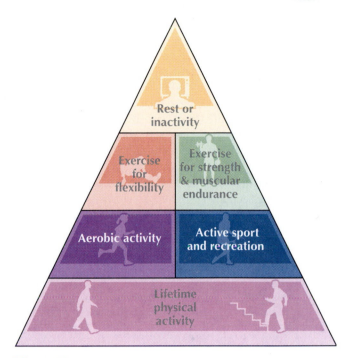

Figure 7
Select activities from level 2 of the pyramid for optimal cardiovascular fitness.

Maximum Oxygen Uptake ($\dot{V}O_2$ max) A laboratory measure held to be the best measure of cardiovascular fitness. Commonly referred to as $\dot{V}O_2$ max or the volume ($\dot{V}$) of oxygen used when a person reaches his or her maximum (max) ability to supply it during exercise.

Resting Oxygen Uptake This is the amount (volume) of oxygen used at rest; also called resting metabolism. One MET is another unit of measure representing resting oxygen uptake.

Oxygen Uptake Reserve ($\dot{V}O_2$R) This is the difference between your maximum oxygen uptake and your resting oxygen uptake. A percentage of this value is often used to determine appropriate intensities for physical activities.

Performance Benefit In this concept, performance benefit refers to an improved score on a cardiovascular fitness test or in performance of activities requiring cardiovascular fitness.

Unfortunately, $\dot{V}O_2R$ is hard to assess in normal day-to-day activities. For this reason, two different heart rate measures have been developed to help you estimate your $\dot{V}O_2R$. The first method is called percentage of **heart rate reserve (HRR),** which is the preferred method because it correlates very well with $\dot{V}O_2R$. A second method is called percentage of maximum heart rate (max HR). Both of these methods will be described in detail later (see Tables 4 and 5).

Ratings of perceived exertion (RPE) have also been shown to be useful in assessing the intensity of aerobic physical activity. This method will also be described in more detail in a later section (see Table 6).

As noted in a previous concept, calorie counting is useful for assessing the intensity of moderate lifestyle physical activities. The American College of Sports Medicine (ACSM) has cautioned against using this technique for determining intensity of aerobic activity for promoting cardiovascular fitness development; instead, they recommend heart rate monitoring and measures of relative perceived exertion.

The duration of physical activity for building cardiovascular fitness is 20 to 60 minutes.

In the past, it was thought that the 20 to 60 minutes of active aerobic activity necessary to promote cardiovascular fitness should be done continuously in one session. Recent ACSM guidelines indicate that activity can be either intermittent or continuous if the total amount of exercise is the same and if the shorter sessions last at least 10 minutes. In other words, three 10-minute exercise sessions appear to give you the same benefit as one 30-minute session if the exercise is at the same intensity level.

There is a FIT formula for building cardiovascular fitness.

Table 2 illustrates the threshold of training and target zones for performing physical activity designed to promote cardiovascular fitness and cardiovascular health.

Your current fitness status and activity patterns should influence the type and amount of activity you do to promote cardiovascular fitness.

Making proper decisions about how much physical activity you should do is an art that is based on science. It is important that you listen to your body and not try to do too much too soon. Part of the art of making good decisions about activity is using the principle of progression. The amount of

Table 2 Threshold of Training and Target Zones for Activities Designed to Promote Cardiovascular Fitness*

	Threshold of Training	Target Zone
Frequency	3 days a week	At least 3 days and no more than 6 days a week
Intensity		
Heart rate reserve (HRR)	40%*	40–85%
Maximum heart rate (max HR)	55%*	55–90%
Relative perceived exertion (RPE)	12*	12–16
Time	20 minutes	20 to 60 minutes

*These values are for beginners—the threshold for fit individuals reaches higher into the target zone.

activity performed by a beginner differs from that performed by a person who is more advanced.

Beginners with low fitness may choose to start with lifestyle physical activity of relatively moderate intensity. Performing this type of activity at about 40 percent of HRR or 12 RPE for several weeks will allow the beginner to adapt gradually. Initial bouts of activity may be less than the recommended 20 minutes, but as fitness increases, at least 20 minutes a day should be accumulated. As fitness improves from the low to marginal range, the frequency, intensity, and time of activity can be increased (see Table 3). Cardiovascular fitness improvements for fit and active people are best when activity is at least 50 percent HRR, 65 percent max HR, and 13 RPE. Your current fitness and activity status will affect how quickly you progress. The type of activity you choose should be appropriate for the intensity of activity at each stage of the progression.

Learning to count heart rate at rest and after activity can help you monitor the intensity of your activity to determine if it is adequate to promote cardiovascular fitness.

To determine the intensity of physical activity for building cardiovascular fitness, it is important to know how to count your pulse. Each time the heart beats, it pumps blood into the arteries. The surge of blood causes a pulse that can be felt by holding a finger against an artery. Major arteries

Table 3 Progression of Activity Frequency, Intensity, and Time Based on Fitness Level

	Low Fitness	Marginal Fitness	Good Fitness
Frequency	3 days a week	3 to 5 days a week	3 to 6 days a week
Intensity			
Heart rate reserve (HRR)	40–50%	50–60%	60–85%
Maximum heart rate (max HR)	55–65%	65–75%	75–90%
Relative perceived exertion (RPE)	12–13	13–14	14–16
Time	10–30	20–40	30–60

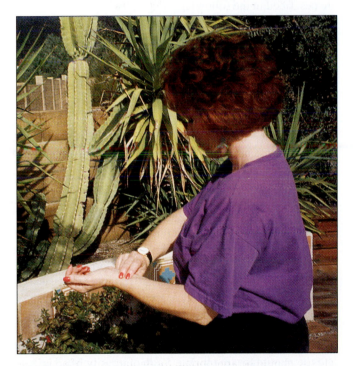

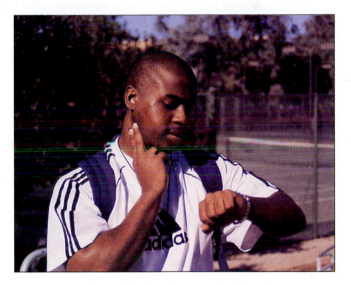

Figure 8

Counting your own pulse: (*A*) wrist (radial) and (*B*) neck (carotid).

that are easy to locate and are frequently used for pulse counts include the carotid on either side of the Adam's Apple, and the radial just below the base of the thumb on the wrist (see Figure 8). In lab 1 you will have the opportunity to practice counting your resting and postexercise heart rates.

To count the pulse rate, simply place the fingertips (index and middle finger) over the artery at one of the previously mentioned locations. Move the fingers around until a strong pulse can be felt. Press gently so as not to cut off the

Heart Rate Reserve (HRR) The difference between your maximum heart rate (highest heart rate in vigorous activity) and your resting heart rate (lowest heart rate at rest).

Ratings of Perceived Exertion (RPE) The assessment of the intensity of exercise based on how the participant feels; a subjective assessment of effort.

blood flow through the artery. Counting the pulse with the thumb is *not* recommended because the thumb has a relatively strong pulse of its own, and it could be confusing when counting another person's pulse.

Counting the pulse at the carotid artery is the most popular procedure, probably because the carotid pulse is easy to locate. Some researchers suggest that caution should be used when taking carotid pulse counts because pressing on this artery can cause a reflex that slows the heart rate. This could result in incorrect heart rate counts. More recent research indicates that carotid palpation, when done properly, can be safely used to count heart rate for most people. Some have suggested that if the carotid pulse is taken on the right side of the neck, it should be taken with the right hand to avoid applying too much pressure to the artery. You may choose to use this procedure, though you can learn to be quite effective with either hand. The key is to press gently no matter which hand you use.

The radial pulse is a bit harder to find than the carotid pulse because of the many tendons near the wrist. Moving the fingers around to several locations on the wrist just above the thumb will help you locate this pulse. For older adults or those with known medical problems, the radial pulse is recommended. Though less popular, the pulse can also be counted at the brachial artery. This is located on the inside of the upper arm just below the armpit.

Once the pulse is located, the heart rate can be determined in beats per minute. At rest, this is done simply by counting the number of beats in one minute. To determine exercise heart rate, it is best to count heart beats or pulses during activity; however, during most activities this is difficult. Machines do exist that can count heartbeats during exercise, but they are not available to most people. The most practical method is to count the pulse immediately after exercise. During physical activity, the heart rate increases but immediately after exercise, it begins to slow and return to normal. In fact, the heart rate has already slowed considerably within one minute after activity ceases. Therefore, it is important to locate the pulse quickly and to count the rate for a short period of time in order to obtain accurate results. For best results, keep moving while quickly locating the pulse, then stop and take a 15-second count. Multiply the number of pulses by 4 to convert heart rate to beats per minute.

You can also count the pulse for 10 seconds and multiply by 6, or count the pulse for six seconds and multiply by 10 to estimate a one-minute heart rate. The latter method allows you to easily calculate heart rates by adding a 0 to the six-second count. However, short duration pulse counts increase the chance of error because a miscount of one beat is multiplied by six or 10 beats rather than by four beats.

The pulse rate should be counted after regular activity, not after a sudden burst. Some runners sprint the last few yards of their daily run and then count their pulse. Such a burst of exercise will elevate the heart rate considerably. This gives a false picture of the actual exercise heart rate. It would be wise for every person to learn to determine resting heart rate accurately and to estimate exercise heart rate by quickly and accurately making pulse counts after activity.

Two different procedures are commonly used to estimate threshold and target zone heart rates. The first involves calculating a percentage of your heart rate reserve, also referred to by some as the working heart rate range or the Karvonen method. The second method, percentage of maximum heart rate, is easier to calculate but is less personalized. The heart rate reserve method is considered by many to be the better of the two because it is more personal in that it uses your true resting heart rate in making the calculations. As noted in Table 2, the percentage of heart rate intensity necessary to get you in the target zone differs depending upon which method of heart rate calculation you use. Both methods of determining threshold and target zone heart rates are described in the following paragraphs.

Percentage of Heart Rate Reserve

To calculate your heart rate reserve, you must know your resting and maximal heart rates.

The resting heart rate is easily determined by counting the pulse for one minute while sitting or lying. Ideally, this should be done early in the morning when you are rested, rather than late in the day when you have been involved in many activities.

Maximum heart rate is harder to determine. It could be measured by an electrocardiogram while exercising to exhaustion; however, for most people, it is safer and better to estimate maximum heart rate by using a formula. This is done by subtracting your age from 220. Maximum heart rates are near 200 in young people but decrease with age. The formula for calculating your maximum heart rate and an example of the calculations for a 22-year-old individual are shown in Table 4.

The heart rate reserve is determined by subtracting the resting heart rate from the maximum heart rate. The heart always works in the range between the resting (the lowest) and the maximum (the highest) rate of your pulse. The formula for calculating the working heart rate and an example for the 22-year-old with a resting heart rate of 68 beats per minute are also shown in Table 4.

The threshold of training, or minimum heart rate, for achieving health benefits, is determined by calculating 40 percent of the working heart rate and then adding it to the resting heart rate. The upper limit of the target zone is 85 percent of the working heart rate added to the resting heart rate. The formula for determining threshold and the upper limit of the target heart rate zone, and examples for a hypothetical exerciser, are shown in Table 4. For best results, begin lower in the target zone and gradually increase exercise intensity (see Table 3).

Table 4 Formula and Example for Calculating Target Heart Rates for Moderate Physical Activity Using Percentage of Heart Rate Reserve*

Formula for Calculating Maximal Heart Rate	Example
220 - Age (in years) = Maximal Heart Rate (beats per minute)	220 - 22 = 198

Formula for Calculating Heart Rate Reserve	Example
Maximal Heart Rate - Resting Heart Rate = Heart Rate Reserve	198 - 68 = 130

Formula for Calculating Threshold of Training Heart Rate	Example
Heart Rate Reserve × 40% + Resting Heart Rate Threshold Heart Rate	130 × .40 = 52 + 68 = 120

Formula for Calculating the Upper Limit Target Heart Rate	Example
Heart Rate Reserve × 85% + Resting Heart Rate Upper Limit Target Zone Heart Rate	130 × .85 =110.5 (111) + 68 = 179

*Example is for a 22-year-old person with a resting heart rate of 68 bpm. The target zone for this twenty-two-year-old is 120–179 bpm.

It is important to note that activities that produce heart rates above 85 percent of heart rate reserve are considered to be **anaerobic activities** for most people. Physical activities of this high intensity may be needed for those in training for competition or for special physical tasks; however, it is not necessary for improving cardiovascular fitness associated with good health and wellness. Threshold and target zone values for anaerobic activities will be discussed in later concepts.

Percentage of Maximum Heart Rate

To use this method, first estimate your maximum heart rate just as you did for the previous method, then determine the threshold heart rate by calculating 55 percent of the maximum heart rate. The upper limit of the target zone is determined by calculating 90 percent of the maximum heart rate. Table 5 gives an example for a hypothetical 22-year-old person. This procedure, using a percentage of maximum heart rate, is deemed an acceptable alternative to the procedure using a percentage of heart rate reserve because it provides

target heart rates similar to those using 40–85 percent of the heart rate reserve (see examples).

The ACSM recently increased the percentage of maximum heart rate values for light-to-moderate activity categories such as the lifestyle physical activity described here. As the examples in Tables 4 and 5 indicate, the threshold and target values for the percentage of heart rate maximum still underestimates by approximately five to 10 beats. The formula is more accurate at higher intensity levels.

You should learn to calculate your threshold and target heart rate values using one of the two methods. (The first method, percentage of heart rate reserve range, is a bit more difficult to calculate.) Regardless of which method you use,

Anaerobic Activity Physical activity performed at high intensity followed by rest periods.

Table 5 Formula and Example for Calculating Target Heart Rates Using the Percentage of Maximum Heart Rate Procedure*

Formula for Calculating Maximal Heart Rate	Example
220 - Age (in years) = Maximum Heart Rate (beats per minute)	220 - 22 = 198

Formula for Threshold Heart Rate	Example
Maximum Heart Rate × 55% Threshold of Training Heart Rate	198 × .55 108.9 (109)

Formula for Upper Limit Heart Rate	Example
Maximum Heart Rate × 90% Upper Limit Target Zone Heart Rate Zone	198 × .90 178.2 (178)

*Example is of a 22-year-old person. The target zone for this person is 109–178 bpm.

you should perform activity with enough intensity to bring your heart rate above threshold and into the target zone to get the health benefits of lifestyle physical activity.

It should be noted that there are several possible sources of error in calculating threshold and target heart rates. First, the method of calculating maximum heart rate is an estimate based on typical values for typical people. Second, errors in counting heart rate are possible. Finally, it is possible that the count you make *after* exercise may not actually reflect your heart rate *during* the activity. For this reason, it is important that you make several estimates of your threshold and target heart rates, especially when you are first starting a cardiovascular fitness program.

The recent development of inexpensive watch-sized heart-rate monitors has provided a reliable method of heart-rate assessment for those who wish to use them. They give you a heart-rate count *during* activity, allowing you to easily and quickly determine your heart rate at any time. Though these computerized monitors are helpful to some, they are not a requirement for accurate assessment of physical activity intensity.

> Ratings of perceived exertion can be used as a method of monitoring the intensity of physical activity designed to promote cardiovascular fitness.

The American College of Sports Medicine suggests that people experienced in physical activity can use ratings of perceived exertion (RPE) to determine if they are exercising

in the target zone (see Table 6). Ratings of perceived exertion have been shown to correlate well with $\dot{V}O_2R$ and HRR. For this reason, RPE can be used to estimate exercise intensity among those who have learned to use the RPE rating categories. This avoids the need to stop and count heart rate during exercise. A rating of 12 (somewhat hard) is equal to threshold, and a rating of 16 (hard) is equal to the upper limit of the target zone. With practice, most people can recognize when they are in the target zone using ratings of perceived exertion.

Strategies for Action: The Facts

> An important step in taking action to develop and maintain cardiovascular fitness is assessing your current status.

www.mhhe.com/hper/physed/clw/student/
For an activity program to be most effective, it should be based on personal needs. Some type of testing is necessary to determine your personal need for cardiovascular fitness. With proper instruction and practice, you can learn to self-assess your cardiovascular fitness.

A person's maximal oxygen uptake ($\dot{V}O_2$ max), commonly referred to as aerobic capacity, is determined in a laboratory by measuring how much oxygen a person can use in maximal exercise. It is a good measure of cardiovascular fitness because you cannot use a great amount of oxygen if

Table 6 Ratings of Perceived Exertion (RPE)

Rating	Description
6	
7	Very, very light
8	
9	Very light
10	
11	Fairly light
12	
13	Somewhat hard
14	
15	Hard
16	
17	Very hard
18	
19	Very, very hard
20	

SOURCE: Data from G. Borg, "Psychological Bases of Perceived Exertion" in *Medicine and Science in Sports and Exercise,* 14:377, 1982, the American College of Sports Medicine.

you do not have good fitness of all systems, including the heart, blood vessels, blood, respiratory system, and muscles. Great endurance athletes can extract 5 or 6 liters of oxygen per minute from the environment during an all-out treadmill run or bicycle ride. An average person extracts only 2 or 3 liters in a one-minute exercise session. $\dot{V}O_2$ max is often adjusted to account for a person's body size because bigger people may have higher scores due to their larger size. Scores are often reported as milliliters (ml) of oxygen per kilogram (kg) of body weight (ml/O_2/kg). This score is calculated by dividing your $\dot{V}O_2$ max value by your weight in kilograms.

www.mhhe.com/hper/physed/clw/student/
$\dot{V}O_2$ max is the gold standard for cardiovascular fitness tests, but it is also impractical for regular use by most people because it must be done in a lab with expensive equipment. It is also a maximum test, so it may not be especially appropriate for those with low levels of fitness. Several tests can be done with a minimum of equipment in or near your home. Commonly used tests are the step test, the 12-minute run, the Astrand-Ryhming bicycle test, and the walking test. With proper instruction, you can learn to measure your own cardiovascular fitness using one of these methods (see lab resource materials). These tests have been shown to estimate $\dot{V}O_2$ max with

reasonable accuracy. Since these tests are not as accurate as laboratory tests of $\dot{V}O_2$ max, using more than one test is recommended to help you get a valid assessment of your cardiovascular fitness.

www.mhhe.com/hper/physed/clw/student/
The self-assessment you choose depends on your current fitness and activity levels, availability of equipment, and other factors. The walking test is probably best for those at beginning levels because more vigorous forms of activity may cause discomfort and may discourage future participation. The step test is somewhat less vigorous than the running test and takes only a few minutes to complete. The bicycle test is also submaximal or relatively moderate in intensity. It is quite accurate but it does require more equipment than the other tests and requires more expertise. You may need help from a fitness expert to do this test properly. The running test is the most vigorous and for this reason may not be best for beginners. On the other hand, more-advanced exercisers with high levels of motivation may prefer this test.

Results on the walking and running tests are greatly influenced by the motivation of the test taker. If the test taker does not try hard, fitness results are underestimated. The bicycle and step tests are influenced less by motivation because one must exercise at a specified workload and at a regular pace. Because heart rate can be influenced by emotional factors, exercise prior to the test, and other factors, tests using heart rate can sometimes give incorrect results. It is important to do your self-assessments when you are relatively free from stress and are rested.

www.mhhe.com/hper/physed/clw/student/
Prior to performing any of these, be sure that you are physically and medically ready. Prepare yourself by doing some regular physical activity for three to six weeks before actually taking the tests. If possible, take more than one test and use the summary of your test results to make a final assessment of your cardiovascular fitness. In Lab 8B you will have the opportunity to self-assess your cardiovascular fitness using one or more tests.

WebReview

Web review materials for Concept 8 are available are at *www.mhhe.com/hper/physed/clw/student/*.
American College of Sports Medicine
www.acsm.org
American Heart Association
www.amhrt.org

Heart Assessment

www.goodhealth.com

National Stroke Association

www.stroke.org

Suggested Readings

American College of Sports Medicine. *ACSM's Guidelines for Exercise Testing and Exercise Prescription,* 5th ed. Baltimore, MD: Williams and Wilkins, 1995.

American College of Sports Medicine. The Recommended Quantity and Quality of Exercise for Developing and Maintaining Cardiorespiratory and Muscular Fitness, and Flexibility in Healthy Adults. *Medicine and Science in Sports and Exercise,* 30(6), 975–991, 1998.

American Heart Association. "A Statement on Exercise: Benefits and Recommendations for Physical Activity Programs for All Americans," *Circulation* 91(1995):580.

Blair, S. N. et al. "Influences of Cardiorespiratory Fitness and other Precursors on Cardiovascular Disease and All-Cause Mortality in Men and Women." *Journal of the American Medical Association.* 276(3) (1996):205.

Bouchard, C. "Heredity and Health-Related Fitness." In Corbin C. B. and Pangrazi, R.P. *Toward a Better Understanding of Physical Fitness and Activity.* Scottsdale, AZ: Holcomb Hathaway 1999.

Fletcher, G., et al. "American Heart Association: Statement on Exercise." *Circulation* 86(1992):2726.

Franklin, B. A. (1998). "A Common Misunderstanding About Heart Rate and Exercise." *ACSM's Health and Fitness,* 2(1),18–19.

Public Health Service. *Surgeon General's Report on Physical Activity and Health.* Washington, D.C.: U.S. Government Printing Office, 1996.

Lab Resource Materials: Evaluating Cardiovascular Fitness

The Walking Test

- Warm-up, then walk 1 mile as fast as you can without straining. Record your time to the nearest second.
- Immediately after the walk, count your heart rate for 15 seconds, then multiply by 4 to get a 1-minute heart rate. Record your heart rate.
- Use your walking time and your post-exercise heart rate to determine your rating using chart 1.

The Step Test

- Warm-up prior to exercise, and after finishing be sure to cool-down.
- Step up and down on a 12-inch bench for 3 minutes at a rate of 24 steps per minute. One step consists of four beats; that is, "up with the left foot, up with the right foot, down with the left foot, down with the right foot."
- Immediately after the exercise, sit down on the bench and relax. Don't talk.
- Locate your pulse or have another person locate it for you.
- Five seconds after the exercise ends, begin counting your pulse. Count the pulse for 60 seconds.
- Your score is your 60-second heart rate. Locate your score and your rating on chart 2.

Chart 1   Walking Ratings for Males and Females

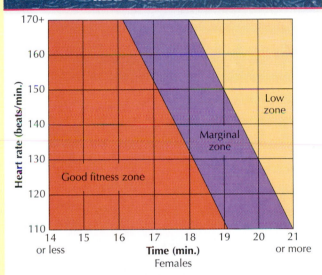

Females

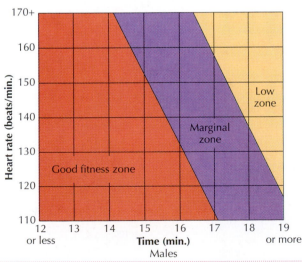

Males

The ratings in chart 1 are for ages 20–29. They provide reasonable ratings for people of all ages.

NOTE: The walking test is not a good indicator of high performace, the running or bicycle tests are recommended.

SOURCE: Test adapted from the *One Mile Walk Test,* with permission of the author, James M. Rippe, M.D.

Chart 2   Step Test Rating Chart

Classification	60-Second Heart Rate
High-performance zone	84 or less
Good fitness zone	85–95
Marginal zone	96–119
Low zone	120 and above

As you grow older, you will want to continue to score well on this rating chart. Because your maximal heart rate decreases as you age, you should be able to score well if you exercise regularly.

SOURCE: Data from F. W. Kasch and J. L. Boyer, *Adult Fitness: Principles and Practices,* 1968, Mayfield Publishing Company, Palo Alto, CA.

The 12-Minute Run Test

- Locate an area where a specific distance is already marked, such as a school track or football field, or measure a specific distance using a bicycle or automobile odometer.
- Use a stopwatch or wristwatch to accurately time a 12-minute period.
- For best results, warm-up prior to the test, then run at a steady pace for the entire 12 minutes (cool-down after the tests).
- Determine the distance you can run in 12 minutes in fractions of a mile. Depending upon your age, locate your score and rating in chart 3.

Chart 3 Twelve-Minute Run Test Rating Chart (Scores in Miles)

	Men (Age)			
Classification	17–26	27–39	40–49	50+
High-performance zone	1.80+	1.60+	1.50+	1.40+
Good fitness zone	1.55–1.79	1.45–1.59	1.40–1.49	1.25–1.39
Marginal zone	1.35–1.54	1.30–1.44	1.25–1.39	1.10–1.24
Low zone	<1.35	<1.30	<1.25	<1.10

	Women (Age)			
Classification	17–26	27–39	40–49	50+
High-performance zone	1.45+	1.35+	1.25+	1.15+
Good fitness zone	1.25–1.44	1.20–1.34	1.15–1.24	1.05–1.14
Marginal zone	1.15–1.24	1.05–1.19	1.00–1.14	.95–1.04
Low zone	<1.15	<1.05	<1.00	<.94

A chart showing the metric equivalents for this chart can be found in Appendix B.

The Astrand-Ryhming Bicycle Test

- Ride a stationary bicycle ergometer for 6 minutes at a rate of 50 pedal cycles per minute (one push with each foot per cycle). Cool-down after the test.
- Set the bicycle at a workload between 300 to 1,200 kpm. For less fit or smaller people, a setting in the range of 300 to 600 is appropriate. Larger or fitter people will need to use a setting of 750 to 1,200. The workload should be enough to elevate the heart rate to at least 125 bpm but no more than 170 bpm during the ride.
- During the sixth minute of the ride (if the heart rate is in the correct range—see previous step), count the heart rate for the entire sixth minute. The carotid or radial pulse may be used.
- Use the nomogram (Chart 4) to determine your predicted oxygen uptake score. Connect the point that represents your heart rate with the point on the right-hand scale that represents the workload you used in riding the bike (use the scale for men and the scale for women). Read your score at the point where a straight line connecting the two points crosses the $\dot{V}O_2$ max line. For example, the sample score the woman represented by the dotted line is 2.55, or nearly 2.6. She had a heart rate of 150 and worked at a load of 600 kpm.
- Determine your score in terms of $\dot{V}O_2$ per kilogram of body weight by dividing your weight in kilograms into the score obtained from the nomogram. To compute your weight in kilograms, divide your weight in pounds by 2.2.
- To determine your cardiovascular fitness rating on the bicycle test, look up your $\dot{V}O_2$ per kilogram of body weight score on the nomogram and your rating in Chart 4.

Chart 4 Nomogram

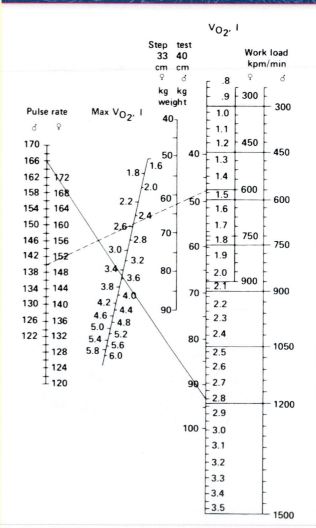

SOURCE: Data from P. O. Astrand and K. Rodahl, *Textbook of Work Physiology*, 1986.

Chart 5   Bicycle Test Rating Scale (ml/O₂/kg)

Women

Age	17–26	27–39	40–49	50–59	60–69
High-performance zone	46+	40+	38+	35+	32+
Good fitness zone	36–45	33–39	30–37	28–34	24–31
Marginal zone	30–35	28–32	24–29	21–27	18–23
Low zone	<30	<28	<24	<21	<18

Men

Age	17–26	27–39	40–49	50–59	60–69
High-performance zone	50+	46+	42+	39+	35+
Good fitness zone	43–49	35–45	32–41	29–38	26–34
Marginal zone	35–42	30–34	27–31	25–28	22–25
Low zone	<35	<30	<27	<25	<22

SOURCE: Data from P. O. Astrand and K. Rodahl, *Textbook of Work Physiology,* 1986.

Chart 6   Threshold of Training and Target Zone Heart Rates

Resting Heart Rate		Age Less than 25	25–29	30–34	35–39	40–44	45–49	50–54	55–59	60–64	Over 65
below 50	Threshold	108	106	104	102	100	98	96	94	92	90
	Target Zone	108–173	106–172	104–167	102–163	100–159	98–155	96–150	94–146	92–142	90–139
50–54	Threshold	111	109	107	105	103	101	99	97	95	93
	Target zone	111–174	109–172	107–168	105–163	103–160	101–155	99–151	97–146	95–143	93–140
55–59	Threshold	114	112	110	108	106	104	102	100	96	96
	Target Zone	114–174	112–173	110–168	108–164	106–160	104–156	102–151	100–147	98–143	96–140
60–64	Threshold	117	115	113	111	109	107	105	103	101	99
	Target Zone	117–175	115–174	113–169	111–165	109–161	107–156	105–152	103–148	101–144	99–141
65–69	Threshold	120	118	116	114	112	110	108	106	104	102
	Target Zone	120–176	118–173	116–170	114–165	112–161	110–157	108–153	106–149	104–144	102–142
70–74	Threshold	123	121	119	117	115	113	111	109	107	105
	Target Zone	123–177	121–173	119–171	117–166	115–162	113–158	111–154	109–150	107–145	105–143
75–79	Threshold	126	124	122	120	118	126	124	112	110	108
	Target Zone	126–177	124–174	122–171	120–167	118–163	116–159	114–154	112–150	110–146	108–143
80–85	Threshold	129	127	125	123	121	129	127	115	113	111
	Target Zone	129–178	127–175	125–172	123–168	121–164	119–159	117–155	115–151	113–147	111–144
86 and over	Threshold	132	130	128	126	124	122	130	118	116	114
	Target Zone	132–179	130–176	128–173	126–169	124–164	122–160	120–156	118–152	116–147	114–145

*Threshold for beginners. Mid target or above recommended after becoming a regular exerciser.

Major Blood Vessels

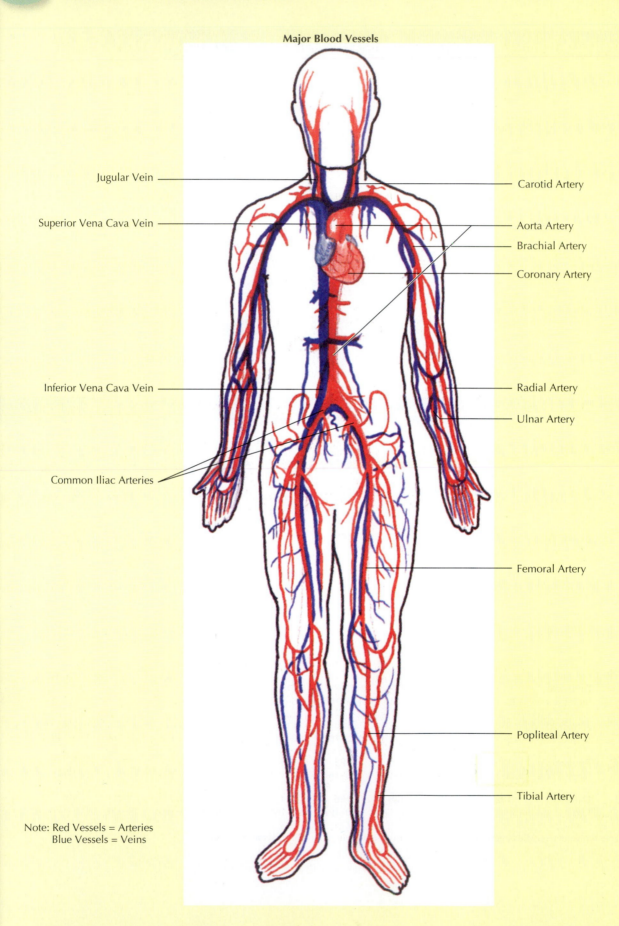

Jugular Vein

Superior Vena Cava Vein

Inferior Vena Cava Vein

Common Iliac Arteries

Carotid Artery

Aorta Artery

Brachial Artery

Coronary Artery

Radial Artery

Ulnar Artery

Femoral Artery

Popliteal Artery

Tibial Artery

Note: Red Vessels = Arteries
Blue Vessels = Veins

Lab 8B: Evaluating Cardiovascular Fitness

Name	**Section**	**Date**

Purpose: To acquaint you with several methods for evaluating cardiovascular fitness and to help you evaluate and rate your own cardiovascular fitness.

Procedure: Perform one or more of the four cardiovascular fitness tests described in the Lab Resource Materials. Determine your ratings on the test(s) using the rating charts provided.

Results: Record the information obtained from taking the cardiovascular fitness test(s) (one or more) in the space provided.

Walking Test

(Time) _____ minutes

Heart rate _____ bpm

Rating _____ (see chart 1, page 119)

The Step Test

Heart rate _____ bpm

Rating _____ (see chart 2, page 119)

Twelve-Minute Run

(Distance) _____ miles

Rating _____ (see chart 3, page 120)

The Bicycle Test

Workload _____ kpm

Heart rate _____ bpm

Weight _____ lbs

Weight in kg* _____

ml/O$_2$/kg _____

Rating _____ (see chart 5, page 121)

*Weight in lbs ÷ 2.2.

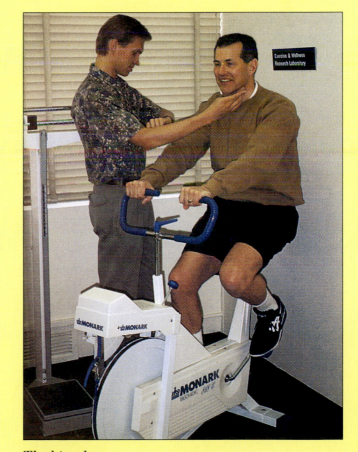

The bicycle test.

Conclusions and Implications:

1. In several sentences, explain why you selected the test or tests you chose. If you only selected one test explain why.

2. In several sentences, explain your results. Discuss your perception of the accuracy of the test results. Also, discuss whether you think you might have gotten different results if you had taken another test, and if so, why.

3. In several sentences, discuss your current level of cardiovascular fitness and steps that you should take in the future to maintain or improve it.

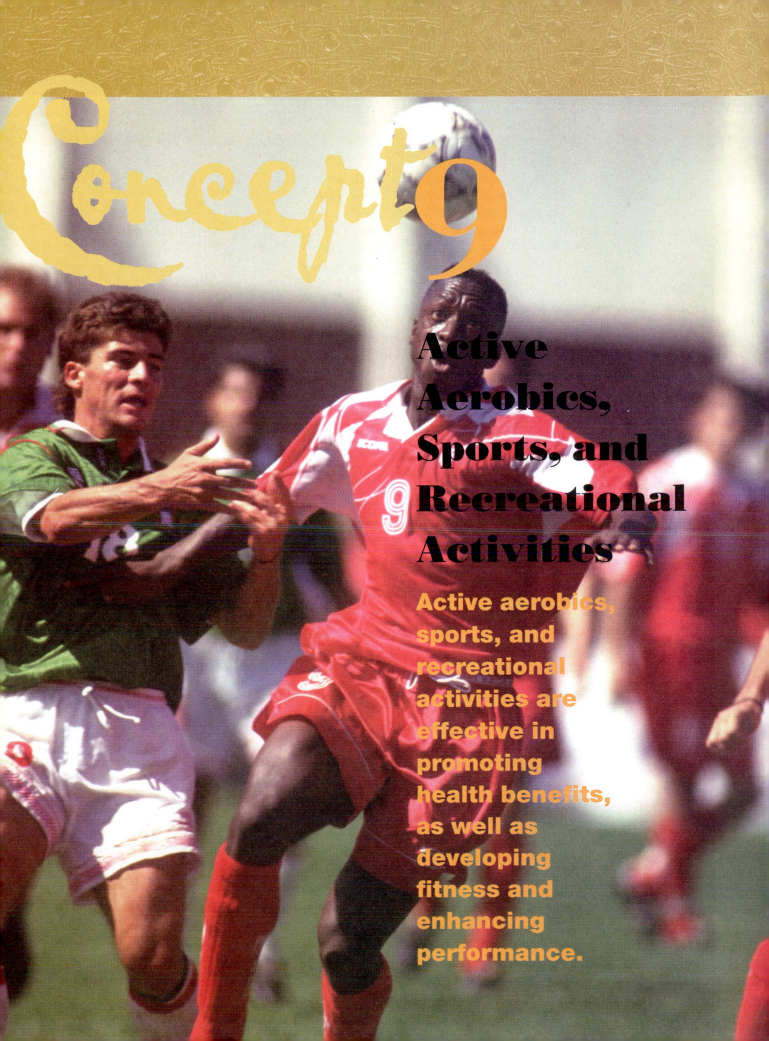

Concept 9

Active Aerobics, Sports, and Recreational Activities

Active aerobics, sports, and recreational activities are effective in promoting health benefits, as well as developing fitness and enhancing performance.

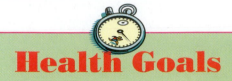

Health Goals

for Year 2010

Increase proportion of people who do vigorous physical activity that promotes cardiovascular fitness 3 or more days a week for 20 minutes per occasion.

Increase the adoption and maintenance of daily physical activity.

Increase incidence of people reporting "active days."

Increase leisure time physical activity.

Decrease incidence of and deaths from heart diseases.

Introduction

The two categories of physical activities at the second level of the physical activity pyramid are active aerobics, and active sports and recreational activities. Some of the more popular activities are described in this concept.

The Facts about the Physical Activity Pyramid: Level 2

Active aerobics are among the most popular physical activities among adults and are included at the second level of the physical activity pyramid.

www.mhhe.com/hper/physed/clw/student/

Active aerobics are placed at the second level of the physical activity pyramid because, next to lifestyle physical activities, they are among the most popular activities among adults (see Figure 1). They are more vigorous than lifestyle physical activities, which are at the base of the pyramid. It is probably because they are more vigorous that active aerobics are not performed as frequently as lifestyle physical activities. According to the *Surgeon General's Report,* the most common active aerobic activities for adults are outdoor and indoor stationary cycling (16 percent for men and 15 percent for women), jogging or running (13 percent for men and 6 percent for

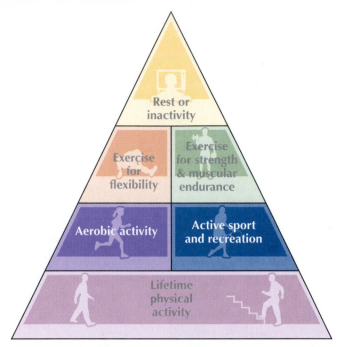

Figure 1
Active aerobics, sports, and recreational activities are included in the second level of the Physical Activity Pyramid.

women), swimming for exercise (7 percent for men and 6 percent for women), and aerobic dance (3 percent for men and 11 percent for women).

It is obvious from the above statistics that gender groups differ in their interest for various active aerobics. Men are much more likely to jog than women, but women are much more likely to do aerobic dance than men. Interest varies considerably with age as well. As people grow older, they decrease in all types of activity, but decreases in active aerobics are more dramatic than in lifestyle physical activities. Twice as many young people cycle as older people. Young men are three times more likely to jog than men 45 years of age, and by 65, men are 10 times less likely to participate than young men. Young women are three times more likely to participate in aerobic dance than those 45 years of age, and young women are five times more likely to participate than those 65 and older.

A list of the 10 most popular physical activities among adults is presented in Table 1.

Active recreational activities done at moderate to vigorous intensity are included in the second level of the physical activity pyramid.

www.mhhe.com/hper/physed/clw/student/

Some experts classify activities such as hiking, boating, fishing, horseback riding, and other outdoor activities as recreational in nature. Recre-

Table 1 Ten Most Popular Physical Activities among Adults

Activity	Rank
Walking	1
Gardening (yard work)	2
Stretching exercises	3
Resistance training	4
Jogging/running	5
Aerobic dance	6
Cycling (outdoor/indoor)	7
Stair climbing	8
Swimming for exercise	9
Tennis	10

Based on the *Surgeon General's Report on Physical Activity and Health*.

Note: Running, cycling, and swimming are considered to be active aerobic activities because most participants do these activities for exercise, not competition. These activities, however, could be considered as sports.

Table 2 Ten Most Popular Sports among Adults[*]

Activity	Participant Rank	Spectator Rank
Tennis	1	4
Bowling	2	9
Golf	3	5
Baseball/softball	4	2
Handball/racquetball	5	Not ranked
Basketball	6	3
Volleyball	7	Not ranked
Soccer	8	Not ranked
Football	9	1
Others	10	Not ranked

Participant rank based on the *Surgeon General's Report on Physical Activity and Health*. Spectator rank is based on the Gallup poll.

ational activities performed at heart rates adequate to build cardiovascular fitness are considered to be **active recreational activities** and are appropriately included at the second level of the physical activity pyramid. Hiking and cross-country skiing are examples. Recreational activities done at less intensity can be considered as lifestyle physical activities.

Though it is not among the activities listed in Table 1, hiking was the sixth most popular physical activity in a recent Gallup poll. Cross-country skiing, on the other hand, is not as common. Only one-half of 1 percent (.5%) of all adults participate in this excellent cardiovascular fitness activity.

Sports done at moderate to vigorous intensity are included in the second level of the physical activity pyramid.

Many **sports** are aerobic in nature—some light to moderate in intensity and some more vigorous in intensity. Sports such as golf, softball, and bowling are aerobic in nature and are light to moderate in intensity. They can be considered as lifestyle physical activities. More vigorous sports such as basketball, handball, and racquetball are typically anaerobic and intermittent in nature. In these activities, short bursts of very hard anaerobic activity are followed by rest periods. When done frequently, intensely enough, and for a long-enough time, these activities can provide benefits similar to active aerobics.

It is for this reason that active sports (those moderate to vigorous in nature) are included at the second level of the pyramid.

www.mhhe.com/hper/physed/clw/student/

 WEB Sports classified as light to moderate in intensity are more popular than more vigorous sports as participation activities. Tennis is moderate in nature for most people but the intensity depends on how it is played. Bowling, golf, and baseball/softball are all light to moderate in nature. The only more-vigorous sport in the top 10 is handball/raquetball. It is interesting that sports performed by youth (football, baseball, and basketball) are ranked in the top three of spectator sports and but not among the top five in actual participation (Table 2). It is also interesting that tennis is the only sport in the 10 most popular participation activities (see Table 1).

Active Aerobics Active aerobic physical activities are those of enough intensity to produce improvements in cardiovascular fitness. They are more intense than lifestyle physical activities that are also aerobic.

Active Recreational Activities Activities done during leisure time that do not meet the characteristics of sports. Many types of active aerobics are recreational activities.

Sports are typically considered to be competitive physical activities that have an organized set of rules and both winners and losers.

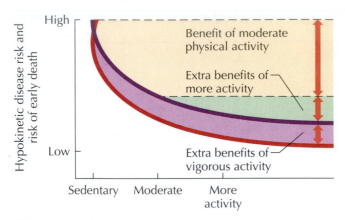

Figure 2

The extra benefits of vigorous physical activities.

Table 3 Risk of Injury in Exercise	
Activity	**Injury per 1,000 Hours of Activity**
Skating	20
Basketball	18
Average competitive sports	16
Running/jogging	16
Racquetball	14
Average aerobic activity	10
Tennis	8
Cycling	6
High-impact dance aerobics	6
Step aerobics	5
Aerobic exercise machines	3
Walking	2
Low-impact dance aerobics	2

Source: Data from the Center for Sports Medicine at St. Francis Hospital, San Francisco, CA.

> **Physical activities at level 2 of the pyramid can produce improvements in cardiovascular fitness and health in addition to those produced by lifestyle physical activities.**

Lifestyle physical activities are a form of light-to-moderate aerobic physical activity that promotes significant health benefits. Active aerobics provide similar health benefits to lifestyle physical activities and are of enough intensity to promote cardiovascular fitness improvement as well. If done on a regular basis, active aerobics actually promote health benefits in addition to those produced by less-intense activity.

The first curve in Figure 2 illustrates the additional benefits that can result if you do active aerobics for the same length of time as less vigorous activity. The more-vigorous activity expends more calories, and this has been shown to produce extra health and fitness benefits. This benefit could occur among those who do less-intense activity if they expended 2,000 to 3,500 calories per week. Studies show, however, that most people who do this much run, cycle, or swim vigorously. One study of runners has shown that running can have significant health benefits over and above those achieved with activity of lesser intensity.

The second curve in Figure 2 is based on a long-term study of a large number of people. It illustrates the fact that vigorous aerobic activity and active sports produce added benefits for *the same amount of energy expenditure*. Clearly, there are health and fitness benefits associated with vigorous physical activity.

> **Activities included in the second level of the activity pyramid can be done less frequently than activities at level 1 of the pyramid.**

The lower the level in the pyramid, the more frequently an activity should performed. Lifestyle physical activities need to be performed all, or most, days of the week. Active aerobics, sports, and recreation can be performed as few as three days a week. They can be done less often because the activities are performed at a more vigorous level. This is important for young people who feel that their time is limited. Performing more vigorous activities provides health and fitness benefits with a relatively small time commitment.

> **Not all activities at level 2 of the pyramid are equally safe.**

Sports medicine experts indicate that certain types of physical activities are more likely to result in injury than others. As shown in Table 3, walking and low-impact dance aerobics are among the least risky activities. Skating, an aerobic activity, is the most risky, followed by basketball and competitive sports. Among the most popular aerobic activities, running has the greatest risk, with cycling, high-impact dance aerobics, and step aerobics having moderate risk of injury. Water activities were not considered in the study on which Table 3 was based. However, swimming and water aerobics are among those least likely to cause muscle and joint injuries because they do not involve impact such as running. There is also less risk of falling or collision as in skating or competitive sports.

The Facts about Active Aerobics

Active aerobics can be done either continuously or intermittently.

We generally think of active aerobics as being continuous in nature. Jogging, swimming, and cycling at a steady pace for long periods are classic examples. Experts have shown that aerobic exercise can be done intermittently as well as continuously. Both **continuous** and **intermittent aerobic activities** can build cardiovascular fitness. For example, recent studies have shown that three 10-minute exercise sessions in the target zone were as effective as one 30-minute exercise session. Still, experts recommend bouts of 20 to 60 minutes in length, with several 10 to 15 minute bouts being an acceptable alternative when longer sessions are not possible.

Aerobic interval training and interval dance exercise are examples of intermittent aerobic exercise. There are advantages and disadvantages of continuous and intermittent exercise, which are presented in Table 4.

There are many popular forms of active aerobics.

www.mhhe.com/hper/physed/clw/student/
Some of the most popular forms of aerobic exercise are discussed briefly here. Active recreational activities such as hiking and cross-country skiing are also discussed in this section.

Aerobic Exercise Machines

There are many kinds of aerobic exercise machines, including stairclimbers, cross-country ski machines, stationary bicycles, and a wide variety of new machines that come on the market periodically. Advantages of such machines are that they can be used in the home. Also they do not require excessive amounts of skill. There is some evidence that use

Table 4	Continuous versus Intermittent Exercise: Advantages and Disadvantages
Continuous	**Intermittent**
• Is done slowly and continuously, rather than in short, vigorous bursts; therefore, many people consider continuous exercise to be less demanding and more enjoyable.	• When done in the target zone, it has the same benefits as continuous exercise. If done intensely, it can increase risk of soreness and injury for beginners.
• Is less intense and because of lower injury risk may be best for beginners, especially for people who are older and who are just starting an exercise program after a long layoff.	• Three 10-minute or two 15-minute exercise sessions might be easier to schedule for busy people than one longer exercise period.
• Provides health benefits associated with cardiovascular fitness.	• May be more interesting to some people.
• May not provide optimal performance benefits for competitors.	• If done at relatively high intensity with alternating rest periods, it can be beneficial in preparing for competition.

of these machines is fun and interesting initially, but that interest decreases with repeated use. Ski machines would seem to be most useful for people who ski on a regular basis, and bicycles would seem to be most interesting to those who do cycling. Aerobic exercise machines can be useful in developing cardiovascular fitness for people who use them to exercise in the target zone for fitness. The key to the effectiveness of the machines is persistent use over long periods of time.

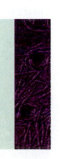

Continuous Aerobic Activity Aerobic activity that is slow enough to be sustained for relatively long periods without frequent rest periods.

Intermittent Aerobic Activity Aerobic activity that is alternated with frequent rest periods; often of relatively high intensity.

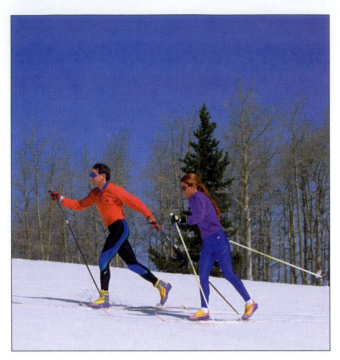

Cross country (Nordic) skiing is an effective type of aerobic exercise.

Recent evidence in a leading scholarly journal suggested that treadmill running was preferable to using other aerobic exercise machines because it was perceived to be less vigorous than other activities. Advertisements on television and in magazines have dramatized these results, and claims have been made that certain machines can expend large numbers of calories in short periods of time. In reality, the type of device you choose should be based on your personal needs and interests. The activity that you personally enjoy is probably the best for you. Machines that actually cause very large calorie expenditures in very short periods of time are exceptionally vigorous and probably do not foster lifetime adherence.

Aerobic Interval Training

Interval training is one of the most common forms of intermittent exercise. Short bursts of energy, commonly referred to as sprints, are alternated with rest periods. Sprints may be in running, swimming, or cycling. For many years, interval training was considered to be exclusively a form of anaerobic training. However, athletes and coaches now feel that aerobic interval training may be very important for competitors in a variety of activities. In aerobic interval training, the pace should be slightly beyond a normal aerobic level, and the rest periods should be fairly short (e.g., 400 meter running followed by rest periods of 10–15 seconds). Even

though this type of activity is aerobic in nature, it is primarily for those interested in competition. For this reason, a more extensive discussion of this type of training is included in the concept on performance.

Bicycling and Spinning

Bicycling, when done in bouts of appropriate length, is a form of aerobic exercise. This activity requires only a bicycle and some safety equipment, such as a helmet and a light and reflectors if done after dark. A tall flag is needed if biking in traffic. To be most effective in building physical fitness, you should pedal continuously, rather than coasting for long periods. Maintaining a steady pace is recommended, though mountain biking often requires hill climbing and faster downhill riding. Periodically, riding a different course can increase enjoyment of the activity. Critical to enjoyable cycling is selecting a bicycle that is of appropriate size. The type of riding you do (touring or off-road) will dictate the type of bicycle you need.

Cycling is more efficient than running and some other aerobic activities because of the mechanical efficiency of the bicycle. Cycling on the level at 5 mph is about three times less intense than running at the same speed. It would take a ride of 13 mph to expend a similar number of calories compared to running at 5 mph. The speed of cycling will give you an indicator of activity intensity, but you should monitor the intensity of the activity using heart rate or perceptions of exertion to determine if it suits your personal needs.

www.mhhe.com/hper/physed/clw/student/

Spinning is a type of stationary cycling that has become popular in some locales. This activity involves alternate bouts of slow cycling followed by faster bouts of low-resistance high-speed pedaling (spinning). Depending on how it is performed, spinning can be either aerobic or anaerobic in nature. It is most likely to be effective for people who like regular cycling. Because it is often relatively high in intensity, it may not be an activity to which large numbers of people are likely to adhere over long periods of time. It may be useful to provide variety for those interested in a change of program.

Circuit Resistance Training (CRT)

Originally, circuit training was a type of physical training involving movement from one exercise station to another. A different type of exercise was performed at each station. In order to complete the circuit, you had to complete all the exercises at all of the stations. The goal was to perform the circuit in progressively shorter periods. Circuit resistance training (CRT) principally promotes muscle fitness development (see level 3 of the pyramid). However, when performed frequently enough and for enough time at the appropriate intensity, CRT can make a significant contribution to cardiovascular fitness. When aerobic exercise, such as riding on stationary bicycles and running on treadmills, is incorporated in the continuous exercise circuit, the contribution of this type of exercise to cardiovascular fitness increases.

If cardiovascular fitness is the goal, the best of programs are ineffective if they cannot be performed properly. Some clubs promote exercise circuits as a method of building both strength and cardiovascular fitness, yet exercise stations are often crowded, and it is next to impossible to perform the circuit without long waiting periods. You may want to add aerobic exercise to your circuit during periods of waiting.

Cooper's Aerobics

www.mhhe.com/hper/physed/clw/student/

Based on the needs of military personnel, Dr. Kenneth Cooper developed a physical activity program that he called "aerobics." In fact, he popularized the term. His program includes a variety of aerobic activities that have point values for the different types of exercise involved. For example, walking a mile in $14^1/_2$ to 20 minutes would earn 1 point, while running a mile in less than 6 minutes and 30 seconds would earn 5 points. Examples of other activities that will earn 1 aerobic point are cycling 2 miles at 10 to 15 mph and swimming 300 yards in 8 to 10 minutes. To develop fitness (especially cardiovascular fitness) using the aerobics point system, it is necessary to earn 30 aerobic points per week. Aerobic points are part of Cooper's system for helping people know when they are exercising frequently enough, intensely enough, and long enough. Though earning 30 points per week is a good way of achieving fitness, we now know that earning less than 30 points can be beneficial to health. For more complete details on the Cooper aerobic points program, the reader is encouraged to read one of Cooper's books (see Suggested Readings).

Continuous Calisthenics

Survey results repeatedly show that calisthenics are among the most frequently performed participant activities. Calisthenics are exercises such as the crunch and push-ups and are designed to build flexibility, strength, or muscular endurance in specific muscle groups. Even though most calisthenics are aerobic, they are usually done intermittently. That is, calisthenic exercises are done a few at a time followed by a rest period. They will do little for cardiovascular fitness or fat control unless they are done continuously.

Continuous calisthenics, or calisthenics that are done without stopping or with walking, jogging, rope jumping, or some other aerobic activity performed during the rest period, can develop virtually all health-related aspects of physical fitness. Fitness pioneer Dr. Thomas Cureton long-advocated

the use of continuous calisthenics, or what he referred to as "continuous rhythmical endurance exercise." An example would be jogging followed by jumping jacks, then walking, then knee push-ups, then jumping rope, then doing crunches. Almost everyone can plan a continuous calisthenic program by selecting exercises for each fitness component that will elevate the heart rate to the optimal level and sustain this intensity an adequate length of time. As is the case with CRT, it is essential that resting between exercises be kept to a minimum. Continuous calisthenics can be done individually, but are also excellent for group use.

Cross-Country Skiing

In Europe, cross-country skiing is one of the most popular aerobic activities. Of course, this sport requires snow and a certain amount of specialized equipment. For those who can cross-country ski on a regular basis, studies show that it is one of the most effective types of cardiovascular fitness exercise. Cross-country skiing uses both the arms and legs, whereas some aerobic activities primarily use the legs. This is one reason for its effectiveness. It is also why this activity is high in caloric expenditure. Cross-country skiing be a fun family activity.

Dance and Step Aerobics

This type of activity was first popularized by Jackie Sorensen in the 1970s as "aerobic dance." Since then, other versions of the activity have been promoted as rhythmic aerobics, Jazzercise, and Dancercize, to note just a few of the popular names. Dance aerobics is a choreographed series of dance steps and exercises done to music. Certified instructors may tailor dance routines to individuals, but many dance routines are preplanned (e.g., dance aerobic videos). Most of the early programs were considered to be high-impact because they included jumping, leaping, and hopping dance steps that resulted in stress on the feet and legs.

In an attempt to reduce the risk of injury or soreness, lower-impact dance aerobics were developed. Now dance aerobic activities are commonly divided into three categories: low-impact aerobics, moderate-impact aerobics, and high-impact aerobics. In low-impact dance aerobics, one foot stays on the floor at all times. Low-impact dance aerobics are an especially wise choice for beginners and older exercisers. Moderate-impact dance aerobics alternates between low- and high-impact steps that allow it to be considerably less stressful than high-impact exercise. It is especially useful for people who want more vigorous activity than low-impact but who do not want the intensity of high-impact aerobics. In high-impact aerobics, both feet leave the ground simultaneously for a good part of the routine. It is recommended only for advanced exercisers. Even for these people high-impact aerobics increases injury risk.

Step aerobics, also known as bench stepping and step training, is an adaptation of dance aerobics. In this activity, the performer steps up and down on a bench when performing various dance steps. In most cases, step aerobics is considered to be low-impact but higher in intensity than many forms of dance aerobics. Step training has been used by professional athletic teams to promote cardiovascular fitness. A major benefit is the ability to change the height of the step to meet the needs of individual participants.

Dance and step aerobics, when planned appropriately for individual participants, can be very effective in building cardiovascular fitness for both men and women. One problem with dance aerobics is that it is often a preplanned exercise program; therefore, it requires all participants to do the same activity regardless of their fitness or activity levels. A vigorous routine can cause unfit people to overextend themselves, whereas an easy routine may not result in fitness gains for those who are already quite fit. Also, some dance aerobic routines have been known to include contraindicated exercises. Good instructors, who are certified by legitimate organizations, know how to adapt dance aerobics to the needs of individuals. Dance and step aerobics do require skill, so instruction from a qualified instructor and practice are necessary for optimal enjoyment.

Fartlek (or Speed Play)

Fartlek is a Swedish word for "speed play." This form of physical activity was developed in Scandinavia where pinewood paths follow curves of lakes and up and down many hills, where the scenery takes your mind off the task at hand. The idea is to get away from the regimen of running or walking on a track and to enjoy the woods, lakes, and mountains. Because of the terrain, the pace is never constant. The uphill path requires a slow pace, while a straight stretch or downhill trail allows for speed. In the speed play, or Fartlek system, you run easily for a time at a steady pace, then sprint for a while, sometimes up or down a hill. Walking typically follows these vigorous bursts. High-intensity Fartlek is typically considered to be an anaerobic type of training. However, when done at a less-vigorous intensity with more modest sprints followed by a walking recovery, the total experience can be considered aerobic. You can plan your own speed play program using your own course, which may include both uphill and downhill running with other variations.

Hiking and Backpacking

Like walking and jogging, hiking is a recreational activity that can promote cardiovascular fitness. Hiking has the advantage of an outdoors setting, often in a very scenic environment. It does require some equipment, such as a rucksack and good hiking shoes, but highly specialized skills are not needed.

Backpacking is a form of hiking that usually covers longer distances and involves an overnight stay, often in the mountains. Backpacking is excellent for building cardiovascular fitness as well as muscular endurance. Like other aerobic activities, it can be helpful in controlling body fatness. In recent years, it has become a popular activity; nearly 11 million American adults report regular involvement in backpacking.

Jogging/Running

A consistently popular form of active aerobics among both adult men and women is jogging or running. Though there is no official distinction between jogging and running, those who run more than a few miles per day, who participate in races, and who are concerned about improving the time in which they run a certain distance often prefer to be called "runners" rather than "joggers." Fifteen to 20 million American adults report that they jog or run on a regular basis.

The major advantage of jogging/running is that it requires only a good pair of running shoes, some inexpensive clothing, and very little skill. With effort, almost anyone can benefit from the activity and even improve performance if that is the goal. There are some techniques that every jogger should be familiar with before starting a jogging program.

- *Foot placement.* The heel of the foot hits the ground first in jogging. Your heel should strike before the rest of your foot (but not hard), then you should rock forward and push off with the ball of your foot. Contrary to some opinions, you should *not* jog on your toes. (A flat-foot landing can be all right as long as you push off with the ball of your foot.) Your toes should point straight ahead. Your feet should stay under your knees and *not* swing out to the sides as you jog.
- *Length of stride.* For efficiency, you should have a relatively comfortable stride length. Your stride should be several inches longer than your walking stride. If necessary, you may have to reach to lengthen your stride. Most older people find it more efficient to run with a shorter stride.
- *Arm movement.* While you jog, you should swing your arms as well as your legs. The arms should be bent and should swing freely and alternately from front to back in the direction you are moving, not from side to side. Keep your arms and hands relaxed.
- *Body position.* While jogging, you should hold your upper body in a relatively erect position with your head and chest up. Don't lean forward, as you would with sprinting or fast running.

Rope Jumping

Rope jumping is aerobic if done at a slow or moderate pace, but is anaerobic if done vigorously. One study shows that typical exercisers jump very briskly, and for this reason cannot maintain the jumping continuously. Even people who are highly trained or who jump at a moderate pace find it difficult to continue this exercise long enough to build cardiovascular fitness because of leg fatigue, high heart rate, or loss of interest in the activity. To be most effective, a continuous routine involving several different jump steps should be used in combination with other forms of exercise. For example, rope jumping could be a part of a circuit resistance training program or a dance aerobics program. Rope jumping is a relatively high-impact activity, and long-term adherence is likely to result in risk of injury similar to other high-impact activities.

Rowing and Canoeing

Rowing and canoeing are recreational activities that can be done at a leisurely pace or at a more vigorous pace. When done continuously for periods of 10 minutes or longer and with an intensity in the target zone, these activities are classified as a type of active recreation that produces similar benefits to active aerobics. When done at a leisurely pace with more floating than paddling or rowing, the activities are more appropriately considered to be similar to lifestyle physical activity.

Skating

Ice skating tends to be regional in its appeal, roller skating is often limited to roller rinks or amusement areas, and roller blading is most frequently done by young people. However, all three are examples of active aerobics that can be useful in promoting cardiovascular fitness when done regularly. In-line (rollerblades) skates, originally developed for training skiers in the off-season, have been improved through recent technology and are now a popular form of aerobic exercise. Because the risk of injury is greater for skating than for many other aerobic activities (see Table 3), special precautions should be taken when doing this activity, including wearing a helmet and knee and elbow pads. Some degree of fitness and skill is necessary to perform skating safely and effectively.

Swimming

Public opinion polls typically rank swimming as the first- or second-most popular form of regular physical activity among adults. Data from the *Surgeon General's Report* show that swimming for exercise ranks ninth among participation activities. The discrepancy is probably because many people swim on an occasional basis but fewer people swim as exercise on a regular basis. When done frequently, intensely enough, and for a long-enough time, swimming is an excellent form of physical activity to promote cardiovascular fitness. When using heart rate to monitor intensity, it is necessary to adjust the target zone heart rate for swimming. Typically, the heart rate does not increase as rapidly in response to swimming as to other activities. Target zone

heart rates are often five to 10 beats less than for other forms of active aerobics.

Walking

Walking is generally considered as a lifestyle physical activity and is very effective in promoting metabolic fitness and health benefits. If cardiovascular fitness is desired, walking must be done intensely enough to elevate the heart rate to target zone levels. As people grow older, walking often provides the intensity necessary for building and maintaining cardiovascular fitness. For younger people, walking would have to be quite brisk to promote cardiovascular fitness.

Water Exercises

Swimming is not the only activity done in the water. Water walking and water exercise are two popular alternatives to swimming. These activities are good for people with arthritis or other musculoskeletal problems and for people relatively high in body fatness. The body's buoyancy in water assists the participant and reduces injury risk. The resistance of the water provides an overload that helps the activity promote health and cardiovascular benefits. Exercises done in shallow water are very low in impact, and deeper-water exercises are considered to be no-impact activities. An advantage of water walking and water exercise is that neither requires the ability to swim. Depending on intensity, they can be classified either as lifestyle activity or active aerobics. Many water exercise programs include activities designed to promote flexibility and muscle fitness development as well as cardiovascular fitness development. Instructors certified by appropriate national organizations, both as water exercise instructors and in water safety, are recommended for optimal benefits and water safety.

The Facts about Active Sports

Some sports are more active than others.

Some sports require more activity than others. Activities that involve muscles from different parts of the body are more active than those that involve fewer muscles. Some are of high intensity and others are less intense. When done vigorously, tennis and basketball involve many different muscle groups and are relatively high in intensity. Soccer is an activity that involves many muscle groups and is high in intensity but does not emphasize the use of the arms. Golf, on the other hand, is less intense, and relies more on skill and technique. The action in basketball, tennis, and soccer involves bursts of activity followed by rest but requires persistent vigorous activity over a relatively long period of time. Golf requires little vigorous activity. Sports that have characteristics similar to those of basketball, tennis, and soccer have similar benefits to active aerobic activities. Of course, any given sport can be more or less active depending on how you perform the activity. Shooting baskets or even playing half-court basketball is not as vigorous as a full-court game.

The most popular sports share characteristics that contribute to their popularity.

The most popular sports (see Table 2) are often considered to be lifetime sports because they can be done at any age. The characteristics that make these sports appropriate for lifelong participation probably contribute significantly to their popularity. Four of the top five are individual sports that do not require a large group of people to perform them. Often the popular sports are adapted so people without exceptional skill can play them. For example, bowling uses a handicap system to allow people with a wide range of abilities to compete. Slow-pitch softball is much more popular than fast pitch or baseball because it allows people of all abilities to play successfully.

Sports are most enjoyable when the challenge is optimal.

One of the primary reasons sports participation is so popular is that sports provide a challenge. For the greatest enjoyment, the challenge of the activity should be balanced by the person's skill in the sport. If you choose to play against a person with lesser skill, you will not be challenged. On the other hand, if you lack skill or your opponent has considerably more skill, the activity will be frustrating. For optimal challenge and enjoyment, the skills of a given sport should be learned before competing. Likewise, choose an opponent who has a similar skill level.

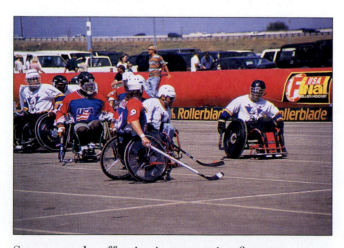

Sports can be effective in promoting fitness and health.

There are benefits to both watching and participating in sports.

Active involvement in sports can have many physical, social, and personal benefits. Though watching sports will not build physical fitness, it does have other benefits. According to recent research, watching sports almost always makes people feel happy when their team wins and gives them a feeling of accomplishment and pride, even though they did not participate. On the downside, when the favorite team loses, feelings of depression and lack of accomplishment may occur. In extreme cases, displays of poor sportsmanship and even violence have occurred. Hooliganism among soccer crowds in world events is an example.

Becoming skillful will help you enjoy sports.

Improving your performance skill can increase the probability that you will perform sports for a lifetime. The following self-management guidelines can help you improve your sport performance.

- *When learning a new activity, concentrate on the general idea of the skill first; worry about details later.* For example, a diver who concentrates on pointing the toes and keeping the legs straight at the end of a flip may land flat on his/her back. To make it all the way over, the diver should concentrate on merely doing the flip. When the general idea is *mastered,* then concentrate on details.
- *The beginner should be careful not to emphasize too many details at one time.* After the general idea of the skill is acquired, the learner can begin to focus on the details, one or two at a time. Concentration on too many details at one time may result in **paralysis by analysis.** For example, a golfer who is told to keep the head down, the left arm straight, and the knees bent cannot possibly concentrate on all of these details at once. As a result, neither the details nor the general idea of the golf swing is performed properly.
- *Once the general idea of a skill is learned, a skill analysis of the performance may be helpful.* Be careful not to overanalyze; it may be helpful to have a knowledgeable person help you locate strengths and weaknesses. Movies and videotapes of performances have been known to be of help to learners.
- *In the early stages of learning a lifetime sport or physical activity, it is not wise to engage in competition.* Beginners who compete are likely to concentrate on beating their opponent rather than on learning a skill properly. For example, in bowling, the beginner may abandon the newly learned hook ball in favor of the sure thing straight ball. This may make the person more

successful immediately, but is not likely to improve the person's bowling skills for the future.

- *To be performed well, sports skills must be overlearned.* Oftentimes, when you learn a new activity, you begin to play the game immediately. The best way to learn a skill is to overlearn it, or practice it until it becomes habit. Frequently, games do not allow you to overlearn skills. For example, during a tennis match is not a good time to learn how to serve because there may be only a few opportunities to do so. For the beginner, it would be much more productive to hit many serves (overlearn) with a friend until the general idea of the serve is well learned. Further, the beginner *should not* sacrifice speed to concentrate on serving for accuracy. Accuracy will come with practice of a properly performed skill.

- *When unlearning an old (incorrect) skill and learning a new (correct) skill, a person's performance may get worse before it gets better.* For example, a golfer with a baseball swing may want to learn the correct golf swing. It is important for the learner to understand that the score may worsen during the relearning stage. As the new skill is overlearned, skill will improve, as will the golf score.

- *Mental practice may aid skill learning.* Mental practice (imagining the performance of a skill) may benefit performance, especially if the performer has had previous experience in the skill. Mental practice can be especially useful in sports when the performer cannot participate regularly because of weather, business, or lack of time.

- *For beginners, practicing in front of other people may be detrimental to learning a skill.* An audience may inhibit the beginner's learning of a new sports skill. This is especially true if the learner feels that his or her performance is being evaluated by someone in the audience.

- *There is no substitute for good instruction.* Getting good instruction, especially at the beginning level, will help you learn skill faster and better. Instruction will help you apply these rules and to use practice more effectively.

Strategies for Action: The Facts

There are steps you can take to become successful in physical activity.

There are three self-management strategies that can be used to help you enjoy sports, active aerobics, and active recreational activities. First, you can make efforts to improve your performance skills by taking lessons and doing regular practice (see guidelines on previous page). Second, you can participate in activities such as swimming, bicycling, jog-

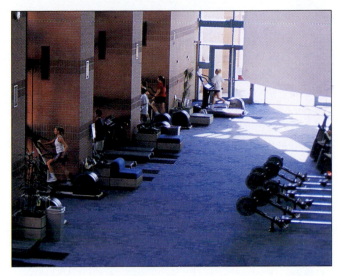

Choose a self-promoting form of physical activity.

ging, or dance exercise. These activities require fewer skills than active sports, and because they can be done individually, you are less likely to make unfavorable comparisons to others. Finally, you can make efforts to change your way of thinking about participation. You can learn *not* to criticize yourself for not being the best at an activity. Accepting yourself for who you are will reduce the self-criticism and make the activity more self-promoting.

Self-promoting activities are especially good for people with special needs.

Because **self-promoting activities** allow you to set your own standards of success and can be done individually or in small groups, they are especially suited to people with special needs. Wheelchair distance events, jogging, weight training, and aquatics are a few examples of these activities. In Lab 9A you have the opportunity to learn more about one type of self-promoting activity—jogging/running.

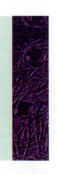

Paralysis by Analysis An overanalysis of skill behavior. This occurs when more information is supplied than a performer can use or when concentration on too many details results in interference with performance.

Self-Promoting Activities Activities that do not require a high level of skill to be successful.

A regular plan for performing active aerobics, sports, or recreation will help you to adhere for a lifetime.

All people are not equally good at all activities, but because there are so many activities from which to choose virtually all people can find something in which they can succeed. In Lab 9A you can set goals and develop a one-week plan for activities in level 2 of the pyramid. In the plan, you can indicate the activities you plan to do and when you plan to do them. You may do these activities instead of lifestyle physical activities or in addition to them.

Self-monitoring your activity can help you stick with it.

Self-monitoring is a self-management skill that can be valuable in encouraging long-term activity adherence. A self-monitoring chart is provided in Lab 9B to help you keep a log of the activities you perform during a one-week period. This is a short-term record sheet. However, charts such as this can be copied to make a log book to allow long-term self-monitoring.

Web Review

Web review materials for Concept 9 are available are at *www.mhhe.com/hper/physed/clw/student/*.

American Council on Exercise

www.acefitness.org

American Association for Active Lifestyles and FItness

www.aahperd/aaalf/aaalf-main.html

National Association for Sports and Physical Education

www.aahperd.org/naspe/naspe-main.html

President's Council on Physical Fitness and Sports

http://www.whitehouse.gov/WH/PCPFS/html/fitnet.html

Running and Fitness Association

www.arfa.org

Disable Sports USA

www.dsusa.org

Special Olympics International

www.specialolympics.org

Women's Sports Foundation

www.lifetimetv.com/wosport/index/html

Suggested Readings

Allsen, P. E., and Witbeck, P. *Racquetball,* 6th ed. Dubuque, IA: Brown & Benchmark Publishers, 1996.

Brown, R., and Henderson, J. *Fitness Running.* Champaign, IL: Human Kinetics Publishers, 1994.

Carmichael, C., and Burke, E. *Fitness Cycling.* Champaign, IL: Human Kinetics Publishers, 1994.

Cooper, K. H. *The Aerobics Program for Total Well-Being.* New York: M. Evans & Co., 1982.

Corbin, C. B. & Pangrazi, R. P. "Physical Activity Pyramid Rebuffs Peak Exercise." *ACSM's Health and Fitness Journal,* 2(1)(1998):12.

Gallup, G., and Newport, F. "Football Remains America's Number One Spectator Sport," *Gallup Poll Monthly,* 325(1992):36.

Johnson, E. "Aquatic exercise for better living on land." *ACSM's Health and Fitness Journal,* 2(3)(1998),16.

Johnson, J. D., and Xanthos, P. *Tennis,* 7th ed. Dubuque, IA: The McGraw-Hill Companies, Inc., 1997.

Kluka, D., and Dunn, P. *Volleyball,* 3d ed. Dubuque, IA: Brown & Benchmark Publishers, 1996.

Magill, R. A. *Motor Learning: Concepts and Applications.* 5th ed. Dubuque, IA: The McGraw-Hill Companies, Inc., 1998.

Olson, M. S. and Williford, H. N. "Step aerobics fulfills its promise: High on fitness, low on impact." *ACSM's Health and Fitness Journal,* 2(2)(1997):2.

Seaborg, E., and Dudley, E. *Hiking and Backpacking,* Champaign, IL: Human Kinetics Publishers, 1994.

Terbizan, D. J. & Strand, B. "How Much Exercise?" *Fitness Management.* 14(9)(1998):32.

White, M. *Water Exercise.* Champaign, IL: Human Kinetics Publishers, 1995.

Lab 9A: Jogging/Running

Name	**Section**	**Date**

Purpose: To give you an opportunity to experience one type of jogging program that can be used to develop and maintain cardiovascular fitness, and to acquaint you with basic jogging techniques.

Procedure:

1. Work with a partner and evaluate each other on jogging techniques.
   a. Stand 20 yards in front of your partner while he/she jogs toward you; watch his/her arm and leg swing and foot placement.
   b. Jog along 10 yards behind your partner while he/she is jogging and watch for arm and leg swing and foot placement.
   c. Stand 10 yards to one side as your partner jogs past you; watch for body position and foot placement.
   d. Change places with your partner and repeat this procedure.
2. Check the appropriate Correct or Incorrect boxes in chart 1.
3. Using proper jogging technique, jog for 15 minutes at your own individual cardiovascular threshold of training.

Results:

Record your target zone heart rate here ☐ bpm

Record your heart rate after the jog ☐ bpm

Have your partner evaluate your jogging technique and then record your results in chart 1.

Chart 1 Jogging Technique

Body Segment	Check Appropriate Circles Below		Technique
	Correct	Incorrect	
Foot placement	◯	◯	Heel hits ground first
	◯	◯	Rock forward, push off ball of foot
	◯	◯	Toes point straight ahead
	◯	◯	Feet under knees, do not swing side to side
Length of stride	◯	◯	Stride is several inches longer than regular step
Arm movement	◯	◯	Elbows bent at 90 degrees
	◯	◯	Arms swing front to back, not side to side
	◯	◯	Arms and legs move in opposition
	◯	◯	Hands and arms are relaxed
Body position	◯	◯	Upper body nearly erect
	◯	◯	Head and chest are up

Conclusions and Implications:

1. In several sentences, give an overall evaluation of your jogging technique.

2. In several sentences, indicate whether jogging is an appropriate activity for you. Indicate your reasons for your answer.

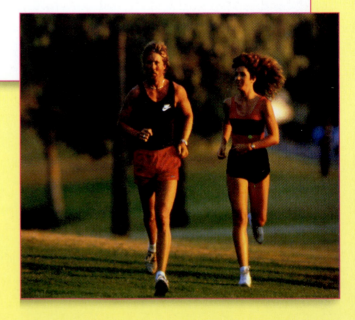

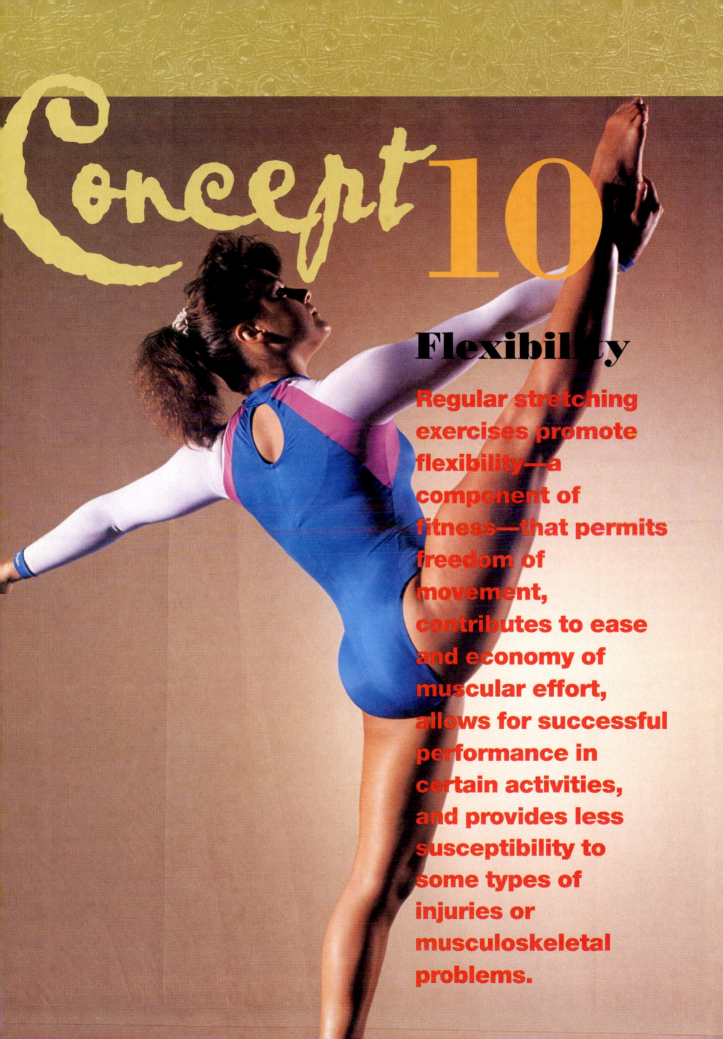

Concept 10

Flexibility

Regular stretching exercises promote flexibility—a component of fitness—that permits freedom of movement, contributes to ease and economy of muscular effort, allows for successful performance in certain activities, and provides less susceptibility to some types of injuries or musculoskeletal problems.

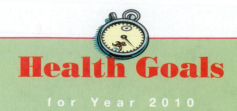

Introduction

Flexibility is a measure of the range of motion available at a joint or group of joints. It is determined by the shape of the bones and cartilage in the joint, and by the length and extensibility of muscles, tendons, ligaments, and fascia that cross the joint. The range of movement at a joint may vary. In some cases, the joint will not bend or straighten, and is said to be tight or stiff, or to have contractures. The deformed hand of an arthritic is an example of this extreme. At the other end of the spectrum is a high degree of flexibility referred to as loose jointedness, hypermobility, or erroneously, as double-jointedness. An example of this extreme is the contortionist seen at the circus. Each person, depending upon his or her individual needs, must have a reasonable amount of flexibility to perform efficiently and effectively in daily life.

Stretching is a type of physical activity done with the intent of improving flexibility. The many types of stretching exercises designed to promote or maintain flexibility are described in this concept.

The Facts about Flexibility

Flexibility is not the same thing as stretching.

Flexibility is a component of health-related physical fitness. It is a state of being. Stretching is the primary technique used to improve the state of one's flexibility.

Long muscle-tendon units are important to flexibility.

Range of motion (ROM) in a joint determines one's flexibility. Having long muscles and tendons allows greater range of joint movement, and for this reason is important to having good flexibility. Together, the muscles and tendon are referred to as a **muscle-tendon unit (MTU).** When you stretch a muscle, you also place stretch on a tendon, and visa versa. Technically, it would be correct to refer to stretching the MTU rather than muscle alone. However, for ease of understanding muscle stretching rather than MTU, stretching will be used.

There is no ideal standard for flexibility.

It is not known how much flexibility any one person should have in a joint. There are norms available that list how hundreds of subjects of various ages, of both sexes, and in many walks of life have performed on different tests. But there is little scientific evidence to indicate that a person who can reach 2 inches past his or her toes on a sit-and-reach test is less fit than a person who can reach 8 inches past the toes. Too much flexibility could be as detrimental as too little. The standards presented in the lab resource materials are based on the best available evidence.

Lack of use, injury, or disease can decrease joint mobility.

Arthritis and calcium deposits can damage a joint, and inflammation can cause pain that prevents movement. Failure to move a joint regularly through its full range of motion can lead to a shortening of muscles and **ligaments.** Static positions held for long periods, such as in poor posture, working postures, and when a body part is immobilized by a cast, lead to shortened tissue and loss of mobility. Improper exercise that overdevelops one muscle group while neglecting the opposing group results in an imbalance that restricts flexibility. For example, body builders who overdevelop their biceps in comparison to the triceps develop a muscle-bound look that is characterized by a restricted range of motion in the elbow joint.

Some people are unusually flexible because of a genetic trait that makes their joints hypermobile.

In some families, the trait for loose joints is passed from generation to generation. This hypermobility is sometimes referred to as joint looseness. Studies show that people with this trait may be more prone to dislocated patellas. There is not much research evidence, but some experts believe that those with hypermobility or **laxity** may also be more susceptible to athletic or dance injuries, especially to the knee and ankle, and may be more apt to develop premature osteoarthritis. One recent study found that subjects

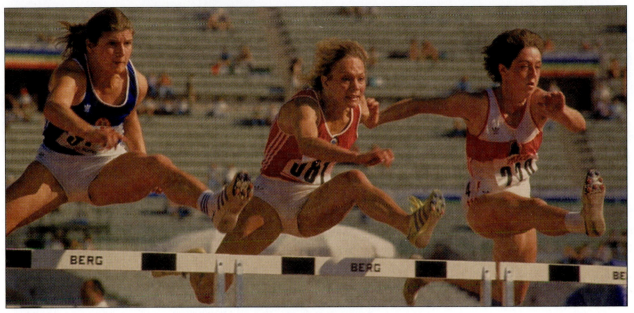

Flexibility aids athletic performance and can help reduce injury risk.

who were loose-jointed used more energy in walking and jogging than those who were medium- or tight-jointed.

In the fifth century, Hippocrates noted the disadvantage of hyperextension of the elbow in archery. The hyperextended position for elbows and knees is not an efficient position from which to move because of a poor angle of muscle pull. For example, it is difficult to perform push-ups when the elbows lock into hyperextension because extra effort is required to unlock the joint. It may be advantageous for loose-jointed people to take extra care to strengthen muscles around the joints most used.

Flexibility is influenced by several factors, including age, sex, and race.

As children grow older, their flexibility increases until adolescence when they become progressively less flexible. As a general rule, girls tend to be more flexible than boys. This is probably due to anatomical differences in the joints, as well as to differences in the type and extent of activities the two sexes tend to choose. In adults, there is less difference between the sexes. Some races and ethnic groups have been reported to have specific joints that are hypermobile. For example, the thumb and finger joints of Middle Eastern people and East Indians tend to be more flexible. Older adults frequently have reduced flexibility, principally because of reduced activity. Studies show that regular stretching can help older people maintain good flexibility throughout life.

It is not necessary to sacrifice flexibility in order to develop strength.

A person with bulging muscles may become muscle-bound or have a restricted range of motion if strength training is done improperly. In any progressive resistance program, both the muscle being strengthened and the

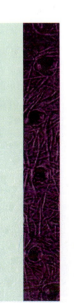

Range of Motion (ROM) The full motion possible in a joint.

Muscle-Tendon Unit (MTU) The skeletal muscles and the tendons that connect them to bones. Stretching to improve flexibility is associated with increased length of the MTU.

Ligaments Bands of tissue that connect bones. Unlike muscles and tendons, overstretching ligaments is not desirable.

Hypermobility Looseness or slackness in the joint and of the muscles and ligaments (soft tissue) surrounding the joint.

Laxity Motion in a joint outside the normal plane for that joint, due to loose ligaments.

antagonist muscles should receive equal training, and all movements should be carried through the full range of motion. Properly conducted strength training does not cause a person to be muscle-bound. A good rule of thumb is: "Stretch what you strengthen and strengthen what you stretch."

The Facts about the Health Benefits of Flexibility

Adequate flexibility may help prevent muscle strain and such orthopedic problems as backache.

Back pain is a leading medical complaint in Western culture. One common cause of backache is shortened lower back muscles and hip flexor muscles. Short hamstrings (muscles in the back of the leg) are also associated with lower back problems. Improving flexibility can decrease risk of back problems.

Adequate flexibility is necessary for achieving and maintaining optimal posture.

When muscles in specific body regions are too short, poor posture can result. Shortness of muscles that can result in back pain is also likely to contribute to a posture problem called swayback. Short shoulder muscles can result in rounded shoulders and forward head.

Adequate flexibility may reduce risk of muscle strain.

Short, tight muscles are more likely to be involuntarily overstretched than are long muscles. Overstretching may result in tearing of muscle fibers, commonly referred to as a muscle strain. Injury to tendons is also more likely if flexibility is limited.

Flexibility is associated with effective daily functioning, including driving ability, among older adults.

Older drivers who perform stretching exercises, to improve their range of motion, are better able to look over their shoulders for blind spots or to parallel park, and back into parking spaces than older drivers with poor flexibility. It is normal for tissue to lose its elasticity with age, but a seden-tary lifestyle is probably the greatest contributor to loss of flexibility with aging. Fortunately, the elderly do respond to training. Spinal mobility is important not only for driving, but also for daily activities such as tying one's shoes and reaching and twisting.

Good flexibility can bring about improved athletic performance.

A hurdler must have good back and hip joint mobility to clear the hurdle. A swimmer requires shoulder and ankle flexibility for powerful strokes. A diver must be able to reach his or her toes in order to assume a pike position. Low back flexibility allows a runner to lengthen the stride. The fencer needs long hamstrings and hip adductors in order to lunge a long distance.

Even weight lifters have been shown to improve their performances by flexibility training. Those who trained were significantly better in the amount of weight they could bench press when it was performed with a rebound (no pause between the lowering and lifting phase) to take advantage of the elastic snap-back force. It has been hypothesized that stretching exercises not only increase the length of the muscle, but can also decrease its stiffness. Power athletes who use ballistic movements, such as baseball pitchers, high jumpers, and shot-putters, may benefit from this type of training.

The Facts about Stretching Methods

To develop flexibility, it is necessary to do exercises from the flexibility exercise section of the physical activity pyramid.

The activities in the first two levels of the physical activity pyramid (see Figure 1) do little to develop flexibility. To build this important part of fitness, stretching exercises from the third level of the pyramid are essential. Three commonly used types of stretching exercises are static stretch, PNF (proprioceptive neuromuscular facilitation) exercise, and ballistic stretch.

Static stretching is widely recommended because most experts believe it is less likely to cause injury.

Static stretching is done slowly and held for a period of several seconds. With this type of stretch, the probability of tearing the

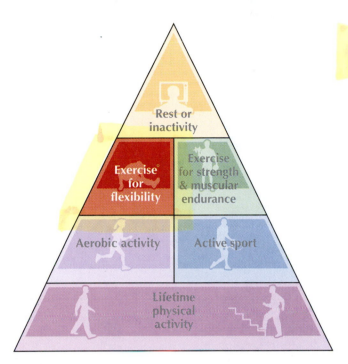

Figure 1
Flexibility or stretching exercises should be selected from level 3 of the Physical Activity Pyramid.

soft tissue is low if performed properly. Static stretch can be performed with **active assistance** or with **passive assistance.**

When active assistance is used, you contract the opposing muscle group to produce a reflex relaxation (**reciprocal inhibition**) in the muscles you are trying to stretch. This enables you to stretch the muscle more easily. For example, when doing a calf stretch exercise (see Figure 2*A*), the muscles on the front of the shin are contracted to assist in the stretch of the muscles of the calf. For this reason, many experts prefer static stretch with active assistance. There is one problem, however, with active assistance to static stretching. It is almost impossible to produce adequate overload by simply contracting the opposing muscles.

When passive assistance (see Figures 2*B, C*) is used, an outside force, such as a partner aids you in stretching. For example, in the calf stretch passive assistance can be provided by another person (Figure 2*B*), another body part (Figure 2*B*), or gravity (Figure 2*C*). This type of stretch does not create the relaxation in the muscle associated with active assisted stretch. A muscle that is not relaxed cannot be stretched as far, and there is potential for injury. Therefore, it is best to combine the active assistance with a passive assistance when performing a static stretch. This gives the advantage of a relaxed muscle and a sufficient force to provide an overload to stretch it.

A good way to begin static stretching exercises is to stretch until you begin to feel tension, back off slightly and hold the position several seconds, then gradually try to stretch a little farther, back off, hold. Decrease the stretch slowly after the hold.

PNF techniques have proven to be most effective at improving flexibility.

www.mhhe.com/hper/physed/clw/student/

PNF has been popular for rehabilitation since the 1960s. It consists of dozens of techniques to stimulate muscles to contract more strongly or to relax more fully so that they can be stretched. Several PNF techniques have become popular in fitness programs to improve the flexibility of healthy people. The contract-relax-antagonist-contract (CRAC) technique is the most popular. CRAC PNF involves three steps: (1) move the limb so the muscle to be stretched is elongated initially, then contract it (**agonist muscle**) isometrically for several seconds (against an immovable object or the resistance of a partner); (2) relax the muscle; and (3) immediately statically stretch the muscle with the active assistance of the antagonist muscle and an assist from a partner, gravity, or other body part.

Antagonist Muscles In this concept, antagonist refers to the muscle group on the opposite side of the limb from the muscle group being stretched (e.g., biceps is antagonist of triceps).

Stiffness Elasticity, or lack of it, in the muscle-tendon unit.

Static Stretch A muscle is slowly stretched and then held in that stretched position for several seconds.

PNF (Proprioceptive Neuromuscular Facilitation) Exercise A type of static stretch most commonly characterized by a precontraction of the muscle to be stretched and a contraction of the antagonist muscle during the stretch.

Ballistic Stretch Muscles are stretched by the force of momentum of a body part that is bounced, swung, or jerked.

Active Assistance Muscles are stretched using an assist from an active contraction of the opposing (antagonist) muscle.

Passive Assistance Stretch imposed on a muscle with the assistance of a force other than the opposing muscle.

Reciprocal Inhibition Reflex relaxation in the muscle being stretched during the contraction of the antagonist.

Agonist Muscles Refers to the muscle group being stretched.

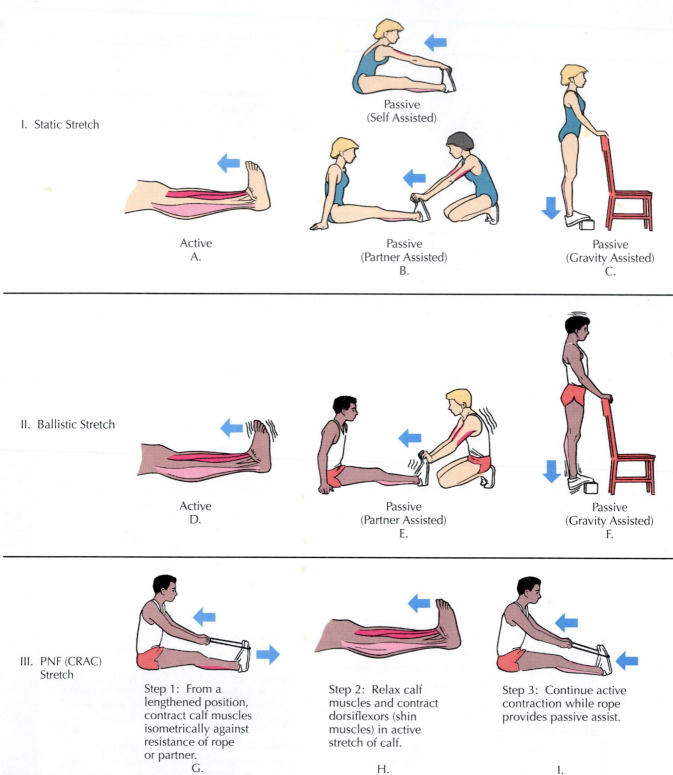

I. Static Stretch

Passive
(Self Assisted)

Active
A.

Passive
(Partner Assisted)
B.

Passive
(Gravity Assisted)
C.

II. Ballistic Stretch

Active
D.

Passive
(Partner Assisted)
E.

Passive
(Gravity Assisted)
F.

III. PNF (CRAC) Stretch

Step 1: From a lengthened position, contract calf muscles isometrically against resistance of rope or partner.
G.

Step 2: Relax calf muscles and contract dorsiflexors (shin muscles) in active stretch of calf.
H.

Step 3: Continue active contraction while rope provides passive assist.
I.

Figure 2

Examples of static, ballistic, PNF, active and passive stretches of the calf muscles (gastrocnemius and soleus). Muscles shown in dark pink are the muscles being contracted. Muscles shown in pink are those being stretched.

Figure 2*G*, *H*, and *I* provide a detailed illustration of how this technique is applied to the calf stretch. Research shows that this and other types of PNF stretch are more effective than a simple static stretch. Additional types of PNF are described in the concept on performance.

Ballistic stretching may be an important technique for active people.

A ballistic stretch uses momentum to produce the stretch. Momentum is produced by vigorous motion, such as flinging a body part (bobbing) or rocking it back and forth to create a bouncing movement. As with static stretching, the ballistic movement can be provided either actively or passively. For example, in the calf stretch shown in Figures 2*D*, *E*, and *F*, the foot is actively bounced forward by the antagonist muscle force or passively by an assist from another person or gravity.

Because ballistic movement often stretches the muscle farther than other methods, there is the potential for injury. Most experts believe that static stretching is the preferred method for beginners, for people with a history of muscle injury, and for people who do not need exceptional levels of flexibility for athletic performances. However, because many athletic activities are ballistic in nature, sport-specific ballistic stretches are appropriate for most athletes. The principle of specificity implies that one should train using the types of movements that are most likely to occur in the activity for which one is training. Since ballistic movement is very much a part of most athletic events (those requiring speed and power), it is appropriate to train using this type of movement. Even among athletes, however, static stretching is recommended prior to ballistic stretching. Passive ballistic stretching is particularly risky and is *not* recommended for use outside of a clinic.

Some opponents argue that the sudden stretch of the ballistic motion elicits a **stretch reflex** (myotatic reflex), which then causes the muscle to contract to prevent injury. Allegedly, this prevents the muscle from being stretched adequately. It is true that a stretch reflex occurs (it also occurs in a static stretch), but except in extreme circumstances the momentum of ballistic stretch occurs just after the bouncing or bobbing, and the stretch reflex is not evident at the time the muscle is actually stretched.

Performing warm-up exercises is not the same as doing a stretching workout for flexibility development.

The warm-up typically includes stretching exercises to prepare you for the workout and to reduce the risk of injury. Modest static stretching exercises done after a general warm-up are recommended by most experts (see concept on preparing for physical activity). Stretching exercises are typically done later in the workout to promote flexibility.

The best time for stretching is when the muscles are warm.

Some studies have shown that increasing the temperature of the muscle through warm-up exercises or applying heat packs has resulted in improved ability to stretch the muscle. Other studies have failed to find a difference between the flexibility of subjects who warmed up and those who did not warm up. Some experts believe that cooling the muscle with ice packs in the final phases of stretching aids in lengthening the muscle, but a recent study has failed to confirm this. Until scientists reach a consensus, it seems wise to perform the stretching phase of your workout when the muscles are warm. This means that stretching can be done in the middle or near the end of the workout. Since some people do not want to interrupt their workout in the middle, they prefer to stretch at the end. Stretching at the end of the workout serves a dual purpose—building flexibility and cooling-down. It is, however, appropriate to stretch at any time in the workout after the muscles have been active and are warm.

Each form of flexibility exercise has its advantages and disadvantages.

The advantages and disadvantages of unassisted ballistic, static, and PNF exercises using active stretch with passive assist are summarized in Table 1. The best method(s) for you may depend upon your physical condition, whether you wish to increase your range of motion or just maintain it, whether you have a partner to assist, and whether you are training for speed or power athletic events.

The Facts about How Much Stretch Is Enough

There is a minimum amount of exercise (threshold of training) and an optimal amount of exercise (target zone) necessary for developing flexibility.

Threshold and target zones for each type of stretching to improve and maintain flexibility are presented in Table 2.

Stretch Reflex Also called the myotatic reflex, the stretch reflex is an automatic reaction of the muscle to excessive stretch to prevent the muscle from becoming overstretched or injured.

Table 1   Comparison of Advantages and Disadvantages of Three Types of Flexibility Exercises

	Static-Active, Assisted	Ballistic-Active	PNF (CRAC), Assisted
Advantages		Rating	
Less danger of overstretch	Good-Excellent	Poor-Fair	Good-Excellent
Relieves muscle cramps or soreness	Excellent	Poor	Good
Strength may be developed	Poor	Poor	Good
Utilizes reflexes to relax the stretched muscle	Good	Fair	Excellent
Specific to most athletics and daily activities such as speed and power skills	Poor	Excellent	Poor
Convenient; less apt to need another person to assist	Fair	Excellent	Poor-Fair
Efficient; requires less time	Fair	Fair	Poor
Effective in lengthening muscles	Good	Good	Excellent

The values in this table illustrate how the principles of overload and progression are best applied to promote and maintain flexibility through regular stretching.

Stretching exercises must be done frequently to improve or maintain flexibility.

It is generally agreed that stretching should be done at least three days a week and preferably daily. After a week without stretching, muscle length decreases, suggesting that stretching one day a week can help maintain muscle length if more frequent stretching is not possible.

To increase the length of a muscle, you must stretch it more than its normal length (overload) but not overstretch it.

There is much that is not known about flexibility, but the best evidence suggests that muscles should be stretched to about 10 percent beyond their normal length to bring about an improvement in flexibility. More practical indicators of the intensity of stretching are to stretch just to the point of tension or just before discomfort. Exercises that do not cause an overload will not increase flexibility. Excessively intense stretching may actually result in decreased flexibility. Once adequate flexibility has been achieved, **range of motion exercises** that do not require stretch greater than normal can be performed to maintain flexibility and joint range of motion.

For flexibility to be increased, muscles must be stretched and held beyond normal length for an adequate amount of time.

www.mhhe.com/hper/physed/clw/student/
Decreased tension in a muscle lasts for about 100 seconds of stretching. However, most of the benefits occurs in the first 15 seconds of the stretch. To get the most benefit for the least effort, most experts now recommend stretching for at least 15 seconds and up to 30 to 60 seconds.

For flexibility to be increased, stretching exercises must be repeated an adequate number of times.

www.mhhe.com/hper/physed/clw/student/
The number of times you perform an exercise before taking a rest is referred to as repetitions, or reps. Most of the benefits of stretching occur in the first repetition of an exercise, though some additional benefits occur when exercises are repeated as many as 10 times. The American College of Sports Medicine recommends three to five repetitions because this number seems to give the most benefits for the amount of time spent in exercise.

Table 2 Flexibility Threshold of Training and Target Zones

	Threshold of Training			Target Zones		
	Static	**Ballistic**	**PNF (CRAC)**	**Static**	**Ballistic**	**PNF (CRAC)**
Frequency	• 3 days per week for all methods			• 3 to 7 days per week for all methods		
Intensity	• Stretch as far as you can go without pain; with slow movement, hold at the end of the range of motion.	• Stretch muscle beyond normal length with gentle bounce or swing, but do not exceed 10 percent of active-static range of motion.	• Same as static except use a maximum isometric contraction of muscle prior to stretch.	• Add assist • Avoid overstretch and pain for all methods.	• Same as threshold	• Same as static • Add assist.
Time	• Hold 15 seconds. • 3 reps. • Rest 30 seconds between reps.	• Continuous reps for 30 seconds (this is 1 set).	• Hold isometric contraction 3 seconds. • Hold stretch 15 seconds. • 3 reps. • Rest 30 seconds between reps.	• Hold 15–60 seconds. • 3–5 reps. • Rest 30 seconds between reps. • Rest 1 minute between sets.	• 1–3 sets. • Rest 1 minute between sets.	• 3–5 reps of 3 second contraction and 15–60 second hold. • Rest 30 seconds between reps. • 1–3 sets. • Rest 1 minute between sets.

Stretching is specific to each muscle or muscle group.

www.mhhe.com/hper/physed/clw/student/

No single exercise can produce total flexibility. For example, stretching tight hamstrings can increase the length of these muscles, but will not lengthen the muscles in other areas of the body. For total flexibility, it is important to stretch each of the major muscle groups of the body and to use the major joints of the body through full range of normal motion.

Overstretching may make a person more susceptible to injury or hamper performance.

Muscles and tendons have the ability to lengthen (extensibility) and to return to their normal length after stretching (elasticity). Ligaments and the joint capsule are extensible but lack elasticity. When stretched, they remain in the lengthened state. If this occurs, the joint may lack stability and is susceptible to chronic dislocation or movement in an undesirable plane. This is particularly true of weight-bearing joints, such as the hip, knee, and ankle. Loose ligaments may allow the joint to twist abnormally, tearing the cartilage and other soft tissue.

There is a correct way to perform flexibility exercises.

Remember that stretching can *cause* muscle soreness, so "easy does it." Start at your threshold if you are unaccustomed to stretching a given muscle group, then increase within the target zone. The list in Table 3 will help you to gain the most benefit from your exercises.

Range of Motion Exercises Exercises used to maintain existing joint mobility (to prevent loss of ROM).

Table 3 Do and Don't List for Stretching

Do	Don't
Do warm muscles before you attempt to stretch them.	Don't stretch to the point of pain. Remember, you want to stretch muscles, not joints!
Do stretch with care if you have osteoporosis or arthritis.	Don't use ballistic stretch if you have osteoporosis or arthritis.
Do use static or PNF stretching rather than ballistic stretching if you are a beginner.	Don't perform ballistic stretches with passive assistance unless you are under the supervision of an expert.
Do stretch weak or recently injured muscles with care.	Don't ballistically stretch weak or recently injured muscles.
Do use great care in applying passive assistance to a partner; go slowly and ask for feedback.	Don't stretch a muscle after it has been immobilized (such as in a sling or cast) for a long period.
Do perform stretching exercises for each muscle group and at each joint where flexibility is desired.	Don't statically bounce a muscle through excessive range of motion. Ballistic stretch should be gentle and should not involve excessive range of motion.
Do make certain the body is in good alignment when stretching.	Don't stretch swollen joints without professional supervision.
Do stretch muscles of small joints in the extremities first, then progress toward the trunk with muscles of larger joints.	Don't stretch several muscles all at one time until you have stretched individual muscles. For example, stretch muscles at the ankle, then the knee, then the ankle and knee simultaneously.
Do precede sport-specific ballistic stretch with static or PNF stretching.	

The Facts about the Benefits of Stretching

Performing stretching exercises has benefits in addition to those that result from having good flexibility.

As noted earlier in this concept, people who do regular stretching exercises receive benefits in addition to those that come from having good flexibility. However, all people with good flexibility do not do stretching exercises on a regular basis. Of course, one of the benefits of stretching is an increase in flexibility, so people who are active get both the benefits of good flexibility and regular exercise.

Static muscle stretching is effective in relieving muscle spasms.

A muscle spasm or cramp may result for a variety of reasons, including overexertion, dehydration, and heat stress. Stretching a cramped (but not a strained) muscle will help relieve the cramp. Stretching should be done statically and can be done with active or passive assistance, though passive assistance should be applied carefully. For example, a person with a cramp or spasm in the calf muscle can pull the toe toward the shin using the shin muscles, or a partner could push the ball of the foot toward the shin to get the same benefit.

Trigger points may sometimes be prevented or inactivated by static or PNF stretching of the muscles involved.

When body parts are held in static positions for long periods, or when muscles are chronically overloaded, fatigued, or chilled, myofascial **trigger points** may cause stiffness and local or referred pain. Often, the trigger point can be deactivated and the pain relieved by gentle but persistent stretching of the muscle, especially if heat or cold packs are applied.

Stretching exercises are useful in preventing and remediating some cases of dysmenorrhea in women.

Painful menstruation (dysmenorrhea) of some types can be prevented or reduced by stretching the pelvic and hip joint fascia. Billig's exercise is an example of an effective exercise for this condition (see exercise 11).

Static stretching is probably *ineffective* in preventing muscle soreness.

In the past, it was suggested that stretching during a cool-down will *prevent* muscular soreness. In a controlled study, muscle soreness was deliberately induced in a group of subjects. When half of the group stretched immediately afterward and at intervals for 48 hours, they had no less soreness than the group who did not stretch.

Strategies for Action: The Facts

> An important step in taking action for developing and maintaining flexibility is assessing your current status.

www.mhhe.com/hper/physed/clw/student/
An important early step in taking action to improve fitness is self-assessment. There are dozens of tests of flexibility. Four tests that assess range of motion in the major joints of the body, that require little equipment, and that can be easily administered are presented in the lab resources materials. In Lab 10A you will get an opportunity to try these self-assessments. It is recommended that you perform these assessments before you begin your regular stretching program and use these assessments to periodically reevaluate your flexibility. A fitness profile is provided on the web as is information about self-assessments.

> Scores on flexibility tests may be influenced by several factors.

Your range of motion at any one time may be influenced by your motivation to exert maximum effort, warm-up preparation, muscular soreness, tolerance for pain, room temperature, and ability to relax. Recent studies have found a relationship between leg or trunk length and the scores made on the sit-and-reach test. The sit-and-reach test used in this book is adapted to allow for differences in body build.

> Select exercises that promote flexibility in all areas of the body.

The American College of Sports Medicine recommends that adults regularly perform 8 to 10 stretching exercises for the major muscle groups of the body. Table 4 provides eight exercises referred to as the Basic 8. These exercises are easy to perform and meet the ACSM guidelines. For most people, these will be adequate for building flexibility for health and leisure-time recreational activities.

www.mhhe.com/hper/physed/clw/student/
Additional exercises are provided for people who may want alternatives to the Basic 8 or who want to do more than the basic exercises (see Table 5).

The exercises presented in Tables 4 and 5 are static stretching exercises that can also be performed using PNF techniques. Ballistic stretching exercises are discussed in more detail in the concept on performance benefits of physical activity.

> Keeping records of progress is important to adhering to a stretching program.

An activity logging sheet is provided in Lab 10B to help you keep records of your progress as you regularly perform stretching exercises to build and maintain good flexibility.

 Web Review

Web review materials for Concept 10 are available are at *www.mhhe.com/hper/physed/clw/student/*.
Flexibility Execises

> *www.mhhe.com/hper/physed/clw/student/*

Suggested Readings

Alter, M. J. *Science of Stretch.* Champaign, IL: Human Kinetics Publishers, 1996.
Fomby, E. W. and Mellon, M. B. Identifying and Treating Myofascial Pain Syndrome. *The Physician and Sports Medicine.* 25(2)(1997):67.
Gleim, G. W. and McHugh, M. P. "Flexibility and Its Effect on Sports Injury and Performance." *Sports Medicine* 24(1997):289–299.
Golding, L. A. (1997). Flexibility, Stretching, and Flexibility Testing. *ACSM's Health and Fitness.* 1(1)(1997):17.
Knudson, D. "Stretching: From Science to Practice." *Journal of Physical Education, Recreation and Dance,* 69 (1998):38–42.
McAtee, R. *Facilitated Stretching.* Champaign, IL: Human Kinetics Publishers, 1993.
Smith, C. A. "The Warm-Up Procedure: To Stretch or Not to Stretch. A Brief Review." *Journal of Orthopaedic and Sport Physical Therapy* 19(1994):12–17.

Trigger Point An especially irritable spot, usually a tight band or knot in a muscle or fascia. This often refers pain to another area of the body.

8 for Stretching Exercises

1. Calf Stretcher

This exercise stretches the calf muscles and Achilles tendon. Face a wall with your feet 2 or 3 feet away. Step forward on your left foot to allow both hands to touch the wall. Keep the heel of your right foot on the ground, toe turned in slightly, knee straight, and buttocks tucked in. Lean forward by bending your front knee and arms and allowing your head to move nearer the wall. Hold. Bend right knee, keeping heel on floor. Stretch and hold. Repeat with other leg.

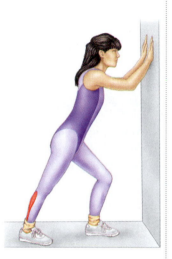

3. Sitting Stretcher

This exercise stretches the muscles on the inside of the thighs. Sit with soles of feet together; place hands on knees or ankles and lean forearms against knees; resist (contract) by attempting to raise knees. Hold; then relax and press the knees toward the floor as far as possible; hold. This exercise is useful for pregnant women and anyone whose thighs tend to rotate inward causing backache, knock-knees, and flat feet.

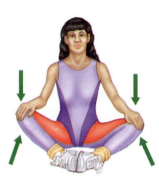

2. Hip and Thigh Stretcher

This exercise stretches the hip (iliopsoas) and thigh muscles (quadriceps) and is useful for people with lordosis and back problems. Place right knee directly above right ankle and stretch left leg backward so knee touches floor. If necessary, place hands on floor for balance.

1. Tilt the pelvis forward by tucking in the abdomen and flattening the back.

2. Then shift the weight forward until a stretch is felt on the front of the thigh; hold. Repeat on opposite side. Caution: Do not bend front knee more than 90 degrees.

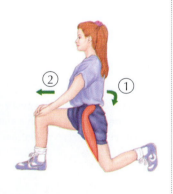

4. Hamstring Stretcher

This exercise stretches the muscles on the back of the hip, thigh, knee, and ankle. Lie on your back with your knees bent. Bring right knee to chest and grasp toes with right hand. Place left hand on back of right thigh. Pull knee toward chest and push heel toward ceiling and pull toes toward shin. Attempt to straighten knee. Stretch and hold. Repeat on left side.

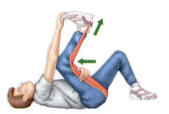

Table 4
The Basic 8 for Stretching Exercises *(continued)*

5. Leg Hug

This exercise stretches the lower back and gluteals. Lie on your back with your knees bent in a hook-lying position. Contract gluteals and lumbar muscles. Lift hips. Hold for 3 seconds. Relax and pull knees to chest with arms as hard as possible; hold. Useful for people with backache and lordosis. Do not place the hands over the knees to apply stretch.

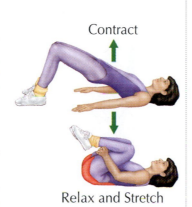

Contract

Relax and Stretch

7. Pectoral stretch

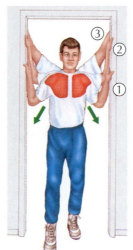

This exercise stretches the chest muscle (pectorals).

1. Stand erect in doorway with arms raised 45 degrees, elbows bent, and hands grasping doorjamb; feet in front-stride position. Press out on door frame, contracting the arms maximally for 3 seconds. Relax and shift weight forward on legs; lean into doorway so muscles on front of shoulder joint and chest are stretched; hold.

2. Repeat with arms raised 90 degrees.

3. Repeat with arms raised 135 degrees. Useful to prevent or correct round shoulders and sunken chest.

6. Trunk Twister

This exercise stretches the trunk muscles and muscles on the outside of hip. Sit with right leg extended, left leg bent and crossed over the right knee. Place right arm on the left side of the left leg and push against that leg while turning the trunk as far as possible to the left. Place left hand on floor behind buttocks. Stretch and hold. Reverse position and repeat on opposite side.

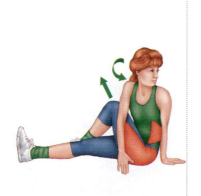

8. Arm Stretcher

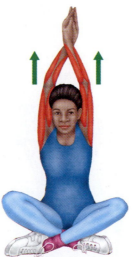

This exercise stretches the arm and chest muscles. Cross arms and turn palms of hands together. Raise arms overhead behind ears. Extend elbows. Stretch as high as possible. Hold.

Table 5
Supplemental Stretching Exercises for Flexibility

1. Lower Leg Stretcher

This exercise stretches the calf muscles and Achilles tendon. Stand with the toes on a stair step or thick book. Use hands to balance by holding a rail or wall. Keep toes pointed straight ahead or slightly inward. Rise up on toes (contract) as far as possible and hold for 3 seconds. Relax and lower heels to floor as far as possible; hold. Static stretch may alleviate spasms or cramps in calf muscles.

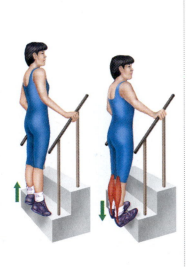

2. Standing Thigh Stretcher

This exercise stretches the hip flexor (iliopsoas) and thigh muscles (quadriceps). Stand near a wall so you can use one hand for balance. Place the top of one foot on a flat surface slightly higher than knee height (use a chair or table). Keep the knee of the elevated foot bent. Slide the leg backward until a stretch is felt on the front of the thigh. Keep the top of the pelvis tilted backward so the back does not arch. Repeat with the opposite leg.

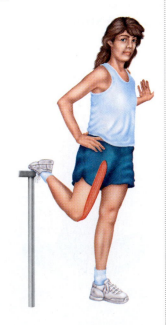

3. Lateral Thigh and Hip Stretch

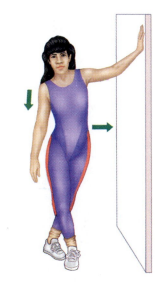

This exercise stretches the muscles and connective tissue on the outside of the legs (iliotibial band and tensor fascia lata). Stand with left side to wall, left arm extended and palm of hand flat on wall for support. Cross the left leg behind right and turn toes of both feet out slightly. Bend left knee slightly and shift pelvis toward wall (left) as trunk bends toward right. Adjust until tension is felt down outside of left hip and thigh. Stretch and hold. Repeat on other side.

4. Back-Saver Hamstring Stretch

This exercise stretches the hamstrings and calf muscles and helps prevent or correct backache caused in part by short hamstrings. Sit on the floor with the feet against the wall or an immovable object. Bend left knee and bring foot close to buttocks. Clasp hands behind back. Contract the muscles of the back of the upper leg (hamstrings) by pressing the heel downward toward the floor; hold; relax. Bend forward from hips, keeping lower back as straight as possible. Let bent knee rotate outward so trunk can move forward. Lean forward keeping back flat; hold and repeat on each leg.

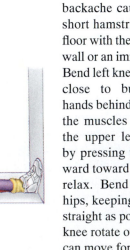

Table 5

Supplemental Stretching Exercises for Flexibility *(continued)*

5. One-Leg Stretcher

This exercise stretches the lower back and hamstring muscles. Stand with one foot on a bench, keeping both legs straight. Contract the hamstrings and gluteals by pressing down on bench with the heel for 3 seconds, then relax and bend the trunk forward, toward the knee. Hold for 10–15 seconds. Return to starting position and repeat with opposite leg. As flexibility improves, the arms can be used to pull the chest toward the legs. Do not allow either knee to lock. This exercise is useful in relief of backache and correction of lordosis (swayback).

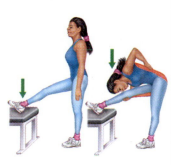

7. Wand Exercise

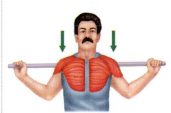

This exercise stretches the front of the shoulders and chest. Sit with wand grasped at ends. Raise wand overhead. Be certain that the head does not slide forward. Keep the chin tucked and neck straight. Bring wand down behind shoulder blades. Keep spine erect. Hold. Press forward on the wand simultaneously by pushing with the hands. Relax, then try to move the hands lower, sliding the wand down the back. Hold again. Hands may be moved closer together to increase stretch on chest muscles. If this is an easy exercise for you, try straightening the elbows and bringing the wand to waist level in back of you.

6. Lateral Trunk Stretcher

This exercise stretches the trunk muscles. Sit on the floor. Stretch the left arm over head to right. Bend to the right at waist, reaching as far to right as possible with left arm and as far as possible to the left with right arm; hold. Do not let trunk rotate. Repeat on opposite side. For less stretch, overhead arm may be bent at elbow. This exercise can be done in the standing position but is less effective.

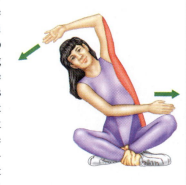

8. Arm Pretzel

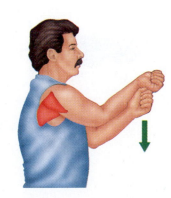

This exercise stretches the shoulder muscles (lateral rotators). Stand or sit with elbows flexed at right angles, palms up. Cross right arm over left; grasp right thumb with left hand and pull gently downward, causing right arm to rotate laterally. Stretch and hold. Reverse arm position and repeat on left arm.

Table 5

Supplemental Stretching Exercises for Flexibility (*continued*)

9. Shin Stretcher

This exercise relieves shin muscle soreness by stretching muscles on front of shin. Kneel on both knees, turn to right, and press down and stretch right ankle with right hand. Move pelvis forward. Hold. Repeat on opposite side. Except when they are sore, most people need to strengthen rather than stretch these muscles.

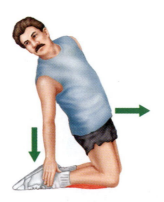

11. Billig's Exercise

This exercise stretches the pelvic fascia, hip flexors, and muscles of the inside thigh. Stand with side to a wall and place the elbow and forearm against the wall at shoulder height. Tilt the pelvis backward, tightening the gluteal and abdominal muscles. Place opposite hand on hip and push the hips toward the wall. Push forward and sideward (45 degrees) with the hips. Do not twist the hips. Hold. Repeat on opposite side. Useful for preventing some cases of dysmenorrhea.

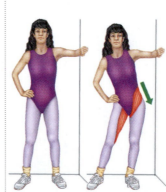

10. Spine Twist

This exercise stretches the trunk rotators and lateral rotators of the thighs. Start in hook-lying position, arms extended at shoulder level. Cross left knee over right; keep arms and shoulders on floor while touching knees to floor on left. Stretch and hold. Reverse leg position and lower knees to right.

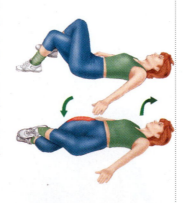

12. Two-Hand Ankle Wrap

This exercise is most useful for athletes or people interested in performance. It should not be done until after individual muscles have been stretched using other exercises. It stretches multiple muscle groups including the back, shoulders, and legs. Stand with heels together. Bend forward and place arms between knees; bend knees and wrap arms around legs, attempting to touch fingers in front of ankles. Hold.

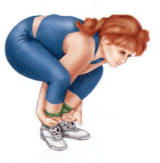

Lab Resource Materials: Flexibility Tests

Directions: It is impractical to test the flexibility of all joints. These tests are for joints used frequently. Follow instructions carefully.

Test

1. *Modified sit-and-reach* (Flexibility Test of Hamstrings)

   a. Remove shoes and sit on the floor. Place the sole of the foot of the extended leg flat against a box or bench, and place the head, back, and hips against a wall; 90-degree angle at the hips.

   b. Place one hand over the other and slowly reach forward as far as you can with arms fully extended; head and back remain in contact with the wall. A partner will slide the measuring stick on the bench until it touches the fingertips.

   c. With the measuring stick fixed in the new position, reach forward as far as possible, three times, holding the position on the third reach for at least 2 seconds while the partner reads the distance on the ruler. Keep the knee of the extended leg straight (see illustration).

   d. Repeat the test a second time and average the scores of the two trials.

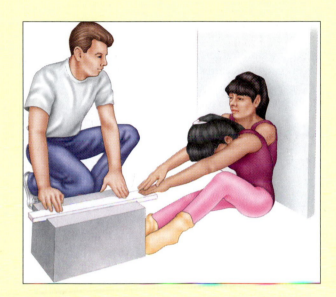

Test

2. *Shoulder Flexibility* ("Zipper" Test)

   a. Raise your arm, bend your elbow, and reach down across your back as far as possible.

   b. At the same time, extend your left arm down and behind your back, bend your elbow up across your back, and try to cross your fingers over those of your right hand as shown in the accompanying illustration.

   c. Measure the distance to the nearest half-inch. If your fingers overlap, score as a plus; if they fail to meet, score as a minus; use a zero if your fingertips just touch.

   d. Repeat with your arms crossed in the opposite direction (left arm up). Most people will find that they are more flexible on one side than the other.

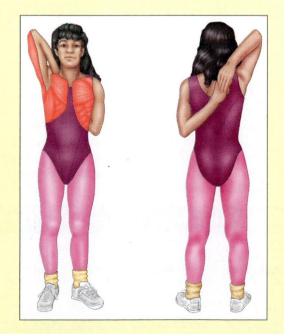

Test

3. *Hamstring and Hip Flexor Flexibility*

   a. Lie on your back on the floor beside a wall.
   b. Slowly lift one leg off the floor. Keep the other leg flat on the floor.
   c. Keep both legs straight
   d. Continue to lift the leg until either leg begins to bend or the lower leg begins to lift off the floor.
   e. Place a yardstick against the wall and underneath the lifted leg.
   f. Hold the yardstick against the wall after the leg is lowered.
   g. Using a protractor, measure the angle created by the floor and the yardstick. The greater the angle, the better your score.
   h. Repeat with the other leg.*

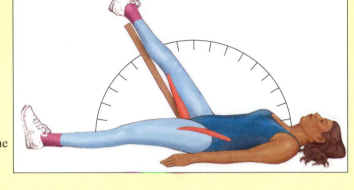

*Note: For ease of testing, you may want to draw angles on a piece of posterboard as illustrated. If you have goniometers, you may be taught to use them instead.

Test

4. *Trunk Rotation*

   a. Tape two yardsticks to the wall at shoulder height, one right side up and the other upside down.
   b. Stand with your left shoulder an arm's length (fist closed) from the wall. Toes should be on the line (which is perpendicular to the wall and even with the 15-inch mark on the yardstick).
   c. Drop the left arm and raise the right arm to the side, palm down, fist closed.
   d. Without moving your feet, rotate the trunk to the right as far as possible, reaching along the yardstick, and hold it 2 seconds. Do not move the feet nor bend the trunk. Your knees may bend slightly.
   e. A partner will read the distance reached to the nearest half-inch. Record your score. Repeat two times and average your two scores.
   f. Next, perform the test facing the opposite direction. Rotate to the left. For this test you will use the second yardstick (upside down) so that the greater the rotation, the higher the score. If you have only one yardstick, turn it right side up for the first test and upside down for the second test.

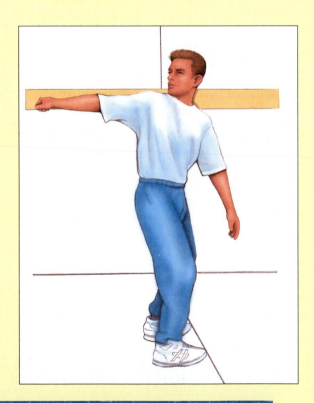

Chart 1 Flexibility Rating Scale for Tests 1–4

Classification	Men					Women				
	Test 1	Test 2		Test 3	Test 4	Test 1	Test 2		Test 3	Test 4
		Right Up	Left Up				Right Up	Left Up		
High-performance*	16+	5+	4+	111+	20+	17+	6+	5+	111+	20.5 or >
Good fitness zone	13–15	1–4	1–3	80–110	16–19.5	14–16	2–5	2–4	80–110	17–20
Marginal zone	10–12	0	0	60–79	13.5–15.5	11–13	1	1	60–79	14.5–16.5
Low zone	<9	<0	<0	<60	13 or less	<10	<1	<1	<60	14 or <

*Though performers need good flexibility, hypermobility may increase injury risk.

Lab 10B: Planning and Logging Stretching Exercises

Name	**Section**	**Date**

Purpose: To set one-week lifestyle goals for stretching exercises, to prepare a stretching for flexibility plan, and to self-monitor progress in your one-week plan.

Procedures:
1.   On chart 1 check the stretching exercises you plan to perform during the next week. Try to do at least eight exercises three times a week. The Basic 8 are listed. You may substitute other exercises by writing them in the "other" blank. See Table 5 for additional exercises.
2.   Keep a one-week log of your actual participation using chart 2. If possible, keep the log with you during the day. Place a check by each of the stretching exercises you perform each day—including ones that you didn't originally have planned. If you cannot keep the log with you, fill in the log at the end of the day. If you choose to keep a log for more than one week, make extra copies of the log before you begin.
3.   Answer the questions in the results section.

Chart 1 Stretching Exercise Plan

Place a check beside the stretching exercises you plan to do and under the days you plan to do them.	Day 1 Date:	Day 2 Date:	Day 3 Date:	Day 4 Date:	Day 5 Date:	Day 6 Date:	Day 7 Date:
1. Calf stretcher							
2. Hip and thigh stretcher							
3. Sitting stretcher							
4. Hamstring stretcher							
5. Back stretcher (leg hug)							
6. Trunk twister							
7. Pectoral stretcher							
8. Arm stretcher							
Other:							
Other:							
Other:							
Other:							

Results:

	Yes	No
Did you do eight exercises at least three days in the week?	○	○
Did you do eight exercises more than three days in the week ?	○	○

Chart 2 Stretching Exercise Log

Place a check beside the stretching exercises you actually performed and the days on which you performed them.	Day 1 Date:	Day 2 Date:	Day 3 Date:	Day 4 Date:	Day 5 Date:	Day 6 Date:	Day 7 Date:
1. Calf stretcher							
2. Hip and thigh stretcher							
3. Sitting stretcher							
4. Hamstring stretcher							
5. Back stretcher (leg hug)							
6. Trunk twister							
7. Pectoral stretcher							
8. Arm stretcher							
Other:							
Other:							
Other:							
Other:							

Conclusions and Interpretations:

1. Do you feel that you will use stretching exercises as part of your regular lifetime physical activity plan, either now or in the future? Use several sentences to explain your answer.

2. Discuss the exercises you feel benefited you and the ones that did not. What exercises would you continue to do and which ones would you change? Use several sentences to explain your answer.

3. Did the logging of your stretching exercise help you to adhere to your program? In several sentences, explain why or why not.

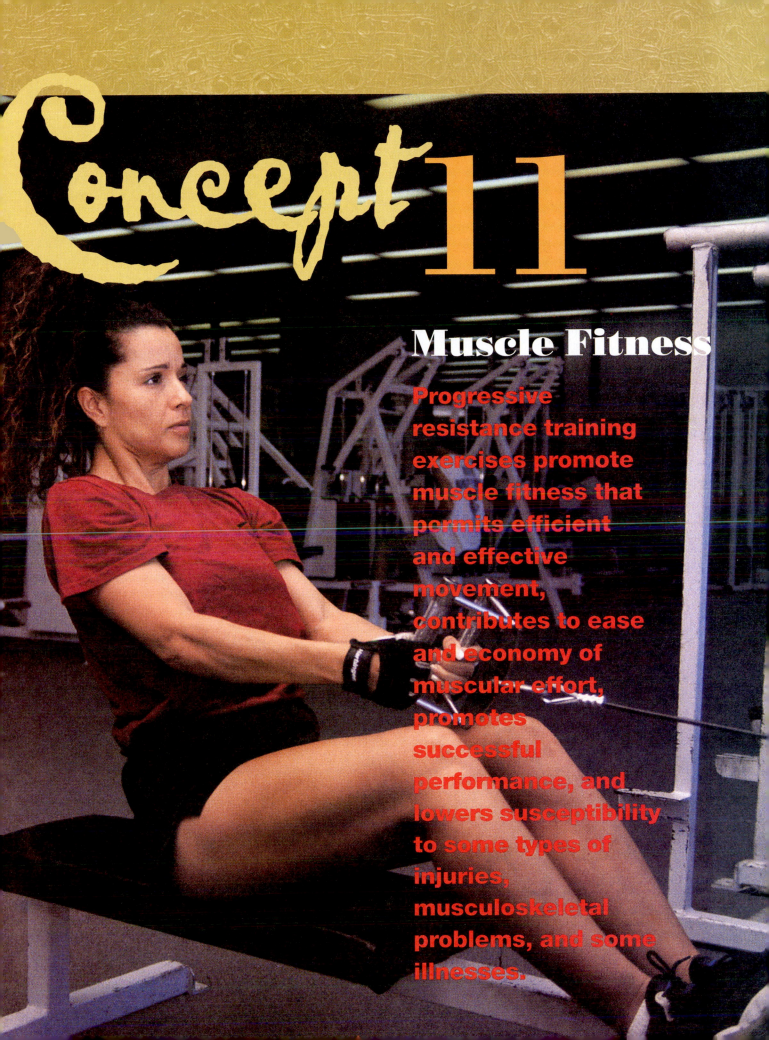

Concept 11

Muscle Fitness

Progressive resistance training exercises promote muscle fitness that permits efficient and effective movement, contributes to ease and economy of muscular effort, promotes successful performance, and lowers susceptibility to some types of injuries, musculoskeletal problems, and some illnesses.

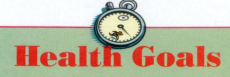

Health Goals

for Year 2010

Increase proportion of people who regularly perform exercises for strength and muscular endurance.

Reduce steroid use especially among youth.

Increase screening and reduce incidence of osteoporosis.

Reduce activity limitation due to chronic back pain.

Introduction

There are two components of muscle fitness: strength and muscular endurance. Strength is the amount of force you can produce with a single maximal effort of a muscle group. Muscular endurance is the capacity of the skeletal muscles or group of muscles to continue contracting over a long period of time. You need both strength and muscular endurance to increase work capacity; to decrease the chance of injury; to prevent low back pain, poor posture, and other hypokinetic conditions; to improve athletic performance; and perhaps to save a life or property in an emergency. Muscle fitness training increases the fitness of the bones, tendons, and ligaments, as well as the muscles. It has been found to be therapeutic for patients with chronic pain.

Progressive resistance training is the type of physical activity done with the intent of improving muscle fitness. The many types of progressive resistance exercises designed to promote or maintain muscle fitness are described in this concept.

The Basic Facts about Strength and Muscular Endurance

There are three types of muscle tissue.

www.mhhe.com/hper/physed/clw/student/

The three types of muscle tissue—smooth, cardiac, and skeletal—have different structures and functions. Smooth muscle tissue consists of long, spindle-shaped fibers with each fiber containing only one nucleus.

The fibers are involuntary and are located in the walls of the esophagus, stomach, and intestines, where they function to move food and waste products through the digestive tract. Cardiac muscle tissue is also involuntary and, as its name implies, it is found only in the heart. These fibers contract in response to demands on the cardiovascular system. The heart muscle contracts at a slow steady rate at rest but contracts more frequently and forcefully during physical activity. Skeletal muscle tissues consist of long, cylindrical, multinucleated fibers. They provide the force needed to move the skeletal system and may be controlled voluntarily. Skeletal muscles are made up of slow- (red), intermediate-, and fast- (white) twitch fibers.

Some experts suggest that strength-training exercises tend to selectively develop fast-twitch muscle fibers, and muscular endurance training selectively develops slow-twitch fibers.

Fast-twitch muscle fibers generate greater tension than slow-twitch fibers, but they fatigue more quickly. They primarily use anaerobic metabolism. These fibers are particularly suited to fast, high-force activities such as explosive weight-lifting movements, sprinting, and jumping. Strength training primarily increases the size (muscle **hypertrophy**) of fast-twitch fibers, though intermediate fibers also increase in size and take on fast-twitch fiber characteristics with training. Slow-twitch fibers generate less tension but are more resistant to fatigue because they rely on aerobic metabolism. As you train specifically for muscular endurance, the muscles adapt primarily through changes in slow-twitch fibers, including increased activity of aerobic enzymes in the muscle.

An example of fast-twitch muscle fiber in animals is the white meat in the flying muscles of a chicken. The chicken is heavy and must exert a powerful force to fly a few feet up to a perch. A wild duck that flies for hundreds of miles has dark meat (slow-twitch fibers) in the flying muscles for better endurance.

People who want large muscles will use progressive resistance exercises designed to build strength (fast-twitch fibers). People who want to be able to persist in activities for a long period of time without fatigue will want to use progressive resistance training programs designed to build muscular endurance (slow-twitch fibers).

Genetics, gender, and age affect muscle fitness performance.

www.mhhe.com/hper/physed/clw/student/

Each person inherits a certain percentage of fast-twitch and slow-twitch muscle fibers. This allocation influences the potential a person has for mus-

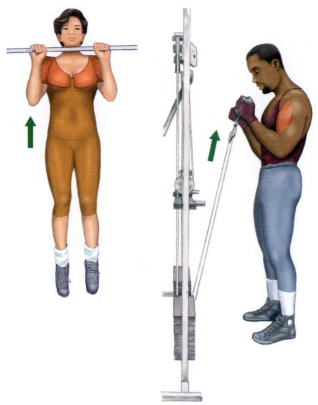

Figure 1
Overcoming a heavy resistance one time requires strength. Repeating an activity with less resistance requires muscular endurance.

cle fitness activities. Individuals with a larger percentage of fast-twitch fibers will generally increase muscle size and strength more readily than individuals endowed with a larger percentage of slow-twitch fibers. People with a larger percentage of slow-twitch fibers have greater potential for muscular endurance performance. Regardless of genetics, all people can improve their strength and muscular endurance with proper training.

Women have smaller amounts of the anabolic hormone testosterone and therefore have less muscle mass than men. Because of this, women typically have 60 percent to 85 percent of the **absolute strength** of men. **Absolute muscular endurance** also favors men over women, though not as dramatically as for strength. When differences in size and muscle mass are taken into consideration, women have **relative strength** and **relative muscular endurance** similar to men.

Maximum strength is usually reached in the twenties and typically declines with age. Though muscular endurance declines with age, it is not as dramatic as decreases in absolute strength. As people grow older, regardless of gen-

der, strength and muscular endurance is better among people who train than people who do not. This suggests that progressive resistance training is one antidote to premature aging.

Some endurance tests penalize the weaker person.

If you are tested on absolute endurance (the number of times you can move a designated number of pounds), a stronger person has an advantage. However, if you are tested on relative muscular endurance (the number of times you can move a designated percentage of your maximum strength), the stronger person does not have an advantage. For this reason, men and women can compete more evenly in relative muscular endurance activities. In fact, on some endurance tasks women have done as well or better than men. For example, the women at the United States Military Academy do as well as the men on tests of abdominal muscular endurance.

Hypertrophy Increase in the size of muscles as the result of strength training; increase in bulk.

Absolute Strength The maximum amount of force one can exert (e.g., maximum number of pounds or kilograms that can be lifted on one attempt. (See Relative Strength.)

Absolute Muscular Endurance (Dynamic Type) Endurance measured by the maximum number of repetitions (muscle contractions) one can perform against a given resistance (e.g., the number of times you can bench press 50 pounds).

Relative Strength Amount of force that can be exerted in relation to one's body weight or per unit of muscle cross-section; that is, if a 100-pound person lifts 250 pounds, he or she has lifted 2.5 pounds per pound of body weight, and thus has more relative strength than a 250-pound person who lifts 500 pounds, or 2 pounds per pound of body weight. The latter has more absolute strength.

Relative Muscular Endurance (Dynamic Type) Endurance measured by the maximum number of repetitions one can perform against a resistance that is a given percentage of one's 1 RM (e.g., the number of times you can lift 50 percent of your 1 RM).

Muscular endurance is related to cardiovascular endurance, but it is not the same thing.

Cardiovascular endurance depends primarily upon the efficiency of the heart muscle, circulatory system, and respiratory system. It is developed with activities that stress these systems, such as running, cycling, and swimming. Muscular endurance depends upon the efficiency of the local skeletal muscles and the nerves that control them. Most forms of cardiovascular exercises such as running require good cardiovascular and muscular endurance. For example, if your legs lack the muscular endurance to continue contracting for a sustained period of time, it will be difficult to perform well in running or other aerobic activities.

The Facts about the Health Benefits of Muscle Fitness

Good muscle fitness is associated with reduced risk of injury.

www.mhhe.com/hper/physed/clw/student/
Experts believe that strong muscles with good endurance are able to resist various injuries. People with good muscle fitness are less likely to suffer joint injuries (e.g., neck, knee, ankle) than those with poor muscle fitness. Weak muscles are more likely to be involuntarily overstretched than are strong muscles.
Muscle balance is important in reducing the risk of injury. Resistance training should build both agonist and **antagonist muscles**. For example, if you do resistance exercise to build the quadriceps muscles (front of the thigh), you should also exercise the hamstring muscles (back of the thigh). In this instance, the quadriceps are the agonist (muscle being used), and the hamstrings are the antagonist. If the quadriceps become too strong relative to the antagonist hamstring muscles, the risk of injury increases (see Figure 2).

Good muscle fitness is associated with good posture and reduced risk of back problems.

www.mhhe.com/hper/physed/clw/student/
When muscles in specific body regions are weak or overdeveloped, poor posture can result. Lack of fitness of the abdominal and low back muscles is particularly related to poor posture and potential back problems. Excessively strong hip flexor muscles can lead to swayback. Poor balance in muscular development can also result in postural problems. For example, the muscles on the sides of the body must be balanced to maintain an erect posture.

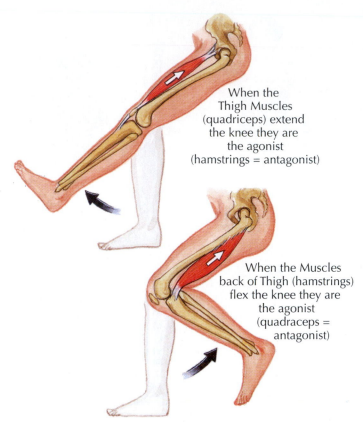

When the Thigh Muscles (quadriceps) extend the knee they are the agonist (hamstrings = antagonist)

When the Muscles back of Thigh (hamstrings) flex the knee they are the agonist (quadraceps = antagonist)

Figure 2
Agonist and antagonist muscles.

Good muscle fitness can bring about improved athletic performance.

Many sports depend on strength and muscular endurance. A football player must have good muscle strength to block and tackle effectively. A swimmer or a wrestler requires good muscular endurance to perform optimally. Athletes and people interested in jobs requiring high-level performance such as law enforcement and fire safety are especially likely to benefit from good muscle fitness.

Good muscular fitness is associated with wellness.

Wellness is reflected in quality of life and well-being. A person with muscle fitness is able to perform for long periods of time without undue fatigue. As a result, the person has energy to perform daily work efficiently and effectively and has reserve energy to enjoy leisure time. Among older people, maintenance of strength is associated with increased balance, less risk of falling, and greater ability to perform the tasks of daily living independently. Muscle fitness also contributes to looking one's best. Muscles can help the abdomen from protruding, and because people with more muscle burn more calories at rest, good muscle fitness helps in the maintenance of a healthy body weight.

cles. All three of these competitive events rely on progressive resistance exercise to improve performance. Weight training is a form of PRE and is a method of improving muscle fitness that is different from weight lifting—the competitive event.

Progressive resistance exercise programs can be performed in a variety of ways and with different equipment.

change **Isotonic** exercise (also called dynamic) refers to such activities as weight training, calisthenics, pulley weights, and resistance machine exercises. When performing isotonic exercise, both **concentric** (shortening) and **eccentric** (lengthening **contractions** should be used. For example, in an overhead press exercise, the muscles on the back of the arm (triceps) shorten (contract concentrically) to lift the weight overhead (see Figure 3a). When the weight is lowered, the muscles lengthen (contract eccentrically) if the weight is lowered slowly. Both concentric and eccentric contractions build the muscle.

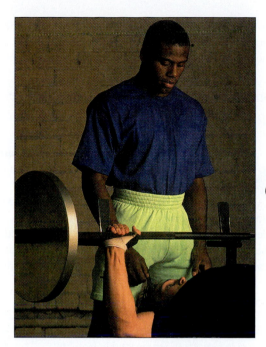

Progressive resistance exercises are methods of training designed to build muscle fitness.

The Facts about Progressive Resistance Exercise

The best type of training for muscle fitness is referred to as progressive resistance exercise.

The type of training most commonly used to promote muscle fitness is referred to as **progressive resistance exercise (PRE)**, or progressive resistance training (PRT). This name is used because the frequency, intensity, and length of time of muscle overload are progressively increased as muscle fitness increases. Progressive resistance exercises are typically done in one to three sets of three to 25 repetitions (also called reps). A set is a group of reps that are done in succession followed by a rest period.

Progressive resistance exercise is not the same thing as weight lifting, powerlifting, or bodybuilding.

Progressive resistance exercise is a method of training to build muscle fitness that provides health and performance benefits. It should not be confused with the following three competitive activities. Weight lifting is a competitive sport that involves two lifts: the snatch and the clean and jerk. Powerlifting is also a competitive sport that includes three lifts: the bench press, the squat, and the dead lift. Bodybuilding is a competition in which participants are judged on the size and **definition** of their mus-

Antagonistic Muscles The muscles that have the opposite action from those that are contracting (agonists); normally, antagonists reflexively relax when agonists contract.

Progressive Resistance Exercise (PRE) Exercise done against a resistance; also referred to as progressive resistance training (PRT).

Definition (of Muscle) The detailed external appearance of a muscle.

Isotonic Type of muscle contraction in which the muscle changes length, either shortening (concentrically) or lengthening (eccentrically). Isotonic exercises are those in which a resistance is raised and then lowered, as in weight training and calisthenics (also called dynamic or phasic).

Concentric Contraction An isotonic muscle contraction in which the muscle gets shorter as it contracts, such as when a joint is bent and two body parts move closer together. An example is the biceps muscle contraction that occurs when pulling up on a chinning bar.

Eccentric Contraction An isotonic muscle contraction in which the muscle gets longer as it contracts; that is, when a weight is gradually lowered and the contracting muscle gets longer as it gives up tension. Lowering the body from a pull-up on a chinning bar is an example of eccentric contraction of the biceps muscle. Eccentric contractions are also called negative exercise.

Eccentric contractions, sometimes called negative contractions, are more likely to cause delayed-onset muscle soreness than concentric contractions. Typically, the stress on the muscle in either concentric or eccentric exercises varies with speed, joint position, and muscle length. Thus, the muscle may work harder at the beginning of a lift than it does near the end of the range of motion.

www.mhhe.com/hper/physed/clw/student/
Isometric exercises involve nonmoving or static contractions (see Figure 3*b*). They are effective for developing strength and muscular endurance and require little or no equipment and only minimal space. Isometric exercises build static strength and static muscular endurance as opposed to dynamic strength or dynamic muscular endurance. They work the muscle only at the angle of the joint used in the exercise and promote less hypertrophy and strength than isotonic resistance exercise. Thus, isometric exercises are probably less effective as an overall training method than isotonic exercises. On the other hand, isometrics have been found to be quite useful for some athletes, such as wrestlers and gymnasts, and work especially well for people in the early stages of some rehabilitation programs. Research has shown that strength can be enhanced significantly by using isometric training at the **sticking points** of isotonic lifts.

Isometrics previously have been thought to be dangerous for people with high blood pressure or cardiovascular disease. Recent evidence suggests that may not be the case for all people with these cardiovascular problems. These people should consult a medical expert before using isometric techniques.

www.mhhe.com/hper/physed/clw/student/
Isokinetic exercises are isotonic-concentric muscle contractions performed on devices such as the Apollo, Exer-Genie, Mini-Gym, Hydra-Fitness (hydraulic machine), or on electromechanical dynamometers, such as the Cybex II. These machines keep the velocity of the movement constant and match their resistance to the effort of the performer, permitting maximal tension to be exerted throughout the range of motion (see Figure 3*c*). For example, on the Cybex II, speeds range from 0 to 300 degrees per second. This rate-limiting mechanism prevents the performer from moving faster no matter how much force is exerted. Thus, isokinetic devices attempt to overcome the basic weakness of isotonics. On the other hand, these devices do not permit acceleration, so it is not possible to train specifically for sports skills, such as throwing or kicking, in which the limb is accelerated while applying maximum force. Another limitation is that some of these devices permit only concentric contractions. Isokinetic exercise has the advantage of being safer than most other forms of exercise and may be better for developing power (see concept on performance benefits of physical activity). It is not better for developing pure strength, however. More research is needed to determine the best training regimen for isokinetic exercise.

Some of the advantages and disadvantages of the various forms of progressive resistance exercises, not including plyometrics, are outlined in Table 1.

Plyometrics is a form of isotonic exercise that promotes athletic performance.

www.mhhe.com/hper/physed/clw/student/
Plyometrics is a form of isotonic exercise that is especially useful for athletes training for power development. High jumpers, long jumpers, volleyball, and basketball players often use this technique, which includes jumping from boxes, hopping on one foot, and similar types of activities. For most people primarily interested in the health benefits of physical activity, plyometrics are not a

---

Isometric A type of muscle contraction in which the muscle remains the same length. Isometric exercises are those in which no movement takes place while a force is exerted against an immovable object (also known as static contraction).

Static Strength A muscle's ability to exert a force without changing length. It is also called isometric strength.

Static Muscular Endurance A muscle's ability to remain contracted for a long period. This is usually measured by the length of time you can hold a body position. It is also called isometric endurance.

Dynamic Strength A muscle's ability to exert force that results in movement. It is typically measured isotonically.

Dynamic Muscular Endurance A muscle's ability to contract and relax repeatedly. This is usually measured by the number of times (repetitions) you can perform a body movement in a given time period. It is also called isotonic endurance.

Sticking Point The point in the range of motion where the weight cannot be lifted any farther without extreme effort or assistance; the weakest point in the movement.

Isokinetic Isotonic concentric exercises done with a machine that regulates movement velocity and resistance.

Plyometrics A training technique used to develop explosive power. Referred to as speed-strength training in Eastern Europe and the former Soviet Union, where it originated. It consists of concentric isotonic muscle contractions performed after a pre-stretch or eccentric contraction of a muscle.

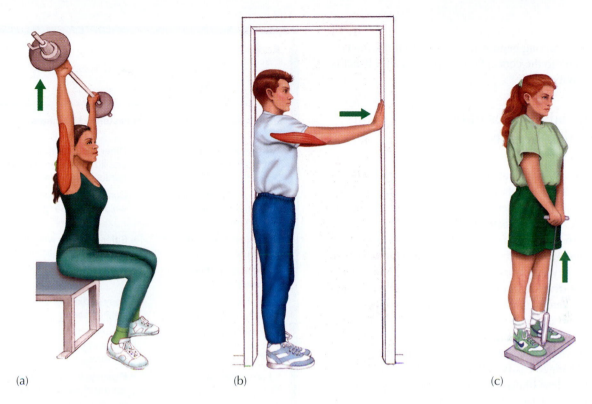

(a)   (b)   (c)

Figure 3
Examples of three types of muscle fitness exercises (*a*) isotonic, (*b*) isometric, and (*c*) isokinetic.

Table 1 Advantages and Disadvantages of Isometric, Isotonic, and Isokinetic Resistance Exercises*			
	Isometrics (Statics)	**Isotonics (Dynamics)**	**Isokinetics**
In small space	E	F-G	F-G
No equipment or low-cost equipment	E	F-G	P
Provides feedback for motivation	P	E	F
Can rehabilitate immobilized joint	E	P	P
Builds strength through full range of motion	P	F-G	E
Less likely to cause soreness	E	F-G	E
Aids dynamic coordination	P	E	G
Safe for hypertensives	P	E	G-E
Amount of strength developed	F	E	E
Dynamic exercises and controlled testing	P	F-G	E
Hypertrophy	P	E	E
Power development	P	G	E
Rapid improvement in strength	E	F-G	F-G
Can accelerate to resemble sport skill	P	E	P

*Key: E = Excellent; G = Good; F = Fair; P = Poor

preferred type of exercise. In fact, they can increase risk of injury, especially among beginners. For more information on plyometrics, refer to the concept on the performance benefits of physical activity.

There are advantages of both free weights and machine weights.

Free weights are weights that are not attached to a machine or exercise device. Typically, they come in the form of a barbell or dumbbell that can be adjusted as necessary for different exercises to provide optimal resistance. Weight training with free weights is very popular because it can be done in the home with inexpensive equipment. Because free weights require balance and technique, they may be somewhat difficult for beginners to use, but competitive weight lifters generally prefer them because they can exercise muscle groups in a very specific way.

Resistance training machines can be effective in developing strength and muscular endurance if used properly. They can save time because, unlike free weights, the resistance can be changed easily and quickly. They may be safer because you are less likely to drop weights. A disadvantage is that the kinds of exercises that can be done on these machines are more limited than free-weight exercises. They also may not promote optimal balance in muscular development since a stronger muscle can often make up for a weaker muscle in the completion of a lift.

www.mhhe.com/hper/physed/clw/student/

Some machines, such as Nautilus and Universal, offer what is called "variable" or "accommodating resistance." The Nautilus, for example, uses a cam to adapt the resistance as the performer moves through the range of motion. The Universal Trainer uses a rolling pivot to do the same thing. These adaptations attempt to compensate for an inherent weakness in isotonic constant-resistance exercises done with free weights and other machines. They are only partially successful, however, in adapting to the shapes, sizes, and torques of individual human bodies. There is no evidence that variable-resistance machines develop more strength or muscular endurance than other devices, although they may offer advantages in muscle fitness by allowing movement through an extended range of motion.

Table 2 provides a comparison of free weights with weight machines (for example, Nautilus, Universal, Marcy, Hydra-Gym, Dynacam, and Paramount). Free weights are compared with other resistance machines in Table 3.

Many resistance training exercises can be done with little or no equipment.

Calisthenics are among the most popular forms of muscle fitness exercise among adults. Calisthenics, such as curl-ups and push-ups, are suitable for people of different ability lev-

Table 2   Advantages and Disadvantages of Free Weights and Resistance Machines

Free Weights	Resistance Machines
• Requires balance and coordination; uses more muscles for stabilization.	• Other body parts are stabilized; easier to isolate particular muscle group.
• Truer to real-life situation, so skills transfer to daily life.	• Controlled path of weight not true to life.
• Creates more possibility of injury.	• Safer because weight cannot fall on participant.
• Requires spotters for safety.	• No spotters required.
• Takes more time to change weights.	• Easy and quick to change weights.
• Unlimited number of exercises possible.	• Restricted to range and angle of movement permitted by the machine.
• Less expensive.	• Expensive; need to go to club if cannot afford equipment; need more than one machine for variety.
• Loose equipment clutters area and may get lost or stolen.	• Machines are stationary but occupy large space.

els, and can be used to improve both strength and muscular endurance. One disadvantage is that this type of exercise does little to increase strength unless resistance in addition to your body weight is added. For example, doing a push-up will build strength to a point. However, once you can do several, adding more repetitions will only build muscular endurance but not strength. To develop additional strength, you can add more weights to increase the resistance or change the body position so there is a greater gravitational effect or more torque. For example, you can elevate your feet or wear a weighted vest while doing push-ups.

Another alternative to expensive resistance training machines or commercially made free weights are homemade weights and elastic exercise bands. Homemade weights can be constructed from pieces of pipe or broom sticks and plastic milk jugs filled with water. Elastic tubes or bands available in varying strengths may be substituted for the weights and for the pulley device used in many resistance training machines to impart resistance.

Muscular endurance can be developed through activities such as running, swimming, circuit training, and aerobic dance if they are designed appropriately. Even games, such as rope climbing, tug-of-war, and hopping races can contribute to muscular endurance.

Table 3 Comparison of Selected Resistance Training Devices

	Free Weights	Weight-Stack Machine	Compressed Air Machine	Hydraulic Machine	Isokinetic Machine
Concentric resistance	+	+	+	+	+
Eccentric resistance	+	+	+	-	+-
Isometric resistance	+	+	+	+	-
Match resistance to effort through range of motion	-	+-	+	+	+
Isolation of all major muscle groups	-	+-	+	+	+
Safety features	-	+	+	+	+
Durability	+	+	+	+	+

From Wayne L. Westcott, "Strength Training" in *Sportcare & Fitness Magazine*, July/August 1988, page 62. Reprinted by permission of Wayne L. Westcott.

The Facts about How Much PRE Is Enough

The overload principle must be applied using progressive resistance exercises such as those in the muscle fitness section of the physical activity pyramid if muscle fitness is to be developed and maintained.

It was in the area of muscle fitness development that the overload principle was first clearly outlined. Centuries ago, Milo of Crotona was said to have recognized the value of progressive overload. His strength increased as he repeatedly lifted a calf. As the calf grew into a bull, its weight increased, and Milo's strength increased as well. We now know that for most people, special exercises referred to as progressive resistance exercises are necessary if muscle fitness is to be developed and maintained (see Figure 4). Activities from other levels of the physical activity pyramid rarely promote adequate muscle fitness.

The amount of overload for strength is different than for muscular endurance.

The stimulus for strength is maximal exertion. Strength training should therefore utilize high resistance overload with low repetitions. The stimulus for muscular endurance is repeated contractions with short rests. Muscular endurance exercises should be performed with a relatively high number of repetitions and lower resistance.

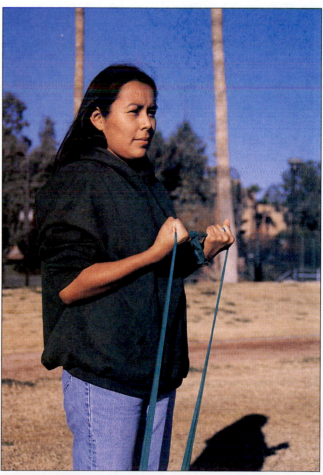

Elastic bands can provide resistance to build muscle fitness.

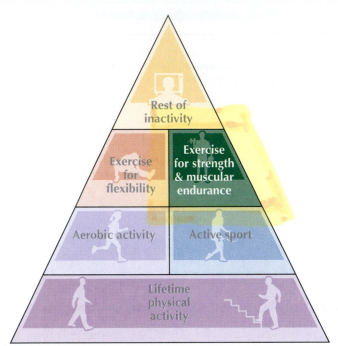

Figure 4

To build muscle fitness, activities should be selected from level 3 of the Physical Activity Pyramid.

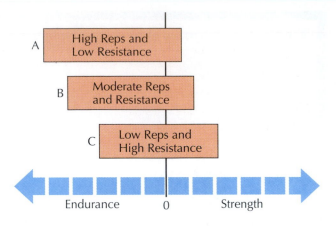

Figure 5

Comparison of muscular endurance to muscle strength developed by different repetitions and resistance.

The graph in Figure 5 illustrates the relationship between strength and muscular endurance. In *A*, the training program calls for a high number of repetitions and light resistance. This results in a small gain in strength (the area of the bar to the right of the line), and a large increase in absolute endurance (the area of the bar to the left of the line). In *B*, the training program calls for a moderate number of repetitions (less than in *A*), and a moderate resistance (more than in *A*). This results in slightly less absolute endurance and slightly more strength than in program *A*. Program *C* uses high resistance and low repetitions. This results in the least gain in endurance but the most gain in strength.

While strength training (program *C*) promotes strength, studies show that the person who is strength-trained will fatigue as much as four times faster than the person who is endurance-trained (program *A*). However, there is a modest correlation between strength and endurance because the person who trains for strength will develop some endurance, and the person who trains for muscular endurance will develop some strength.

Muscular endurance and strength are part of the same continuum.

Though strength and muscular endurance are developed in different ways, strength and muscular endurance are part of the same continuum (Figure 6). This has led some writers to refer to muscular endurance as strength endurance. "Pure" strength is approached as one nears the end (right) of the continuum, where only one maximum contraction is made. As the number of repetitions increases and the force of the contractions decreases, one nears the other end (left) of the continuum and approaches "pure" endurance. In between the two extremes, varying degrees of strength and endurance are combined. The activities listed along the continuum are examples that might represent points along the scale. You will note that most of the activities of daily living are at the middle of the continuum, indicating that they take a combination of strength and muscular endurance.

The intensity of muscle fitness training is determined using a percentage of the amount of weight you can lift one time (1 RM).

The maximum amount of resistance you can move (or weight you can lift) one time is called your one **repetition maximum (RM)**. The amount of resistance you use in a progressive resistance exercise program is based on a percentage of your 1 RM. The percentage of 1 RM used in a program depends on the program goals. For strength, the percentages vary from 60 to 80 percent depending on a person's current strength level. More experienced strength trainers often exercise at a higher percentage of 1 RM than beginners. For muscular endurance, the percentages vary from 20 to 40 percent. People interested in a combination of strength and muscular endurance should use 40 to 60 percent of 1 RM in their training.

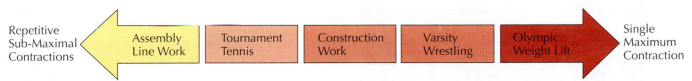

Figure 6
Muscle strength-endurance continuum.

The principle of specificity applies to progressive resistance exercise.

Depending on the specific muscle that you want to develop, you will use different types of resistance training programs. Factors that can be varied in your program are the type of muscle contraction (isometric or isotonic), the speed or cadence of the movement, and the amount of resistance being moved. For example, if you want strength in the elbow extensor muscles (e.g., triceps) so that you could more easily lift heavy boxes onto a shelf, you would train using isotonic contractions, at a relatively slow speed, with a relatively high resistance. If you want muscle fitness of the fingers to grip a heavy bowling ball, much of your training should be done isometrically using the fingers the same way you normally hold the ball. If you are training for a particular skill that requires explosive power, such as in throwing, striking, kicking, or jumping, your strength exercises should be done with less resistance and greater speed. If you are training for a skill that uses both concentric and eccentric contractions or is plyometric, you should perform strength exercises using these characteristics. More information on these techniques is included in the concept on the performance benefits of physical activity.

If you are not training for a specific task, but merely wish to develop muscle fitness for daily living, consider the advantages and disadvantages of isometrics, isotonics, and isokinetics listed in Table 1. You may wish to use a variety of methods.

The principle of diminishing returns applies to resistance training.

To get optimal strength gains from progressive resistance training, one or more sets of exercise repetitions is performed. Some high-level performers use as many as five sets of a particular exercise. Research indicates that most of the fitness and health benefits, however, are achieved in one set. As much as 80 to 90 percent of the benefits may result in the first set, with each additional set producing less and less benefit. Because compliance with resistance training programs is less likely as the time needed to complete the program increases, the American College of Sports Medicine recently recommended single-set programs for most adults. They acknowledge that additional benefits are likely with more multiset routines, but they believe that adults are more

likely to participate if they can get most of the benefits in a relatively short amount of time. In sports or competition where very small performance differences make big differences, doing multiple sets is important.

The principle of rest and recovery especially applies to strength development.

Progressive resistance training for strength development done every day of the week does not allow enough rest and time for recovery. Recent studies have shown that the greatest proportion of strength is accomplished in two days of training per week. Exercise done on a third day does result in additional increases, but the amount of gain is relatively small compared to gains resulting from two days of training per week. For people interested in health benefits rather than performance benefits, two days a week saves time and may result in greater adherence to a strength-training program. For people interested in performance benefits, more frequent training may be warranted. Rotating exercises so that certain muscles are exercised on one day and other muscles are exercised the next allows for more frequent training.

The amount of exercise necessary to maintain strength is less than the amount needed to develop it.

Recent evidence suggests that once strength is developed, it may be maintained by performing fewer sets or exercising fewer days per week. For example, if you have performed three sets of an exercise three days a week to build strength, you may be able to maintain current levels of strength with one set a week. Also you may be able to maintain strength by exercising one or two rather than three days per week. If schedules of fewer sets or fewer days per week result in strength loss, frequency must be increased.

Repetitions Maximum (RM) The maximum amount of resistance one can move a given number of times; for example: 1 RM = maximum weight lifted one time; 6 RM = maximum weight lifted six times.

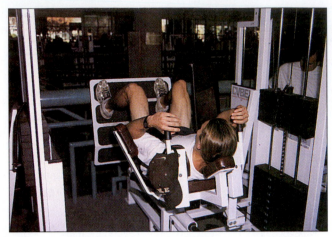

The repetition maximum (1 RM) is a good measure of strength.

Some muscle groups seem to need training less often to maintain strength levels. For example, evidence suggests that muscle fitness of the back can be maintained using one-day-a-week single-set exercises. Smaller muscles seem to need more frequent exercise.

There is a threshold of training and a target zone for strength development.

The FIT formula for strength defines the threshold and target values for strength development. Table 4 illustrates the FIT formulae for isometrics, isotonics, and isokinetic resistance training for typical people. People interested in advanced progressive resistance training, such as body builders or competitive weight lifters, will need special training programs to excel at these activities (refer to the concept on the performance benefits of physical activity).

There is a threshold of training and a target zone for muscular endurance development.

There is a frequency, intensity, and time at which a training effect for muscular endurance will begin to take place (threshold). There is also an optimal range, or target zone, where the most effective and efficient improvement will occur (see Table 5). We do not know the exact range, but studies suggest that it has wide limits. The intensity, or resistance (load), is less important than the number of repetitions or the length of time the muscle contracts.

The Facts about Using PRE Effectively

The muscle fitness workout should be based on the principle of progression.

Many beginning resistance trainers experience extreme soreness after the first few days of training. The reason for the sore-

Table 4 Strength Threshold of Training and Fitness Target Zones

	Threshold of Training			Target Zone		
	Isometrics	**Isotonics**	**Isokinetics**	**Isometrics**	**Isotonics**	**Isokinetics**
Frequency	• 2 days a week for each muscle group.			• 2 to 3 days per week		
Intensity	• Use 60–65% of maximum contraction (1 RM).	• 60–65% of 1 RM for every rep.	• 90% of 1 RM at set speed.	• Maximum contractions.	• 60–80% 1 RM (for number of reps on every set.)	• Maximum effort at set speed.
Time	• 1 set. • 1 rep held for 2–5 seconds. • Repeat once a day.	• 1 set. • 3–8 reps.	• 2 sets. • 3 reps lasting 3–4 seconds (30–60 degrees per second). • Rest 1 minute between sets.	• 1 set. • 6 reps held 6–8 seconds (or 2 sets of 3 reps each). • Rest 30 seconds between reps.	• 1–3 sets. • 3–8 reps. • Rest 1 minute between sets.	• 3–5 sets. • 3–8 reps lasting 1–2 seconds (70–120 degrees per second). • Rest 1 minute between sets.

Table 5 Muscular Endurance Threshold of Training and Fitness Target Zones

	Threshold of Training	Target Zone
Dynamic Endurance		
Frequency	• 2 days per week.	• Every other day.
Intensity	• Move 20%–30% of the maximum resistance you can lift.	• Move 40%–60% of the maximum resistance you can lift.
Time	• One set of 9 repetitions of each exercise.	• 2–5 sets of 9–25 repetitions.
		• Rest 15–60 seconds between sets.
Static Endurance		
Frequency	• 3 days per week.	• Every other day.
Intensity	• Hold a resistance 50%–100% of the weight you ultimately will need to hold in your work or leisure activity.	• Hold a resistance equal to and up to 50% greater than the amount you will need to hold in your work or leisure activity.
Time	• Hold for lengths of time 10%–50% shorter than the time you plan to do the activity. Repeat 10–20 times.	• Hold for lengths of time equal to and up to 20% greater than the time you plan to do the activity. For longer times, use fewer repetitions (5–10).
	• Rest 30 seconds between reps.	• Rest 30–60 seconds between reps.

titions in one set. As the repetitions become easy, additional repetitions are added. When you have progressed to eight repetitions, increase the resistance and decrease the repetitions in each set back to three and begin the progression again.

There are various systems available regarding the order and progression of exercises in a workout.

www.mhhe.com/hper/physed/clw/student/

There are numerous variables that could be manipulated within a training session to alter the training effect. Some recommend a "light to heavy" system (Delorme system) in which progressively heavier weights are lifted with each set. Others recommend the "heavy to light" system (Oxford system) in which the heaviest weight is used on the first set when the muscles are most rested. Still others advocate a pre-exhaust routine in which small accessory muscle groups are fatigued before the exercises for major muscle groups are performed. Various other systems are covered in the performance concept.

Circuit resistance training (CRT) is an effective way to build muscular endurance and cardiovascular endurance.

Circuit resistance training consists of the performance of high repetitions of an exercise with low to moderate resistance, progressing from one station to another, performing a different exercise at each station. The stations are usually placed in a circle to facilitate movement. CRT typically employs about 20 to 25 reps against a resistance that is 30 to 40 percent of 1 RM for 45 seconds. Fifteen seconds of rest is provided while changing stations. Approximately 10 exercise stations are used, and the participant repeats the circuit two to three times (sets). Because of the short rest periods, significant cardiovascular benefits have been reported, in addition to muscular endurance gains.

Circuit training on weight or hydraulic machines has been found to be more effective than standard set weight training for caloric consumption during and after exercise and for improving cardiovascular endurance, although it is not as effective as aerobic exercises, such as cycling or bench stepping.

Programs intended to slim the figure/physique should be of the muscular endurance type.

Many men and women are interested in exercises designed to decrease girth measurements. High-repetition, low-resistance exercise is suitable for this because it usually brings about some

ness is that the principle of progression has been violated. Soreness can occur with even modest amounts of training if the volume of training is considerably more than normal. In the first few days or weeks of training, the primary adaptations in the muscle are due to motor learning factors rather than to muscle growth. Because these adaptations occur no matter how much weight is used, it is prudent to start your program slowly with very light weights. After these adaptations occur and the rate of improvement slows down, it would be necessary to follow the appropriate target zone to achieve proper overload.

The most common progression used in resistance training is the double progressive system, so-called because this system periodically adjusts both the resistance and the number of repetitions of the exercise performed. For example, if you are training for strength, you may begin with three repe-

strengthening and may decrease body fatness, which in turn, changes body contour. Exercises do not spot-reduce fat but they do speed up metabolism so more calories are burned. However, if weight or fat reduction is desired, aerobic (cardiovascular) exercises are best. To increase girth, use strength exercises.

Endurance training may have a negative effect on strength and power.

Some studies have shown that for athletes who rely primarily on strength and power in their sports event, too much endurance training can cause a loss of strength and power because of modification of different muscle fibers. Strength and power athletes need some endurance training, but not too much, just as endurance athletes need some strength and power training, but not too much.

Is There Strength in a Bottle? The Facts

Anabolic steroids are used by some athletes and a significant number of nonathletes to enhance performance and build muscular bodies.

Anabolic steroids are prescription drugs—a synthetic reproduction of the male hormone testosterone. They may be taken orally or injected. Physicians prescribe them to treat such conditions as muscle diseases, breast cancer, severe burns, rare types of anemia, and kidney disease. Steroids have also been used to help people with AIDS and muscle-wasting diseases retain muscle mass. Because of their dangerous side effects, doctors prescribe minimal doses. At first, research showed steroids to be ineffective in promoting muscle gain. This was because the doses used in the studies were much smaller than those taken today for performance enhancement. Many athletes and people interested in muscle development have reportedly taken massive doses 20 to 100 times the normal therapeutic dose used for medical conditions. Studies now show that when taken in large doses by people doing regular strength training, gains in muscle mass and strength can be considerable. The best evidence indicates that steroids allow the muscles to recover faster, allowing more frequent training. Taking anabolic steroids without doing progressive resistance training would be counterproductive.

Anabolic steroids can be obtained on the black market or illegally from unethical physicians, coaches, trainers, body builders, athletes, and other entrepreneurs. While athletes use the drugs in an attempt to enhance performance, an increasing number of nonathletes use steroids to enhance their strength or improve their physique or appearance. Two

million people are estimated to be using "roids." Steroid use has leveled off among males, but the levels among females has increased dramatically. As many as 175,000 high school girls have used steroids primarily to look leaner.

A popular product in recent years is androstendione, also called "andro." This product causes the body to produce testosterone and has similar effects as taking artificial testosterone. It is controversial because it has not been banned by all athletic governmental groups and can be purchased legally. It has also been used by popular athletes. More than a few young athletes and nonathletes have begun using the product assuming that it must be okay if it is legal and popular athletes use it. Most experts, however, indicate that "andro" has dangers similar to anabolic steroids.

Taking anabolic steroids is illegal and a dangerous way to build muscle fitness.

The adverse side effects of taking anabolic steroids far outweigh any benefits that result from taking them. In women, unlike men, some of these effects are irreversible (see Table 6). As can be seen in the table, steroids (like all drugs) are dangerous. They can be addictive and produce more than 70 serious side effects, some of which may be fatal. More than a few deaths have been attributed to their use. Twenty-five athletes from the former Soviet Union who competed in the 1980 Olympics died because of conditions attributed to steroid use, and the deaths of several American professional athletes have also been attributed to anabolic steroid use. The death of Lyle Alzado, a former professional football star, was one of those attributed to steroid use. Unfortunately, some studies show that many athletes who use anabolic steroids are familiar with the adverse effects, but say, "I don't care, I will use them anyway."

Steroids have also been linked to other dangerous and unhealthy behaviors. Violent behavior, sometimes referred to as "roid rage," has been found to accompany steroid use. Recent research suggests that "roid rage" is most likely to result in people who are mentally unstable prior to use. Evidence indicates that steroid users are at greater risk of hepatitis or HIV/AIDS infections from shared needles.

Steroids taken in pill form are especially dangerous to the kidneys and other organs of the body. This is one reason why many medical experts are especially concerned about "andro," which is sometimes taken in pill form.

Injuries happen more easily and last longer in people who use steroids.

Though steroids may make muscles stronger, tendons and ligaments do not proportionally increase in strength. Therefore, a strong muscle contraction can tear a tendon and/or a ligament. This is made more serious because steroids make the injury heal more slowly. When steroids increase muscle

Table 6 Adverse Effects of Anabolic Steroids

Gender	Physical	Psychological
M/F	• Cancer of liver	• Total personality changes
M/F	• Cardiac disease/early heart attacks	• Hostile and aggressive; violent behavior; sexual crimes
M/F	• Hypertension and increased risk of strokes	• Addiction (both psychological and physiological)
M/F	• Edema (puffy face)	• Inability to accept failure
M/F	• Scalp hair loss** (baldness in men)	• Sleep disturbance (when cycled off drug)
M/F	• Nosebleeds	• Depression
M/F	• Premature closure of growth plates of long bones	• Apathy
M/F	• Immune system may be suppressed	• Wide mood swings
M/F	• Decreased HDL	• "Reverse anorexia" (eating compulsion)
M/F	• Decreased aerobic capacity	
M/F	• Altered glucose tolerance	
M/F	• Severe acne (face, chest, upper back, and thighs)*	
M/F	• Oily skin*	
M/F	• Muscle or bone injuries	
M/F	• Injuries take longer to heal	
M/F	• Fever	
M/F	• Frequent headaches	
M/F	• Sterility	
M/F	• Death	
M	• Testicular atrophy	
M	• Prostate enlargement	
M	• Decreased sperm count	
M	• Impotence	
M	• Feminine breast characteristics	
F	• Uterine atrophy	
F	• Decreased breast size	
F	• Menstrual irregularities	
F	• Clitoral enlargement	
F	• Deepening voice**	
F	• Dark facial hair**	

Key: M = Males; F = Females

*In women, only partially reversible when drug is stopped.

**In women, irreversible when drug is stopped.

size, the extra muscle can grow around the bones and joints, causing them to break more easily.

Human growth hormone (HGH), taken to increase strength, may be even more dangerous than anabolic steroids.

HGH is produced by the pituitary gland but is made synthetically. Some athletes are taking it in addition to anabolic

Anabolic Steroid A synthetic hormone similar to the male sex hormone testosterone. It functions androgenically to stimulate male characteristics and anabolically to increase muscle mass, weight, bone maturation, and virility.

steroids or in place of anabolic steroids because it is difficult to detect in urine tests of competitors. It is believed to increase muscle mass and bone growth and hasten healing of tendons and cartilage; however, its adverse effects can be deforming and life-threatening. They include the danger of irreversible acromegaly (giantism) and gross deformities, cardiovascular disease, goiter, menstrual disorder, excessive sweating, lax muscles and ligaments, premature bone closure, decreased sexual desire, and impotence. In addition, the life span can be shortened by as much as 20 years. Like steroids, there are some medical uses for HGH. People deficient in HGH can benefit from it, though a recent well-controlled study shows that many of the health benefits for HGH were overstated and that side effects such as swelling of the ankles and legs as well as aching of the joints and hands were common.

Another hormone being used by some male athletes is human chorionic gonadotropin (HCG), a substance found in the urine of pregnant women. It is being used to stimulate testosterone production before competition. The International Olympic Committee (IOC) has banned its use, but no test has been developed to detect it.

> **Creatine use is becoming increasingly popular among people training for strength development.**

www.mhhe.com/hper/physed/clw/student/
Creatine is produced naturally by your body from foods containing protein such as meat and fish. It is stored in the muscles and helps supply energy for muscle contraction. Because it is classified as a food supplement and not a drug, it is legal for people in competition. Users typically consume creatine as a powder that is dissolved in a liquid. Creatine supplements increase the creatine level in the muscle above the amount possible from normal food intake. The theory is that extra creatine in the muscle will allow quicker recovery from intense exercise such as vigorous strength training and sprinting. A review of many studies indicates that creatine supplements can keep muscle creatine levels higher than normal, and this may result in faster recovery from vigorous short-duration exercise bouts. This, in turn, may allow more intense workouts.

An important point is that strength gains resulting from creatine supplementation occur as a result of the increased training stimulus and not from the supplement itself. Results indicate that creatine causes relatively immediate increases in body weight, but it is mostly a result of water retention. The ability to train harder may benefit strength trainers and people interested in very short intense performances such as sprinting, but few benefits would occur for those who do not do this type of intense training. There is no evidence of mus-

cular endurance benefits or benefits to performance in swimming and distance running events. In fact, the extra weight resulting from water retention may actually impair endurance performance and may also negatively affect sports such as high jumping because the body has to lift the extra weight over the bar.

Recently, the deaths of three college wrestlers led the FDA to study creatine to determine if it was in some way associated with these deaths. No evidence of creatine involvement was found, though the various organizations have warned that creatine supplementation may precipitate dehydration. This could be a problem among athletes who are trying to lose weight by losing body water. The long-term effects of creatine supplementation are unknown, and public health officials are concerned. Short-term side effects include stomach distress and cramping. Many people using the supplement take doses far in excess of those recommended for optimal saturation in the muscles. Doses of 20 to 25 grams per day for five days followed by much smaller doses of 2 to 3 grams per day will result in maximal muscle saturation. Though not recommended for most people, if you are going to take creatine, it should not be taken in doses greater than those listed above. Further, changes in the law in 1994 leave quality-control issues up to the manufacturer rather than the government. For this reason, the quality of any food supplement (which creatine is considered) is only as good as the integrity of the supplier.

> **Some people have turned to other dietary supplements and glandular extracts, which have been promoted as substitutes for anabolic steroids.**

In an effort to avoid the undesirable side effects of anabolic steroids or the detection of its use by sports-governing bodies who have banned it, some athletes or body builders are taking chemicals and supplements such as boron, chromium picolinate, gamma oryzanol and L-carnitine (see concept on quackery). There is also a considerable market for "glandulars" such as ground-up bull testes, hypothalamus and pituitary glands, hearts, livers, spleens, and brains. These products have been advertised as "steroid alternatives." Dietitians, the FDA, and the National Council for Reliable Health Information are alarmed and consider these products potentially dangerous because they have not been tested on humans or animals for safety and effectiveness. Very little is known about some of them. There is no published scientific evidence to substantiate claims for improved human performance. An article in the *Journal of the American Medical Association* has cautioned people concerning the use of such "body-building" supplements.

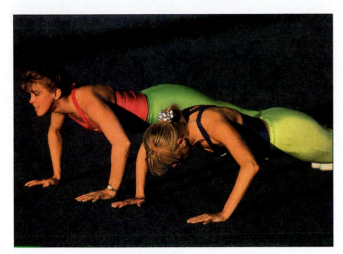

Resistance training can reduce the risk of osteoporosis.

The Facts about the Health Benefits of PRE

PRE is associated with reduced risk of osteoporosis.

PRE stresses the bones of the body. Together with good diet, including adequate calcium intake, this stress on the bones reduces the risk of osteoporosis. Evidence suggests that young people who do PRE develop a high bone density. As we grow older, bone mass decreases, so people who have a high bone density when they are young have a "bank account" from which to draw as they grow older. These people have bones that are less likely to fracture or be injured. Injuries to the bones, particularly the hip and back, are common among older adults. Regular PRE can reduce the risk of these conditions. For postmenopausal women, adequate estrogen is important in preventing osteoporosis.

PRE contributes to weight control and looking your best.

Regular PRE results in muscle mass increases. Muscle or lean body mass takes up less space than fat, contributing to attractive appearance. Further, muscle burns calories at rest so extra muscle built through PRE can contribute to increased resting and basal metabolism. Recent studies indicate that muscle mass decreases as people grow older, resulting in lower metabolism and gradual increase in body fatness. PRE can help people retain muscle mass as they grow older.

A combined strength/muscular endurance program provides most of the health benefits associated with PRE.

The *Surgeon General's Report on Physical Activity and Health* clearly identifies the benefits of muscle fitness training to good health. Recent research has shown that most of these benefits can be achieved using a combined strength/muscular endurance program. For young adults, one set of eight to 12 repetitions performed two days a week provides most of the health benefits of PRE. For older adults (50 and older), less intense exercises performed 10–15 times appears to be most effective. For both age groups, eight to 10 basic exercises are recommended so that muscle fitness of the total body is accomplished. Those who want pure strength or high-level muscular endurance for performance will benefit from extra sets and from the specific protocols outlined in tables 4 and 5. For people interested primarily in health benefits, the FIT formula outlined in Table 7 is recommended.

The Facts about PRE Methods

There is a proper way to perform resistance training.

The following are some guidelines for safe and effective strength training for beginners:

* When beginning a weight program, start with weights that are too light so you can learn proper technique and avoid soreness and injury. Novices might, for example, start with one-fourth of their body weight for the military press; 10 pounds less than the press for the curl; 10 pounds more than the press for the bench press; and half of the body weight for back and leg exercises.

Table 7	The FIT Formula for PRE Designed to Achieve Health Benefits	
Frequency	Young adults	2 to 3 days a week
	Adults over 50	2 to 3 days a week
Intensity	Young adults	40 to 60% of 1 RM
	Adults over 50	30 to 50% of 1 RM
Time	Young adults	1 set of 8 to 12 reps
	Adults over 50	1 set of 10 to 15 reps

- Progress gradually. For strength training, use one set of three repetitions with a light weight to begin; add one or two repetitions when it gets easy, then another, until you reach eight repetitions; then drop back to three repetitions and add a second set. Repeat until you can do three sets. After this, the double progressive system (previously described) can be used, increasing the weight and the repetitions.
- Beginning exercisers should probably begin with endurance training. For example, a reasonable goal might be 10 to 15 repetitions at 20 to 40 percent of the maximum amount of weight they can lift for one repetition.
- For health purposes, most people will benefit from the combined strength and endurance program.
- Beginners should not attempt to use advanced techniques. After training for several months, you may wish to experiment with such things as supersets, split routines, and plateau systems used by advanced trainers.
- To ensure overall development, include all body parts and balance the strength of antagonistic muscles. For example, the ratio of quadriceps strength to hamstring strength should be 60:40. Exercise large muscles before small muscles.
- Athletes should train muscles the way they will be used in their skill, employing similar patterns, range of motion, and speed (the principle of specificity). This applies to anyone who knows the precise skill for which he or she is training.
- If you wish to develop a particular group of muscles, remember that the muscle group can be worked harder when isolated than when worked in combination with other muscle groups.
- Sports participants should include some eccentric training, such as plyometrics, to prevent injury to decelerating muscles during sports events and to develop power in accelerating muscles. Choose an exercise sequence that alternates muscle groups so muscles have a rest period before being used in another exercise.
- Make all movements through the full range of motion.
- Isometric training should be done at several joint angles.
- To avoid boredom, especially when you reach a plateau or sticking point, use such motivating techniques as music, record keeping, partners, competition, and variation in routine.
- To avoid overtraining, take a break by resting or choosing some other activity after eight to 10 weeks. Also, try varying your training days so one is light, one is medium, and one is heavy. It has been estimated that motivation can account for 10 to 15 percent of the score on a strength test. Varying the routine helps motivation.
- Lifters may reduce spinal and abdominal injury by using a belt that supports the back and abdomen.
- Unilateral training allows a muscle to exert more force than is possible when both sides of the body work simultaneously (bilaterally).

There are many fallacies, myths, and superstitions associated with strength training.

Some common misconceptions about strength training are described below:

- It is *not* true that you will become muscle-bound and lose flexibility just because you do strength training. This could only happen if you train improperly. It has been found, however, that powerlifters are less flexible than other weight lifters.
- It is *not* true that women will become masculine looking if they develop strength. Contrary to popular belief, most women will not be able to develop as large and bulky muscles as men, nor will their muscles be as well defined. On a heavy resistance training program, women and men make about the same percentage change in strength and hypertrophy. The greater percentage of fat in most women prevents the muscle definition possible in men and camouflages the increase in bulk. (Until CAT scans were used in research studies, it was not evident that women achieved hypertrophy at the same rate as men.)
- Strength training does *not* make you move more slowly or make you more uncoordinated. Up to a point, increased strength may help to increase speed.
- The expression *"no pain, no gain"* is a fallacy. It may be helpful to strive for a burning sensation in the muscle, but this is not painful. If it hurts, you are probably harming yourself.
- Protein supplements are not ergogenic aids and do *not* benefit muscle mass or strength building. You do need a balanced diet, however.
- Drugs do *not* make you fit. Anabolic steroids, growth hormones, diuretics, narcotics, and other drugs taken to enhance performance are extremely dangerous and ultimately produce an unhealthy person rather than a fit one.
- Strength training is *not* effective in building cardiovascular fitness and flexibility. Gains in muscle mass do cause an increase in resting metabolism so muscle fitness training can aid in controlling body fatness.
- It does *not* require two hours to complete a workout in weight training—unless you are a competitive lifter or bodybuilder. If you are training for athletics, you will need 45 to 90 minutes; the beginner or the person training for fitness or recreation can complete a circuit in 30 to 45 minutes.
- It is *not* true that progressive resistance training is only for young people. Studies have shown that even people in the 80s and 90s can benefit from regular PRE training.

Table 8   How to Prevent Injury (for the Beginner)

- Warm up 10 minutes before the workout and stay warm during the workout.
- Do not hold your breath while lifting. This may cause blackout or hernia.
- Avoid hyperventilation before lifting a weight.
- Avoid dangerous or high-risk exercises.
- Progress slowly.
- Use good shoes with good traction.
- Avoid arching your back. Keep the pelvis in normal alignment.
- Keep the weight close to the body.
- Do not lift from a stoop (bent over with back rounded).
- When lifting from the floor, do not let the hips come up before your upper body.
- For bent-over rowing, lay your head on a table and bend the knees, or use one-arm rowing and support the trunk with the free hand.
- Stay in a squat as short a time as possible and do not do a full squat.
- Be sure collars on free weights are tight.
- Use a moderately slow, continuous, controlled movement and hold the final position a few seconds.
- Overload but don't overwhelm! A program that is too intense can cause injuries.
- Do not pause between repetitions.
- Try to keep a steady rhythm.
- Do not allow the weights to drop or bang.
- Do not train without medical supervision if you have a hernia, high blood pressure, fever, infection, recent surgery, heart disease, or back problems.
- Use chalk or a towel to keep hands dry when handling weights.

Most injuries can be prevented by using correct technique and proper care.

Refer to Table 8 for some tips on injury prevention.

Strategies for Action: The Facts

An important step in taking action for developing and maintaining muscle fitness is assessing your current status.

www.mhhe.com/hper/physed/clw/student/
An important early step in taking action to improve fitness is self-assessment. There are many different tests of muscle fitness. A 1 RM

test of isotonic strength is described in the lab resource materials. This test allows you to determine both absolute and relative strength for the arms and legs. In addition, the 1 RM values can be used to help you select the appropriate resistance for your muscle fitness training program. A grip strength test of isometric strength is also provided in the resource materials for Lab 11A. In addition to descriptions of the 1 RM test, a body weight test for isotonic strength is provided in the Web Review for people who do not have the equipment to perform the 1 RM assessment.

www.mhhe.com/hper/physed/clw/student/
Three tests of muscular endurance are described in the lab resource materials for Lab 11B. It is recommended that you perform the assessments for both strength and muscular endurance before you begin your progressive resistance training program. Periodically reevaluate your muscle fitness using these assessments.

Many factors other than your own basic abilities affect muscle fitness test scores.

If muscles are warmed up before lifting, more force can be exerted, and heavier loads can be lifted. Muscle endurance performance may also be enhanced by a warm-up. It is important, however, not to perform your self-assessments after vigorous exercise because that exercise can cause fatigue and result in less-than-optimal test results. It is appropriate to practice the techniques involved in the various tests on days preceding the actual testing. People who have good technique achieve better scores than those who do not have good technique and are less likely to be injured when performing tests. It is best to perform the strength and muscular endurance tests on different days.

Choose exercises that build muscle fitness in the major muscle groups of the body.

www.mhhe.com/hper/physed/clw/student/
The American College of Sports Medicine recommends eight to ten basic exercises for muscle fitness. The Basic 8 exercises for free weights and resistance machines should be supplemented with one or both of the exercises presented in Table 9.) To aid the reader, four different sets of basic exercises have been prepared for free weights (Table 10), resistance machines (Table 11), isometrics (Table 12), and calisthenics (Table 13). For most people performing the Basic 8, using any of the four types of exercises will produce the majority of benefits associated muscle fitness.

People interested in additional exercises that serve as alternates exercises or that focus on improving fitness in other muscle groups are referred to the supplemental exercises in Webshow. Webshow also includes eight basic exercises using elastic bands as well as many of the exercises described in Table 13.

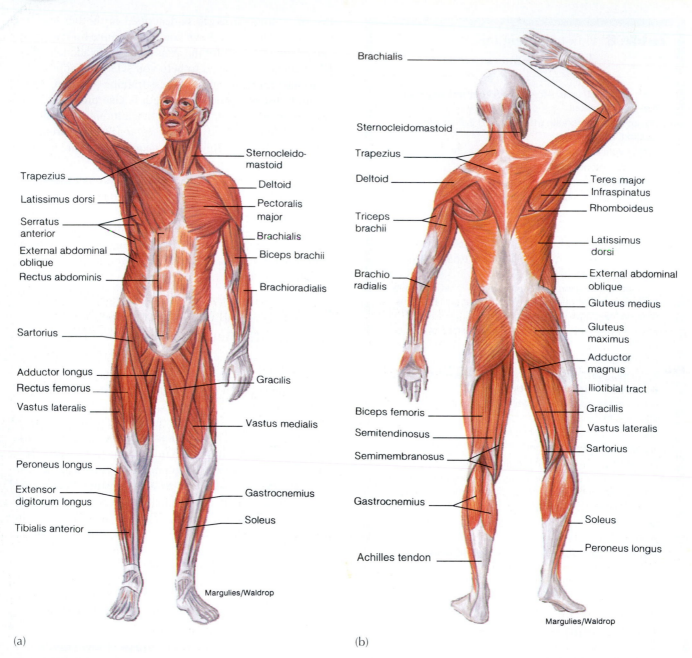

Trapezius

Latissimus dorsi

Serratus anterior

External abdominal oblique

Rectus abdominis

Sartorius

Adductor longus

Rectus femorus

Vastus lateralis

Peroneus longus

Extensor digitorum longus

Tibialis anterior

Sternocleido-mastoid

Deltoid

Pectoralis major

Brachialis

Biceps brachii

Brachioradialis

Gracilis

Vastus medialis

Gastrocnemius

Soleus

Margulies/Waldrop

(a)

Brachialis

Sternocleidomastoid

Trapezius

Deltoid

Triceps brachii

Brachio radialis

Biceps femoris

Semitendinosus

Semimembranosus

Gastrocnemius

Achilles tendon

Teres major

Infraspinatus

Rhomboideus

Latissimus dorsi

External abdominal oblique

Gluteus medius

Gluteus maximus

Adductor magnus

Iliotibial tract

Gracillis

Vastus lateralis

Sartorius

Soleus

Peroneus longus

Margulies/Waldrop

(b)

Figure 8

Muscles in the body.

> Keeping records of progress is important to adhering to a PRE program.

An activity logging sheet is provided in Lab 11C to help you keep records of your progress as you regularly perform PRE to build and maintain good muscle fitness. A guide to the different muscles of the body is presented in Figure 8.

 Web Review

Web review materials for Concept 11 are available are at *www.mhhe.com/hper/physed/clw/student/*.

American College of Sports Medicine
   www.acsm.org
Muscle Fitness Exercises
   www.mhhe.com/hper/physed/clw/student/
National Athletic Trainers Association
   www.nata.org
National Strength and Conditioning Association
   www.nsca-cc.org/aboutnsca.htm

Suggested Readings

Ebbens, W. P., and Jensen, R. L. Strength Training for *and Sports Medicine*. 26(5)(1998):86.

Feigenbaum, M. S., and Pollock, M. L. Strength Training: Rationale for Current Guidelines for Adult Fitness Programs. *Physician and Sports Medicine*. 25(2)(1997):44.

Franklin, B. A. Pumping Iron: Rationale, Benefits, Safety, and Prescription. *ACSM's Health and Fitness Journal*. 2(5)(1998):12.

Franks, B. D., Welsch, M. A., and Wood, R.H. "Physical Activity Intensity: How Much Is Enough?" *ACSM's Health and Fitness Journal* 1(6)(1998): 14–19.

Philen, R., et al. Survey of Advertising for Nutritional Supplements in Health and Body Building Magazines. *Journal of the American Medical Association* 268(1992):1008.

Physician and Sportsmedicine. Androstenedione et al: Nonprescription Steroids. *Physician and Sports Medicine*. 26(11)(1998):15.

Pollock, M. L., and Vincent, K. R. "Resistance Training for Health." *President's Council on Physical Fitness and Sports Research Digest* 2(8) (1996): 1996.

Pope, H. G., et al. Muscle Dysmorphia: An Underrecognized Form of Body Dysmorphic Disorder. *Psychosomatics*. 38(6)(1997):548.

Volek, J. S. Creatine Supplementation and Its Possible Role in Improving Physical Performance. *ACSM's Health and Fitness Journal*. 1(4)(1997):23.

Westcott, W., *Strength Fitness*, 4th ed. Dubuque, IA: Brown & Benchmark Publishers, 1995.

Westcott, W. L., and Baechle, T. R. *Strength Training for Seniors*. Champaign, IL: Human Kinetics, 1999.

Yesalis, C. E., and Cowart, V. S. *The Steroids Game*. Champaign, IL: Human Kinetics, 1998.

Table 9
Exercise for the Abdominals

1. Crunch (Curl-Up)

This exercise develops the upper abdominal muscles. Lie on the floor with the knees bent and the arms extended or crossed with hands on shoulders or palms on ears. If desired, legs may rest on bench to increase difficulty. For less resistance, place hands at side of body (do not put hands behind neck). For more resistance, move hands higher. Curl up until shoulder blades leave floor, then roll down to the starting position. Repeat. Note: Twisting the trunk on the curl-up develops the oblique abdominals.

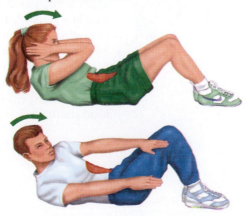

2. Reverse Curl

This exercise develops the lower abdominal muscles. Lie on the floor. Bend the knees, place the feet flat on the floor, and place arms at sides. Lift the knees to the chest, raising the hips off the floor; do not let the knees go past the shoulders. Return to the starting position. Repeat.

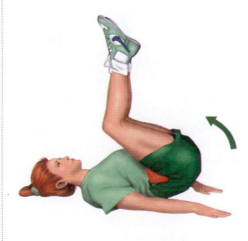

Table 10

The Basic 8 for Free Weights

1. Bench Press

This exercise develops the chest (pectoral) and triceps muscles. Lie supine on bench with knees bent and feet flat on bench or flat on floor in stride position. Grasp bar at shoulder level. Push bar up until arms are straight. Return; repeat; do not arch lower back. Note: Feet may be placed on floor if lower back can be kept flattened. Do not put feet on the bench if it is unstable.

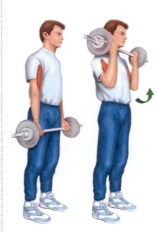

3. Biceps Curl

This exercise develops the muscles of the upper front part of the arms (biceps). Stand erect with back against a wall, palms forward, bar touching thighs. Spread feet in comfortable position. Tighten abdominals and back muscles. Do not lock knees. Move bar to chin, keeping body straight and elbows near the sides. Lower bar to original position. Do not allow back to arch. Repeat. Spotters are usually not needed. Variations: Use dumbbell and sit on end of bench with feet in stride position, work one arm at a time; or use dumbbell with the palm down or thumb up to emphasize other muscles.

2. Overhead (Military Press)

This exercise develops the muscles of the shoulders and arms. Sit erect, bend elbows, palms facing forward at chest level, hands spread (slightly more than shoulder width). Have bar touching chest, spread feet (comfortable distance). Tighten your abdominal and back muscles. Move bar to overhead position (arms straight). Lower bar to chest position. Repeat. Caution: Keep arms perpendicular and do not allow weight to move backward or wrists to bend backward. Spotters are needed.

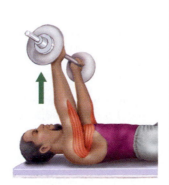

4. Triceps Curl

This exercise develops the muscles on the back of the upper arms (triceps). Sit erect, elbows and palms facing up, bar resting behind neck on shoulders, hands near center of bar, feet spread. Tighten abdominal and back muscles. Keep upper arms stationary. Raise weight overhead, return bar to original position. Repeat. Spotters are needed. Variation: Substitute dumbbells (one in each hand, or one held in both hands, or one in one hand at a time).

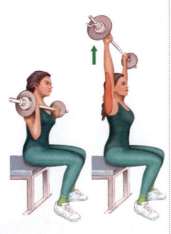

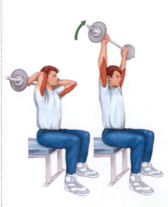

Table 10
The Basic 8 for Free Weights *(continued)*

5. Wrist Curl

This exercise develops the muscles of the fingers, wrist, and forearms. Sit astride a bench with the back of one forearm on the bench, wrist and hand hanging over the edge. Hold a dumbbell in the fingers of that hand with the palm facing forward. To develop the flexors, lift the weight by curling the fingers then the wrist through a full range of motion. Slowly lower and repeat. To strengthen the extensors, start with the palm down. Lift the weight by extending the wrist through a full range of motion. Slowly lower and repeat. Note: Both wrists may be exercised at the same time by substituting a barbell in place of the dumbbell.

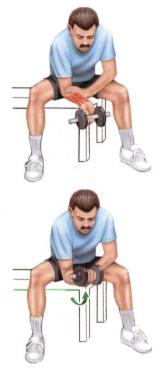

6. Half-Squat

This exercise develops the muscles of the thighs and buttocks. Stand erect, feet turned out 45 degrees. Rest bar behind neck on shoulders. Spread hands in a comfortable position. Squat slowly, keeping back straight, eyes ahead. Bend knees to approximately 90 degrees; keep knees over feet. Pause, then stand. Repeat. Spotters are needed. Variations: Substitute dumbbell in each hand at sides.

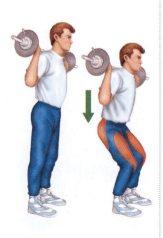

7. Lunge

This exercise develops the thigh and gluteal muscles. Place a barbell (with or without weight) behind your head and support with hands placed slightly wider than shoulder-width apart. In a slow and controlled motion, take a step forward and allow the leading leg to drop so that it is nearly parallel with the ground. The lower part of the leg should be near vertical and the back should be maintained in an upright posture. Take stride with opposite leg to return to standing posture. Repeat with other leg, remaining stationary or moving slowly in a straight line with alternating steps.

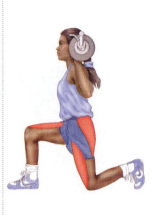

8. Heel Raise

This exercise develops the muscles of the legs (calf). Stand erect with palms facing forward, hands wider than shoulder-width apart, bar resting behind neck on shoulders. Rest balls of feet on 2-inch block with heels on floor. Toes together, heels apart. Rise on toes quickly, hold for 1 second. Lower heels to floor. Repeat. Keep toes turned in slightly. Spotters are needed. Note: Some people do this with toes straight ahead or turned out; however, this tends to weaken the foot muscles.

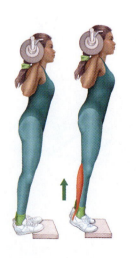

Table 11
The Basic 8 for Resistance Machine Exercises

1. Chest Press

This exercise develops the chest (pectoral) and tricep muscles. Position seat height so that arm handles are directly in front of chest. Position backrest so that hands are at a comfortable distance away from the chest. Push handles forward to full extension and return to starting position in a slow and controlled manner. Repeat. Note: Machine may have a foot lever to help position, raise, and lower the weight.

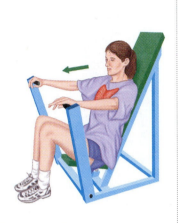

2. Seated Press

This exercise develops the muscles of the shoulders and arms. Position seat so that arm handles are slightly above shoulder height. Grasp handles with palms facing away and push lever up until arms are fully extended. Return to starting position and repeat. Note: Some machines may have an incline press.

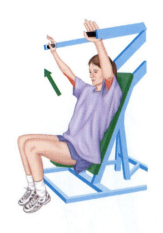

3. Bicep Curl

This exercise develops the elbow flexor muscles on the front of the arm—primarily the biceps. Adjust seat height so that arms are fully supported by pad when extended. Grasp handles palms up. While keeping the back straight, flex the elbow through the full range of motion.

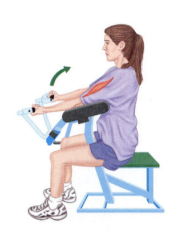

4. Tricep Press

This exercise develops the extensor muscles on the back of arm—primarily the triceps. Adjust seat height so that arm handles are slightly above shoulder height. Grasp handles with thumbs toward body. While keeping the back straight, extend arms fully until wrist contacts the support pad (arms straight). Return to starting position and repeat.

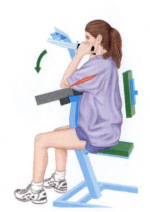
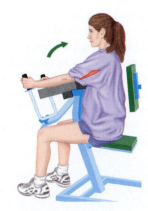

Table 11
The Basic 8 for Resistance Machine Exercises (*continued*)

5. Lat Pull Down

This exercise primarily develops the latissmus dorsi, but the biceps, chest, and other back muscles may also be developed. Sit on the floor. Adjust seat height so that hands can just grasp bar when arms are fully extended. Grasp bar with palms facing away from you and hands shoulder-width (or wider) apart. Pull bar down to chest and return. Repeat.

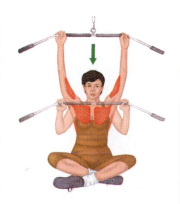

7. Knee Extension

This exercise develops the thigh (quadriceps) muscles. Sit on end of bench with ankles hooked under padded bar. Grasp edge of table. Extend knees. Return; repeat. Alternative: Leg press (similar to half-squat). Note: The knee extension exercise isolates the quadriceps but places greater stress on the structures of the knee than the leg press or half-squat.

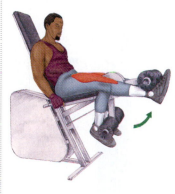

6. Seated Rowing

This exercise develops the muscles of the back and shoulder. Adjust the machine so that arms are almost fully extended and parallel to the ground. Grasp handgrip with palms turned down and hands shoulder-width apart. While keeping the back straight, pull levers straight back to chest. Slowly return to starting position and repeat.

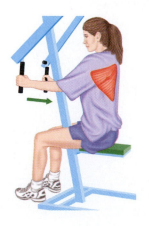
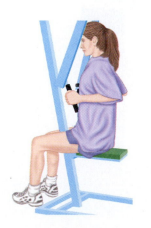

8. Hamstring Curl

This exercise develops the hamstrings (muscles on back of thigh) and other knee flexors. Lie prone on bench with ankles hooked under padded bar. Rest chin on hands or grasp bench. Flex knees as far as possible without allowing hips to raise. Return; repeat. Caution: Do not hyperextend the knees while assuming the starting position. If necessary, ask a partner to raise the pads while you place the heels under the bar.

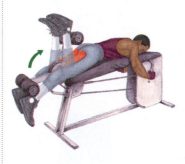

Table 12
The Basic 8 for Isometric Exercises

1. Arm Press in Doorway

This exercise develops the tricep and pectoral muscles. Stand in doorway, back flat on one side of doorway, hands placed on other side. Push with maximum force.

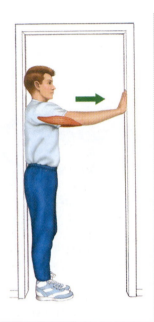

3. Curls

This exercise develops the muscles on the front of the arms. Place rope or towel loop behind thighs while standing in a half-squat position. Grasp loop, palms up, shoulder-width apart. Lift upward with maximum effort. Variation: Repeat, gripping with palms down.

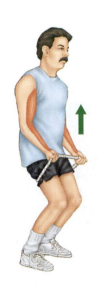

2. Overhead Press in Doorway

This exercise develops the muscles of the arms and shoulders. Stand in doorway, face straight ahead, hands shoulder-width apart, elbows bent. Tighten leg, hip, and back muscles. Push upward as hard as possible.

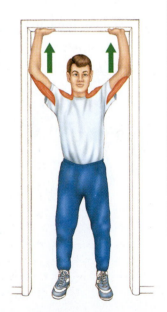

4. Triceps Press

This exercise develops the muscles on the back of the upper arm (triceps). Grasp towel or rope at both ends. Hold left hand at small of back, right hand over shoulder. Pull hands apart with maximum force; repeat exercise, reversing position of hands.

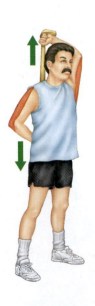

Table 12
The Basic 8 for Isometric Exercises (continued)

5. Pelvic Tilt

This exercise develops the muscles of the abdomen and buttocks. Assume a supine position with the knees bent and slightly apart. Press the spine down on the floor and hold for several seconds. Keep abdominal and gluteal muscles tightened.

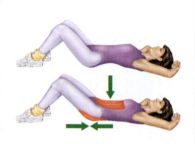

7. Wall Seat

This exercise develops the muscles of the legs and hips. Assume a half-sit position, back flat against wall, knees bent to 90 degrees. Push back against wall with maximum force and hold for several seconds.

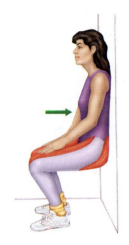

6. Leg Press in Doorway

This exercise develops the muscles of the legs and hips. Sit in doorway facing side of door frame. Grasp molding behind head. Keep back flat on side of doorway, feet against other side. Push legs with maximum force and hold for several seconds.

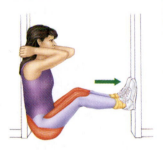

8. Hamstring Curl

This exercise develops the muscles on back of legs. Stand on rope or towel loop with left foot. Place loop around right ankle. Flex knee until taut. Apply maximum force upward.

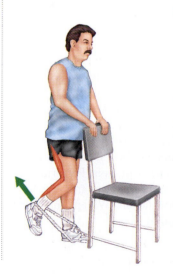

Table 13
The Basic 8 for Calesthenics

1. Bent Knee Push-Ups and Let-Down

This exercise develops the muscles of the arms, shoulders, and chest. Lie on the floor face down with the hands under your shoulders. Keep your body straight from the knees to the top of the head. Push up until the arms are straight. Slowly lower chest (let-down) to floor. Repeat. Variation: full push-up and let-down performed the same way except body is straight from the toes to the top of head. Variation: Start from the up position and lower until the arm is bent at 90 degrees; then push up until arms are extended. Caution: Do not arch back.

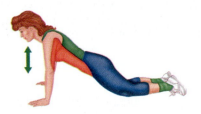

2. Modified Pull-Ups

This exercise develops the muscles of the arms and shoulders. Hang (palms forward and shoulder-width apart) from a low bar (may be placed across two chairs), heels on floor, with the body straight from feet to head. Bracing the feet against a partner or fixed object is helpful. Pull up, keeping the body straight, touch the chest to the bar, then lower to the starting position. Repeat. Note: This exercise becomes more difficult as the angle of the body approaches horizontal and easier as it approaches the vertical. Variation: Perform so that the feet do not touch the floor (full pull-up). Variation: Perform with palms turned up. When palms are turned away from the face, pull-ups tend to use all the elbow flexors. With palms facing the body, the biceps are emphasized more.

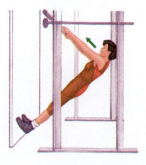

3. Dips

This exercise will develop the latissimus dorsi (on the back) and also the tricep. Start in a fully extended position with hands grasping the bar (palms facing in). Slowly drop down until the upper part of the arm is horizontal or parallel with the floor. Extend the arms back up to the starting position and repeat. Note: Many gyms have a dip/pull-up machine with accommodating resistance that provides a variable amount of assistance to help you complete the exercise.

4. Crunch (Curl-Up)

This exercise develops the upper abdominal muscles. Lie on the floor with the knees bent and the arms extended or crossed with hands on shoulders or palms on ears. If desired, legs may rest on bench to increase difficulty. For less resistance, place hands at side of body (do not put hands behind neck). For more resistance, move hands higher. Curl up until shoulder blades leave floor, then roll down to the starting position. Repeat. Note: Twisting the trunk on the curl-up develops the oblique abdominals.

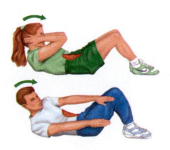

Table 13
The Basic 8 for Calesthenics (continued)

5. (Trunk) Lift

This exercise develops the muscles of the upper back and corrects round shoulders. Lie face down with hands clasped behind the neck. Pull the shoulder blades together, raising the elbows off the floor. Slowly raise the head and chest off the floor by arching the upper back. Return to the starting position; repeat. For less resistance, hands may be placed under thighs. Caution: Do not arch the lower back; lift only until the sternum (breastbone) clears the floor. Variations: arms down at sides (easiest), hands by head, arms extended (hardest).

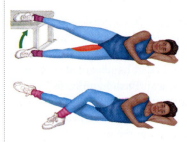

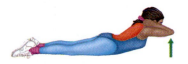

7. Lower Leg Lift

This exercise develops the muscles on the inside of thighs. Lie on the side with the upper leg (foot) supported on a bench. Note: If no bench is available, bend top leg and cross it in front of bottom leg for support. Raise the lower leg toward the ceiling; repeat. Roll to opposite side and repeat. Keep knees pointed forward. Variation: An ankle weight may be added for greater resistance.

6. Side Leg Raises

This exercise develops the muscles on the outside of thighs. Lie on your side. Point knees forward. Raise the top leg 45 degrees, then return. Do the same number of repetition with each leg. Caution: Keep knee and toes pointing forward. Variation: Ankle weights may be added for greater resistance.

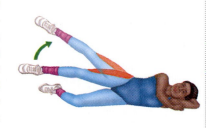

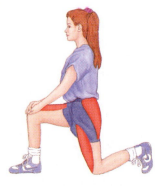

8. Alternate Leg Kneel

This exercise develops the muscles of the legs and hips. Stand tall, feet together. Take a step forward with the right foot, touching the left knee to the floor. The knees should be bent only to a 90-degree angle. Return to the starting position and step out with the other foot. Repeat, alternating right and left. Variation: Dumbbells may be held in the hands for greater resistance.

Lab Resource Material

Table 14
IRM Tests

1. Seated Press (Chest Press)

This test can be performed using a seated press (see picture) or using a bench press machine. When using the seated position the seat height so that arm handles are directly in front of the chest. Position backrest so that hands are at comfortable distance a way from the chest. Push handles foreward to full extension and return to starting position in a slow and controlled manner. Repeat. Note: machine may have a foot lever to help position raise, and lower the weight.

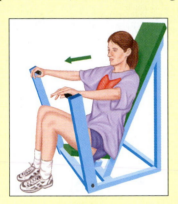

2. Leg Press

To perform this test use a leg press machine. Typically, the beginning position is with the knees bent at right angles with the feet placed on the press machine pedals or a foot platform. Extend the legs and return to beginning position, Do not lock the knees when the legs are straightened. Typically handles are provided. Grasp the handles with the hands when performing this test.

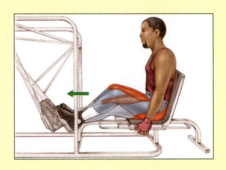

Lab Resource Material

Evaluating Isotonic Strength: 1 RM

1. Use a weight machine for the leg press and seated arm press (or bench press) for the evaluation.
2. Estimate how much weight you can lift two or three times. Be conservative; it is better to start with too little weight than too much. If you lift the weight more than 10 times, the procedure should be done again on another day when you are rested.
3. Using correct form, perform a leg press with the weight you have chosen. Perform as many times as you can up to 10.
4. Use chart 1 to determine your 1 RM for the leg press. Find the weight used in the left-hand column and then find the number of repetition you performed across the top of the chart.
5. Your 1 RM score is the value where the weight row and the repetitions column intersect.
6. Repeat this procedure for the seated arm press.
7. Record your 1 RM scores for the leg press and seated arm press in the Results section.
8. Next, divide your 1 RM scores by your body weight in pounds to get a "strength per pound of body weight" (str/lb/body wt.) score for each of the two exercises.
9. Finally, determine your strength rating for your upper body strength (arm press) and lower body (leg press) using chart 2.

Chart 1 Predicted 1 RM Based on Reps-to-Fatigue

Wt	\multicolumn{10}{Repetitions}										Wt	\multicolumn{10}{Repetitions}								
	1	2	3	4	5	6	7	8	9	10		1	2	3	4	5	6	7	8	9	10
30	30	31	32	33	34	35	36	37	38	39	170	170	175	180	185	191	197	204	211	219	227
35	35	37	38	39	40	41	42	43	44	45	175	175	180	185	191	197	203	210	217	225	233
40	40	41	42	44	46	47	49	50	51	53	180	180	185	191	196	202	209	216	223	231	240
45	45	46	48	49	51	52	54	56	58	60	185	185	190	196	202	208	215	222	230	238	247
50	50	51	53	55	56	58	60	62	64	67	190	190	195	201	207	214	221	228	236	244	253
55	55	57	58	60	62	64	66	68	71	73	195	195	201	206	213	219	226	234	242	251	260
60	60	62	64	65	67	70	72	74	77	80	200	200	206	212	218	225	232	240	248	257	267
65	65	67	69	71	73	75	78	81	84	87	205	205	211	217	224	231	238	246	254	264	273
70	70	72	74	76	79	81	84	87	90	93	210	210	216	222	229	236	244	252	261	270	280
75	75	77	79	82	84	87	90	93	96	100	215	215	221	228	235	242	250	258	267	276	287
80	80	82	85	87	90	93	96	99	103	107	220	220	226	233	240	247	255	264	273	283	293
85	85	87	90	93	96	99	102	106	109	113	225	225	231	238	245	253	261	270	279	289	300
90	90	93	95	98	101	105	108	112	116	120	230	230	237	244	251	259	267	276	286	296	307
95	95	98	101	104	107	110	114	118	122	127	235	235	242	249	256	264	273	282	292	302	313
100	100	103	106	109	112	116	120	124	129	133	240	240	247	254	262	270	279	288	298	309	320
105	105	108	111	115	118	122	126	130	135	140	245	245	252	259	267	276	285	294	304	315	327
110	110	113	116	120	124	128	132	137	141	147	250	250	257	265	273	281	290	300	310	321	333
115	115	118	122	125	129	134	138	143	148	153	255	256	262	270	278	287	296	306	317	328	340
120	120	123	127	131	135	139	144	149	154	160	260	260	267	275	284	292	302	312	323	334	347
125	125	129	132	136	141	145	150	155	161	167	265	265	273	281	289	298	308	318	329	341	353
130	130	134	138	142	146	151	156	161	167	173	270	270	278	286	295	304	314	324	335	347	360
135	135	139	143	147	152	157	162	168	174	180	275	275	283	291	300	309	319	330	341	354	367
140	140	144	148	153	157	163	168	174	180	187	280	280	288	296	305	315	325	336	348	360	373
145	145	149	154	158	163	168	174	180	186	193	285	285	293	302	311	321	331	342	354	366	380
150	150	154	159	164	169	174	180	186	193	200	290	290	298	307	316	326	337	348	360	373	387
155	155	159	164	169	174	180	186	192	199	207	295	295	303	312	322	332	343	354	366	379	393
160	160	165	169	175	180	186	192	199	206	213	300	300	309	318	327	337	348	360	372	386	400
165	165	170	175	180	186	192	198	205	212	220	305	305	314	323	333	343	354	366	379	392	407

This chart is reprinted with permission from the *Journal of Physical Education, Recreation & Dance*, January 1993, p. 89. *JOPERD* is a publication of the American Alliance for Health, Physical Education, Recreation and Dance, 1900 Association Drive, Reston, VA 22091.

Evaluating Isometric Strength

Test: *Grip Strength*

Adjust a hand dynamometer to fit your hand size. Squeeze it as hard as possible. You may bend or straighten the arm, but do not touch the body with your hand, elbow, or arm. Perform with both right and left hands. *Note:* When not being tested, perform the basic 8 isometric strength exercises, or try to squeeze and indent a new tennis ball (*after* completing the dynamometer test).

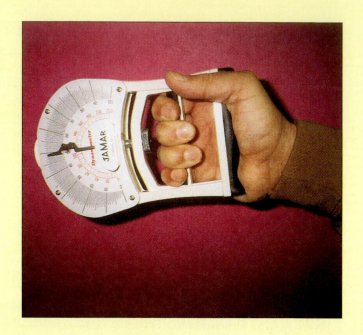

Evaluating Muscular Endurance

1.   Curl-Up (Dynamic)

Sit on a mat or carpet with your legs bent more than 90 degrees so your feet remain flat on the floor (about halfway between 90 degrees and straight). Make two tape marks 4-1/2 inches apart or lay a 4-1/2 inch strip of paper or cardboard on the floor. Lie with your arms extended at your sides, palms down and the fingers extended so that your fingertips touch one tape mark (or one side of the paper or cardboard strip). Keeping your heels in contact with the floor, curl the head and shoulders forward until your fingers reach 4-1/2 inches (second piece of tape or other side of strip). Lower slowly to beginning position. Repeat one curl-up every 3 seconds. Continue until you are unable to keep the pace of one curl-up every 3 seconds.

Two partners may be helpful. One stands on the cardboard strip (to prevent movement) if one is used. The second assures that the head returns to the floor after each repetition.

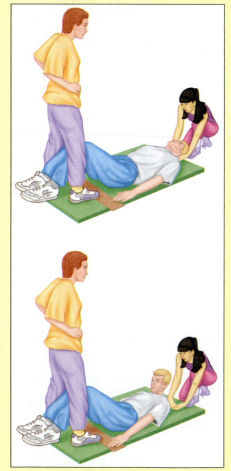

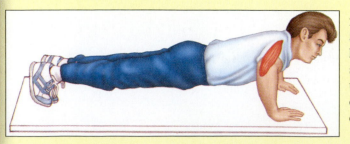

2.   Ninety-Degree Push-Up (Dynamic)

Support the body in a push-up position from the toes. The hands should be just outside the shoulders, the back and legs straight, and the toes tucked under. Lower the body until the upper arm is parallel to the floor or the elbow is bent at 90 degrees. The rhythm should be approximately one push-up every 3 seconds. Repeat as many times as possible up to 35.

3.   Flexed-Arm Support (Static)

Women: Support the body in a push-up position from the knees. The hands should be outside the shoulders, and the back and legs straight. Lower the body until the upper arm is parallel to the floor or the elbow is flexed at 90 degrees.

Men: Use the same procedure as for women except support the push-up position from the toes instead of the knees. (Same position as for 90-degree push-up, see previous page.) Hold the 90-degree position as long as possible, up to 35 seconds.

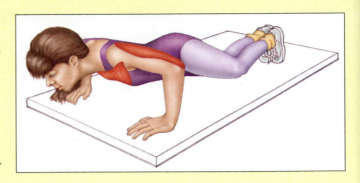

Chart 2 Strength Per Pound of Body Weight Ratings

Rating:	Leg Press			Arm Press		
Age:	30 or Less	31–50	51+	30 or Less	31–50	51+
Men						
High-performance	2.06+	1.81+	1.61+	1.26+	1.01+	.86+
Good fitness	1.96–2.05	1.66–1.80	1.51–1.60	1.11–1.25	.91–1.00	.76–0.85
Marginal	1.76–1.95	1.51–1.65	1.41–1.50	.96–1.10	.86–0.90	.66–0.75
Low fitness	1.75 or less	1.50 or less	1.40 or less	.96 or less	.80 or less	.65 or less
Women						
High-performance	1.61+	1.36+	1.16+	.75+	.61+	.51+
Good fitness	1.46–1.60	1.21–1.35	1.06–1.15	.65–0.75	.56–0.60	.46–0.50
Marginal	1.31–1.45	1.11–1.20	.96–1.05	.56–0.65	.51–0.55	.41–0.45
Low fitness	1.30 or less	1.10 or less	.95 or less	.55 or less	.50 or less	.40 or less

Chart 3 Isometric Strength Rating Scale (Pounds)

Classification	Left Grip	Right Grip	Total Score
Men			
High-performance zone	125+	135+	260+
Good fitness zone	100–124	110–134	210–259
Marginal zone	90–99	95–109	185–209
Low zone	less than 90	less than 95	less than 185
Women			
High-performance zone	75+	85+	160+
Good fitness zone	60–74	70–84	130–159
Marginal zone	45–59	50–69	95–129
Low zone	less than 45	less than 50	less than 95

Suitable for use by young adults between 18 and 30 years of age. After 30, an adjustment of 0.5 of 1 percent per year is appropriate because some loss of muscle tissue typically occurs as you grow older.

Chart 4 Rating Scale for Dynamic Muscular Endurance

Age:	17–26		27–39		40–49		50–59		60+	
Classification	Curl-Up	Push-Ups	Curl-Up	Push-Ups	Curl-Up	Push-Ups	Curl-Up	Push-Ups	Curl-Up	Push-Ups
Men										
High-performance zone	35+	29+	34+	27+	33+	26+	32+	24+	31+	22+
Good fitness zone	24–34	20–28	23–33	18–26	22–32	17–25	21–31	15–23	20–30	13–21
Marginal zone	15–23	16–19	14–22	15–17	13–21	14–16	12–20	12–14	11–19	10–12
Low zone	<15	<16	<14	<15	<13	<14	<12	<12	<11	<10
Women										
High-performance zone	25+	17+	24+	16+	23+	15+	22+	14+	21+	13+
Good fitness zone	18–24	12–16	17–23	11–15	16–22	10–14	15–21	9–13	14–20	8–12
Marginal zone	10–17	8–11	9–16	7–10	8–15	6–9	7–14	5–8	6–13	4–7
Low zone	<10	<8	<9	<7	<8	<6	<7	<5	<6	<4

Chart 5 Rating Scale for Static Endurance (Flexed-Arm Support)

Classification	Score in Seconds
High-performance zone	30+
Good fitness zone	20–29
Marginal zone	10–19
Low zone	10

Lab 11A: Evaluating Muscle Strength: 1 RM and Grip Strength

Brandie Marett	10	10/26
Name	**Section**	**Date**

Purpose: To evaluate your muscle strength using 1 RM and to determine the best amount of weight to use for various strength exercises.

Procedure: 1 RM refers to the maximum amount of weight you can lift for a specific exercise. Testing yourself to determine how much you can lift only one time using traditional methods can be fatiguing and even dangerous. The procedure you will perform here allows you to estimate 1 RM based on the number of times you can lift a weight that is less than 1 RM.

Evaluating Strength Using Estimated 1 RM

1. Use a resistance machine for the leg press and arm or bench bench press for the evaluation part of this lab.
2. Estimate how much weight you can lift two or three times. Be conservative; it is better to start with too little weight than too much. If you lift a weight more than 10 times, the procedure should be done again on another day when you are rested.
3. Using correct form, perform a leg press with the weight you have chosen. Perform as many times as you can up to 10.
4. Use Chart 1 to determine your 1 RM for the leg press. Find the weight used in the left-hand column and then find the number of repetitions you performed across the top of the chart.
5. Your 1 RM score is the value where the weight row and the repetitions column intersect.
6. Repeat this procedure for the arm or bench press using the same technique.
7. Record your 1 RM scores for the leg press and bench press in the Results section.
8. Next divide your 1 RM scores by your body weight in pounds to get a "strength per pound of body weight" (str/lb/body wt.) score for each of the two exercises.
9. Determine your strength rating for your upper body strength (arm press) and lower body (leg press) using Chart 2 in the lab resource materials. Record in the Results section. If time allows, assess 1 RM for other exercises you choose to perform (see Lab 3).
10. If a grip dynamometer is available, determine your right- and left-hand grip strength using the procedures in the lab resource materials. Use chart 3 to rate your grip (isometric) strength.

Results:

Arm press
(or bench press):   Wt. selected [ ]   Reps [ ]   Estimated 1 RM [ ]
(chart 1, lab resource materials)

Strength per lb. body weight [ ]   Rating [ ]
(1 RM ÷ body weight)   (chart 2, lab resource materials)

Leg press: Wt. selected [ ]   Reps [ ]   Estimated 1 RM [ ]
(chart 1, lab resource materials)

Strength per lb. body weight [ ]   Rating [ ]
(1 RM ÷ body weight)   (chart 2, lab resource materials)

Grip strength: Right grip score [ ]   Right grip rating [ ]

Left grip score [ ]   Left grip rating [ ]

Total score [ ]   Total rating [ ]

Conclusion and Implications: In several sentences, discuss your current strength, whether you believe it is adequate for good health, and whether you think that your "strength per pound of body weight" scores are really representative of your true strength.

Lab 11C: Planning and Logging Muscle Fitness Exercises: Free Weights or Resistance Machines

Name	**Section**	**Date**

Purpose: To set lifestyle goals for muscle fitness exercise, to prepare a muscle fitness exercise plan, and to self-monitor progress for the one-week plan.

Procedures:

1. The Basic 8 exercises are listed for free weights and resistance machines. Use Chart 1 to select 8 exercises to represent your Basic 8 exercises. If you would like to add other exercises to your program, then list them on the lines at the bottom of the chart. Descriptions of the exercises are provided in Tables 10 and 11.
2. In Chart 1, also indicate the days of the week that you plan on performing the exercises and the number of reps and the number of sets. Be sure to base your program on your goals (strength/endurance). If you are just starting out it is best to start with one set of 12–15 repetitions. Use the 1 RM procedure described in Lab 11A, to help you determine the amount of weight or resistance to use. Plan to do at least eight exercises, two or three times a week. Note: All exercises do not have to be performed on the same day, but many people find this more convenient.
3. Though abdominal exercises are not typically done using free weights or resistance machines, an abdominal exercise is recommended as part of a resistance exercise program. Two abdominal exercises are provided in the "other" category for you to consider (see Table 9).
4. In Chart 2, keep a one-week log of your actual participation. For best results, keep the log with you during your workout session. Indicate the exercises you performed, including any that you didn't plan on performing when you developed your schedule. If you would like to keep a log for more than one week, make extra copies of the log before you begin.
5. Answer the questions in the Results section.

Chart 1 Muscle Fitness Exercise Plan

What is your goal? Check one or more: Strength ☐   Endurance ☐   General Fitness ☐
Check boxes beside at least 8 exercises, note days, reps, sets and resistance to be used.

Primary Body Parts to Be Exercised	Free Weight Exercises (Basic 8)	Machine Weight Exercises (Basic 8)	Day 1 Date	Day 2 Date	Day 3 Date	How Many Reps?	How Many Sets?	Weight or Setting
Chest	Bench press	Chest press						
Shoulder	Overhead press	Seated press						
Arm (bicep)	Bicep curl	Bicep curl						
Arm (tricep)	Tricep curl	Tricep press						
Arm (wrist)	Wrist curl	(No equivalent*)						
Back	(No equivalent*)	Lat pull down						
Back (lower)	(No equivalent*)	Seated rowing						
Hip/leg (thigh)	Lunge	(No equivalent*)						
Leg (thigh)	Half squat	Knee extension						
Leg (hamstring)	(No equivalent*)	Hamstring curl						
Leg (calf)	Heel raise	(No equivalent*)						
Other exercises								
Abdominal	Crunch	Reverse curl						

*Note: Some free weight and machine exercises do not have equivalents.

Chart 2 Muscle Fitness Exercise Log

Check the exercises you performed and the days you performed them.

Primary Body Parts to Be Exercised	Free Weight Exercises (Basic 8)	Machine Weight Exercises (Basic 8)	Day 1 Date	Day 2 Date	Day 3 Date
Chest	Bench press	Chest press			
Shoulder	Overhead press	Seated press			
Arm (bicep)	Bicep curl	Bicep curl			
Arm (tricep)	Tricep curl	Tricep press			
Arm (wrist)	Wrist curl	(No equivalent*)			
Back	(No equivalent*)	Lat pull down			
Back (lower)	(no equivalent*)	Seated rowing			
Hip/leg (thigh)	Lunge	(No equivalent*)			
Leg (thigh)	Half squat	Knee extension			
Leg (hamstring)	(No equivalent*)	Hamstring curl			
Leg (calf)	Heel raise	(No equivalent*)			
Other exercises					
Abdominal	Crunch	Reverse curl			

*Note: Some free weight and machine exercises do not have equivalents.

Results:

Were you able to do your Basic 8 exercises at least two days in the week?   ◯ Yes ◯ No

Conclusions and Implications:

1. Do you feel that you will use muscle fitness exercises as part of your regular lifetime physical activity plan, either now or in the future? Use several sentences to answer.

2. Discuss the exercises you feel benefited you and the ones that did not. What modifications would you make in your program for it to work better for you? Use several sentences to answer.

Lab 11D: Planning and Logging Muscle Fitness Exercises: Calisthenics or Isometric Exercises

Name	**Section**	**Date**

Purpose: To set lifestyle goals for muscle fitness exercises that can easily be performed at home, to prepare a muscle fitness exercise plan, and to self-monitor progress for a one-week plan.

Procedures:

1. The Basic 8 exercises are listed for calisthenics and isometric exercises. Use Chart 1 to select eight exercises to represent your Basic 8. If you would like to add other exercises to your program, then list them on the lines at the bottom of the chart. Descriptions of the exercises are provided in Tables 12 and 13.
2. In Chart 1, indicate the days of the week that you plan to perform the exercises and the number of reps and the number of sets. Plan to do at least eight exercises, two or three times a week. Note: All exercises do not have to be performed on the same day, but many people find this more convenient. Do what is best for your schedule.
3. In Chart 2, keep a one-week log of your actual participation. For best results, keep the log with you during your workout session. Indicate the exercises you performed, including any that you didn't plan on. If you would like to keep a log for more than one week, make extra copies of the log before you begin.
4. Answer the questions in the Results section.

Chart 1 Muscle Fitness Exercise Log

What is your goal? Check one or more: Strength ☐   Endurance ☐   General Fitness ☐
Check boxes beside at least 8 exercises, note days, reps, sets and resistance to be used.

Primary Body Parts to Be Exercised	Calisthenic Exercises (Basic 8)	Isometric Exercises (Basic 8)	Day 1 Date	Day 2 Date	Day 3 Date	How Many Reps?	How many Sets?
Chest	Knee pushup	Arm press in door					
Shoulder	(No equivalent*)	Overhead press in door					
Arm (bicep)	Modified pullup	Bicep curl					
Arm (tricep)	Dips	Tricep press					
Trunk/back	Trunk lift	(No equivalent*)					
Abdominals	Crunch	Pelvic tilt					
Leg (outer)	Side leg raise	(No equivalent*)					
Leg (inner)	Lower leg lift	(No equivalent*)					
Leg (thigh)	Leg kneel	Leg press					
Leg (thigh)	(No equivalent*)	Wall seat					
Leg (hamstring)	(No equivalent*)	Hamstring exercise					
Other							

*Note: Calisthenics and isometric exercises may not have exact equivalents.

Chart 2 Muscle Fitness Exercise Log

Check the exercises you performed and the days you performed them.

Primary Body Parts to Be Exercised	Calisthenic Exercises (Basic 8)	Isometric Exercises (Basic 8)	Day 1 Date	Day 2 Date	Day 3 Date
Chest	Knee pushup	Arm press in door			
Shoulder	(No equivalent*)	Overhead press in door			
Arm (bicep)	Modified pullup	Bicep curl			
Arm (tricep)	Dips	Tricep press			
Trunk/back	Trunk lift	(No equivalent*)			
Abdominals	Crunch	Pelvic tilt			
Leg (outer)	Side leg raise	(No equivalent*)			
Leg (inner)	Lower leg lift	(No equivalent*)			
Leg (thigh)	Leg kneel	Leg press			
Leg (thigh)	(No equivalent*)	Wall seat			
Leg (hamstring)	(No equivalent*)	Hamstring exercise			
Other					

*Note: Calisthenics and isometric exercises may not have exact equivalents.

Results:

Were you able to do your Basic 8 exercises at least two days in the week?   ◯ Yes   ◯ No

Conclusions and Implications:

1. Do you feel that you will use these muscle fitness exercises as part of your regular lifetime physical activity plan, either now or in the future? Would the convenience of being able to do these exercises anywhere make it easier for you to stick with your program? Use several sentences to answer.

2. Discuss the exercises you feel benefited you and the ones that did not. What modifications would you make in your program for it to work better for you? Use several sentences to answer.

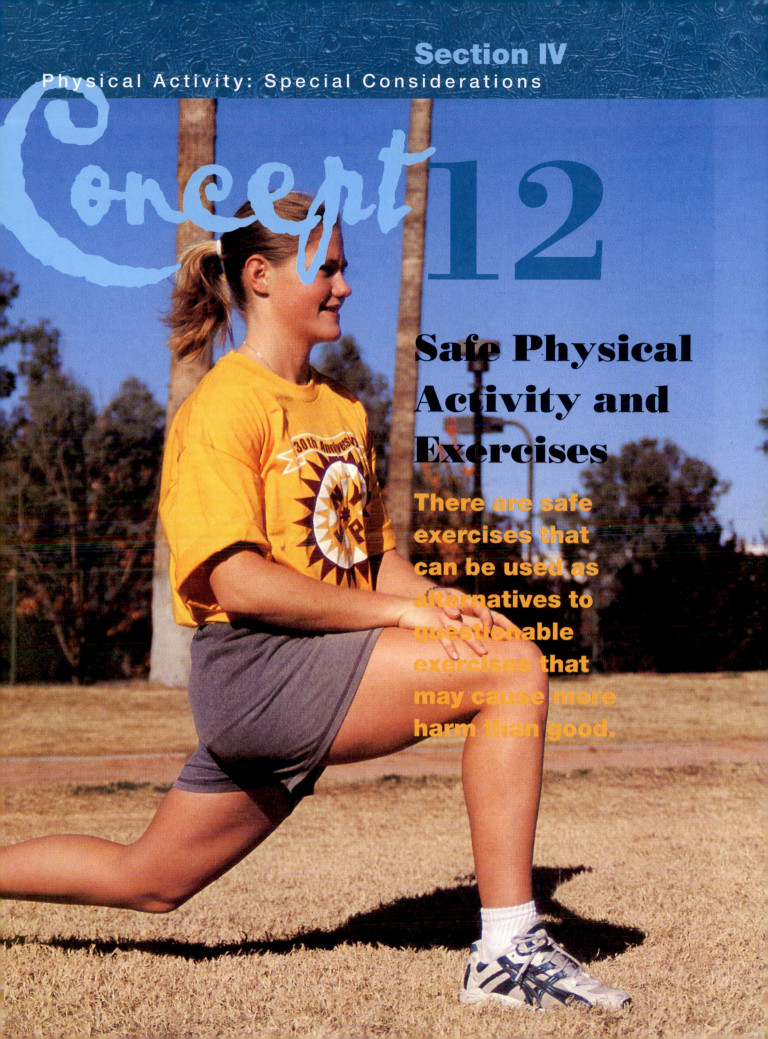

Concept 12

Safe Physical Activity and Exercises

There are safe exercises that can be used as alternatives to questionable exercises that may cause more harm than good.

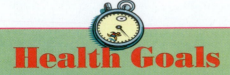

Health Goals

for Year 2010

Increase incidence of people reporting "healthy days."

Increase incidence of people reporting "active days."

Increase "active days" without pain.

Reduce activity limitations.

Introduction

There are literally thousands of exercises from which one can choose, but they must be chosen carefully because not all exercises are good for all people. Some exercises should be avoided because there is some risk of injury. We term these exercises "questionable" or "hazardous." Some of these exercises so drastically violate the mechanics of the human frame that they are dangerous and should never be used by anyone.

Studies indicate that many fitness centers and health clubs do not employ properly trained instructors. Those most likely to be qualified to advise you about exercise have college degrees and four to eight years of study in such courses as anatomy, physiology, kinesiology, preventive and therapeutic exercise, and physiology of exercise. These qualified individuals are most likely to be physical educators, biomechanists, kinesiotherapists, and physical therapists. On-the-job training, a certificate, a good physique or figure, or good athletic or dancing ability are not sufficient qualifications for teaching or advising about exercise.

If you have had knowledgeable instructors, you may recognize some questionable exercises, but others listed here may set off a protest such as: "I've been doing that all my life and it never has hurt me!"

This concept explains the difference between individually prescribed exercise and mass prescription; what is good for you may not be good for me. The difference between microtrauma and acute injury, and the significance of the number of repetitions, will also be discussed. Exercises that are believed to be potentially hazardous for most people are presented with the reasons for classifying them as such. Safer alternative exercises are suggested. The old saying "when in doubt, don't do it" is a good philosophy when choosing exercises, because there are always safe, effective alternative exercises for any specific muscle group.

The Facts: Rationale

There is a difference between exercises that are good when prescribed for a particular individual and those that are good for everyone (mass prescription).

Individual Prescription

In the clinical setting, a therapist works with one patient. A case history is taken and tests made to determine which muscles are weak or strong, short or long. Exercises are then prescribed for that specific person. The patient is supervised in the correct execution of the exercises.

For example, in a back-care program for an individual with lumbar lordosis, back hyperextension exercises might

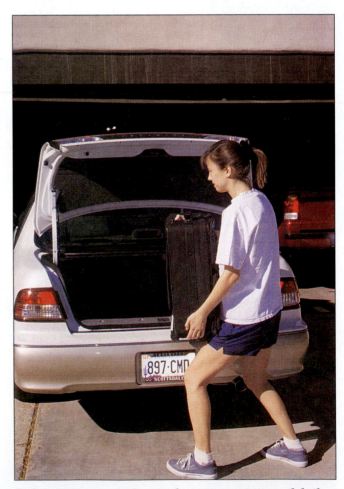

Safe exercise includes performing activites of daily living properly.

be **contraindicated**. However, another client might have a flat lumbar spine with limited range of motion, in which case, a set of back hyperextension exercises would be indicated. Thus, the classification of exercises in this concept does not necessarily apply to the setting where individual prescription is done by a qualified professional. A qualified professional is one who is expert in applied anatomy, kinesiology, therapeutic exercise, and functional tests as well as being knowledgeable about pathomechanics and other acute and chronic conditions. Typically, this includes physical therapists, kinesiotherapists, biomechanists, and physical educators with graduate specialization in corrective/remedial/therapeutic physical education.

Mass Prescription

When a physical educator, aerobics instructor, or coach leads a group of people in exercises, or a book or magazine describes a great exercise to "slim and trim," and all participants in the group or all readers perform the same exercise, this is a mass prescription. There is little if any consideration for individual differences except perhaps some allowance made in the number of repetitions or in the amount of weight (resistance) used.

Some of the exercises that would be appropriate for an individual would not be appropriate for all individuals in the group. Since it is not practical to prescribe individually for everyone, it is necessary to consider what the needs of the majority may be and choose the least harmful (but most effective) exercises for the group.

> Some exercises can produce microtrauma, and some may cause acute injuries.

www.mhhe.com/hper/physed/clw/student/
Microtrauma refers to "a silent injury"; that is, an injury that results from chronic, repetitive motions such as the ones we use in calisthenics or sports. These injuries also occur in occupations. Other terms that frequently appear in the scientific literature include repetitive motion syndrome, repetitive strain injury (RSI), cumulative trauma disorder (CTD), and overuse syndrome. They all refer to injury caused by repetitive movement. We may violate the integrity of our joints by performing, for example, 40 backward arm circles with the palms down three days per week for 10 or 20 years. The wear and tear is usually not noticed by the participant until the friction over time wears down the tendon, ligament, and/or bone, resulting in tendonitis, faciitis, bursitis, arthritis, and nerve compression. The injury may not become apparent until later in life. Chances are, when the injury reaches an acute stage in later life, the cause of the injury is never really identified and it will be attributed to old age. Because

the injury is unseen and unfelt, the participant views the exercise as harmless. Note: Many of the changes in the musculoskeletal system normally attributed to aging are found in young athletes. Degenerated disks are not an uncommon finding.

The term *acute injury* as used here refers to the stress, strain, or sprain that produces pain at the time it occurs or within a few hours of performing the exercise. For example, violating the integrity of the knee joint by placing torque on it during a toe touch or knee bend can tear the ligament and cartilage on the inside of the knee so the participant knows immediately that an injury occurred during that exercise. Some of the exercises considered questionable in this concept are capable of producing this kind of injury, whereas others in the list are more apt to produce the "silent" microtrauma. Some exercises can produce both types of injury.

> Some exercises may be reasonably safe for most people when performed only once but may become hazardous when done repetitively.

An acute exercise injury in any hazardous activity may occur the first time you place yourself at risk, or it may never happen. The odds of performing a hazardous activity safely decrease as the number of repetitions increases. It is like playing Russian roulette! You may have performed bilateral straight leg raises for years and never had a backache but, as the saying goes, "You are living on borrowed time." Microtrauma, on the other hand, occurs with each repetition of an exercise that violates physiologic movements or normal joint mechanics. It is true that we cannot avoid all wear and tear on the body, and it is true that we must "use it or lose it," but we can reduce wear and tear by eliminating hazardous activities, because if we do not use it correctly, then we will also lose it! Some of the exercises that are considered questionable because of microtrauma can probably be performed safely when the number of repetitions is very small and they are rarely used. For example, if it feels comfortable, hyperextending the back in the prone press-up is probably safe when done once as a static stretch after a series of abdominal strengthening exercises, but repetitive hyperextension exercises, even if comfortable, are hazardous.

Contraindicated A term used to describe treatments or exercises that are not recommended because of the potential for harm.

Microtrauma Injury so small it is not detected at the time it occurs.

Table 1   Guidelines for Exercising Safely

- Avoid stretching ligaments and joint capsules.
- Do *not* hyperflex the neck.
- Do *not* hyperextend the neck.
- Avoid compression on disks (e.g., neck circling, double-leg lift).
- Avoid movements that may damage cartilage (e.g., forward palm-down arm circles).
- Do stretch the chest, hip, calf, hamstring, low back and thigh rotator muscles.
- Do *not* stretch the abdominal muscles.
- Do strengthen the abdominals, shoulders, low back, lateral hip, and shin muscles.
- Avoid fast forceful flexion of the spine.
- Do *not* hyperextend the lower back except when individually prescribed.
- Avoid simultaneous flexion of the hip and rotation (twisting) of the spine.
- Do *not* twist or bend the knee laterally.
- Do *not* hyperflex the knee.
- Do *not* hyperextend the knee.

Some Guidelines for Avoiding Hazardous Exercises

> Most hazardous exercises can be avoided.

The human body is made to move. Nevertheless, there are certain movements that put the joints and musculoskeletal system at risk and should therefore be avoided. Most of the contraindicated exercises involve positions at the extreme ranges of motion. General guidelines for exercising safely are presented in Table 1. These guidelines are appropriate except when a physician or qualified professional has prescribed otherwise for you.

Other Important Facts

> If sports or special jobs require dangerous movements or exercises, it is especially important to develop and maintain high levels of physical fitness.

In baseball, the catcher has to assume and maintain a deep squat position for long periods of time. This causes micro-trauma to the knee. Gymnasts frequently perform double-leg raises and movements that result in hyperextension of the back. These movements cause microtrauma to the spine. Some workers (e.g., postal workers and construction workers) may also perform movements that produce microtrauma, even when adhering to guidelines for efficient and safe exercise. It is especially important that these people develop muscle fitness and flexibility in the regions of the body that are exposed to the dangerous movements. Baseball catchers should be sure to strengthen the muscles around the knee and stretch the hamstring and quadriceps muscles. Gymnasts should exercise to build strong abdominal and back muscles as well as stretch to lengthen the back, hamstring, and hip flexor muscles. Workers should similarly strengthen and lengthen the muscles associated with the movements commonly used in their jobs.

> Manual stretching of the shoulders as done by some competitive swimmers has been found to create instability in the shoulder joint.

The practice of some athletes of using the passive assistance of a partner can cause excessive stretch. Examples of such exercises are pulling the arms backward at shoulder level until they cross each other behind the back or pulling the bent elbows together making them touch while the hands are on the back of the head. Competitive swimmers sometimes begin such practices while they are in children's swimming programs and continue them through their competitive years. Such overstretching has resulted in painful shoulders and disability.

> Repeatedly rising on the toes and heels may weaken the long arches of the feet.

Tiptoeing exercises will develop the calf muscles, but at the same time, they will overstretch the muscles and ligaments that help support the long arch of the foot. Heel walking may have the same effect; that is, it may develop strong shin muscles while further weakening the arch. The potential harm is lessened if these exercises are performed with the toes turned in slightly.

> Jogging and aerobic dance exercise may not be appropriate activities for all people.

www.mhhe.com/hper/physed/clw/student/
Jogging and aerobic dance exercises are excellent for cardiovascular conditioning, weight control, and improvement of a variety of conditions; however, reasonable caution should be observed. Jogging has

been used successfully in rehabilitating cardiac patients and a variety of other health problems. Like many other exercises, jogging should not be done without a physician's approval for people with arthritis, osteoporosis, and heart and circulatory diseases. The pounding from repeated strides can lead to shin splints, blisters, and a variety of foot, ankle, knee, and hip problems. Wearing the proper footwear and learning how to jog correctly will minimize these hazards. If you have poor leg or foot alignment, you would be wise to jog only three or four days per week because studies show that the risk of injury is greatest for those who jog every day. Or you should choose another activity such as cycling or swimming. The same fitness levels will result with less risk of injury.

Aerobic dance exercise has some of the same hazards as jogging; these include the overstress syndromes from too many hours of high-impact landings on the floor. The most common problems are shin splints, Achilles tendon injuries, arch strains, and pain under the knee cap. Most of these problems can be prevented by warming up and stretching properly before exercising, by using low-impact movements, and by avoiding hazardous exercises such as those described in this concept. More recently, there have been increasing reports of dizziness, hearing loss, and impaired balance—in pupils and in teachers. Loud music can cause hearing loss, and high-impact landings may cause inner ear damage, but the causes are not now understood. Some women may need to wear a special bra as a comfort measure for either jogging or dance exercise.

Equipment that can be hazardous for some people is the gravity inversion boot and similar devices designed to allow a person to hang upside down.

These devices are marketed to assist with body alignment and for the treatment of backache. However, studies have shown that during hanging (inactively or while oscillating), systemic blood pressure significantly increases; intraocular and retinal arterial pressure (in the eye) doubles; and pulse and other heart irregularities occur. Therefore, this type of equipment is potentially dangerous to the elderly and medically compromised, and to people with high blood pressure, glaucoma, diabetes, and heart abnormalities.

Exercise can alter the effect of drugs in the body, as well as the effect of certain disorders.

The effect of drugs used to treat thyroid disease may be altered by exercise. Likewise, patients taking certain medicine for asthma and collagen diseases may not be able to perform exercises that require moderate or heavy exertion in

a normal fashion. Exercise alters the effect of nonsteroidal analgesics and anti-inflammatory drugs (like aspirin). During exercise, these drugs can cause oxygen consumption and carbon dioxide production to increase, as well as promote sweating and dehydration. Muscle relaxants may cause depression and hinder coordination.

The valsalva maneuver should be avoided when exerting great force in weight lifting, calisthenics, and isometrics.

Dizziness, blackouts, and inguinal hernias may result from the **valsalva maneuver**. This can be prevented in heavy weight lifting by avoiding **hyperventilation**, squatting as briefly as possible, and raising the weight as rapidly as possible to a position where it can be supported while breathing normally. In all other activities, breathe normally! Do not hold your breath during exercise.

Strategies for Action: The Facts

Common exercises when misused or abused are potentially harmful.

www.mhhe.com/hper/physed/clw/student/
Unless a qualified person evaluates the individual participant and determines one of the exercises listed as questionable in this book to be indicated for that individual, it is prudent to choose a safer exercise to accomplish the same purpose. On the pages that follow, many questionable exercises are presented with safer alternatives. Because of space limitations, this concept does not include every possible questionable exercise; however, some of the more commonly misused exercises are presented.

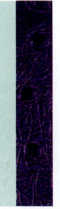

Valsalva Maneuver Exerting force with the epiglottis closed. This action increases pressure in the thorax and raises arterial blood pressure. When released, arterial pressure drops rapidly, blood vessels expand and are then filled, causing a lag in blood flow to the left ventricle. When this occurs, the subject may become dizzy or feel faint. May be caused by holding the breath while exerting force.

Hyperventilation Overbreathing; forced, rapid, or deep breathing.

Questionable Exercises and Safe Alternatives

Questionable Exercise: The Swan

This exercise (Figure 1) hyperextends the lower back and stretches the abdominals. These muscles are too long and weak in most people and should not be lengthened farther. It can be harmful to the back, potentially causing an impingement on the nerve, compression, and even herniation of the disc, and myofascial trigger points. Other exercises in which this occurs include: cobras, backbends, straight-leg lifts, straight-leg sit-ups, prone-back lifts, donkey kicks, fire hydrants, prone swans, backward trunk circling, weight lifting with the back arched, and landing from a jump with the back arched.

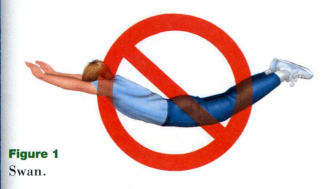

Figure 1
Swan.

Questionable Exercise: Back-Arching Abdominal Stretch

This exercise (Figure 3) can stretch the hip flexors, quadriceps, and shoulder flexors (such as the pectorals), but it also stretches the abdominals, which is not desired. Because of the armpull, it can potentially hyperflex the knee joint.

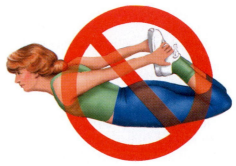

Figure 3
Back-arching abdominal stretch.

Safer Alternative Exercise: Back Extension

Lie prone over a roll of blankets or pillows and extend the back to a neutral or horizontal position (Figure 2).

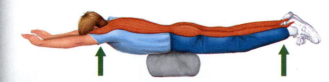

Figure 2
Back extension.

Safer Alternative Exercise: PNF Pectoral Stretch

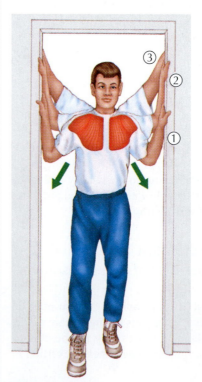

Stand erect in the doorway with arms raised 45 degrees, elbows bent, and hands grasping door jambs; feet in front stride position. Press forward on door frame, contracting the arms maximally for several seconds. Relax and shift weight on legs so muscles on front of shoulder joint and chest are stretched; hold. Repeat with arms at 90 and 135 degrees. If your goal is stretching the hip flexors and quadriceps, try substituting the hip and thigh stretcher (Figure 24).

Figure 4
Pectoral stretch.

Questionable Exercise: Donkey Kick

This exercise (Figure 5) may involve touching the nose with the knee followed by a ballistic backward kick, hyperextending the neck and the lower back when the leg is lifted above the horizontal.

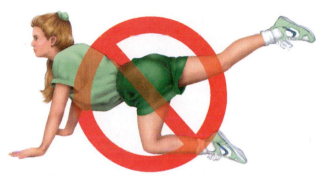

Figure 5
Donkey kick.

Safer Alternative Exercise: Knee-to-Nose

Kneel on all fours. While looking forward, pull the knee up under the chest, then extend the leg backward, being sure not to raise leg higher than the horizontal; change legs (Figure 6).

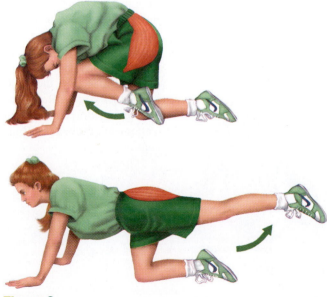

Figure 6
Knee-to-nose touch.

Questionable Exercise: Double-Leg Lift

This exercise (Figure 7) is usually used with the intent of strengthening the lower abdominals, when in fact it is primarily a hip flexor (iliopsoas) strengthening exercise. Most people have overdeveloped the hip flexors and do not need to further strengthen those muscles because this may cause forward pelvic tilt. Even if the abdominals are strong enough to contract isometrically to prevent hyperextension of the lower back, the exercise produces excess compression on the discs.

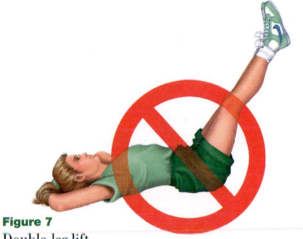

Figure 7
Double-leg lift.

Safer Alternative Exercise: Reverse Curl

This exercise strengthens the lower abdominals. Lie on your back on the floor and bring your knees in toward the chest. Place the arms at the sides for support. For movement, pull the knees toward the head, raising the hips off the floor. Do not let knees go past the shoulders. Return to starting position and repeat (Figure 8).

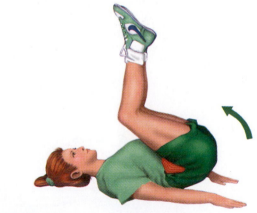

Figure 8
Reverse curl.

Questionable Exercises and Safe Alternatives (*continued*)

Questionable Exercise: The Windmill

This exercise (Figure 9) involves simultaneous rotation and flexion (or extension) of the lower back, which is contraindicated. Because of the shape of the facet joints in the lumbar spine, these movements violate normal joint mechanics, placing tremendous torsional stress on the joint capsule.

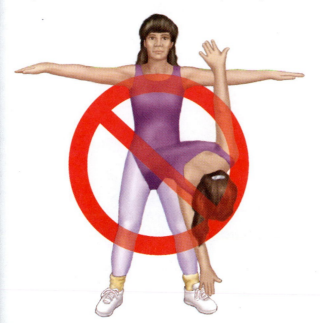

Figure 9
The windmill.

Questionable Exercise: Neck Circling

This exercise (Figure 11) and other exercises that require neck hyperextension (e.g., neck bridging) can pinch arteries and nerves in the neck and at the base of the skull, grind down the discs, and produce dizziness or myofascial trigger points. In persons with degenerated discs, it can cause dizziness, numbness, or even precipitate strokes. It also aggravates arthritis and degenerated discs.

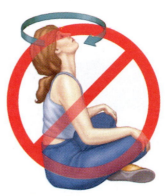

Figure 11
Neck circling.

Safer Alternative Exercise: Back-Saver Hamstring Stretch

This exercise stretches the hamstring and lower back muscles. Sit with one leg extended and one knee bent, foot turned outward and close to the buttocks. Clasp hands behind back. Bend forward from the hips, keeping the low back as straight as possible. Allow bent knee to move laterally so trunk can move forward. Stretch and hold. Repeat with the other leg (Figure 10).

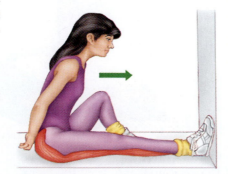

Figure 10
Back-saver hamstring stretch.

Safer Alternative Exercises: Head Clock

This exercise relaxes the muscle of the neck. Assume a good posture (seated with legs crossed or in a chair), and imagine that your neck is a clock face with the chin at the center. Flex the neck and point the chin at 6:00, hold, lift the chin; repeat pointing chin to 4:00, then to 8:00, then 3:00 and finally 9:00. Return to center position with chin up after each movement (Figure 12).

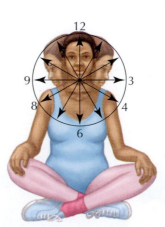

Figure 12
Head clock.

Questionable Exercise: Shoulder Stand Bicycle

This exercise (Figure 13) and the yoga positions called the plough and the plough shear (not shown) force the neck and upper back to hyperflex. It has been estimated that 80 percent of the population has forward head and kyphosis (humpback) with accompanying weak muscles. This exercise is especially dangerous for these people. Neck hyperflexion results in excessive stretch on the ligaments and nerves. It can also aggravate preexisting thin discs and arthritic conditions. If the purpose for these exercises is to reduce gravitational effects on the circulatory system or internal organs, try lying on a tilt board with the feet elevated. If the purpose is to warm up the muscles in the legs, try a slow jog in place. If the purpose is to stretch the lower back, try the leg hug exercise.

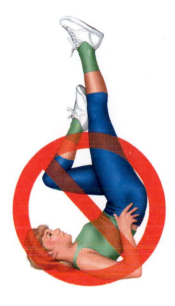

Figure 13
Shoulder stand bicycle.

Safer Alternative Exercise: Leg Hug

Lie on your back with the knees bent at about 90 degrees. Bring both knees to the chest and wrap the arms around the back of the thighs. Pull knees to chest and hold (Figure 14).

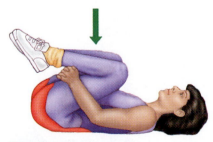

Figure 14
Leg hug.

Questionable Exercise: Straight-Leg and Bent-Knee Sit-Ups

There are several valid criticisms of the sit-up exercise. Straight-leg sit-ups can displace the fifth lumbar vertebra causing back problems. A bent-knee sit-up (Figure 15) creates less shearing force on the spine, but some recent studies have shown it produces greater compression on the lumbar discs than the straight-leg sit-up. Placing the hands behind the neck or head during the sit-up or during a crunch results in hyperflexion of the neck.

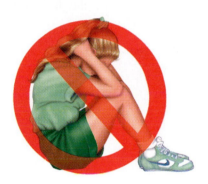

Figure 15
Hands-behind-the-head sit-up.

Safer Alternative Exercise: Crunch

Lie on your back with the knees bent more than 90 degrees. Curl up until the shoulder blades lift off the floor, then roll down to starting position and repeat. There are several safe arm positions. The easiest is with the arms extended straight in front of the body. Alternatives are with the arms crossed over the chest or the palms or fist held beside the ears (Figure 16).

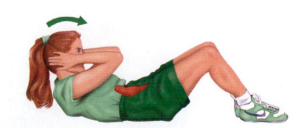

Figure 16
Crunch (hands on ears).

Questionable Exercises and Safe Alternatives (*continued*)

Questionable Exercise: Standing Toe Touches or Double-Leg Toe Touches

These exercises—especially when done ballistically—can produce degenerative changes at the lumbosacral joint. They also stretch the ligaments and joint capsule of the knee. Bending the back while the legs are straight (Figure 17) may cause back strain, particularly if the movement is done ballistically. If performed only on rare occasions as a test, there is less chance of injury than if incorporated into a regular exercise program. Safer stretches of the lower back include the leg hug, the single knee-to-chest, the hamstring stretcher, and the back-saver toe touch.

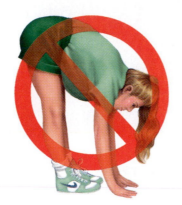

Figure 17
Standing toe touch.

Questionable Exercise: Bar Stretch

This type of stretch may be harmful (Figure 19). Some experts have found that when the extended leg is raised 90 degrees or more and the trunk is bent over the leg, it may lead to **sciatica** and **pyriformis syndrome,** especially in the person who has limited flexibility.

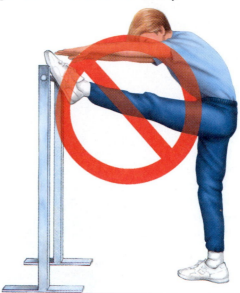

Figure 19
Bar stretch.

Safer Alternative Exercise: Back-Saver Toe Touch

Sit on the floor. Extend leg and bend the other knee, placing the foot flat on the floor. Bend at the hip and reach forward with both hands. Grasp one foot, ankle, or calf depending upon the distance you can reach. Pull forward with your arms trying to touch your head to your knee. Slight bend in the knee is acceptable. Hold. Repeat with the opposite leg (Figure 18).

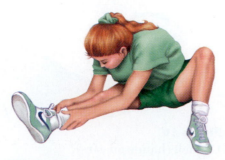

Figure 18
Back-saver toe touch.

Safer Alternative Exercise: Hamstring Stretcher

Lie on your back with the knees bent at about 90 degrees. Draw one knee to the chest by pulling on the thigh with the hands, then extend the knee toward the ceiling; hold. Pull to chest again and return to the starting position. Repeat with the other leg (Figure 20).

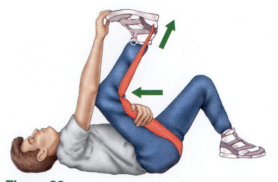

Figure 20
Hamstring stretcher.

Questionable Exercise: Shin and Quadriceps Stretcher and the Hero

These exercises (Figure 21 and 22) cause hyperflexion of the knee. When the knee is hyperflexed to 120 degrees or more, the ligaments and joint capsule are stretched and the cartilage may be damaged. The hero hyperflexes the knee and places the knee in a rotated position with **torque** on the flexed knee, which stretches the ligaments and capsule, and may damage the cartilage. The shin and quadriceps stretcher may also cause knee rotation. Note: One of the quadriceps, the rectus femoris, is not stretched by these exercises because it crosses the hip as well as the knee joint. If the exercise is used to stretch the quadriceps, substitute the hip and thigh stretcher (Figure 24). It is usually not necessary to stretch the shin muscles, since they tend to be weak and elongated; however, if you need to stretch the shin muscles to relieve muscle soreness, try the shin stretcher (Figure 23).

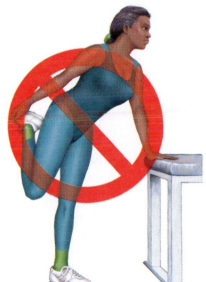

Figure 21
Shin and quadriceps stretch.

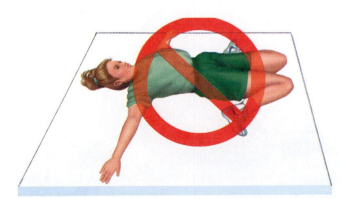

Figure 22
The hero.

Safer Alternative Exercise: Shin Stretcher

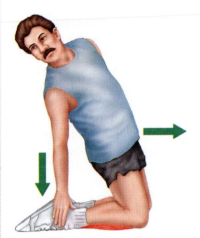

Kneel on both knees, turn to right and press down on right ankle with right hand. Hold. Keep hips thrust forward to avoid hyperflexing the knees. Do not sit on the heels. Repeat on the left side.

Figure 23
Shin stretcher.

Safer Alternative Exercise: Hip and Thigh Stretcher

Kneel so that the front leg is bent at 90 degrees (front knee directly above the front ankle). The knee of the back leg should touch the floor well behind the front foot. Press the pelvis forward and downward. Hold. Repeat with the opposite leg forward. Do not bend the front knee more than 90 degrees.

Figure 24
Hip and thigh stretcher.

Sciatica Pain along the sciatic nerve in the buttock and leg.

Pyriformis Syndrome Muscle spasm and nerve entrapment in the pyriformis muscle of the buttocks region causing pain in the buttock and referred pain down the leg (sciatica).

Torque A twisting or rotating force.

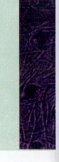

Questionable Exercises and Safe Alternatives (*continued*)

Questionable Exercise: Deep Squatting Exercises

This exercise (Figure 25), with or without weights, places the knee joint in hyperflexion, tends to "wedge it open," stretching the ligaments, irritating the synovial membrane, and possibly damaging the cartilage. There is even greater stress on the joint when the lower leg and foot are not in straight alignment with the knee. If you are performing squats to strengthen the knee and hip extensors, then try substituting the alternate leg kneel or half-squat with free weight or leg presses on a resistance machine.

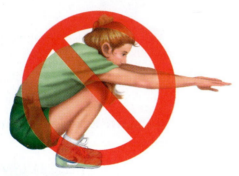

Figure 25
Deep knee bends.

Safer Alternative Exercise: Alternate Leg Kneel

From a standing position, with or without a free weight, take a step forward with right foot, touching left knee to floor. The front knee should be bent only to a 90-degree angle. Return to start and lunge forward with other foot. Repeat, alternating right and left (Figure 26).

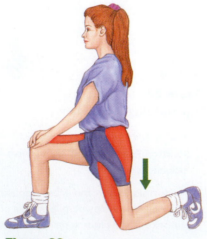

Figure 26
Alternate leg kneel (lunge).

Questionable Exercise: Knee Pull-Down

This exercise (Figure 27) can result in hyperflexion of the knee. The arms or hands placed on top of the shin places undue stress on the knee joint.

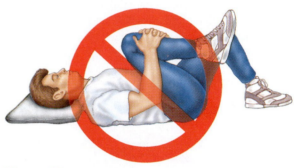

Figure 27
Knee pull-down.

Safer Alternative Exercise: Single Knee-to-Chest

From the hook-lying position, draw one knee to the chest by pulling on the thigh with the hands, then extend the knee toward the ceiling; hold. Pull to chest again and return to starting position. Repeat with other leg (Figure 28).

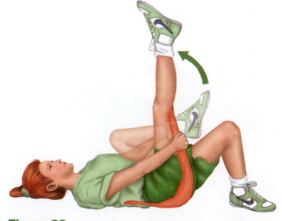

Figure 28
Single knee-to-chest.

Questionable Exercise: Seated Forward Arm Circles with Palms Down

This exercise (arms straight out to the sides) (Figure 29) may cause the bony knob in the shoulder to squeeze the muscles and the **bursa** in the shoulder every time the arm is lifted. In addition, there is a tendency to emphasize the use of the stronger chest muscles (pectorals) rather than to stretch those muscles and emphasize the weaker upper back muscles.

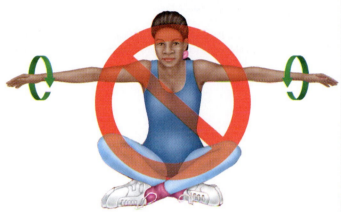

Figure 29
Forward arm circles (palms down).

Safer Alternative Exercise: Seated Backward Arm Circles with Palms Up

Sit, turn palms up and pull in chin, contract abdominals. Circle arms backward (Figure 30).

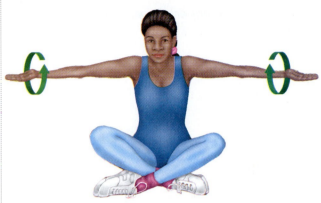

Figure 30
Backward arm circles (palms up).

Bursa Small sac filled with fluid and situated between muscles, or between muscles and bones, to prevent friction.

WebReview

WebReview materials for Concept 12 are available at *www.mhhe.com/hper/physed/clw/student/*.

American Academy of Orthopaedic Surgeons

www.aaos.org/wordhtml/press/prevent.htm

Safe Exercises

www.mhhe.com/hper/physed/clw/student/

Suggested Readings

Almkinders, L. C., et al. "An In Vitro Investigation Into the Effects of Repetitive Motion and Nonsteroidal Antiinflammatory Medication on Human Tendon Fibroblasts." *American Journal of Sports Medicine* 23(1995):119.

Knudson, D. Stretching: From Science to Practice. *Journal of Physical Education, Recreation and Dance*. 69(3)(1998):38.

Macfarlane, P. "Out With the Sit-up, in With the Curl-up!" *Journal of Physical Education, Recreation and Dance* (August 1993):62.

Reeves, R. K., Laskowski, E. R., & Smith, J. Weight Training Injuries: Part I. *Physician and Sportsmedicine*. 26(2)(1998):67.

Reeves, R. K., Laskowski, E. R., & Smith, J. Weight Training Injuries: Part II. *Physician and Sportsmedicine*. 26(3)(1998):54.

Signorile, J., et al. "An Electromyographical Comparison of the Squat and Knee Extension Exercises." *Journal of Strength and Conditioning Research* 8(1994):178.

Wallman, H. Low Back Pain: Is It Really All Behind You? An Excellent 7-Step Abdominal Strengthening Program. ACSM's Health and Fitness. 2(5)(1998):30.

Lab 12A: Safe Exercises

Name	**Section**	**Date**

Purpose: To perform safe exercises that are good alternatives to commonly performed questionable exercises and to self-monitor progress in your one-week plan.

Procedures:
1. On chart 1 check the questionable exercises you have performed.
2. Perform the safe exercises listed in the chart. Use the descriptions in this concept to help you perform them properly.
3. Place a check by the exercises you think you might consider using as part of your regular program.
4. Answer the questions in the Results section.

Chart 1 Questionable Exercises and Safe Alternatives

Place a check beside the questionable exercises you have performed in the past.

1. The swan
2. Back-arching abdominal stretch
3. Donkey kick
4. Double-leg lift
5. The windmill
6. Neck circling
7. Shoulder stand bicycling, plough, or plough shear
8. Straight-leg or bent-knee sit-ups
9. Standing toe touches
10. Bar stretch
11. Shin and quadriceps stretcher
12. Hero
13. Deep squatting exercise
14. Knee pull-down
15. Forward arm circles (palms down)

Place a check beside the safe exercises you think you might include in your exercise program.

1. Back extension
2. Pectoral stretch
3. Knee-to-nose
4. Reverse curl
5. Back-saver hamstring stretch
6. Head clock
7. Leg hug
8. Crunch
9. Back-saver toe touch
10. Hamstring stretcher
11. Shin stretcher
12. Hip and thigh stretcher
13. Alternate leg kneel
14. Single knee-to-chest
15. Backward seated arm circles (palms up)

Results: How many of the questionable exercises listed above have you performed?

Conclusions and Interpretations:

1. In most cases, it takes a considerable amount of time for a questionable exercise and the microtrauma they cause to result in noticeable damage to the body. To what extent do you think that you might be effected by questionable exercises you have done in the past? Use several sentences to explain.

2. Will you change your way of exercising as a result of learning about questionable exercises and safe alternatives? Use several sentences to explain your answer.

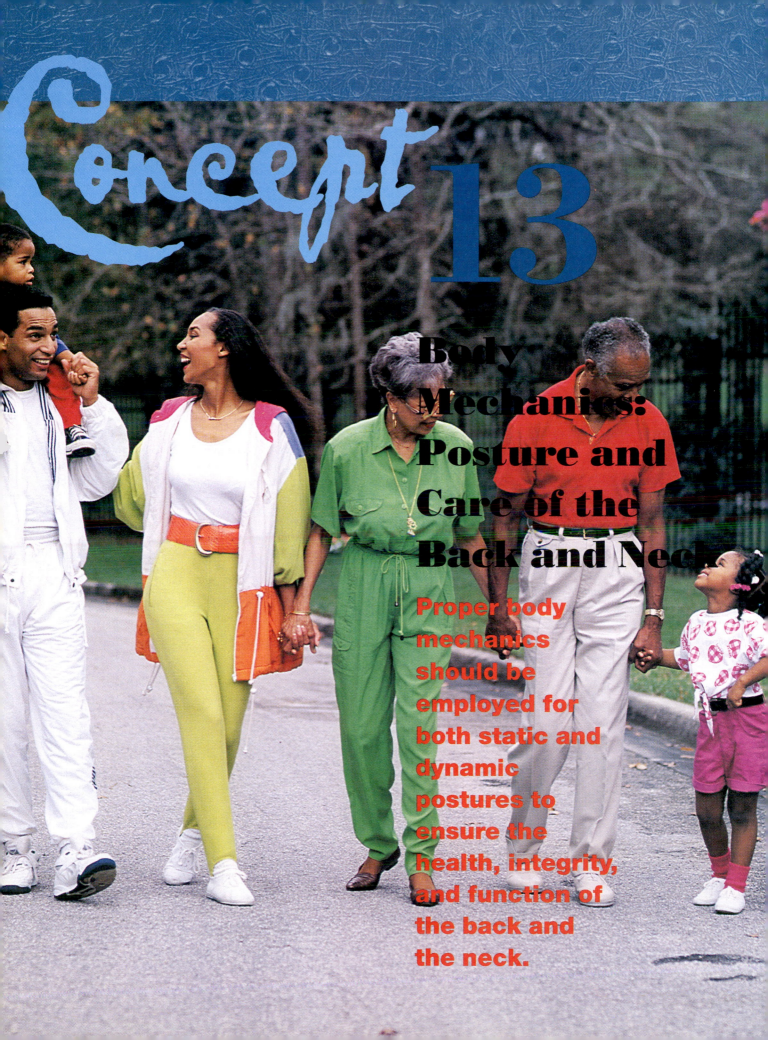

Concept 13

Body Mechanics: Posture and Care of the Back and Neck

Proper body mechanics should be employed for both static and dynamic postures to ensure the health, integrity, and function of the back and the neck.

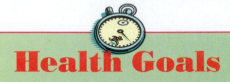

Health Goals
for year 2010

Increase healthy and active days.

Reduce days with pain and activity limitations.

Increase assistance to those with pain and activity limitations.

Increase proportion of people who regularly perform exercises for strength and muscular endurance.

Increase proportion of people who regularly perform exercises for flexibility.

Introduction

Body mechanics is the application of physical laws to the human body. The bones of the body act as levers or simple machines, with the muscles supplying the force to move them. Therefore, mechanical laws can be applied to the body to aid in performing more and better work with less energy while avoiding strain or injury.

This concept focuses on four aspects of body mechanics. The first part of the concept discusses the mechanics of body alignment while sitting or standing (static postures). The second part of the concept emphasizes the prevention of low back and neck pain through proper body mechanics. The third section of the concept stresses dynamic postures for activities of daily living. The fourth section includes exercises that are effective in correcting postural problems and removing the cause of neck and back pain.

The Facts about Posture

Good posture has aesthetic benefits.

The first impression a person makes is usually a visual one. Good **posture** can help convey an impression of alertness, confidence, and attractiveness.

Proper posture allows the body segments to be balanced.

www.mhhe.com/hper/physed/clw/student/
The body is made in segments that are balanced in a vertical column by muscles and ligaments. Proper posture helps to maintain this balance. In the standing position, the head should be centered over the trunk, the shoulders should be down and back, but relaxed, with the chest high and the abdomen flat. The spine should have gentle curves when viewed from the side (**lordotic curve**), but should be straight as seen from the back. When the pelvis is tilted properly, the pubis falls directly underneath the lower tip of the sternum. The knees should be relaxed, with the kneecaps pointed straight ahead. The feet should point straight ahead, and the weight should be borne over the heel, on the outside border of the sole, and across the ball of the foot and toes (see Figure 1).

If one part of the body is out of line, other parts must compensate to balance it, thus increasing the strain on muscles, ligaments, and joints.

If gravity or a short muscle pulls one segment out of line, other portions of the body will move out of alignment to compensate (see Figure 1). For example, if the abdomen sticks out over the belt line, the pelvis can tip forward, increasing strain on the low back. Chronic strain from poor alignment can lead to other postural deviations, producing

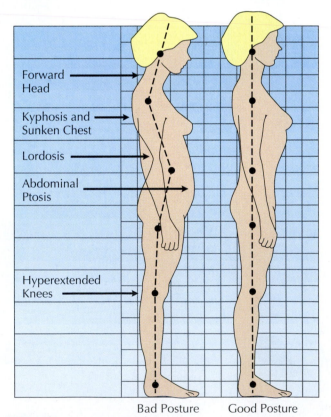

Forward Head

Kyphosis and Sunken Chest

Lordosis

Abdominal Ptosis

Hyperextended Knees

Bad Posture   Good Posture

Figure 1
Comparison of bad and good posture.

worse posture, more stress and strain, and possible deformity of the musculoskeletal system.

Chronic postural problems can lead to a variety of health problems.

With proper posture, there should be a slight inward curvature of the lower spine (lordotic curve). This curve helps support the body weight and promote balance about the trunk. If the lower back curve is too great (lumbar lordosis), the muscles of the low back are more easily fatigued, more likely to suffer muscle spasms, and more prone to injury. If the lower back curve is absent, problems associated with "flat back" posture (lumbar kyphosis) can occur. Some examples of specific health problems that result from these or other postural problems are described in Table 1.

Maintaining proper alignment requires a balance of flexibility and strength in muscles supporting the trunk.

Muscles of the legs, trunk, and neck work in combination to maintain body alignment and posture (Figure 2). The abdominal muscles pull the bottom of the pelvis upward and help keep the top of the pelvis tipped backward, eliminating excessive back curve. Strong hamstring muscles also help keep the pelvis tipped backward. If the hip flexor muscles are too strong, or not long enough, they have the opposite effect of strong abdominal muscles; that is, they tip the top of the pelvis forward, causing excessive low back curve (lordosis). (See Figure 3.) This is why it is important to have long, but not too strong, hip flexor muscles. As a general rule, flexibility exercises are needed to lengthen the hip flexor muscles, and strength and endurance exercises are recommended for the abdominal muscles. Sample exercises are provided later in this concept. For obvious reasons,

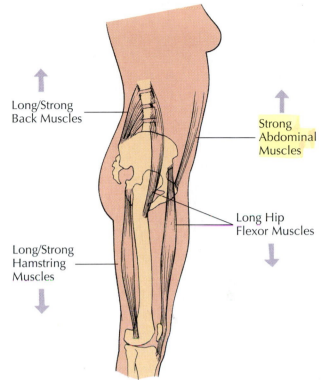

Long/Strong Back Muscles

Strong Abdominal Muscles

Long Hip Flexor Muscles

Long/Strong Hamstring Muscles

Figure 2

Balanced muscle strength and length permit good postural alignment.

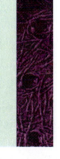

Posture The relationship of body parts, whether standing, lying, sitting, or moving. Good posture is the relationship of body parts that allows you to function most effectively, with the least expenditure of energy and with a minimum amount of strain on muscles, tendons, ligaments, and joints.

Lordotic Curve Normal curvature of the spine that is necessary for good posture and body mechanics.

Table 1 Health Problems Associated with Poor Posture		
Posture Problem	**Definition**	**Health Problem**
Forward head	The head is aligned in front of the center of gravity; also called "poke neck."	Headache, dizziness, and pain in the neck, shoulders, or arms.
Kyphosis	Excessive curvature (flexion) in the upper back; also called "hump back."	Impaired respiration as a result of sunken chest and pain in the neck, shoulders, and arms.
Lumbar lordosis	Excessive curvature (hyperextension) in the lower back (lumbar region), with a forward pelvic tilt; commonly known as "swayback."	Back pain and/or injury, protruding abdomen, low back syndrome, and painful menstruation.
Abdominal ptosis	Excessive protrusion of abdomen, also called "protruding abdomen."	Back pain and/or injury, lordosis, low back syndrome, and painful menstruation.
Hyperextended knees	The knees bend backward excessively.	Greater risk of knee injury and excessive pelvic tilt (lordosis).

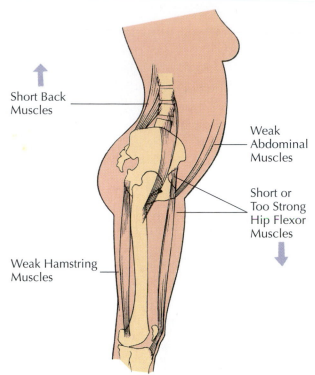

Short Back Muscles

Weak Abdominal Muscles

Short or Too Strong Hip Flexor Muscles

Weak Hamstring Muscles

Figure 3
Unbalanced muscular development may cause poor posture or back problems.

exercises to increase the strength of the hip flexor muscles are not recommended for people with back pain.

In addition to body alignment problems, hereditary, congenital, and disease conditions, as well as certain environmental factors, can cause poor posture.

Some environmental factors that may contribute to poor posture include ill-fitting clothing and shoes, chronic fatigue, improperly fitting furniture (including poor chairs, beds, and mattresses), emotional and personality problems, poor work habits, lack of physical fitness due to inactivity, and lack of knowledge relating to good posture. Some posture problems, such as **scoliosis,** may be congenital, hereditary, or acquired, but may be corrected with exercise, braces, and/or other medical procedures. Early detection is critical in treating scoliosis.

Approximately 80 percent of the adult population suffers from acquired foot defects.

Most foot defects are acquired and are preventable. They are most often caused by improperly fitting shoes and socks;

excessive hard use (such as in athletics); long standing or walking on hard surfaces; obesity or rapid weight gain (as in pregnancy); and improper bearing of weight through poor foot and leg alignment.

The Facts about Backaches and Neck Aches

Most people (more than half) will see a physician about a backache during their lifetimes.

Backache is second only to headaches as a common medical complaint. An estimated 30 to 70 percent of Americans have recurring back problems, and 2 million of these people cannot hold jobs as a result. The nation's medical bill for backaches is $24 billion annually. It is the most frequent cause of inactivity in individuals under the age of 45. It most often affects people between the ages of 25 and 60. Even teenagers have backaches. (One study indicated that 26 percent of teenagers have backaches.) Athletes also have backaches, but the condition is more common in people who are not highly fit.

The causes of backache are varied, but it is rarely a dramatic event such as trauma in a diving or an automobile accident.

Incorrect posture when standing, sitting, lying, or working is responsible for many back problems. Compounding this are weak muscles and muscular imbalance. Other causes of low back pain include improper exercises; incorrect techniques in lifting and in sports; repetitive, forced hyperextension of the back; and other preventable causes. Some of these are reflected in Table 1. This list excludes some uncontrollable causes such as trauma, tumors, and congenital abnormalities. You will have the opportunity to assess your back and neck risk factors in the questionnaire in Lab 13A. You may be familiar with many of the causes listed in Table 1, but what you may not know is that in 80 percent of the cases, physicians are unable to pinpoint the exact cause of back and neck problems.

The overwhelming majority of backaches and neckaches are avoidable.

A common cause of backache is muscular strain, frequently precipitated by poor body mechanics in daily activities or during exercise. When lifting improperly, there is great pressure on the lumbar discs and severe stress on the lumbar muscles and ligaments. Many popular exercises place great strain on the back (see concept on safe physical activity).

Sleeping flat on the back or abdomen on a soft mattress can also cause lower back strain.

> **Poor posture, especially lordosis, can cause back strain and pain and can make the back more susceptible to injury.**

The forward tilt of the pelvis may cause the sacral bone or one of the lumbar vertebrae to press on nerve roots with consequent low back pain and **sciatica**. To be on the safe side, some authorities advise people who have lordosis and weak abdominals to eliminate all exercises that hyperextend the spine. Incidence of lordosis is about the same for men as it is for women, except that women experience an added back strain during pregnancy.

> **Some people have a "flat back" (lumbar kyphosis) in the lower back region that can lead to backaches.**

www.mhhe.com/hper/physed/clw/student/
There is an increased interest among therapists in patients who lack a normal lordotic curve in the lumbar spine. Robin McKenzie's theories and exercises have become increasingly popular in the treatment of people who sit for long periods with the back flat and pelvis tilted backward or of people who engage in prolonged bending, heavy lifting, and standing for long periods of time with flat back postures (see Kuritzky and White, suggested readings).

These people may need to regain a normal lordotic curve and probably need to perform relaxed static stretches with the back in hyperextension, such as the press-up exercise. They may also benefit from the use of lumbar support (rolls or pillows) during sitting.

> **There is no such thing as a slipped disc.**

Disc problems are frequently misunderstood. **Intervertebral discs** may herniate or rupture, but they do not slip (Figure 4). Material from the pulpy center part of the disc (the nucleus pulposus) may bulge outward and press on spinal nerves, causing pain, and a protective reflex muscle spasm may occur to protect it. This causes a lack of circulation to the muscle and more pain, and more muscles tense up to prevent movement. Stiffness results and the muscles become weaker; chronic back pain may set in unless this vicious pain cycle can be stopped (see Figure 5). If it persists, bones may develop spurs, discs may degenerate, the patient may go to bed and worry and tense up, and the cycle may go on indefinitely.

The discs in the lumbar area are subjected to greater compression and torque because they are at the bottom of the spine. They are, therefore, more apt to be damaged. Sudden

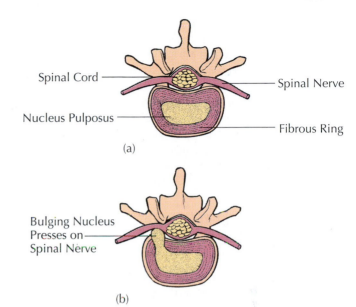

Figure 4
Normal disc (*a*) and herniated disc (*b*).

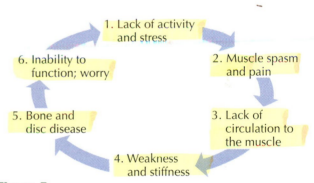

Figure 5
The vicious cycle of back pain.

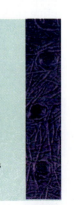

Scoliosis A lateral curvature with some rotation of the spine; the most serious and deforming of all postural deviations.

Sciatica Pain radiating along the course of the sciatic nerve in the back of the hip and leg.

Intervertebral Disc Spinal disc; a cushion of cartilage between the bodies of the vertebrae. Each disc consists of a fibrous outer ring (annulus fibrosus) and a pulpy center (nucleus pulposus).

twisting and flexion or extension movements, such as suddenly reaching for a ball in tennis or racquetball, may precipitate a **herniated disc**. It is more apt to happen when the disc is degenerated from overuse (Figure 6). It is more common in men than women and in people who do heavy manual labor. Degenerated discs are normal with aging, but not uncommon in athletes. One study shows gymnasts' discs were comparable to the discs of 65-year-old men. However, in spite of what popular literature and certain unethical "back doctors" may tell you, studies show that a herniated disc is rarely the cause of back pain—occurring in only 5 to 10 percent of the cases.

The neck is probably strained more frequently than the lower back.

The neck is constructed with the same curve and has the same mechanical problems as the lower back. The postural fault of forward head places a chronic strain on the posterior neck muscles. Tension in these muscles can lead to **myofascial trigger points**, causing headache or **referred pain** in the face, scalp, shoulder, arm, and chest.

Kyphosis is a contributing factor in neck pain.

The more the upper back is flexed, the greater the compensating curve (**cervical lordosis**) in the neck. The sharpest angle is between the fourth and sixth cervical vertebrae, creating wear and tear (microtrauma) that accelerates disc degeneration and arthritic changes, which can ultimately result in nerve and artery impingement.

The exact causes of chronic neck pain are many, and because they vary from individual to individual diagnosis is difficult.

Some of the causes of chronic neck pain (and the often accompanying shoulder pain) include workplace design, poor posture, work habits, and physical fitness, and too much stress. The risk factors that predispose a person to suffering neck pain are listed in Table 2.

Facts about Prevention and Intervention

Practicing good body mechanics and posture can help prevent back problems.

www.mhhe.com/hper/physed/clw/student/
Several practical suggestions for modifying everyday activities to improve posture and reduce the risk of back and neck problems are illustrated and described in Table 2.

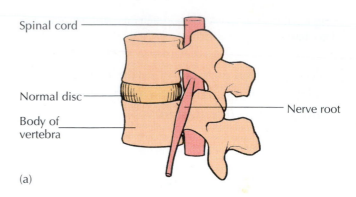

Spinal cord

Normal disc

Body of vertebra

Nerve root

(a)

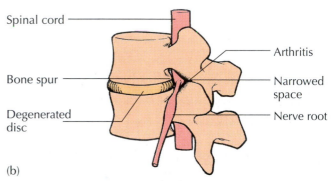

Spinal cord

Bone spur

Degenerated disc

Arthritis

Narrowed space

Nerve root

(b)

Figure 6
Normal disc (*a*) and degenerated disc with nerve impingement and arthritic changes (*b*).

There are some additional general guidelines that will help in preventing posture, back, and neck problems.

In addition to the suggestions for improving body mechanics noted in the previous sections, these guidelines should be helpful.

Herniated Disc The soft nucleus of the spinal disc that protrudes through a small tear in the surrounding tissue; also called prolapse.

Myofascial Trigger Points A sensitive spot in the muscle and muscle fascia caused by muscle spasms.

Referred Pain Pain that appears to be located in one area, although it actually originates in another area.

Cervical Lordosis Excessive hyperextension in the neck region ("swayback of the neck").

Table 2   Body Mechanics Guidelines for Posture and Back/Neck Care

Sitting
- Use a hard chair with a straight back and armrests, placing the spine against the back of the chair. A foot rest reduces fatigue (see Figure 7).
- Keep one or both knees higher than the hips by crossing the legs (alternate sides) or by using a foot rest.
- If your back flattens when you sit, place a lumbar roll behind your lower back.
- When sitting at a table, keep the back and neck in good alignment.
- Do not sit in front-row theater seats so you don't have to tip your head back.
- When driving a car, pull the seat forward so the legs are bent when operating the pedals. If your back flattens when you drive, use a lumbar support pillow.
- Whenever possible, sit while working, but stand occasionally.

Standing
- When standing for long periods of time, keep the lower back flat by propping one foot on a stool or rail; alternate feet occasionally.
- Avoid tilting the head backward (when shaving or washing your hair).

Lying
- Avoid lying on the abdomen.
- When lying on the back, a pillow or lift should be placed under the knees.
- When lying on your side, keep both knees and the hips bent; avoid using thick pillows.

Lifting and Carrying
- When lifting, avoid bending at the hips. Keep the back straight, bend the knees, and lift with the legs. Assume a side-stride position with the object between the feet to allow you to get low and near the object (see Figure 7).
- When performing a one-hand lift, use the same technique as for two-hand lifting but support the trunk with the non-lifting hand (see Figure 7).
- When lifting, do not twist the spine. This can be more damaging from a sitting position than from a standing position.
- When lifting, keep the object close to the body; do not reach to lift. Tighten the back muscles before lifting.
- If possible, avoid carrying objects above waist level.
- When objects must be carried above the waist, carry them in the midline of the body, preferably on the back (use a backpack).
- Push or pull heavy objects, rather than lifting them. It takes 34 times more force to lift than to slide an object across the floor.
- Do not try to lift or carry loads too heavy for you. The most economical load for the average adult is about 35 percent of the body weight. Obviously, with strength training, you can lift a greater load, but heavy loads are a backache risk factor.
- Divide the load if possible, carrying half in each hand/arm. If the load cannot be divided, alternate it from one side of the body to the other (see Figure 7).
- When lifting and lowering an object from overhead, avoid hyperextending the neck and the back. Any lift above waist level is inefficient.
- When objects must be carried in front of the body above the level of the waist, lean backward to balance the load, and avoid arching the back.

Working
- When working above head level, get on a stool or ladder to avoid tipping the head backward.
- Work at eye level; for example, computer monitors should not be too high or low.
- To avoid back and neck strain, climb a ladder or stand on a stool so you don't have to raise your arms over your head.
- When working with the hands, the workbench or kitchen cabinet should be about 2 to 4 inches below the waist. The office desk should be about 29 to 30 inches high for the average man and about 27 to 29 inches high for the average woman.
- Tools most often used should be the closest to reach.
- Avoid constant arm extension, whether forward or sideward.
- The arms should move either together or in opposite directions. When the conditions allow, use both hands in opposite and symmetrical motions while working.
- Organize work to save energy. Vary the working position by changing from one task to another before feeling fatigued. When working at a desk, get up and stretch occasionally to relieve tension.
- Use proper tools and equipment to reduce neck strain; for example, use a paint roller with an extension to reach overhead, thus reducing the need to hold the arms overhead and to hyperextend the neck.
- Avoid stooping or unnatural position that cause strain.

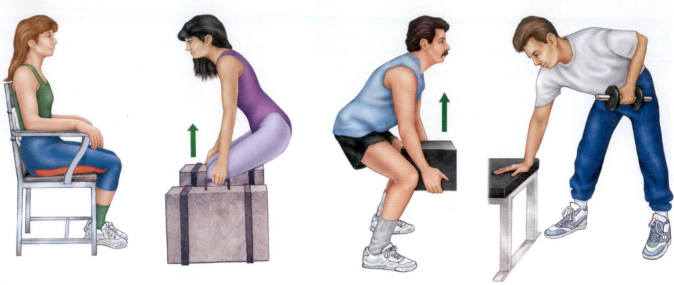

Figure 7
Good body mechanics can help prevent back and neck ache.

- Do exercises to strengthen abdominal and hip extensors, and to stretch the hip flexors and lumbar muscles if they are tight (see Tables 3–9).
- Avoid hazardous exercises (see concept on safe physical activity).
- Do regular physical activity for the entire body, such as walking, jogging, swimming, and bicycling.
- Warm up before engaging in strenuous activity.
- Get adequate rest and sleep. Avoid pushing yourself mentally or physically to the point of exhaustion.
- Sleep on a firm mattress or place a 3/4-inch-thick plywood board under the mattress.
- Avoid sudden, jerky back movements, especially twisting.
- Avoid obesity. The smaller the waistline, the lesser the strain on the lower back.
- Use appropriate back and seat supports when sitting for long periods.
- Maintain good posture when carrying heavy loads; don't lean forward, sideways, or backward.
- Adjust sports equipment to permit good posture; for example, adjust bicycle seat and handle bars to permit good body alignment.
- When you have a neck ache, lie down; apply heat or ice; massage the neck, and shoulders; and stretch the neck muscles.
- Avoid long periods of sitting at a desk or driving; take frequent breaks and adjust the seat and headrest for maximum support.
- To avoid injury, use safe sports equipment and techniques (e.g., proper helmet and cervical collar, if indicated); look before you dive in water.

The Facts about Exercises for Posture and Back/Neck Care

Exercise is one of the most frequently prescribed treatments for back or neck pain.

www.mhhe.com/hper/physed/clw/student/
Treatments range from surgical removal of a disc or fusion, to more conservative measures such as injections, electrical stimulation, muscle relaxants, anti-inflammatory drugs, vapo-coolant spray, bracing, traction, bed rest, heat, cryotherapy, massage, and therapeutic exercise. Regardless of the treatment used, 70 to 85 percent of back patients recover spontaneously. Of those, 70 percent will have no symptoms by the end of three weeks, and 90 percent will recover in two months. The various treatment modalities may simply make patients more comfortable or they may hasten the recovery.

Exercise has been found to be helpful in treating all kinds of chronic pain. (Resistance exercises and aerobic exercises have been particularly helpful in pain clinics.) Aerobic exercise is also known to help nourish the spinal discs.

Exercise can prevent or correct some of the underlying causes of back and neck pain by strengthening weak muscles and stretching short ones. In the process of creating

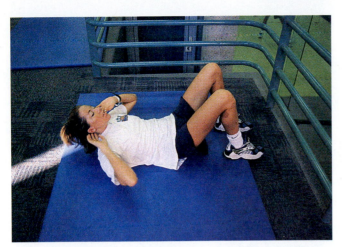

Some exercises that help prevent back problems are also therapeutic

muscle balance, exercise improves postural alignment and body mechanics and relaxes muscle spasms.

Exercise can often correct muscle imbalances that are the underlying cause of many postural and back problems.

If the muscles on one side of a joint are stronger than the muscles on the opposite side, the body part is pulled in the direction of the stronger muscles. Corrective exercises are usually designed to strengthen the long, weak muscles and to stretch the short, strong ones in order to have equal pull in both directions. For example, people with lumbar lordosis may need to strengthen the abdominals and hamstrings, and stretch the lower back and hip flexor muscles (see Figures 2 and 3).

Some people are unable to lift loads safely because tight and/or weak muscles may prevent them from using proper body mechanics.

Some people have backaches because they lift improperly. In many instances, the poor technique is caused by muscle imbalance. Examples include: hamstrings or gluteals that are too tight to permit the lower back to retain its normal curve during lifting; calf muscles that are too tight to allow the heels to remain on the floor during squatting; abdominal muscles that are too weak to support the back; or quadriceps and gluteals that are too weak to lift. Proper exercise can correct these problems.

Strategies for Action: The Facts

An important step in taking action to assure good posture and good back and neck care is assessing your current status.

www.mhhe.com/hper/physed/clw/student/
An important early step in taking action is self-assessment. The Healthy Back Test consists of eight pass or fail items that will give you an idea of the areas in which you might need improvement. The Healthy Back Test is described in the lab resource materials. You will have the opportunity to take this test in Lab 13A.

A posture test is included in Lab 13B to help you determine if you have any of the posture problems described in Table 1. Rating charts for both the back and posture tests are included in the lab resource materials.

It is possible to assess risk factors associated with potential back and neck problems.

Experts have identified behaviors that are associated with potential future back and neck problems. In addition to the back and posture tests, it may be useful to assess your risk factors. A questionnaire is provided in Lab 13A for assessing these risk factors.

Specific exercises are sometimes needed to prevent or help rehabilitate posture, neck, and back problems.

www.mhhe.com/hper/physed/clw/student/
Exercises included in previous concepts were presented with health-related fitness in mind. The exercises included in this concept are not really so different. They are either flexibility or strength/muscle endurance exercises for specific muscle groups; however, each is selected specifically to help correct a postural problem or to remove the cause of neck and back pain. To that extent, these exercises may be classified as therapeutic. These same exercises may be called preventive because they can be used to prevent postural or spine problems. Whether therapeutic or preventive, the exercises will not be effective unless they are done faithfully and with the FIT formula applied. People who have back and neck pain should seek the advice of a physician to make certain that it is safe for them to perform the exercises.

The exercises in Tables 3–9 are not necessarily intended for all people. Rather you should choose exercises based on your own individual circumstances. Use your results on the Healthy Back Test and the Posture Test to determine the exercises that are most appropriate for you.

ng Exercises for the Hip Flexors and Hamstrings

1. Back-Saver Hamstring Stretch

This exercise stretches the hamstrings and calf muscles and helps prevent or correct backache caused in part by short hamstrings. Sit on the floor with the feet against the wall or an immovable object. Bend left knee and bring foot close to buttocks. Clasp hands behind back. Bend forward from hips, keeping lower back as straight as possible. Let bent knee rotate outward so trunk can move forward keeping back flat; hold and repeat on each leg.

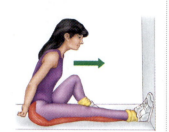

3. Low Back Stretcher

This exercise stretches the hip flexors, gluteals, and lumbar muscles and helps prevent or correct lumbar lordisos and backache. Lie on your back. Draw one knee up to the chest and pull thigh down tightly with the hands, then slowly return to the original position. Repeat with other knee. Do not grasp knee—grasp thigh. If a partner or a weight stabilizes the extended leg, the hip flexor muscles on that leg will be stretched.

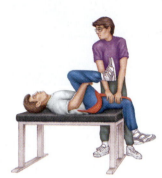

2. Single Knee-to-Chest

This exercise stretches the lower back, gluteals, and hamstring muscles and helps prevent or correct lordosis and backache. Lie on your back with knees bent. Use hands on back of thigh to draw one knee to the chest, then extend the knee and point the foot toward the ceiling; hold. Return to the starting position by drawing the knee back to the chest before sliding the foot to the floor. Repeat with other leg.

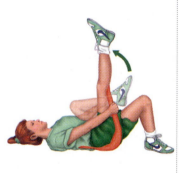

4. Hip and Thigh Stretcher

This exercise stretches the hip flexor muscles and helps prevent or correct forward pelvic tilt, lumbar lordosis, and backache. Place right knee directly above right ankle and stretch left leg backward so knee touches floor. If necessary, place hands on floor for balance. Press pelvis forward and downward; hold. Repeat on opposite side. Caution: Do not bend front knee more than 90 degrees.

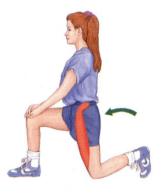

Stretching exercises for the hip flexor and hamstring muscles can benefit most people, including those with lumbar lordosis.

The exercises in Table 3 are designed to stretch the hip flexors since longer hip flexors will make it easier to maintain a "neutral" pelvis. Additional exercises for the hamstrings are provided as they may be effective in combating low back pain caused by lordosis. These exercises are useful for most people because long hip flexors and hamstring muscles are beneficial even to those who do not have lordosis.

Table 4
Postural Training Exercises for Pelvic Stabilization

1. Pelvic Tilt

This exercise strengthens the abdominals and helps prevent or correct lumbar lordosis, abdominal ptosis, and backache. Lie on your back with knees bent. Tighten the abdominal muscles and tilt the pelvis backward; try to flatten the lower back against the floor. At the same time, tighten the hip and thigh muscles; do not push with the legs. Hold, then relax. Breathe normally during the contraction; do not hold your breath.

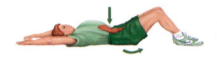

2. Bridging

This exercise strengthens the hip extensors, especially the gluteal muscles, and helps prevent and correct lordosis and forward pelvic tilt. Lie on your back with knees bent and feet close to buttocks. Contract gluteals, lifting buttocks, and lower back off floor. Hold; relax; repeat. Do not allow the lower back to arch.

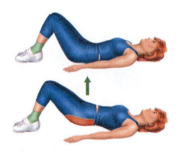

3. Wall Slide

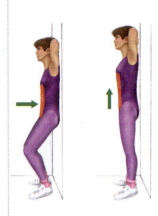

This exercise helps prevent or correct poor spinal alignment by teaching the feel of flattening the neck and back, and tilting the pelvis. Stand with heels 4 to 6 inches from wall, arms at sides. Flatten neck and lumbar region to wall by flexing knees and sliding down wall until spine can be forced against it. Slide up wall, maintaining flat spine. Walk away from wall, keeping curves flat. Return to wall and check alignment. Repeat with hands behind neck and elbows touching wall. Repeat with arms at sides and sandbag on head. Repeated flexion and extension of the knees can develop strength in the quadriceps muscles on the front of the thigh.

4. Pelvic Stabilizer

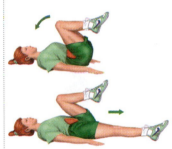

This exercise strengthens the postural muscles needed to maintain a pelvic tilt. Lie on your back. Bend both knees up to chest. Place arms on floor for support. Perform pelvic tilt by flattening the back against the floor. Slowly extend one leg as far as possible without arching the back. Return knee to chest.

> Muscle fitness exercises that train the muscles of the trunk, stabilize the pelvis, and maintain good posture can help prevent and alleviate back problems.

The exercises in Table 4 are designed to train the muscles that provide postural stability. These muscles must be fit to stabilize posture throughout the day. Performing these exercises will also help maintain a **neutral pelvis** and reduce lumbar lordosis. Once the postural muscles have been developed, it is important to be aware of your posture and use these muscles to maintain it.

Neutral Pelvis Proper position of the pelvis to maintain a normal lordotic curve. The pelvis is neither tipped forward nor backward but is in stable, neutral position.

Table 5
Exercises for Muscle Fitness of the Abdominals

1. Reverse Curl

This exercise develops the lower abdominal muscles, corrects abdominal ptosis, and helps prevent backache. Lie on your back. Bend the knees and bring knees in toward the chest. Place arms at sides for balance and support. Pull the knees toward the chest, raising the hips off the floor; do not let the knees go past the shoulders. Return to the starting position. Repeat.

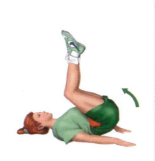

2. Crunch (Curl-Up)

This exercise develops the upper abdominal muscles, corrects abdominal ptosis and lordosis, and aids in backache prevention. Lie on your back with your knees bent and the arms extended or crossed with hands on shoulders or palms on ears. If desired, legs may rest on bench to increase difficulty. For less resistance, place hands at side of body (do *not* put hands behind neck). For more resistance, move hands higher. Curl up until shoulder blades leave floor, then roll down to the starting position. Repeat.

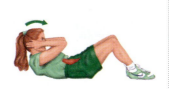

3. Crunch with Twist (on Bench)

This exercise strengthens the oblique abdominals and helps prevent or correct lumbar lordosis, abdominal ptosis, and backache. Lie on your back with your feet on a bench, knees bent at 90 degrees. Arms may be extended or on shoulders or hands on ears (the most difficult). Same as crunch except twist the upper trunk so the right shoulder is higher than the left. Reach toward the left knee with the right elbow. Hold; return and repeat to the opposite side.

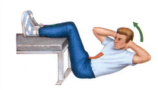

4. Sitting Tucks

This exercise strengthens the lower abdominals, increases their endurance, improves posture, and prevents backache. (This is an advanced exercise and is not recommended for people who have back pain.) Sit on floor with feet raised, arms extended for balance. Alternately bend and extend legs without letting back or feet touch floor.

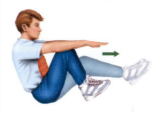

Fit abdominal muscles are important to good posture and prevention of backache.

The exercises in Table 5 are designed to increase the muscle fitness of the abdominal muscles. Strong abdominal muscles are important for maintaining a neutral pelvis, maintaining good posture, and preventing backache associated with lordosis.

Table 6
Stretching and Strengthening Exercises for the Muscles of the Neck

1. Neck Rotation Exercise

This PNF exercise strengthens and stretches the neck rotators. It should always be done with the head and neck in axial extension (good alignment). It is particularly useful for relieving **trigger point** pain and stiffness. Place palm of left hand against left cheek; point fingers toward ear and point elbow forward. Try to turn head and neck to the left while resisting with left hand. Hold 6 seconds. Relax and turn head to right as far as possible; hold 10 seconds. Repeat four times; repeat on opposite side.

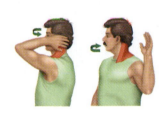

2. Isometric Neck Exercises

This exercise strengthens the neck muscles and prevents or corrects forward head and cervical lordosis, as well as upper back and neck trigger points and pain. Sit; place one or both hands on the head as shown. Assume good head and neck posture by tucking the chin, flattening the neck, and pushing the crown of the head up (axial extension). Apply resistance (a) sideward, (b) backward, and (c) forward. Contract the neck muscles to prevent the head and neck from moving. Hold 6 seconds; repeat each exercise up to six times. Note: For neck muscles, it is probably best to use a little less than a maximal contraction, especially in the presence of arthritis, degenerated discs, or injury.

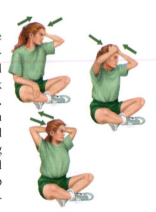

3. Chin Tuck

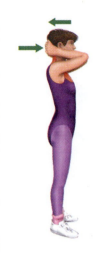

This exercise stretches the muscles at the base of the skull and reduces headache symptoms. Place hands together at the base of the head. Tuck in the chin and gently press head backward into your hands, while looking straight ahead. Hold.

4. Upper Trapezius Stretch

This exercise stretches the upper trapezius muscle and relieves neck ache and headache. Place right hand behind back and place left hand on back of head. Gently move chin towards your chest, turning head toward the left underarm. Gently press head forward with left hand for more stretch. Hold. Repeat to the opposite side.

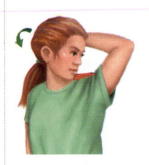

> Stretching and strengthening exercises for the neck can help prevent and relieve neck pain.

The exercises in Table 6 are designed to increase strength in the neck muscles and to improve neck range of motion. They are helpful in preventing and resolving symptoms of neck pain.

Trigger Point An especially irritable spot, usually a tight band or knot in a muscle or fascia. It often refers pain to another area of the body. For example, a trigger point in the shoulder might cause a headache. This condition is referred to as myofascial pain syndrome and is often caused by muscle tension, fatigue, or strain.

Table 7
Exercises for the Trunk and Mobility

1. Upper Trunk Lift

This exercise develops upper back strength. Lie on a table, bench, or a special-purpose bench designed for trunk lifts with the upper half of the body hanging over the edge. Have a partner stabilize the feet and legs while the trunk is raised parallel to the floor, then lower the trunk to the starting position. Place hands behind neck or on ears. Do not raise past the horizontal or arch the back or neck.

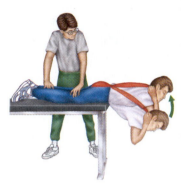 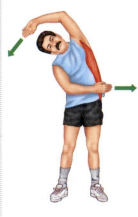

3. Side Bender

This exercise stretches the trunk lateral flexors and helps prevent and correct backaches by maintaining flexibility in the spine. Stand with feet shoulder-width apart. Stretch left arm overhead to right. Bend to right at waist reaching as far to right as possible with left arm; reach as far as possible to the left with right arm; hold. Do not let trunk rotate or lower back arch. Repeat on opposite side. Note: This exercise is made more effective if a weight is held down at the side in the hand opposite the side being stretched. More stretch also occurs if the hip on the stretched side is dropped and most of the weight is borne by the opposite foot.

2. Trunk Lift

This exercise develops the muscles of the upper back and corrects round shoulders. Lie face down with hands clasped behind the neck. Pull the shoulder blades together, raising the elbows off the floor. Slowly raise the head and chest off the floor by arching the upper back. Return to the starting position; repeat. For less resistance, hands may be placed under thighs. Caution: Do not arch the lower back; lift only until the sternum (breastbone) clears the floor. Variations: arms down at sides (easiest), hands by head, hands extended (hardest).

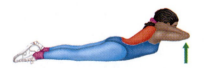

4. Supine Trunk Twist

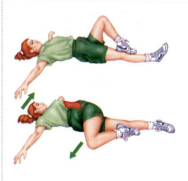

This exercise increases the flexibility of the spine and stretches the rotator muscles. Lie on your back with your arms extended at shoulder level; place left foot on right knee cap. Twist the lower body by lowering left knee to touch floor on right. Turn head to left; try to keep shoulders and arms on floor. Hold for several seconds.

> **Exercises that strengthen the trunk can help prevent backache.**

The exercises in Table 7 are designed to increase the strength and mobility of muscles that move the trunk. Recent research shows that exercises that strengthen these muscles are especially effective for people who have chronic back pain. The exercises in Table 7 can be performed without expensive equipment. Exercises using relatively expensive equipment that stabilize the pelvis and isolate the trunk extensors may be helpful for people who have chronic back pain. For more information on these specific exercises, consult with a physician or physical therapist (see Pollock and Vincent in suggested readings).

Table 8
Stretching and Strengthening Exercises for Round Shoulders

1. Arm Lift

This exercise strengthens the scapular adductors and helps prevent or correct round shoulders and kyphosis. Lie on stomach with arms in reverse-T; rest forehead on floor. Maintain the arm position and contract the muscles between the shoulder blades, lifting the arms as high as possible without raising head and trunk. Hold; relax and repeat. Note: If the arms are first pressed against the floor before lifting, this becomes a PNF exercise and range of motion may be greater. Variation: This more-advanced exercise is performed in the same way except the arms are extended overhead.

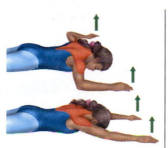

2. Seated Rowing

This exercise strengthens the scapular adductors (rhomboid and trapezius) and prevents or corrects kyphosis, round shoulders, head forward or cervical lordosis, and neck pain. Sit facing pulley, feet braced and knees slightly bent. Grasp bar, palms down with hands shoulder-width apart. Pull bar to chest, keeping elbows high, and return.

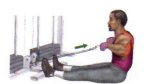

3. Wand Exercise

This exercise helps prevent and correct round shoulders and kyphosis by stretching the muscles on the anterior side of the shoulder joint. Sit with wand grasped at ends. Raise wand overhead. Be certain that the head does not slide forward into a "poke neck" position. Keep the chin tucked and neck straight. Bring wand down behind shoulder blades. Keep spine erect; hold. Hands may be moved closer together to increase stretch on chest muscles.

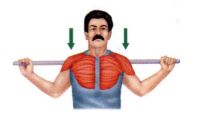

4. Pectoral Stretch

This exercise stretches the chest muscle (pectorals) and prevents or corrects round shoulders and sunken chest.

1. Stand erect in doorway with arms raised 45 degrees, elbows bent, and hands grasping doorjambs; feet in front stride position. Press out on door frame, contracting the arms maximally for 3 seconds. Relax and shift weight forward on legs; lean into doorway so muscles on front of shoulder joint and chest are stretched; hold.
2. Repeat with arms raised 90 degrees.
3. Repeat with arms raised 135 degrees.

> There are exercises that stretch and strengthen muscles to prevent and remediate **round shoulders**.

The exercises in Table 8 are designed to stretch the muscles of the chest and strengthen the muscles that keep the shoulders pulled back in good alignment (scapular adduction).

Round Shoulders The tips of the shoulders are drawn forward in front of the line of gravity.

Table 9
Exercises for Flat Back

1. Lower Trunk Lift

This exercise develops low back and hip strength. Lie on your stomach on bench or table with legs hanging over the edge. Have a partner stabilize the upper back or grasp the edges of the table with hands. Raise the legs parallel to the floor and lower them. Do not raise past the horizontal or arch the back. Suggested progression: (1) Begin by alternating legs; (2) when you can do 25 reps, add ankle weights; (3) when you can do 25 reps, lift both legs simultaneously (no weights).

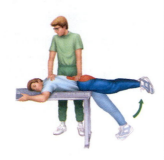

2. Press-Up (McKenzie Extension Exercise)

This exercise increases flexibility of the lumbar spine, reduces tension on posterior discs and longitudinal ligaments, and restores normal lordotic curve, especially for people with a flat lumbar spine. Lie on your stomach with hands under the face. Slowly press up to a rest position on forearms; keep pelvis on floor. Relax and hold 10 seconds. Repeat once; do several times a day. Progress to gradually straightening the elbows while keeping the pubic bone on the floor. Caution: Do not perform if you have lordosis or if you feel any pain or discomfort in the back or legs. Note: A prone press-up will feel good as a stretch after doing abdominal strength or endurance exercises. This relaxed lordotic position can be performed while standing. Place the hands in the small of the back and gently arch the back and hold. This should feel good after sitting for a long period with the back flat.

There are exercises that are therapeutic for people with flat back.

The exercises in Table 9 are designed to strengthen and restore normal curve to the back. They are *not* recommended for people with lordosis.

Web Review

Web review materials for Concept 13 are available are at *www.mhhe.com/hper/physed/clw/student/*.

American Back Care Company
   www.americanback.com

Back Care
   www.backandbodycare.com

National Safety Council: back care
   www.nsc.org

Suggested Readings

Boyce, R., and Jackson, S. One-Arm Lifting for a Healthy Back. *Strategies* (Jan. 1991):19–22.
Kuritzky, L., and White, J. Low Back Pain. *Physician and Sportsmedicine*. 25(1)(1998):56.
Kuritzky, L., and White, J. Extend Yourself for Back Relief. *Physician and Sportsmedicine*. 25(1)(1998):65.

Keeping records of progress is important to adhering to a back care program.

An activity logging sheet is provided in Lab 13C to help you keep records of your progress as you regularly perform exercises to build and maintain good back and neck fitness.

Malvivaara, A., et al. The Treatment of Acute Low Back Pain—Bed Rest, Exercise or Ordinary Activity. *New England Journal of Medicine* 332(6)(1995):351–335.
Nelson, B., et al. The Clinical Effects of Intensive, Specific Exercise on Chronic Low-back Pain: A Controlled Study of 895 Consecutive Patients with One Year Follow-up. *Orthopedics*. 18(1995):971.
Plowman, S. A. Physical Fitness and Healthy Low Back Function. In Corbin, C. B., and Pangrazi, R. P. (ed.). *Towards a Better Understanding of Physical Fitness and Activity*. Scottsdale, AZ: Holcomb-Hathaway, 1999, Chapter 13.
Pollock, M. L., and Vincent, K. R. Resistance Training for Health. In Corbin, C. B., and Pangrazi, R. P. (ed.). *Towards a Better Understanding of Physical Fitness and Activity*. Scottsdale, AZ: Holcomb-Hathaway, 1999, Chapter 14.
Teitz, C. C., and Cook, D. M. Rehabilitation of Neck and Low Back Injuries. *Clinics in Sports Medicine: Rehabilitation of Injured Athletes* 4(1985):456.
U.S. Department of Health and Human Services. (1998). Healthy People 2010 Objectives: Draft for Comment. Washington, DC: U.S. Department of Health and Human Services, Objectives Chapter 16: Arthritis, Osteoporosis, and Chronic Back Conditions.
Wallman, H. Low Back Pain: Is It Really All Behind You? An Excellent 7-Step Abdominal Strengthening Program. *ACSM's Health and Fitness Journal*. 2(5)(1998):30.

Lab Resource Materials

Chart 1 Healthy Back Tests

These tests are among the ones used by physicians and therapists to make differential diagnoses of back problems. You and your partner can use them to determine if you have muscle tightness that may put you at risk for back problems. Discontinue any of these tests if they produce pain, numbness, or tingling sensations in the back, hips, or legs. Experiencing any of these sensation may be an indication that you have a low back problem that requires diagnosis by your physician. Partners should use *great caution* in applying force. Be gentle and listen to your partner's feedback.

Test 1—Back to Wall

Stand with your back against a wall with head, heels, shoulders, and calves of legs touching the wall as shown in the diagram. Try to flatten your neck and the hollow of your back by pressing your buttocks down against the wall. Your partner should just be able to place a hand in the space between the wall and the small of your back.

- If this space is greater than the thickness of his/her hand, you probably have lordosis with shortened lumbar and hip flexor muscles.

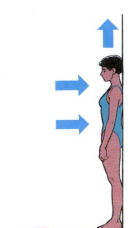

Test 2—Straight-Leg Lift

Lie on your back with hands behind your neck. The partner on your left should stabilize your right leg by placing his/her right hand on the knee. With the left hand, your partner should grasp the left ankle and raise your left leg as near to a right angle as possible. In this position (as shown in the diagram), your lower back should be in contact with the floor. Your right leg should remain straight and on the floor throughout the test.

- If your left leg bends at the knee, short hamstring muscles are indicated. If your back arches and/or your right leg does not remain flat on the floor, short lumbar muscles or hip flexor muscles (or both) are indicated. Repeat the test on the opposite side. (Both sides must pass in order to pass the test.)

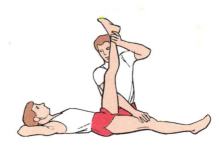

Test 3—Thomas Test

Lie on your back on a table or bench with your right leg extended beyond the edge of the table (approximately one-third of the thigh off the table). Bring your left knee to your chest and pull the thigh down tightly with your hands. Lower your right leg to the table. Your lower back should remain flat against the table as shown in the diagram. Your right thigh should remain on the table.

- If your right thigh lifts off the table while the left knee is hugged to the chest, a tight hip flexor (iliopsoas) on that side is indicated. Repeat on the opposite side. (Both sides must pass in order to pass the test.)

Test 4—Ely's Test

Lie prone: flex right knee. Partner *gently* pushes right heel toward the buttocks. Stop when resistance is felt or when partner expresses discomfort.

- If pelvis leaves the floor or hip flexes or knee fails to bend freely (135 degrees) or heel fails to touch buttocks, there is tightness in the quadriceps muscles. Repeat with left leg. (Both sides must pass in order to pass the test.)

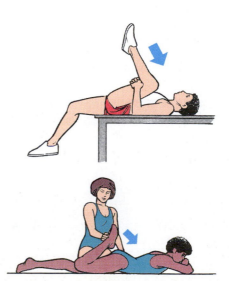

Chart 1 Healthy Back Tests (*Continued*)

Test 5—Ober's Test

Lie on left side with left leg flexed 90 degrees at the hip and 90 degrees at the knee. Partner places right hip in neutral position (no flexion) and right knee in 90-degree flexion; partner then allows the weight of the leg to lower it toward the floor.

- If there is no tightness in the iliotibial band (fascia and muscles on lateral side of leg), the knee touches the floor without pain and the test is passed. Repeat on the other side. (Both sides must pass in order to pass the test.)

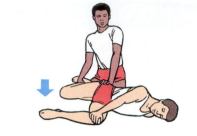

Test 6—Press-Up (Straight Arm)

Perform the press-up.

- If you can press to a straight-arm position, keeping your pubis in contact with the floor, and if your partner determines that the arch in your back is a continuous curve (not just a sharp angle at the lumbosacral joint), then there is adequate flexibility in spinal extension.

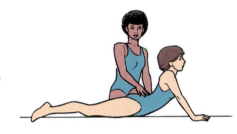

Test 7—Knee Roll

Lie supine with both knees and hips flexed 90 degrees, arms extended to the sides at shoulder level. Keep the knees and hips in that position and lower them to the floor on the right and then on the left.

- If you can accomplish this and still keep your shoulders in contact with the floor, then you have adequate rotation in the spine, especially at the lumbar and thoracic junction. (Both sides must pass in order to pass the test.)

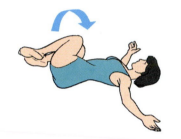

Test 8—Leg Drop Test*

Lie on your back on a table or on the floor with both legs extended overhead. Flatten the low back against the table or floor. Slowly lower legs while keeping the back flat.

- If your back arches before you reach a 45-degree angle, the abdominal muscles are too weak. A partner should be ready to support your legs if needed to prevent lower back arching or strain to the back muscles.

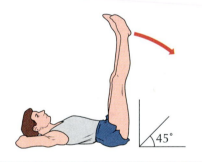

*The double leg drop is suitable as a diagnostic test when performed one time. It is not a good exercise to be performed regularly by most people. If it casuses pain, stop the test.

Chart 2 Healthy Back Test Ratings

Classification	Number of Tests Passed
Excellent	7–8
Very good	6
Good	5
Fair	4
Poor	1–3

Lab 13A: The Healthy Back Test and Back/Neck Questionnaire

Name	Section	Date

Purpose: To self-assess your potential for back problems using the Healthy Back Test and the Back/Neck Questionnaire.

Procedures:

1. Answer the questions in the Back/Neck Questionnaire below. Count your points for nonmodifiable factors, modifiable factors, and total score and record these scores in the Results section. Use chart 1 to determine your rating for all three scores and record them in the Results section.
2. With a partner, administer the Healthy Back Test to each other (see lab resource materials). Determine your rating using chart 2. Record your score and rating in the Results section. If you did not pass a test, list the muscles you should develop to improve on that test.
3. Answer the questions in the Conclusions and Implications section.

Risk Factor Questionnaire for Back and Neck Problems

Directions: Place an X in the appropriate circle after each question. Add the scores for each of the circles you checked to determine your modifiable risk, nonmodifiable risk, and total risk scores.

Nonmodifiable:

1. Do you have a family history of osteoporosis, arthritis, rheumatism, or other joint disease? — (0) No (☑) Yes
2. What is your age? — (☑) < 40 (1) 40–50 (2) 51–60 (3) 61+
3. Did you participate extensively in these sports when you were young (gymnastics, football, weight lifting, skiing, ballet, javelin, or shot put)? — (☑) No (1) Some (3) Extensive
4. How many previous back or neck problems have you had? — (0) None (☑) 1 (2) 2 (5) 3+

Modifiable:

5. Does your daily routine involve heavy lifting? — (☑) No (1) Some (3) A lot
6. Does your daily routine require you to stand for long periods? — (☑) No (1) Some (3) A lot
7. Do you have a high level of job-related stress? — (☑) No (1) Some (3) A lot
8. Do you sit for long periods of time (computer operator, typist, or similar job)? — (0) No (1) Some (☑3) A lot
9. Does your daily routine require repetitive movements or holding objects for long periods of time (e.g., baby, briefcase, sales suitcase)? — (☑) No (1) Some (3) A lot
10. Does your daily routine require you to stand or sit with poor posture (e.g., poor chair, reaching required while standing)? — (☑) No (1) Some (3) A lot
11. What is your score on the Healthy Back Test? — (0) 6–7 (1) 5 (3) 4 (5) 0–3
12. What is your score on the posture test in Lab 13B? — (0) 0–2 (1) 3–4 (3) 5–7 (4) 8+

Results:

Test	Pass	Fail	If you failed, what exercise should you do?
1. Back to wall	◯	◯	
2. Straight-leg lift	◯	◯	
3. Thomas test	◯	◯	
4. Ely's test	◯	◯	
5. Ober's test	◯	◯	
6. Press-up	◯	◯	
7. Knee roll	◯	◯	
8. Leg drop	◯	◯	

Total _____ _____

Chart 1 Back/Neck Questionnaire Ratings

Rating	Alterable Score	Unalterable Score	Total Score
Very high risk	7+	12+	19+
High risk	5–6	6–11	11–18
Average risk	3–4	4–6	7–10
Low risk	0–2	0–3	0–6

Chart 2 Healthy Back Test Ratings

Classification	Number of Tests Passed
Excellent	7–8
Very good	6
Good	5
Fair	4
Poor	1–3

Conclusions and Implications: In several sentences, discuss your need to do exercises for care of the back and neck. Include in your discussion whether you think your muscles are fit enough to prevent problems, the areas in which you are most likely to experience problems, and steps you might take to prevent future problems. Use your test results to answer.

Lab 13B: Evaluating Posture

Name	Section	Date

Purpose: To learn to recognize postural deviations and thus become more posture conscious and to determine your posture limitations in order to institute a preventive or corrective program.

Procedures:
1. Wear as little clothing as possible (bathing suits are recommended) and remove shoes and socks.
2. Work in groups of two or three, with one person acting as the subject while partners serve as examiners, then alternate roles.
   a. Stand by a vertical plumb line.
   b. Using chart 1, check any deviations and indicate their severity (see points scale below).
   c. Total the score and determine your posture rating from the Posture Rating Scale (chart 2).
3. If time permits, perform back and posture exercises (see Lab 13C).

Results:

Record your posture score [ ]

Record your posture rating from the Posture Rating Scale below [ ]

Chart 1 Posture Evaluation

Side View	Points	Back View	Points
Head forward	___	Tilted head	___
Sunken chest	___	Protruding scapulae	___
Round shoulders	___	Symptoms of scoliosis	
		Shoulders uneven	___
Kyphosis	___	Hips uneven	___
Lordosis	___	Lateral curvature of spine (Adam's position)	___
Abdominal ptosis	___	One side of back high (Adam's position)	___
Hyperextended knees	___		
Body lean	___	Total score	[ ]

Rate each using this point system:
- 0 = none
- 1 = slight
- 2 = moderate
- 3 = severe

Chart 2 Posture Rating Scale

Classification	Total Score
Excellent	0–2
Very good	3–4
Good	5–7
Fair	8–11
Poor	12 or more

Conclusion and Implications:

Were you aware of the deviations that were found? Yes ◯   No ◯

1. List the deviations that were moderate or severe.

2. In several sentences, describe your current posture status. Include in this discussion your overall assessment of your current posture, whether you think you will need special exercises in the future, and the reasons why your posture rating is good or not so good.

Lab 13C: Planning and Logging Exercises:
Care of the Back and Neck

Name   **Section**   **Date**

Purpose: To select several exercises for the back and neck that meet your personal needs and to self-monitor progress for one of these.

Procedures:

1. On chart 1 check the tests from the Healthy Back Test that you did *not* pass. Select at least one exercise from the group associated with those items. In addition, select several more exercises (a total of 8 to 10) that you think will best meet your personal needs. If you passed all of the items, select 8 to 10 exercises that you think will best prevent future back and neck problems. Check the exercises you plan to perform in chart 1.
2. Perform each of the exercises you select three days in one week.
3. Keep a one-week log of your actual participation using the last 3 columns in chart 1. If possible, keep the log with you during the day. Place a check by each of the exercises you perform for each day—including ones that you didn't originally have planned. If you cannot keep the log with you, fill in the log at the end of the day. If you choose to keep a log for more than one week, make extra copies of the log before you begin.
4. Answer the questions in the Results section.

Chart 1 Back and Neck Exercise Plan

Check the tests you failed:	√	Place a check beside the exercises you plan to do. In the last 3 columns, check the exercises done and the days done.	√	Day 1 Date:	Day 2 Date:	Day 3 Date:
1. Back to wall		Pelvic tilt				
		Bridging				
		Wall slide				
		Pelvic stabilizer				
2. Straight-Leg lift		Back-Saver hamstring stretch				
		Calf stretcher				
3. Thomas test		Hip and thigh stretcher				
4. Ely's test		Single knee-to-chest				
5. Ober's test		Lateral hip and thigh stretcher				
6. Press-up		Upper trunk lift				
		Trunk lift				
7. Knee roll		Side bender				
		Supine trunk twist				
8. Leg drop		Reverse curl				
		Crunch				
Choose other exercises for the neck and shoulders:		Chin tuck				
		Neck rotation				
		Arm lift				
		Pectoral stretch				

Results:

Did you do 8 to 10 exercises at least three days in the week?

Yes   No

○   ○

Conclusion and Interpretations:

1. Do you feel that you will use back and neck exercises as part of your regular lifetime physical activity plan, either now or in the future? Use several sentences to explain your answer.

2. Discuss the exercises you did. What exercises would you continue to do and which ones would you change? Use several sentences to explain your answer.

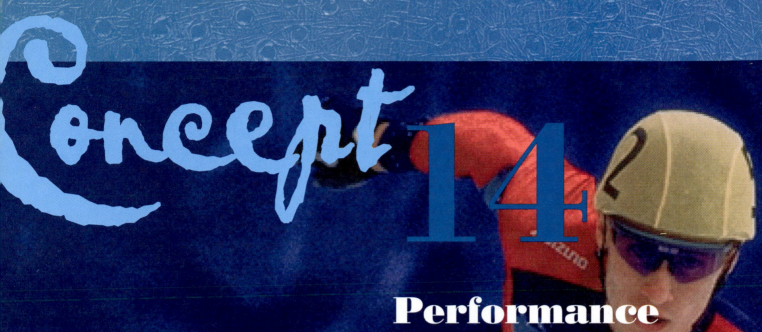

Concept 14

Performance Benefits of Physical Activity

Physical activity provides performance benefits above and beyond the benefits to health. These performance benefits can promote quality of life for the typical person and enhance the abilities of athletes and people in jobs requiring high levels of performance.

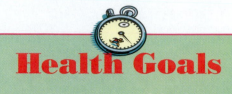

Health Goals
for year 2010

Increase leisure time physical activity.

Increase adoption and maintenance of regular daily physical activity.

Increase proportion of people who participate in employee sponsored activity programs.

Reduce steroid use especially among young people.

Introduction

As described in previous concepts, physical activity can produce many benefits to fitness, health, and wellness. For most people, achieving health-related fitness in the good fitness zone is adequate. However, for some people, high-level performance is an important goal. Professional athletes need more fitness than the person interested primarily in fitness for life or health and wellness for optimal functioning. Nonprofessionals who want to run a marathon or to perform at a high level in recreational sports also require high-performance levels of physical fitness, as well as high-level performance skills. In addition, nonathletes in high-performance jobs can benefit from advanced training techniques. Examples are fire safety, military service, and police work. To improve performance in these activities, more advanced training techniques are warranted. In this concept, information is presented for those interested in training for high-level performance.

The Facts about Performance

Many people pursue physical activity for reasons other than health and wellness.

Sports and competitive athletics are compelling challenges to many individuals. Participation in physical activity provides opportunities for individuals to explore the limits of their ability and to challenge themselves in competition. Some individuals enjoy challenges associated with competitive aerobic activities such as running, cycling, swimming, and triathlons. Others enjoy the challenges associated with competitive resis-

tance training activities, such as powerlifting or bodybuilding. Competitive opportunities are also available in a variety of sport activities. While competitive activities provide health benefits and recreation opportunities, many individuals are more interested in improving their performance. High-level performance is also a requirement for some types of work. Methods of **training** appropriate for sport are also appropriate for enhancing performance for work.

Improving performance requires more specific training than the type needed to improve health.

High levels of performance require good genetics, high levels of motivation, and a commitment to regular training. The effort and training required to excel in sports, competitive athletics, or work requiring high-level performance are greater than the amount required for good health and wellness. Because adaptations to exercise are specific to the type of activity that is performed, training should be matched to the specific needs of a given activity.

High-level performance requires health-related, skill-related fitness and specific motor skills necessary for the performance.

People who possess good fitness levels for each of the five health-related fitness components have enhanced health and wellness, as well as reduced risk of disease. To succeed in sports and certain jobs, high performance levels of health-related physical fitness are necessary, over and above what the normal person needs to enhance health. This is illustrated in Figure 1. Training (regular physical activity) builds health-related fitness to enhance health and high-level performance. This is why arrows in Figure 1 extend from health-related fitness to both health and high-level performance. To some extent, it can be said that high-level health-related fitness is much like skill-related fitness. High performance levels are not necessary for all people, only those who need exceptional performances. A distance runner needs exceptional cardiovascular fitness and muscular endurance, a lineman in football needs exceptional strength, a volleyball player needs power for jumping, and a gymnast needs exceptional flexibility.

Exceptional performance also requires high-level skill-related physical fitness. Skill-related physical fitness is especially affected by heredity. For example, speed is influenced greatly by the number of fast-twitch fibers you inherit, and reaction time is associated with the innate characteristics of your nervous system. With specific training, you can make modest modifications in your skill-related fitness, but most experts believe that it is more important to do regular prac-

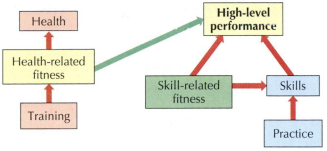

Figure 1
Factors influencing high-level performance.

tice to enhance performance skills associated with the specific tasks of your sport or job. It is important to understand that skill-related fitness and skills are not the same thing! Skill-related fitness components are abilities that help you learn skills faster and better, thus the arrow in Figure 1 from skill-related fitness to skills. Skills, on the other hand, are things like throwing, kicking, catching, and hitting a ball.

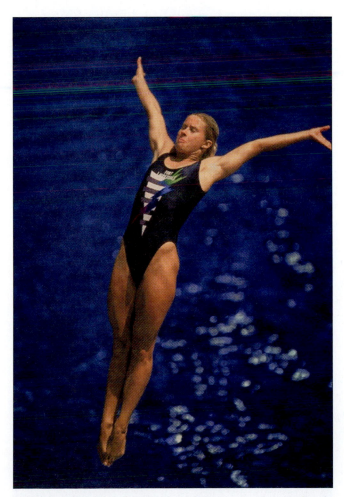

High-level performers need high-performance levels of fitness.

Practice enhances skills (see arrow from practice to skills). Therefore, practicing the specific skills of a sport or a job is more productive to performance enhancement than more general drills associated with changing skill-related fitness. The most successful performers will be those who inherit good potential for health and skill-related fitness, who train to improve their health-related fitness, and who do extensive practice to improve the skills associated with the specific activity in which they hope to excel.

In the following sections, several types of training associated with high-level performance will be discussed, including aerobic training, anaerobic training, special forms of resistance training, and special forms of training that build high performance levels of health-related components (cardiovascular fitness, strength, muscular endurance, and flexibility). Methods for maximizing skill-related fitness and skill will also be presented.

The Facts about Training for High-Level Performance: Aerobic and Anaerobic

Many types of high-level performance require aerobic capacity.

Regardless of the type of activity you perform, you derive energy from high-energy fuel that must be available to the muscle fibers. The breakdown of this high-energy fuel in the muscle cells allows you to perform all types of exercise. People interested in high-level performance are especially in need of fuel for performance.

For some performers, success depends on the ability to sustain activity for long periods of time without stopping. Distance runners and swimmers are good examples. These types of performers are in special need of high levels of cardiovascular fitness or aerobic capacity. In aerobic exercise, adequate oxygen is available to use the carbohydrates and fats available in the body to rebuild the high-energy fuel the muscles need to sustain performance. Aerobic exercise increases aerobic capacity (cardiovascular fitness) by enhancing the body's ability to supply oxygen to the muscles as well as their ability to use it. Slow-twitch muscle fibers appear to benefit most from aerobic exercise. Any performance that involves long sustained performance places special demands on the

Training A term typically used to describe the type of physical activity performed by people interested in high-level performance (e.g., athletes, people in specialized jobs).

slow-twitch fibers and requires a high level of aerobic capacity (cardiovascular fitness). The best measure of cardiovascular fitness is $\dot{V}O_2$ max (see cardiovascular fitness concept).

Many types of high-level performance require anaerobic capacity.

www.mhhe.com/hper/physed/clw/student/

If adequate oxygen is supplied, activity can be sustained for long periods of time. Unfortunately, the energy resulting from the breakdown of the body's high-energy fuel is used in a matter of seconds if adequate oxygen is not supplied. Carbohydrates stored in the cells can be broken down to replenish the high-energy fuel supply to allow performance to continue for an additional time (30 to 40 seconds for most people). Short-term, vigorous exercise performed in the absence of an adequate oxygen supply is called **anaerobic exercise**. Anaerobic exercise results in **lactic acid** build-up in the process of energy production. Muscle fatigue occurs when anaerobic energy supplies are depleted, and lactic acid build-up occurs. Regular anaerobic exercise seems to allow the muscle to tolerate higher lactic acid levels before fatigue occurs. Also, anaerobic exercise improves anaerobic energy production capabilities, primarily in the fast-twitch fibers. These fibers appear to benefit most from anaerobic exercise.

Anaerobic capacity, or the ability to perform vigorous, short-term bouts of exercise, and repeat them after relatively short rest periods, is necessary for success in many sports and jobs that require high-level performance. Anaerobic capacity is often measured in the laboratory using the Wingate test, an all-out, 30-second stationary bicycle ride at high resistance.

Interval training is effective in building anaerobic capacity.

www.mhhe.com/hper/physed/clw/student/

In anaerobic **interval training**, the goal is to challenge the anaerobic energy systems. This is typically accomplished with repeated high-intensity bouts of activity. In response to this training, the body improves its ability to produce energy anaerobically and also improves its ability to tolerate and remove lactic acid from the blood.

www.mhhe.com/hper/physed/clw/student/

Anaerobic interval training can be performed with either short or long intervals. Short-interval workouts should use maximum speed with rest intervals lasting from 10 seconds to 2 minutes. These should be repeated eight to 30 times. Long-interval training should use 90 to 100 percent speed with rest intervals lasting from 3 to 15 minutes. These should be repeated 4 to 15 times. A sample short anaerobic interval program and a sample long interval

running program are presented in Table 1. These plans could be modified for use with other types of activities.

Principles of interval training can be modified for different activities.

The principles of interval training can be applied to specific sports or specific jobs that require high levels of anaerobic performance. Basketball, for example, requires anaerobic sprints up and down the court. Simulated games that required repeated sprints with appropriate rest periods between intervals is a form of interval training that is very specific to the needs of basketball performers. Similar specific types of interval training can be developed for virtually any activity.

Recently, interval training has also been adapted to different forms of exercise such as dance exercise. A recent increase in interest in high-level performance in this area has resulted in the development of dance interval training. This involves vigorous dance exercise alternated with frequent rest periods. In some cases, other forms of exercise, such as running, are alternated with dance exercise bouts.

Fartlek training is a modified form of interval training.

As noted in an earlier concept, *Fartlek* is a Swedish word for "speed play." This exercise was developed in Scandinavia where pinewood paths follow curves of lakes and up and down many hills. The idea is to get away from the regimen of running on a track and to enjoy the woods, lakes, and mountains. Because of the terrain, the pace is never constant. The uphill path requires a slow pace, while a straight stretch or downhill trail allows for speed. In the "speed play," or fartlek system, you run easily for a time at a steady, hard speed, walk

Table 1 Sample Anaerobic Interval Training Program (Moderate Intensity)	
Short Intervals	**Long Intervals**
1. Do a flexibility and cardiovascular warm-up.	1. Do a flexibility and cardiovascular warm-up.
2. Run at 100% speed for 10 seconds (approximately 70 to 100 yards).	2. Run at 90% speed for one minute (approximately 300 to 500 yards).
3. Rest for 10 seconds by walking slowly.	3. Rest for 4 minutes by walking slowly.
4. Alternately repeat steps 2 and 3 until 20 runs have been completed.	4. Alternately repeat steps 2 and 3 until 5 runs have been completed.

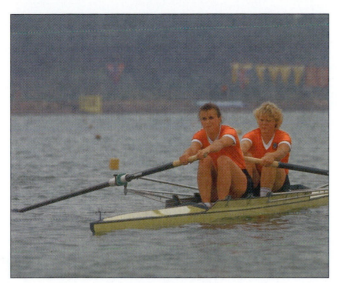
Interval training can be adapted for performers in a variety of activities.

tions that will improve aerobic capacity ($\dot{V}O_2$ max). The use of repeated mile runs at a faster-than-normal training pace would provide this type of challenge to the aerobic system. Alternately, shorter exercise bouts can be performed with brief rest periods to achieve the same goal. For example, a series of quarter-mile repeats with short rests would be suitable as long as the total time at a high intensity was similar. In this case, the rest intervals must be short enough to only allow partial recovery between intervals.

Aerobic intervals are typically conducted at paces slower than the pace an individual would use in a race. An example of a schedule of aerobic interval training for a 10-km runner is illustrated in Table 2. To use the schedule, locate your typical 10-km time in the left-hand column. Perform 400-meter runs at the time specified in the "pace" column. Repeat 20 times with intervals of 10 to 15 seconds between runs. Similar schedules can be developed with other activities such as swimming and cycling. This activity, however, is not recommended for those just beginning exercise.

rapidly following that, alternate short sprints with walking, go full speed uphill, and perhaps at a fast pace for a while. You can plan your own speed-play program using your own course, which may include both uphill and downhill running with other variations.

Training for activities requiring high levels of aerobic capacity can be achieved using a variety of techniques.

WEB

www.mhhe.com/hper/physed/clw/student/
The ability to perform sustained aerobic performance can be enhanced using a variety of techniques. The most common procedure is to perform the activity in which you plan to participate. For example, people who plan to run a marathon or a 10K race will commonly perform regular distance running at speed similar to those required for their specific event. This type of training is also supplemented with aerobic interval training and long slow-distance training. Some training to enhance anaerobic capacity is also performed by most people interested in aerobic activities. Performers in other activities such as swimming and cycling will use similar schedules of training.

Interval training can be done aerobically.

Many people think only of interval training as an anaerobic method of training. In fact, aerobic interval training can be very effective in performance enhancement. In aerobic interval training, the goal is to challenge the aerobic system to work near maximal levels for extended periods of time. Research suggests that a period of 4–6 minutes of activity is needed to cause the aerobic system to elicit maximal adapta-

Table 2   Aerobic Interval Training Schedules for a 10-Kilometer Runner

Best 10-km Times (Min:Sec)	Reps	Distance (Meters)	Rest (Sec)	Pace (Min:Sec)
46:00	20	400	10–15	2:00
43:00	20	400	10–15	1:52
40:00	20	400	10–15	1:45
37:00	20	400	10–15	1:37
34:00	20	400	10–15	1:30

From Jack H. Wilmore and David L. Costill, *Training for Sport and Activity*, 3d ed. Copyright ©1988 Times Mirror Higher Education Group, Inc., Dubuque, Iowa. All Rights Reserved. Reprinted by permission.

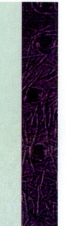

Anaerobic Exercise Anaerobic means "in the absence of oxygen." Anaerobic exercise is performed at an intensity that is greater than the body's ability to provide energy through the aerobic system.

Lactic Acid Substance that results from the process of supplying energy during anaerobic exercise; a cause of muscle fatigue.

Interval Training A training technique often used for high-level aerobic and anaerobic training; uses repeated bouts of activity followed by rest to maximize the quality of the workout.

If your heart rate exceeds your target zone, you will need to modify the running time for each interval.

Long slow-distance training is important for enhancing performances requiring aerobic capacity.

The training techniques described in previous sections are necessary to achieve high-level aerobic performance. However, there is evidence that **long slow-distance training (LSD)** is also needed to promote high-level aerobic performances (such as long-distance running, cycling, or swimming). The reason for this is that there are specific adaptations that take place within the muscles when used for long periods of time. These adaptations improve the muscles' ability to take up and use the oxygen in the bloodstream. Adaptations within the muscle cell also improve the body's ability to produce energy from fat stores. Long slow-distance training involves performances longer than the event for which you are performing but at a slower pace. For example, a mile runner will regularly perform 6–7 mile runs (at 50–60% of racing pace) to improve aerobic conditioning even though the event is much shorter. A marathoner may perform runs of 20 miles or more to achieve even higher levels of endurance. While this 20-mile distance is shorter than the marathon race distance, research suggests that ample adaptations occur from this volume of exercise. Excess mileage in this case may just wear the body down. Long slow-distance training should be performed once every 1 to 2 weeks, and a rest day is recommended on the subsequent day to allow the body to fully recover.

Improved anaerobic capacity can contribute to performance in activities considered to be aerobic.

Many physical activities commonly considered to be aerobic—such as tennis, basketball, and racquetball—have an anaerobic component. These activities require periodic vigorous bursts of exercise. Regular anaerobic training will help you resist fatigue in these activities. Even participants in activities such as long-distance running can benefit from anaerobic training, especially if performance times or winning races is important. A fast start may be anaerobic, a sprint past an opponent may be anaerobic, and a kick at the end will no doubt be anaerobic. Anaerobic training can help prepare a person for these circumstances.

Some training methods can interfere with performance.

Some research studies have shown that certain techniques may actually cause a decrease in performance. For example, when distance runners were trained with weighted wristlets, anklets, and belts, they performed worse than runners who did not wear weights in training. In another study, people who were running and bicycling for aerobic endurance six days per week combined those exercises with a strength training program five days per week. The results suggest that doing intense training for aerobic capacity and muscle fitness simultaneously had somewhat limited muscle fitness benefits.

The Facts about Training for High-Level Performance: Muscle Fitness

The amount of progressive resistance training for high-level performance differs from techniques used to build strength for health.

In the concept on muscle fitness, basic training techniques were described. The focus was on health enhancement. Training techniques for people interested in health differ from those who want high-level performance. For example, there are three competitive sports associated with resistance training. Olympic weight-lifting competitors use free weights and compete in two exercises: the snatch, and the clean and jerk. Powerlifting competitors use free weights and compete in three lifts: the bench press, squat, and dead lift. Bodybuilding competitors use several forms of resistance training, and are judged on muscular hypertrophy and **definition of muscle**. Performers in these activities as well as those in a variety of other activities use advanced resistance training techniques, some of which are described in the sections that follow.

Advanced lifters use heavier resistance than most people during strength training; therefore, they use some techniques not recommended for the beginner.

www.mhhe.com/hper/physed/clw/student/
The compressive force on the lumbar discs during a half-squat can be six to 10 times the body weight. To reduce the spinal compression, prevent abdominal hernias, and aid in lifting more weight, advanced lifters are encouraged to wear a belt with a rigid abdominal pad and a wide band across the lumbar spine. At the same time, they hold their breath until they get past the "sticking point" of a lift. The belt must be loosened between reps to breathe and to allow the blood to return to the heart. Holding the breath permits trunk cavity pressurization to relieve the load on the spine, while the belt helps hold in the abdominal contents. Advanced lifting requires advanced training in

proper techniques to avoid injury. Beginners should not attempt these lifts nor hold the breath, but they may wish to use the belts if they have a history of back problems.

Performers training for bulk and definition often use extra reps and/or sets.

www.mhhe.com/hper/physed/clw/student/
Most bodybuilders use three to seven sets of 10 to 15 repetitions, rather than the three sets of three to eight repetitions recommended for most weight lifters. Bodybuilders are more interested in definition and hypertrophy (large muscles) than strength. Sometimes definition is difficult to obtain because it is obscured by fat. It should be noted that people with the largest-looking muscles are not always the strongest.

"Negative" exercise has no advantage over other types of exercise for muscle fitness development.

Contrary to the claims of some enthusiasts, there does not seem to be any difference between eccentric (negative) exercise and concentric (positive) exercise in terms of their effectiveness in developing strength or muscular endurance. Weight can be handled more comfortably with eccentric exercise, but this type of exercise has a tendency to cause more muscle soreness. This type of exercise also requires the assistance of another person or the use of a special

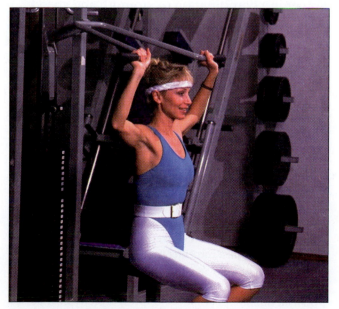

Strength training for high-level performance differs from strength training for health.

machine such as the Kin Com Biodex or Keiser dynamometers. The most common application of eccentric exercise has been in rehabilitation settings where it has been found to be useful in promoting muscle function and recovery from injury.

Eccentric contractions are combined with concentric contractions in most sports. For example, if you lift something, you also lower it. Thus, to apply the law of specificity, progressive resistance exercises should generally include both types of contractions. This can be accomplished with a slow, steady concentric lifting phase and a slower, eccentric, lowering phase (see discussion of technique later in the concept).

Periodization of training may help prevent overtraining.

www.mhhe.com/hper/physed/clw/student/
When a person trains for a single performance or perhaps several competitive events such as games or matches during a sport season, it requires careful planning to reach peak performance at the right time and to avoid overtraining and injuries. Periodization is a modern concept of manipulating repetition, resistance, and exercise selection so there are periodic peaks and valleys during the training program. The peaks are needed to challenge the body, and the valleys are needed to allow the body to fully recover and adapt. Over the course of the season, there should be a gradual progression that allows the person to peak at just the right time. To accomplish this, training normally begins with an emphasis on base training in which the volume of training is gradually increased (increasing reps or performing large numbers of sets). As the season progresses, the focus shifts to an emphasis on the intensity of training (going faster or lifting heavier weights). Because higher intensity exercise requires more time for recovery, the volume of training should be reduced at these times. A key concept in periodization is to provide opportunities for the body to fully adapt and recover prior to competition. Thus, the phase immediately prior to competition (**tapering**) is characterized by a reduced volume and intensity of training. By applying periodization to their training, athletes are able to

LSD Training A training technique that emphasizes long, slow, distance. It is used by marathon runners and other endurance performers.

Definition (of Muscle) The detailed external appearance of a muscle.

Tapering A reduction in training volume and intensity that is used prior to competition to elicit peak performance.

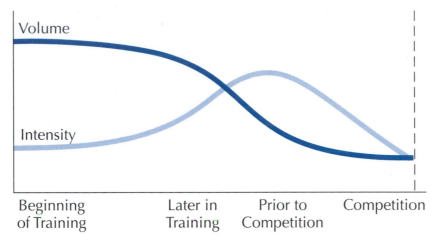

Figure 2
Volume and Intensity of Training During Periodization.

optimize performance and minimize the risk of overtraining. (See Figure 2.)

> **Training for cardiovascular fitness at the same time as strength training may prevent maximum results in both.**

Studies have shown that training simultaneously for strength and cardiovascular fitness may not produce the same result as one could obtain while training for either one separately. Some people have interpreted this to mean that they interfere with each other. The cause of this is not clear. It may be that the time spent on each one is less or that overtraining occurs rather than the fact that one inhibits the other. Whatever the cause, the differences are relatively minor and it should not prevent an individual from doing both concurrently.

> **Muscular endurance is important to high-level performance.**

Muscular endurance training (see muscle fitness concept) is necessary for performers in a variety of activities. For people training for distance events, muscular endurance training can complement cardiovascular fitness training and enhance performance. Resistance training for this type of performance would focus on high repetitions rather than high resistance. For performers in activities requiring strength, the amount of muscular endurance training depends on the specific nature of the activity. For example, if the activity requires only very short duration and has a high strength requirement, muscular endurance training involving high repetitions may actually impair performance. The sport of weight lifting would be an example. On the other hand, activities such as blocking in football require repeated strength performance. For performers doing this type of activity, the ability to persist (muscular endurance) is important so training should use a relatively high number of repetitions.

The Facts about Training for High-Level Performance: Power

> **Power is a combination of strength and speed, and is both health-related and skill-related.**

Most experts classify power as a skill-related component of fitness because it is partially dependent on speed. On the other hand, power is also dependent on strength and can be classified as a health-related component to the extent that strength is involved. Thus, power falls somewhere in between the two distinct groups of fitness attributes. Certainly its use is not limited to sports and dance. We use power extensively in our daily activities every time we apply a force to move something quickly. Power is important in protective movements, such as a pedestrian jumping to dodge a car or a driver jerking the steering wheel to avoid a collision or slamming on the brakes to stop in an emergency. A worker heaves a heavy load from a truck to a dock, and a carpenter uses force to hammer a nail.

Power is usually neglected in fitness literature. Some experts consider power to be the most functional mode in which all human motion occurs. Still, if the typical person builds adequate muscle fitness using the guidelines described earlier in this text, adequate power for daily living will occur. This is not true of people interested in high-level performance of many types. Power is exceptionally important in activities such as hitting a baseball, blocking in football, putting the shot, or throwing the discus. Clearly people interested in high-level performances should consider appropriate exercises that develop power.

The stronger person is not necessarily the more powerful.

Power is the amount of work per unit of time. To increase power, you must do more work in the same time or the same work in less time. If you extend your knee and move a 100-pound weight through a 90-degree arc in 1 second, you have twice as much power as a person who needs 2 seconds to complete the same movement. Power requires both strength and speed. Increasing one without the other limits power. Some power athletes (for example, football players) might benefit more by achieving less strength and more speed.

There is probably no one best training program for developing power, but the law of specificity applies.

If you need power for an activity in which you are required to move heavy weights, then you need to develop *strength-related power* by working against heavy resistance at slower speeds. (See Figure 3.) If you need to move light objects at great speed, such as in throwing a ball, you need to develop *speed-related power* by training at high speeds with relatively low resistance. There must be trade-offs between speed and power because the heavier the resistance, the slower the movement.

There is a target zone for optimum power.

Studies show that power is best developed when the force is between 30 and 60 percent of maximum. But the optimum is probably when the load and the speed are about one-third of maximum. (See Figure 3.) The following example illustrates the relationship between speed, strength, and power. If your maximum strength is represented by 2 and maximum speed by 2, then your power is $2 \times 2 = 4$. If you double your strength ($4 \times 2 = 8$), your power would be doubled. However, if your strength and speed were each increased by only 50 percent, even more power results ($3 \times 3 = 9$).

The principle of specificity should be applied to training programs for power events.

Performers who need explosive power to perform their events should use training that closely resembles the event.

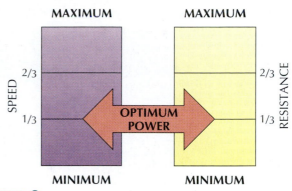

Figure 3
Optimum power is produced when the load and speed are each about one-third of maximum.

Jumpers, for example, should jump as a part of their training programs in order to learn correct timing at the same time they are developing power. This also applies to Olympic weight lifters, shot-putters, jumpers, ballet dancers, and others. These athletes need both strength and endurance; however, studies show that too much of either can have a negative effect on performance. If they use machines, it is better to use the leg press than a knee extension machine because the press more nearly resembles the leg action of the jump.

The performer's program should use similar speed, force, angle, and range of motion, as the activity. However, if a performer is unable to do the specific skill because of weather or injury or is seeking variety, then plyometrics, isokinetics, and weight training (especially with free weights or pulleys if simulating a sport skill) are effective means of developing power.

Plyometrics may be useful in training for tasks or events requiring power.

www.mhhe.com/hper/physed/clw/student/
A quick prestretch, or eccentric contraction of a muscle, immediately followed by an isometric or concentric contraction, produces power. This has been called "pre-exertion countermovement," "wind up," or "**plyometrics**." Former Soviet Olympic coaches pioneered this technique, developing drills for their athletes. Track and

Plyometrics A training technique used to develop explosive power. Referred to as "speed-strength training" in Eastern Europe and the former Soviet Union, where it originated, it consists of concentric isotonic contractions performed after a prestretch or eccentric contraction of a muscle.

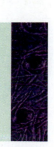

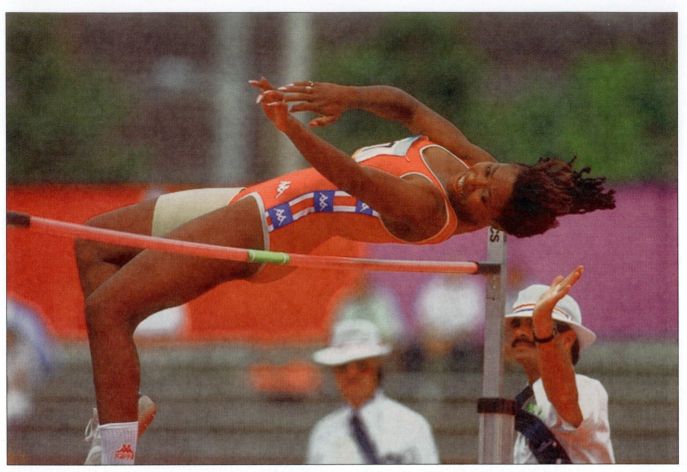

Plyometrics is a technique used to produce high-level power performance.

field athletes may do a hopping drill for 30 to 100 meters or alternate jumping from a box to the floor and back to the box (called "depth jumping," "drop jumping," or "bounce loading"). As the body lands, some of the major leg muscles lengthen in an eccentric contraction, then follow immediately with a strong concentric contraction as the legs push off for the next jump or stride. The prestretch of the muscle during landing adds an elastic recoil that provides extra force to the push-off.

Plyometrics are used to apply the specificity principle to training for certain skills. Because eccentric exercise tends to result in more muscular soreness, it would be wise to proceed slowly with this type of training. It would also be important to have good flexibility before beginning a plyometrics program. Some guidelines are listed in Table 4.

Power exercises can increase muscular endurance or strength.

Power exercises done at high speeds have been shown to increase muscular endurance. Likewise, power exercises that use heavy resistance at lower speeds will increase strength.

The Facts about Training for High-Level Performance: Flexibility

Stretching for performance may differ from stretching for good health.

Guidelines for building flexibility using a variety of stretching exercises are presented in the concept on flexibility. It was noted in that concept that static stretching techniques are recommended for the warm-up, even for high-level performers. Ballistic stretching is appropriate for high-level performers because many of the motions of the activities in which they perform require ballistic movements. Nevertheless, it is recommended that ballistic stretch used as a training technique should be performed after initiating the workout with static or PNF stretch.

After the static stretching phase of the workout, the ballistic stretching phase should use stretches that closely approximate the performance activity. Examples of ballistic stretching exercises for specific performances are presented in Table 5.

Table 4 Safety Guidelines for Plyometrics

- Adolescents whose bones are still growing should avoid plyometric exercise (to avoid permanent growth-stunting damage to the growth plates).
- Progression should be gradual to avoid extreme muscle soreness.
- Adequate strength should be developed prior to plyometric training. (As a general rule, you should be able to do a squat with one-and-a-half times your body weight.)
- Get a physician's approval prior to doing plyometrics if you have a history of injuries or if you are recovering from injury to the body part being trained.
- The landing surface should be semiresilient, dry, and unobstructed.
- Shoes should have good lateral stability, be cushioned with an arch support, and have a nonslip sole.
- Obstacles used for jumping-over should be padded.
- The training should be preceded by a general and specific warm-up.
- The training sequence should:
  - precede all other workouts (while you are fresh);
  - include at least one spotter;
  - be done no more than twice per week, with 48 hours rest between bouts;
  - last no more than 30 minutes;
  - (for beginners) include 3 or 4 drills, with 2 or 3 sets per drill, 10–15 reps per set and 1–2 minutes rest between sets.

SOURCE: Data from G. Brittenham, "Plyometric Exercise: A Word of Caution" in *Journal of Physical Education, Recreation, and Dance*, January 1992: 20–23. American Alliance for Health, Physical Education, Recreation, and Dance, Reston, VA.

The Facts about Training for High-Level Performance: Skill-Related Fitness and Skill

There are many factors that contribute to high-level performance.

Possessing high levels of the six primary components of skill-related physical fitness (agility, coordination, balance, reaction time, speed, and power) make it easier to learn the skills important to high-level performance. However, there are other abilities that also contribute to performing skills. For example, many experts consider various perceptual abilities such as depth and distance perception (ability to judge depth and distances accurately) and visual tracking (ability to visually follow a moving object) to be skill-related parts of physical fitness. Skill-related physical fitness is also sometimes referred to as **motor fitness** or **sports fitness**.

There are sub-components of each component of skill-related physical fitness.

Most of the six parts of skill-related physical fitness have sub-components. For example, coordination includes foot-eye coordination and hand-eye coordination, which are measured quite differently. The tests in this concept were chosen to measure some of the skill-related fitness aspects most important to sports performance.

An individual might possess ability in one area and not in another. For this reason, general motor ability probably does not really exist—individuals do not have one general capacity for performing. Rather, the ability to play games or sports is determined by combined abilities in each of the separate skill-related components. It is, however, possible and even likely that some performers will be above average in many areas.

Exceptional performers tend to be outstanding in more than one component of skill-related fitness.

Though people possess skill-related fitness in varying degrees, great athletes are likely to be above average in

Motor Fitness A term commonly used for skill-related physical fitness.

Sports Fitness A term commonly used for skill-related fitness.

Table 5
Examples of Ballistic Stretch to Enhance Performance

Ballistic Stretch for Throwing and Striking

This exercise is to improve flexibility to aid one-handed throwing and striking skills (for example, racket sports forehand, backhand, and serve; baseball throw, or discus and shot put); and/or two-handed throwing or striking skills (for example, batting a softball or executing a golf drive or hammer throw). Assume a position at the end of the backswing for any skill listed above. Partner grasps hand(s) and resists movement while the performer turns the trunk away from the partner, making a series of gentle bouncing movements, attempting to rotate the trunk as if performing the skill. Alternate roles with the partner. Note: Avoid overstretching by too vigorous bouncing. If no partner is available, use a door frame for resistance, or these sports actions can be practiced using elastic bands or inner tubes (attached to fixed objects) as resistance.

Ballistic Stretch for Golf Swing

This exercise is to improve flexibility for the golf swing. A similar exercise can be performed using one-handed throwing and striking skills (for example, racket sports forehand, backhand, and serve; baseball throw, or discus and shot put); and/or two-handed throwing or striking skills (for example, batting a softball or hammer throw). Stand and swing the club with or without a weight on the implement or on the wrist. Start by swinging backward and forward rhythmically and continuously. Gradually increase the speed and vigor of the swing to finally resemble the actual skill.

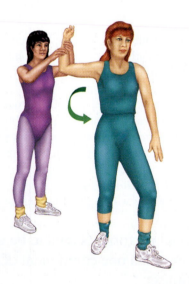

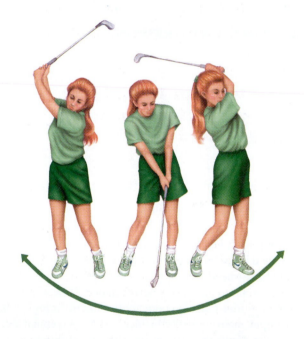

most, if not all, aspects. Indeed, exceptional athletes must be exceptional in many areas of skill-related fitness. Different sports require different skills, each of which requires varying degrees of the six components of skill-related fitness.

> **Excellence in one skill-related fitness component may compensate for a lack in another.**

Each individual possesses a specific level of each skill-related fitness aspect. The performer should learn his or her other strengths and weaknesses in order to produce optimal performances. For example, a tennis player may use good coordination to compensate for lack of speed.

> **Excellence in skill-related fitness may compensate for a lack of health-related fitness when playing sports and games.**

As you grow older, health-related fitness potential declines much more rapidly than many components of skill-related fitness. You may use superior skill-related fitness to compensate. For example, a baseball pitcher who lacks the strength and power to dominate hitters may rely on a pitch such as a knuckle ball, which is more dependent on coordination than on power.

> **Practice can help skill-related fitness but is probably not as effective as practice to improve the specific skills of the activity you expect to perform.**

As noted in a previous section, power is the component of fitness especially likely to be changed with training. Drills for enhancing other aspects of skill-related physical fitness can help improve these abilities. For example, agility drills can improve scores on the specific agility drill that is practiced. Speed in running can be improved by increasing strength. However, experts generally agree that skill-related fitness is highly influenced by heredity.

As illustrated in Figure 1, learning specific skills (not skill-related fitness) through regular practice is the preferred method of improving performance. To achieve high-level performance, lengthy practice of the appropriate kind is essential.

The Facts about Hyperkinetic Conditions

> **Just as too little physical activity can result in health problems, too much can also contribute to illness and injury.**

"Hypokinetic" means too little physical activity. Conversely, "hyperkinetic" means too much. Just as reasonable amounts of physical activity can help reduce the risk of hypokinetic health problems, it has become apparent that excessive exercise can lead to **hyperkinetic conditions** that have negative effects on health and wellness. High-level performance requires high-level training.

Many athletes push themselves too hard in their pursuit of high-level performance, not allowing adequate time for rest. This overtraining results in "overload" syndrome characterized by fatigue, irritability, and sleep problems, as well as one or more hyperkinetic conditions. Some types of common hyperkinetic conditions are presented in the sections that follow.

> **One type of hyperkinetic condition is musculoskeletal overuse injuries.**

As documented in the *Surgeon General's Report*, evidence suggests that periodic rest is necessary to allow the body to recover from the stress of continuous and vigorous training. For example, runners who train seven days a week have more muscle and joint injuries than runners who take off at least one day a week or reduce training levels several days a week. The most common overuse injuries are joint injuries to the foot, ankle, and knee; stress fractures in the lower extremities; and muscle/connective tissue injuries such as shin splints, strained hamstring muscles, and calf pain. These injuries are apparent among exercisers who overdo it. For example, dance aerobics instructors are particularly likely to have overuse injuries. Tennis and baseball players often have similar problems, but their problems occur in different parts of the body (the arm and shoulder). The best way to prevent this type of hyperkinetic condition is periodic rest. Pain, the body's warning signal, is a good clue that the body needs rest.

Hyperkinetic Conditions Condition caused by too much physical activity and/or insufficient rest.

Compulsive physical activity is referred to as activity neurosis.

People with activity neurosis become irrationally concerned about their exercise regimen. They may exercise more than one time a day, rarely take a day off, or feel the need to exercise even when ill or injured. Musculoskeletal overuse injuries are especially common among activity neurotics. The excessive desire to be active can also be the source of poor performance in other aspects of life, as well as a source of stress. Competitive athletes with this condition may have reduced performance, and among females, amenorrhea (no menstrual flow).

Anorexia nervosa can be considered as a hyperkinetic condition.

Anorexia nervosa is an eating disorder associated with an obsessive desire to be lean. There is increasing evidence that many anorexics use compulsive exercise, as well as undereating, to keep body fat at low levels. For this reason, anorexia nervosa can often be considered a hyperkinetic condition. Recent data suggest that at least 25 percent of people with anorexia do compulsive exercise.

A recently defined type of hyperkinetic condition is body neurosis.

Body neurosis is an obsessive concern for having an attractive body. Among females, it is associated with an extreme desire to be lean. In some cases, it can lead to anorexia. Among males, this condition is associated with an extreme desire to be muscular. Recent research indicates that increasing numbers of males are interested in leanness, and a number of females are now compulsive about muscle mass gains. People with body neurosis are often compulsive exercisers, though they are also more likely to be subject to nutritional quackery (using quack dietary supplements) and in some cases resort to the use of anabolic steroids.

The Facts about Ergogenic Aids

Many athletes look to ergogenic aids as an additional way to improve performance.

Athletes are always looking for a competitive edge. In addition to pursuing rigorous training programs, many athletes look for alternative ways to improve their performance. Substances, strategies, or treatments that are designed to improve physical performance beyond the effects of normal training are collectively referred to as **ergogenic aids.** Recent information suggests that many people interested in improving their appearance (including those with body neurosis) also abuse products they think will enhance their appearance.

Mechanical ergogenics may improve mechanical efficiency and performance.

Most competitive activities require equipment or special clothing. As technology and research increase, there are regular improvements in design that improve mechanical efficiency or performance in different activities. An example of mechanical ergogenics is the improved aerodynamics resulting from advances in bicycling clothing and equipment. Another example is the improved performance resulting from oversized, composite tennis racquets. While these types of aids are not required to enjoy or participate in an activity, some may provide an advantage in competition.

Psychological ergogenics improve concentration and focus during competitive activities.

Many competitive activities require extreme levels of concentration and focus. Athletes who are able to maintain this mental edge during an event are at a clear advantage over athletes who cannot. Psychological ergogenics are strategies such as mental imagery and hypnosis, which have been shown to help athletes achieve peak performance. Athletes are encouraged to use these psychological aids but to be wary of untested or unproven techniques since quackery is prominent in this area.

Physiological ergogenics are designed to improve performance by enhancing biochemical and physiological processes in the body.

Physiological ergogenics refer primarily to nutritional supplements that are thought to have a positive effect on various metabolic processes. An example is fluid replacement drinks, that athletes consume during endurance exercise. Consumption of these drinks has been shown to maintain blood sugar levels and delay fatigue in exercise lasting over one hour. While the ergogenic benefit of fluid replacement beverages is clearly established, the safety and effectiveness of most other supplements are questionable. Because the supplement industry is largely unregulated, many products are developed and marketed with little or no research to document their effects. These products prey on an athlete's lack of knowledge and concern over performance. Table 6 summarizes the potential

Ergogenic Aids Substances, strategies, or treatments that are theoretically designed to improve performance in sports or competitive athletics.

Table 6   Effectiveness and Safety of Various Physiological Ergogenic Aids

Ergogenic Aids with Strong Evidence for a Performance Benefit

Name of Supplement	Proposed Effect (Claims)	Safe?
Alkaline salts (e.g., sodium bicarbonate, sodium citrate)	Buffer metabolic acidosis produced from lactic acid buildup	Yes
Caffeine	Increases rate of fat metabolism and sparing glycogen depletion	Yes, in moderation, can dehydrate
Carbohydrates (e.g., glucose, fructose)	Maintain blood glucose levels and delay glycogen depletion	Yes
Creatine	Muscular strength	Questionable safety; side effects include dehydration and cramps
Water	Minimizes dehydration during endurance exercise in the heat	Yes

Ergogenic Aids with Some Evidence for a Performance Benefit

Name of Supplement	Proposed Effect (Claims)	Safe?
Aspartate salts (e.g., potassium, magnesium aspartate)	Mitigate the accumulation of ammonia during exercise	Probably safe
Carbohydrate metabolites (e.g., DHAP, pyruvate)	Maintain blood glucose levels and delay glycogen depletion	Probably safe
Glycerol	Promotes hyperhydration and improves thermoregulation during exercise in the heat	Probably safe
Phosphates	Phosphates are a component of 2,3-DPG, which is essential for the release of oxygen from hemoglobin	Not clear

Ergogenic Aids with Little or No Evidence for a Performance Benefit

Name of Supplement	Proposed Effect (Claims)	Safe?
Amino acids (general)	Alleged increase in muscle mass, prevents protein catabolism	Probably, unless consumed in extremely high doses
Amino acids (e.g., arginine, ornithine)	Alleged increase in strength by increasing levels of human growth hormone and insulin	Probably safe; however, extreme protein consumption is harmful
Androstenedione	Alleged hormone precursor to testosterone	Not established
L-carnitine	Allegedly facilitates the transport of fatty acids, and oxidation of amino acids and pyruvate, which delays glycogen depletion	Not established
Choline	Allegedly maintains acetylcholine levels during exercise; acetylcholine is thought to be related to onset of fatigue	Not established
Chysin	Allegedly prevents conversion of excess testosterone to estrogen, which would allow higher testosterone levels	Not established
Coenzyme Q10 (Ubiquinone)	Allegedly improves oxygen uptake in the mitochondria	Not established
Dehydroepiandrosterone	Alleged hormone precursor to testosterone	Not established
Hydroxy beta-methylbutyrate (HMB)	Allegedly a metabolite of leucine, thought to improve cellular repair of muscle	Not established
Inosine	A nucleic acid found in DNA that is purported to increase energy production	Not established
Lipid metabolites (medium chain triglycerides)	Allegedly increases fat metabolism by increasing the availability of dietary fats in the circulation	Yes, if consumed as a part of diet
Protein metabolites (e.g., tryptophan and branched chain amino acids [BCA])	Alter the formation of serotonin, a neurotransmitter alleged to influence central nervous system fatigue	Yes, if consumed as a part of diet

Adapted from Williams, M. H. Nutritional Ergogenics and Sports Performance, PCPFS Research Digest, 2(10)(1998). Copyright © 1998.

Table 7 Skill-Related Requirements of Sports and Other Activities

Activity	Balance	Coordination	Reaction Time	Agility	Power	Speed
Archery	***	****	*	*	*	*
Backpacking	**	**	*	**	**	*
Badminton	**	****	***	***	**	***
Baseball	***	****	****	***	****	***
Basketball	***	****	****	****	****	***
Bicycling	****	**	**	*	**	**
Bowling	***	****	*	**	**	**
Canoeing	***	***	**	*	***	*
Circuit training	**	**	*	**	***	**
Dance, aerobic	**	****	**	***	*	*
Dance, ballet	****	****	**	****	***	*
Dance, disco	**	***	**	****	*	**
Dance, modern	****	****	**	****	***	*
Dance, social	**	***	**	***	*	**
Fencing	***	****	****	***	***	****
Fitness calisthenics	**	**	*	***	**	*
Football	***	***	****	****	****	****
Golf (walking)	**	****	*	**	***	*
Gymnastics	****	****	***	****	****	**
Handball	**	****	***	****	***	***
Hiking	**	**	*	**	**	*
Horseback riding	***	***	**	***	*	*
Interval training	**	**	*	*	*	**
Jogging	**	**	*	*	*	*
Judo	***	****	****	****	****	****
Karate	***	****	****	****	****	****
Mountain climbing	****	****	**	***	***	*
Pool; billiards	**	***	*	**	**	*
Racquetball; paddleball	**	****	***	****	**	***
Rope jumping	**	***	**	***	**	*
Rowing, crew	**	****	*	***	****	**
Sailing	***	***	***	***	**	*
Skating, ice	****	***	**	***	**	***
Skating, roller	****	***	*	***	**	***
Skiing, cross-country	**	****	*	***	****	**
Skiing, downhill	****	****	***	****	***	*
Soccer	**	****	***	****	***	***
Softball (fast pitch)	**	****	****	***	***	***
Softball (slow pitch)	**	****	***	**	***	***
Surfing	****	****	***	****	**	*
Swimming (laps)	**	***	*	***	**	*
Table tennis	**	***	**	**	**	**
Tennis	**	****	***	***	***	***
Volleyball	**	****	***	***	**	**
Walking	**	**	*	*	*	*
Waterskiing	***	***	*	***	**	**
Weight training	**	**	*	*	**	*

* = minimal needed; **** = a lot needed.

effectiveness of many commercially available supplements. Because safety of many of these supplements has not been established, consumers should be cautious about using them in their training. It should be pointed out that the products with little or no evidence of benefits also have questionable safety. You should also know that supplements are unregulated so it is often impossible to know if the product you buy is really what it is advertised to be.

Strategies for Action: The Facts

You can maximize your chances for success by selecting activities that match your abilities.

Whether your goal is high-level performance or finding an activity that you can enjoy during your leisure time, your choice of activity is important. To give yourself the best chance of being successful, you should consider choosing an activity that matches your abilities. Assessing your skill-related physical fitness abilities can help you determine your areas of strength. In Lab 14A, you have the opportunity to assess your skill-related fitness and build a fitness profile. Using Table 7, you can determine the sports and activities that best match your individual abilities.

It should be noted that the assessments provided in Lab 14A are but a few of the many tests that can be done for each of the skill-related fitness parts. You may want to try other tests if you want more information about your abilities. If you have a personal desire to train for a specific sport or activity, but do not have a fitness profile that predicts success, you should not be deterred. Lab 14A will help you find an activity that you will enjoy and in which you have a good chance of success. People with good motivation, who persist in training, can often excel over others with greater ability.

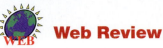

Web Review

Web review materials for Concept 14 are available are at *www.mhhe.com/hper/physed/clw/student/*.

Disabled Sports USA

www.dsusa.org

National Athletic Trainers Association

www.nata.org

National Collegiate Athletic Association

www.ncaa.org

National Strength and Conditioning Association

www.nsca-cc.org/aboutnsca.htm

Special Olympics International

www.specialolympics.org

United States Olympic Committee

www.usoc.org

Women's Sports Foundation

www.lifetimetv.com/wosport/index.html

Suggested Readings

ACSM. (1997). Position Stand on the Female Athlete Triad. *Medicine and Science in Sports and Exercise*. 29(5)(1997):i.

Chu, D. A. *Jumping Into Plyometrics*. Champaign, Il.: Human Kinetics, 1998.

Fleck, S. J., and Kraemer, W. J. *Designing Resistance Training Programs*, 2nd ed. Champaign, IL: Human Kinetics, 1997.

Kreider, R. B., Fry, A. C., and O'Toole, M. L. *Overtraining in Sport*. Champaign, IL: Human Kinetics, 1998.

Morgan, G. T., and McGlynn, G. H. *Cross-Training for Sports*. Champaign, IL: Human Kinetics, 1997.

Otis, C. Too Slim, Amenorrheic, Fracture Prone: The Female Athlete Triad. *ACSM's Health and Fitness Journal*. 2(1)(1998):20.

Tofler, I. R., et al. Physical and Emotional Problems of Elite Female Gymnasts. *New England Journal of Medicine*. 335(4)(1998):281.

Volek, S. "Creatine Supplementation and Its Possible Role in Improving Physical Performance." *ACSM's Health and Fitness Journal* 1(4)(1997):23.

Williams, M. H. "Nutritional Ergogenics and Sports Performance." *PCPFS Research Digest* (10)(1998):1.

Lab Resource Materials

Important Note: Because skill-related physical fitness does not relate to good health, the rating charts used in this section differ from those used for health-related fitness. The rating charts that follow can be used to compare your scores to those of other people. You *do not* need exceptional scores on skill-related fitness to be able to enjoy sports and other types of physical activity; however, it is necessary for high-level performance. After the age of 30, you should adjust ratings by 1 percent per year.

Evaluating Skill-Related Physical Fitness

I. Evaluating agility: The Illinois agility run
An agility course using four chairs 10 feet apart, and a 30-foot running area will be set up as depicted in this illustration. The test is performed as follows:
1. Lie prone with your hands by your shoulders and your head at the starting line. On the signal to begin, get on your feet and run the course as fast as possible.
2. Your score is the time required to complete the course.

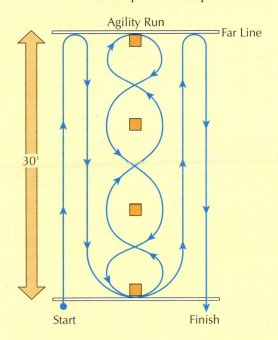

Agility Run
Far Line
30'
Start   Finish

II. **Evaluating balance: The Bass test of dynamic balance**
Eleven circles (9 1/2-inch) are drawn on the floor as shown in the illustration. The test is performed as follows:
1. Stand on the right foot in circle X. *Leap* forward to circle 1, then circle 2 through 10, alternating feet with each leap.
2. The feet must leave the floor on each leap and the heel may not touch. Only the ball of the foot and toes may land on the floor.
3. Remain in each circle for 5 seconds before leaping to the next circle. (A count of five will be made for you aloud.)
4. Practice trials are allowed.
5. The score is 50, plus the number of seconds taken to complete the test, minus the number of errors.
6. For every error, deduct three points each. Errors include touching the heel, moving the supporting foot, touching outside a circle, or touching any body part to the floor other than the supporting foot.

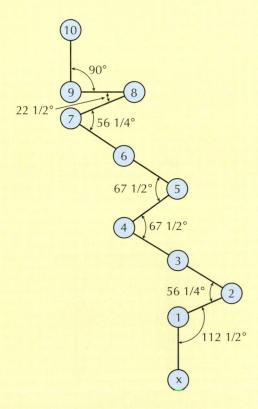

Chart 1 Agility Rating Scale

Classification	Men	Women
Excellent	15.8 or faster	17.4 or faster
Very good	16.7–15.9	18.6–17.5
Good	18.6–16.8	22.3–18.7
Fair	18.8–18.7	23.4–22.4
Poor	18.9 or slower	23.5 or slower

SOURCE: Data from Adams, et al., *Foundations of Physical Activity*, 1965, p. 111.

Chart 2 Balance Test Rating Scale

Rating	Score
Excellent	90–100
Very good	80–89
Good	60–79
Fair	30–59
Poor	0–29

Chart 3 Coordination Rating Scale

Classification	Men	Women
Excellent	14–15	13–15
Very good	11–13	10–12
Good	5–10	4–9
Fair	3–4	2–3
Poor	0–2	0–1

III. Evaluating coordination: The stick test of coordination

The stick test of coordination requires you to juggle three wooden sticks. The sticks are used to perform a one-half flip and a full flip as shown in the illustrations.

1. *One-half flip*—Hold two 24-inch (one-half inch in diameter) dowel rods, one in each hand. Support a third rod of the same size across the other two. Toss the supported rod in the air so that it makes a half turn. Catch the thrown rod with the two held rods.
2. *Full flip*—Perform the preceding task, letting the supported rod turn a full flip.

The test is performed as follows:

1. Practice the half-flip and full flip several times before taking the test.
2. When you are ready, attempt a half-flip five times. Score one point for each successful attempt.
3. When you are ready, attempt the full flip five times. Score two points for each successful attempt.

IV. Evaluating power: The vertical jump test

The test is performed as follows:

1. Hold a piece of chalk so its end is even with your fingertips.
2. Stand with both feet on the floor and your side to the wall and reach and mark as high as possible.
3. Jump upward with both feet as high as possible. Swing arms upward and make a chalk mark on a 5´ × 1´ wall chart marked off in half-inch horizontal lines placed 6 feet from the floor.
4. Measure the distance between the reaching height and the jumping height.
5. Your score is the best of three jumps.

Chart 4 Power Rating Scale

Classification	Men	Women
Excellent	25 1/2" or more	23 1/2" or more
Very good	21"–25"	19"–23"
Good	16 1/2"–20 1/2"	14 1/2"–18 1/2"
Fair	12 1/2"–16"	10 1/2"–14"
Poor	12" or less	10" or less

Metric conversions for this chart appear in Appendix B.

V. Evaluating reaction time: The stick drop test

To perform the stick drop test of reaction time, you will need a yardstick, a table, a chair, and a partner to help with the test. To perform the test, follow these procedures:

1. Sit in the chair next to the table so that your elbow and lower arm rest on the table comfortably. The heel of your hand should rest on the table so that only your fingers and thumb extend beyond the edge of the table.
2. Your partner holds a yardstick at the very top, allowing it to dangle between your thumb and fingers.
3. The yardstick should be held so that the 24-inch-mark is even with your thumb and index finger. No part of your hand should touch the yardstick.
4. Without warning, your partner will drop the stick, and you will catch it with your thumb and index finger.

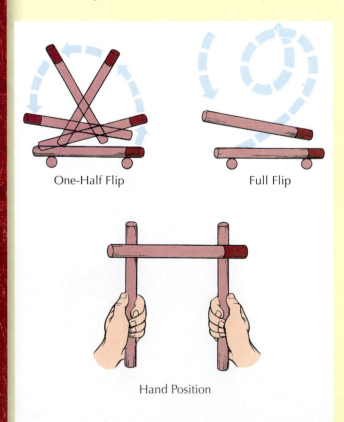

One-Half Flip　　　　　Full Flip

Hand Position

5. Your score is the number of inches read on the yardstick just above the thumb and index finger after you catch the yardstick.
6. Try the test three times. Your partner should be careful not to drop the stick at predictable time intervals so that you cannot guess when it will be dropped. It is important that you react only to the dropping of the stick.
7. Use the middle of your three scores (example: if your scores are 21, 18, and 19, your middle score is 19). The higher your score, the faster your reaction time.

Chart 5 Reaction Time Rating Scale		
Classification		**Score**
Excellent		More than 21"
Very good		19"–21"
Good		16"–18 3/4"
Fair		13"–15 3/4"
Poor		Below 13"

Metric conversions for this chart appear in Appendix B.

VI. Evaluating speed: Running test of speed

To perform the running test of speed, it will be necessary to have a specially marked running course, a stopwatch, a whistle, and a partner to help you with the test. To perform the test, follow this procedure:

1. Mark a running course on a hard surface so that there is a starting line and a series of nine additional lines, each 2 yards apart, the first marked at a distance 10 yards from the starting line.

2. From a distance 1 or 2 yards behind the starting line, begin to run as fast as you can. As you cross the starting line, your partner starts a stopwatch.
3. Run as fast as you can until you hear the whistle that your partner will blow exactly 3 seconds after the stopwatch was started. Your partner marks your location at the time when the whistle was blown.
4. Your score is the distance you were able to cover in 3 seconds. You may practice the test and take more than one trial if time allows. Use the better of your distances on the last two trials as your score.

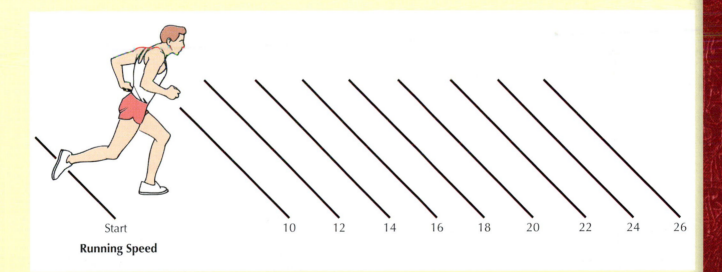

Start 10 12 14 16 18 20 22 24 26

Running Speed

Chart 6 Speed Rating Scale		
Classification	**Men**	**Women**
Excellent	24–26 yards	22–26 yards
Very good	22–23 yards	20–21 yards
Good	18–21 yards	16–19 yards
Fair	16–17 yards	14–15 yards
Poor	Less than 16 yards	Less than 14 yards

Metric conversions for this chart appear in Appendix B.

Lab 14A: Evaluating Skill-Related Physical Fitness

Name	Section	Date

Purpose: To help you evaluate your own skill-related fitness, including agility, balance, coordination, power, speed, and reaction time. This information may be of value in helping decide which sports match your skill-related fitness abilities.

Procedure:
1. Read the direction for each of the skill-related fitness tests presented in the lab resource materials.
2. Take as many of the tests as possible, given the time and equipment available.
3. Be sure to warm-up before and to cool-down after the tests.
4. It is all right to practice the tests before trying them. However, you should decide ahead of time which trial you will use to test your skill-related fitness.
5. After completing the tests, write your scores in the appropriate places in the Results section.
6. Determine your rating for each of the tests from the rating charts in the lab resource materials.

Results:
Place a check in the circle for each of the tests you completed.

Agility (Illinois run) ○

Balance (Bass test) ○

Coordination (stick test) ○

Power (vertical jump) ○

Reaction time (stick drop test) ○

Speed (three-second run) ○

Record your score and rating in the following spaces.

	Score	Rating	
Agility			(chart 1)
Balance			(chart 2)
Coordination			(chart 3)
Power			(chart 4)
Reaction time			(chart 5)
Speed			(chart 6)

Conclusion and Implications:

In two or three paragraphs, discuss the results of your skill-related fitness tests. Comment on the areas in which you did well or did not do well, the meaning of these findings, and the implications of the results with specific reference to the activities you will perform in the future.

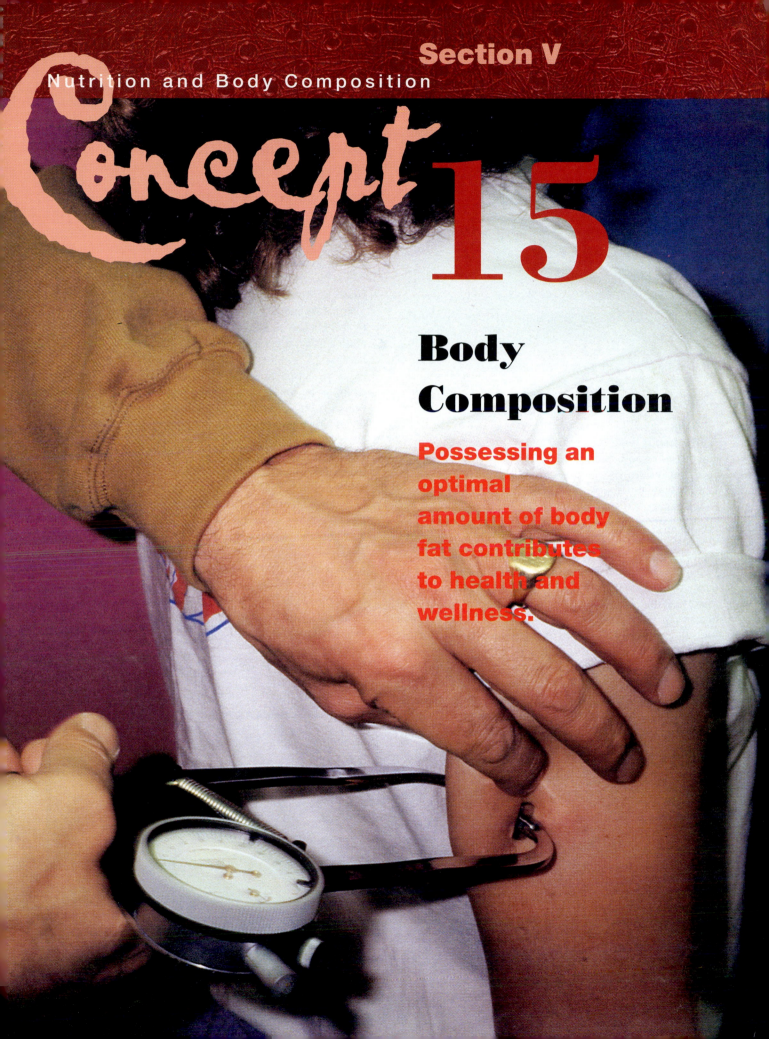

Concept 15

Body Composition

Possessing an optimal amount of body fat contributes to health and wellness.

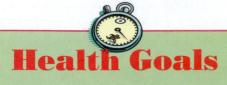

Introduction

Body composition refers to the relative percentage of muscle, fat, bone, and other tissue of the body. Of primary concern, because of its association with various health problems, is body fatness. Being overfat or underfat can result in health concerns.

Our national health goals were designed to encourage a decrease in the prevalence of obesity, yet recent statistics indicate that we have been ineffective in meeting this goal. Regardless of the measurement technique used, the evidence suggests that more adults are considered to be heavier than is healthy and the problem has increased in the last two decades. More women than men and more low-income than high-income people are classified as obese. Even the most conservative figures indicate that children have increased in body fatness in recent years. Since eating disorders such as anorexia nervosa and bulimia are also a significant health concern, especially among teens, the national goal is to keep the percentage of overfat teens from increasing while at the same time reducing the incidence of those who have too little fat associated with eating disorders.

The Facts about the Meaning and Measurement of Fatness

There are standards that can be used to determine how much body fat an individual should possess.

Every person should possess at least a minimal amount of fat (**percent body fat**) for good health. This fat is called

essential fat and is necessary for temperature regulation, shock absorption, and regulation of essential body nutrients, including vitamins A, D, E, and K. The exact amount of fat considered essential to normal body functioning has been debated, but most experts agree that males should possess no less than 5 percent and females no less than 10 percent. For females, an exceptionally low body fat percentage (**underfat**) is especially of concern. **Amenorrhea** may occur at fat levels higher than 10 percent (11 to 16 percent for many women). Some people feel that amenorrhea, when associated with low body fat levels, is a reversible condition that is merely the body's method of preventing pregnancy. However, low body fat levels, accompanied by amenorrhea, places a woman at risk of bone loss (osteoporosis). A body fat level below 10 percent is one of the criteria often used by clinicians for diagnosing eating disorders such as anorexia nervosa.

Close inspection of Table 1 reveals an overlap between essential fat, borderline, and high-performance classifications for body fatness. As noted previously, essential fat levels are those necessary for normal body functioning. Because individuals differ in their response to low fatness, a borderline range is provided. There appear to be no particular health benefits associated with being in the borderline range, and for some people there are health risks. Even though low body fat levels (borderline range) are not generally recommended, there are some individuals who are interested in high-level performance and seek low body fatness in an attempt to enhance performance. Standards for high-level performers are typically lower than for normally active people primarily interested in good health. Performance levels considered to be in the borderline area for nonperformers can be acceptable if the performer eats well, avoids overtraining, and practices a healthy lifestyle. If symptoms such as amenorrhea, bone loss, and frequent injury occur, then levels of body fatness should be reconsidered, as should training tech-

Table 1 Standards for Body Fatness (Percent Body Fat)

Classification	Males	Females
Essential Fat	No less than 5%	No less than 10%
Borderline	5%–9%	10%–16%
High performance	5%–15%	10%–23%
Good fitness (healthy)	10%–20%	17%–28%
Marginal	21%–25%	29%–35%
Overfat	25%+	35%+

niques and eating patterns. For many people in training, maintaining performance levels of body fatness is temporary, thus the risk of long-term health problems is diminished.

Nonessential fat is fat above essential fat levels that accumulates when you take in more calories than you expend. When nonessential fat accumulates in excessive amounts, **overfatness** or even **obesity** can occur. Just as the percent of body fat should not drop too low, it should not get too high either. There is a desirable range of fatness that is associated with good metabolic fitness, good health, and wellness. It is referred to as the good fitness or healthy fatness range. People with more than healthy fat levels but who are not considered obese have scores in the marginal zone. While it is desirable to reach the healthy fitness zone, it will be harder for some people. Most experts agree that fat levels in the marginal zone are healthier than those in the overfatness zone.

Decisions about body composition should be based on more than one measurement.

In Lab 15A, you will have the opportunity to do several different measurements of body composition. Using only one of the methods may result in misinformation and unrealistic goals, which is why it is wise to use several techniques when making decision about personal body composition goals. As you read about the various ways to assess body composition, consider the strengths and weaknesses of each technique and learn to use the techniques that provide the most information to you personally.

Overfat is more important than overweight in making decisions about health and wellness.

Many of the measures described in the following sections of this concept are indicators of the amount of body fat a person possesses. Others focus primarily on body weight. People who do regular physical activity and possess a large muscle mass can be high in body weight without being too fat. This is one of the limitations of measures based primarily on weight. Also, weight measures vary greatly based on your state of hydration or dehydration. You can lose weight merely by losing body water (becoming dehydrated) or gain weight by gaining body water (becoming hydrated). For this reason, measures that use weight as the primary indicator of body composition should be viewed with caution.

There are many ways to assess body fatness.

www.mhhe.com/hper/physed/clw/student/
Underwater weighing, also referred to as "hydrostatic weighing," is considered the gold standard for assessing body fatness. In this lab-

oratory procedure, a person is weighed underwater and out of the water. Corrections are made for the amount of air in the lungs when the underwater weight is measured. Using Archimedes' principle, the body's density can be determined. Because the density of various body tissues is known, the amount of the total body fat can be determined. Body fatness is usually expressed in terms of a percentage of the total body weight. Most of the other techniques for assessing body composition are based on predicting body fatness as assessed using underwater weighing.

Because underwater weighing takes considerable time, equipment, and specialized training, it is not practical for use except in well-equipped laboratories. Other methods of measuring body fatness or body weight are skinfold measurements, bioelectrical impedance, near-infrared interactance, X-ray absorptiometry, dual energy X-ray absorptiometry (DEXA) measurements, height/weight measurements, body mass index (BMI), and body circumference measurements. Table 2 presents a summary of the effectiveness of several of the more commonly used measures. Not all of these have been shown to be equally reliable and valid.

Skinfold measurements are a preferred, practical method of assessing body fatness.

Body fat is distributed throughout the body. About one-half of the body's fat is located around the various body organs and in the muscles. The other half of the body's fat is located just under the skin, or in skinfolds (Figure 1). A skinfold is two thicknesses of skin and the amount of fat that lies just under the skin. By measuring skinfold thicknesses of various sites around the body it is possible to estimate total body

Percent Body Fat The percentage of total body weight that is composed of fat.

Essential Fat The minimum amount of fat in the body necessary to maintain healthful living.

Underfat Too little of the body weight composed of fat (see Table 1).

Amenorrhea Absence of, or infrequent, menstruation.

Nonessential Fat Extra fat or fat reserves stored in the body.

Overfat Too much of the body weight composed of fat (see Table 1).

Obesity Extreme overfatness.

Table 2 Ratings of the Validity and Objectivity of Body Composition Methods

Method	Precise	Objective	Accurate	Valid Equations	Overall Rating
Skinfold measurement	4.0	3.5	3.5	3.5	3.5
Bioelectric impedance	4.0	4.0	3.5	3.5	3.5
Circumferences	4.0	4.0	3.0	3.0	3.0
Near-infrared interactance	5.0	4.5	2.0	2.0	2.5
Body mass index	5.0	5.0	1.5	1.5	2.0

Precise: Can the same person get the same results time after time?   Objective: Can two different people get the same results consistently?

Accurate: Do values compare favorably to underwater weighing?   Valid: Is the formula accurate for predicting fat from measurements?

5 = excellent; 4 = very good; 3 = good; 2 = fair; 1 = unacceptable.

Adapted from Lohman, T.G., Houtkooper, L.H., and Going, S.B. "Body Fat Measurement Goes Hi Tech." *ACSM's Health and Fitness Journal.* 1(1)(1998).

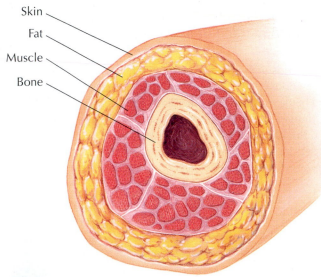

Figure 1
Location of body fat.

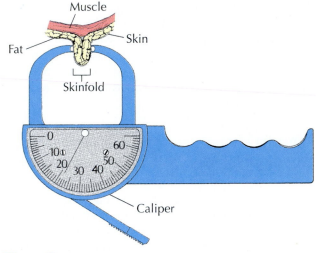

Figure 2
Measuring skinfold thickness.

fatness (Figure 2). Skinfold measurements are often used because they are relatively easy to do. They are not nearly as costly as underwater weighing and other methods that require expensive equipment. A set of calipers is used to make the measurements (Figure 3). The better, more accurate calipers cost several hundred dollars. However, considerably less expensive calipers are now available.

www.mhhe.com/hper/physed/clw/student/

WEB

In general, the more skinfolds measured, the more accurate the body fatness estimate. However, measurements with two or three skinfolds have been shown to be reasonably accurate and can be done in a relatively short period. Two skinfold techniques are used in Lab 15A. You are encouraged to try both. With adequate training, most anyone can learn to use calipers to get a

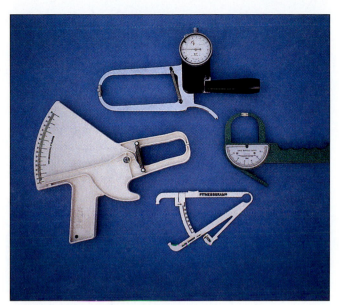

Figure 3
Skin-fold calipers.

good estimate of fatness. When performed by a trained person, skinfold techniques are rated very favorably by experts (see Table 2), but it is a skill that takes practice. Measurements made by an untrained person can be quite inaccurate.

Body circumference measures can be used to assess body fatness.

www.mhhe.com/hper/physed/clw/student/

Body circumference, or girth measurements, can be used to determine body fatness using various weight, height, waist, thigh, hip, and other girth measurements. They are not rated as favorably as skinfold measurements (see Table 2), but they are easy to do. One weakness of circumference measures is they may misclassify people who have a large muscle mass. For this reason, they are not as useful as skinfold measures for active people who have a relatively large muscle mass compared to inactive people. As the sole measure of fatness, they should be used with caution. They can provide a useful second or third source of information about body fatness, however. Another technique that uses body circumferences—the waist-to-hip ratio—will be discussed in a later section.

A variety of technology-based assessments are available to estimate body fatness.

Recently, experts have rated the various techniques for assessing body fatness (see Table 2). Bioelectric impedance analysis (BIA) ranks quite favorably for accuracy. Overall, bioelectric impedance has a similar ranking to skinfold measurement techniques. The advantage of this technique is that it can be performed by a relatively untrained person, it is effective for people high in body fatness (a limitation of skinfold measurements), and it can be done relatively quickly.

Bioelectric impedance measurements are taken while the patient is lying down. Electrodes are placed on the body. A low dose of current is passed through the individual, and the resistance of the current is measured. The amount of resistance and your body size are used to predict your fatness. Accurate measures using this technique require a relatively expensive machine, regular accurate calibration of the machine, and standard placement of electrodes. Measures should not be done within three to four hours of a meal or when you are dehydrated.

Near-infrared interactance machines were originally designed to measure the fat content of meats and grains. They are now used commercially to measure body fatness. These techniques are not as accurate as skinfolds and bioelectrical impedance measures. Various types of X-ray and magnetic resonance machines (MRI) have been used to assess body fatness. They can be quite useful, especially in determining body fatness in specific body locations. Unfortunately, these procedures require very expensive machines and are not practical for personal use. One relatively new procedure uses air displacement to assess fatness. Like X-ray and MRI, this technique requires special equipment, which makes it impractical for most people. One machine that uses this technique is called the BodPod. Preliminary evidence has shown it to be an acceptable alternative to underwater weighing, especially for special populations (obese, older people, and the physically challenged).

The body mass index (BMI) is considered to be a better measure than height-weight charts, but it has its limitations.

www.mhhe.com/hper/physed/clw/student/

Individuals who are interested in controlling their weight often consult height-weight tables to determine their "desirable" weight. Being 20 percent or more above the recommended table weight is one commonly used indicator of obesity. New tables adopted by the federal government are now based on relative risk of health problems rather than normative comparisons to other people. Even the new "healthy weight range tables" have limitations because they do not give an accurate estimate of the amount of fat a person has. A person who has a large muscle mass as a result of regular physical activity could appear to be **overweight** using a height-weight table and still not be too fat. Some experts have criticized the new tables for not adjusting for age, sex, or fitness level. Others defend the fact that the tables encourage maintenance of weight over the lifespan rather than "allowing" weight gain with age.

The **body mass index (BMI)** is probably the best way to use height and weight to assess fatness. The BMI is calculated using a special formula and has a higher correlation with true body fatness than weights determined from height-weight tables. Nevertheless, the BMI may misclassify active people who have a large muscle mass. You can calculate your BMI using the procedures described in the lab resource materials. Just as height and weight standards have changed, the standards for BMI have also been modified recently. The National Institutes for Health now uses a BMI of 25 as the standard for overweight, 30 as the standard for obesity, and 40 as the standard for severe obesity. Prior to the establishment of these standards, different values for men and women were used and a value of approximately 27 was used as the indicator of overweight.

The revised standards are now consistent with those of the Department of Agriculture and the World Health Organization. These organizations have used the more stringent standards for a number of years. Still, the change results in an increase in the number of people classified as overweight by 29 million people. More than a few people have suggested that the changes are arbitrary, but health experts note that the new standards are based on differences in disease risk for those who exceed the standards compared to those who fall below the standards.

www.mhhe.com/hper/physed/clw/student/

Advantages of the BMI are that it is easy to measure objectively and inexpensively. This type of measure is very useful for studying large groups of people over long periods of time. This is why the BMI is often used for research. The BMI is less valuable for making measurements for one specific individual at one particular point in time. Because the BMI is widely cited in news reports, it is important for all people to know how to calculate it and how to use it (and how not to misuse it). Plotting changes in BMI over time can be useful in tracking personal changes. Together with other techniques, the BMI can provide useful information, but the risk of misclassification is high among active people with a high amount of muscle if the BMI is used by itself.

> The waist-to-hip ratio is a body circumference measurement technique that can be used in determining health risk.

www.mhhe.com/hper/physed/clw/student/

Several research studies have shown that a relationship exists between the amount of abdominal fat and various health problems. For this reason, it is important to keep both your total body fat and abdominal fat levels low, especially as you grow older. Other studies have shown that upper body fatness (from the waist up) produces a greater

health risk than lower body fatness (from the waist down). Skinfold measures could help you monitor abdominal and upper body fatness. Another useful measurement that can be done at home is called the waist-to-hip circumference ratio. A high ratio between the waist and hip has been shown to be correlated with a high incidence of heart attack, stroke, chest pain, breast cancer, and death. Recent evidence indicates that people who exercise regularly accumulate less fat in the upper central regions of the body as they get older. This suggests that regular physical activity throughout life will result in a smaller waist-to-hip ratio and a reduced risk of various lifestyle diseases.

> Body composition is considered a component of health-related fitness but can also be considered a component of metabolic fitness.

Body composition is generally considered to be a health-related component of physical fitness. Most national fitness tests include either a skinfold test or the BMI as an indicator of this component. Like the other parts of health-related physical fitness, body composition is related to good health.

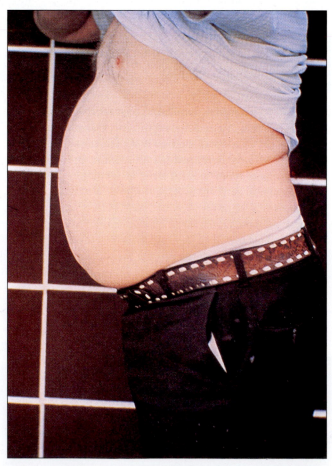

Abdominal fat is associated with increased disease risk.

However, body composition is unlike the other parts of health-related physical fitness in that it is not a performance measure. Cardiovascular fitness, strength, muscular endurance, and flexibility can be assessed using some type of movement or performance such as running, lifting, or stretching. Body composition requires no movement or performance. This is one reason why some experts prefer to consider body composition as a component of metabolic fitness.

Metabolic fitness includes other nonperformance measures associated with increased risk of health problems, such as high blood fat, high blood pressure, and high blood sugar levels. Some experts have hypothesized that metabolic fitness is really one syndrome that is characterized by body composition (body fatness) and the other highly related nonperformance measures described above. Whether you consider body composition to be a part of health-related or metabolic fitness, it is an important health-related factor.

Assessing body weight too frequently can result in making false assumptions about body composition changes.

Taking body weight measurements too frequently can provide incorrect information and lead to false assumptions. For example, people vary in body weight from day to day and even hour to hour based solely on their level of hydration. Short-term changes in weight are often due to water loss or gain, yet many people attribute the weight changes to their diet, a pill they have taken, or the exercise they are doing. In fact, short-term weight changes are more likely water changes than real body composition changes. We know this to be true because it takes a relatively long period of time for diet or exercise to affect weight changes. Monitoring your weight less frequently, once a week for example, is more useful than daily or multiple daily measures because it is more likely to represent real changes in body composition. Weighing at the same time of day, preferably early in the morning, is best because it reduces the chances that your weight variation will be a result of body water changes. Of course, it is best to use body composition assessments in addition to those based on body weight if accurate evaluations are expected.

Health Risks Associated with Overfatness: The Facts

Obesity has recently been elevated from a secondary to a primary risk factor for heart disease.

Prior to 1998, obesity was considered to be a secondary risk factor for heart disease. The reason for this was that the effects of obesity were thought to be mediated by other risk

factors such as blood pressure and blood lipids. Because of the mounting evidence of the relationship of obesity to health risk, especially risk of heart disease, the American Heart Association now classifies obesity as a primary risk factor along with high blood lipids, high blood pressure, tobacco use, and sedentary living.

Overfatness or obesity can contribute to degenerative diseases, health problems, and even shortened life.

Some diseases and health problems are associated with overfatness and obesity. In addition to the higher incidence of certain diseases and health problems, there is evidence that people who are moderately overfat have a 40 percent higher than normal risk of shortening their lifespan. More severe obesity results in a 70 percent higher than normal death rate. This is evidenced by the exorbitant life insurance premiums paid by obese individuals.

Heart disease is not the only disease that is associated with obesity. Diabetes is another leading killer that is associated with all components of metabolic fitness including obesity. The incidence of diagnosis of this disease has increased sixfold in the last 40 years. Recent studies also indicate a significant increase in risk of breast cancer among the obese. High blood pressure and asthma are examples of other conditions associated with obesity.

It should be noted that statistics indicate that underweight people also have a higher than normal risk of premature death. Though there is adequate evidence that extreme leanness can be life threatening (e.g., anorexia nervosa), many underweight people included in these studies have lost weight because of a medical condition such as cancer. It appears that the medical problems are often the reason for low body weight rather than low body weight being the source of the medical problem. Most experts agree that people who are free from disease and who have lower than average amounts of body fat have a lower than average risk of premature death.

Excessive abdominal fat and excessive fatness of the upper body can increase the risk of various diseases.

As noted earlier, research studies have shown that a relationship exists between the amount of abdominal fat and various

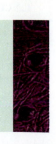

Overweight Weight in excess of normal; not harmful unless it is accompanied by overfatness.

Body Mass Index (BMI) A measure of body composition using a height-weight formula. High BMI values have been related to increased disease risk.

health problems. Fat in the upper part of the body is sometimes called "Northern hemisphere" fat and is considered more risky than "Southern hemisphere" fat, such as in the hips and upper legs. People who have abdominal fatness are sometimes considered to have the "apple" fat pattern, while people with lower body fatness are considered to have the "pear" fat pattern. Regardless of the name used, it is clear that people who distribute fat around their middle as opposed to in the limbs are at greater risk of various health problems. The waist-to-hip ratio described in the previous section provides a means of assessing central body fatness. In general, men have higher waist-to-hip ration than women and postmenopausal women have higher ratios than premenopausal women. As you grow older, it is especially important to monitor your waist-to-hip ratio.

> High weight, and even relatively high body fat levels, may not increase risk of health problems if other indicators of poor health are not present.

www.mhhe.com/hper/physed/clw/student/

Recent research suggests that people who are above normal standards for BMI are not especially at risk if they participate in regular physical activity and possess relatively high levels of cardiovascular fitness. In fact, active people who have a high BMI are at less risk than inactive people with normal BMI levels. Even high levels of body fatness may not be especially likely to increase disease risk if a person has good metabolic fitness as indicated by healthy blood fat levels, normal blood pressure, and normal blood sugar levels. It is when several of these factors are present at the same time that risk levels increase dramatically. For this reason, it is important to consider your cardiovascular and metabolic fitness levels before drawing conclusions about the effects of high body weight or high body fat levels on health and wellness. This information also points out the importance of periodically assessing your cardiovascular and metabolic fitness levels.

Health Risks Associated with Excessively Low Body Fatness: The Facts

> Excessive desire to be thin or low in body weight can result in health problems.

In Western society, the near obsession with thinness has been, at least in part, responsible for health conditions now referred to as eating disorders. Eating disorders, or altered eating habits, involve extreme restriction of food intake and/or regurgitation of food to avoid digestion. The most common disorders are anorexia nervosa, bulimia, and anorexia athletica. All of these disorders are most common among highly achievement-oriented girls and young women, although they affect virtually all segments of the population.

Anorexia nervosa is the most severe of the three disorders. In fact, if not treated, it is life-threatening. Anorexics restrict food intake so severely that their bodies become emaciated. Among the many characteristics of the anorexic are fear of maturity and inaccurate body image. The anorexic starves herself/himself and may exercise compulsively or use laxatives to prevent the digestion of food in an attempt to attain excessive leanness. The anorexic's self-image is one of being too fat even when the person is too lean for good health. Assessing body fatness using procedures such as skinfolds and observation of the eating habits may help identify people with anorexia. Among anorexic girls and women, development of an adult figure is often feared. It is important that people with this disorder obtain medical and psychological help immediately, as the consequences are severe. People with anorexia may also have some of the characteristics of the person with bulimia. About 25 percent of those with anorexia do compulsive exercise in attempt to stay lean.

Bulimics may or may not be anorexic. It may not be possible to use measures of body fatness to identify bulimia, as the bulimic may be lean, normal, or excessively fat. The most common characteristics of bulimia are bingeing and purging. Bingeing means the periodic eating of large amounts of food at one time. A binge might occur after a relatively long period of dieting and often consists of junk foods containing empty calories. After a binge, the bulimic purges the body of the food by forced regurgitation or the use of laxatives. Another form of bulimia is bingeing on one day and starving on the next. The consequences of bulimia are not as severe as anorexia, but can result in serious mental, gastrointestinal, and dental problems.

Anorexia athletica is a recently identified eating disorder that appears to be related to participation in sports and activities, such as ballet, that emphasize excessive body leanness. Studies show that participants in sports such as gymnastics, wrestling, body building, and activities such as ballet and cheerleading are most likely to develop anorexia athletica. This disorder has many of the symptoms of anorexia nervosa, but not of the same severity. In some cases, anorexia athletica can lead to anorexia nervosa.

Female athlete triad is an increasingly common condition among female athletes. The three health concerns (the triad) that characterize the condition are eating disorders, amenorrhea, and osteoporosis. The disordered eating pat-

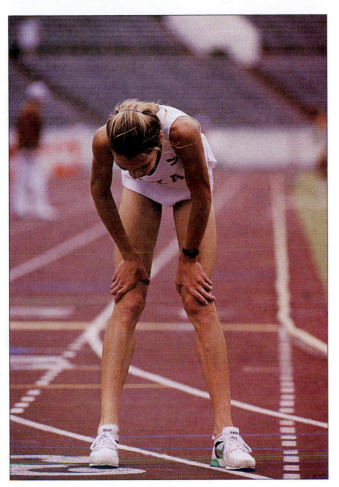

Excessively low levels of body fatness pose health problems.

terns may be extreme as in anorexia or bulemia, or less severe as evidenced by poor eating habits. Because they are athletes, females with this condition are very active. Together, the poor eating habits and high levels of activity typically result in low body fat levels. The triad of symptoms is often accompanied by considerable pressure to perform well, resulting in high stress levels. In addition to the triad of symptoms, the combination of poor eating, over-exercise, and competitive stress can result in other problems, such as depression and anxiety, and even risk of suicide. Many female athletes train extensively and have relatively low body fat levels but experience none of the symptoms of the triad. Eating well, training properly, using stress-management techniques, and monitoring health symptoms are the keys to their success.

Fear of obesity is a less severe condition but it can still have negative health consequences. This condition is most common among achievement-oriented teenagers who impose a self-restriction on caloric intake because they fear obesity. Consequences include stunting of growth, delayed puberty, delayed sexual development, and decreased physical attractiveness. It is important to avoid excessive eating and inactivity to prevent the problems associated with over-fatness and obesity; however, an excessive concern for leanness can also result in serious health problems.

Society can help reduce the incidence of the problems associated with disordered eating and desire to be thin by changing its image of attractiveness, especially among young women. Many of the models and movie stars who convey the "ideal" image are anorexic or are exceptionally thin. Teachers and athletic coaches can help by educating people about these disorders, by not placing too much emphasis on leanness, and by screening students for extreme leanness using procedures such as skinfolds and body mass index. Parents and friends can help by looking for excessive changes in body weight and lack of eating. Once an eating disorder is identified, it is important to help the individual obtain treatment for the problem. While regular physical activity is good, excessive activity can be harmful. It is important to help athletes learn not to overdo it and to keep competition in perspective so that it does not become excessively stressful.

Conflicting news reports should not deter efforts to maintain a healthy body fat level.

One recent headline said "Excess pounds deadly." One week later the headline read "It may be better to be a little fat." Adding to the confusion is that body mass index standards have been lowered in recent years so that more people are now classified as overweight using this measurement technique. At the same time, some of the standards for body fatness are now more lenient than they were in the past. In both cases, the changes are made based on new scientific evidence.

Sometimes people read conflicting headlines and adopt a defeatist attitude. It is important not to let one headline influence your overall plan of fat control. There will be a continuing debate in the years ahead as to just how much you should weigh or how much fat you should have for your good health and wellness. In the meantime, the message is clear! If possible, make several different assessments and consider all of the results before making decisions (see charts in lab resource materials). For some people, meeting the standards described in this book may be difficult. It is far better to be close to the standard than to say "I can't meet the standard, so I won't even try." Some experts feel that many people are overfat because they have repeatedly failed to meet unrealistic body fatness or weight goals. Adopting a realistic personal standard of fatness is very important. Using many different self-assessments and adopting realistic goals based on personal information rather than comparisons to others can help you make informed decisions about your body composition.

The Facts about the Origin of Fatness

Heredity plays a role in fatness.

Some people have suggested that every individual is born with a predetermined weight (sometimes called your set-point). This implies that you have little control over your weight or body fat levels. In fact, you do have considerable control over your weight and level of fatness as evidenced by the fact that calories taken in (diet) and calories expended (activity) are the two most important factors associated with fat control. Nevertheless, research suggests that people are born with a predisposition toward fatness or leanness. For years, some scholars have suggested that your body type, or **somatotype,** is inherited. Clearly, some people will have more difficulty than others controlling fatness because of their body types and because they come from families with a history of obesity. In fact, very recent research by a well-respected team of scholars indicates that the body has a "natural" fatness range, which is influenced by heredity. If you deviate more than 10 to 15 percent from this range, your body may actually alter its metabolism in an attempt to maintain your "natural" fatness level. But even these changes are temporary. If you continue the behavior that caused the weight gain (eating more or exercising less), after a period of time your body accepts your new weight as your "natural" level. Scientists caution people not to overgeneralize the importance of heredity to body fatness. Such overgeneralizations could lead to incorrect conclusions about regulation of body fat levels.

Recently the "ob-gene" (or gene responsible for obesity) was discovered. It is true that this is an important scientific discovery but it is unlikely that it will result in a "cure" for overfatness in the near future. In the meantime, more conventional methods of fat control must be used. Even if you come from a family with a history of obesity, you should not conclude that nothing can be done to prevent obesity. Virtually all people have a natural fatness below obese levels. Those with a predisposition to high fatness will have a harder time having a low body fatness level, but with healthy lifestyles, even these people can maintain body fat levels within normal ranges. Research shows that regular physical activity is especially effective in the control of genetically determined predispositions to fatness.

Glandular disorders are not a cause of overfatness for most people.

Glandular disorders can cause or contribute to overfatness. For example, thyroid problems can cause a low metabolic rate that results in fat gain. However, most experts suggest that only 1 to 2 percent of all overfatness is directly caused

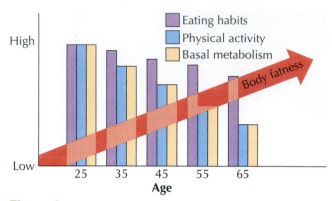

Figure 4
The creeping obesity.

by problems of this type. Medical treatment is necessary for people suffering from these problems.

Fatness early in life leads to adult fatness.

Retention of baby fat is not a sign of good health. On the contrary, excess body fat in the early years is a health problem of considerable concern. There is evidence that childhood overfatness results in hyperplasia, or an increased number of fat cells, and people with extra fat cells may have a greater tendency to become overfat. It was previously thought that only adult obesity was related to health problems. We now know that teens (ages 13–18) who are too fat are at greater risk of heart problems and cancer than their lean peers.

Changes in basal metabolic rate can be the cause of overfatness.

The amount of energy you expend each day must be balanced by your energy intake if you are to maintain your body fat and body weight over time. Your energy intake is determined by the calories you eat. Expenditure is determined by a combination of several factors. You expend calories just to exist—even when you are inactive. Your **basal metabolic rate (BMR)** is the indicator or your energy expenditure when your are totally inactive. You also expend calories digesting food and, of course, in the activities of daily living.

Basal metabolic rate is highest during the growing years. The amount of food eaten increases to support this increased energy expenditure. When growing ceases, if eating does not decrease or activity level increase, fatness can result. Basal metabolism also decreases gradually as you grow older. One major reason for this is the loss of muscle mass associated with inactivity. Regular physical activity throughout life helps keep the muscle mass higher, resulting in a higher BMR. Very recent evidence suggests that regular exercise can contribute in other ways to increased BMR. The higher BMR of active people helps them prevent overfatness, particularly in later life.

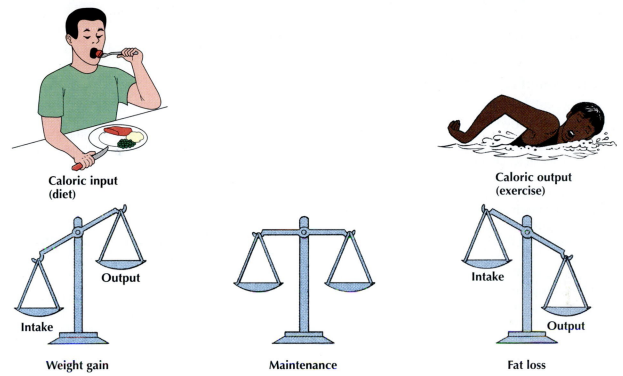

Figure 5
Balancing calorie input and output.

"Creeping obesity" is a problem as you grow older.

People become less active and their BMR gradually decreases with age. Calorie intake does seem to decrease somewhat with age, but the decrease does not adequately compensate for the decreases in BMR and activity levels. For this reason, body fat increases gradually for the typical person as he or she ages (see Figure 4). This increase in fatness over time is commonly referred to as "creeping obesity" because the increase in fatness is gradual. For a typical person, creeping obesity could result in a gain of one-half to one pound per year. People who stay active can keep muscle mass high and delay changes in BMR. For those who are not active, it is suggested that caloric intake should decrease by 3 percent each decade after 25 so that by age 65, caloric intake is at least 10 percent less than it was at age 25. The decrease in calorie intake for active people need not be as great.

The principal cause of most overfatness is the intake of more calories than are expended.

Though fatness may be associated with any of the factors mentioned previously, and overfatness is no doubt the result of multiple causes, excessive food energy intake (food calories) and/or lack of energy expenditure (physical activity) are responsible for most overfatness. (See Figure 5.)

Excess caloric intake or calorie expenditure results in an increase in fat cell size.

Overfatness can result in an increase in the number of fat cells among children. For adults, overfatness is a result of the increase in size of fat cells (hypertrophy). When fat cells become excessively large, they can cause dimples or lumps under the skin. Some people refer to these large fat cells as cellulite. Quacks say that this type of fat is different from other types of fat and is removed from the body in different ways than regular fat. This is not true. All fatness among adults is a result of enlarged fat cells. All fat is lost as a result of reduction in fat cell size.

Somatotype Inherent body build: ectomorph (thin), mesomorph (muscular), and endomorph (fat).

Basal Metabolic Rate (BMR) Your energy expenditure in a basic or rested state.

The Facts about Diet, Physical Activity, and Fatness

A combination of regular physical activity and dietary restriction is the most effective means of losing body fat.

Studies indicate that regular physical activity combined with dietary restriction is the most effective method of losing fat. One study of adult women indicated that diet alone resulted in loss of weight, but much of this loss was lean body tissue. Those who were dieting as well as exercising experienced similar weight losses, but this loss included more body fat. For optimal results, all weight loss programs should combine a lower caloric intake with a good physical exercise program. Thresholds of training and target zones for body fat reduction, including information for both physical activity and **diet** are presented in Table 3.

Good physical activity and diet habits can be useful in maintaining desirable body composition.

Table 3 illustrates how fat can be lost through regular physical activity and proper dieting. However, not all people want to lose fat. For those who wish to maintain their current body composition, a **caloric balance** between intake and output is effective. For people who want to increase their lean body weight, increased caloric intake with increased exercise can result in the desired changes.

Physical activity is one effective means of controlling body fat.

Though physical activity or exercise will not result in immediate and large decreases in body fat levels, there is increasing evidence that fat loss resulting from physical activity may be more lasting than fat loss from dieting. Vigorous exercise can increase the resting energy expenditure up to 13 times (13 **METs**).

Table 3 Threshold of Training and Target Zones for Body Fat Reduction

	Threshold of Training*		Target Zones*	
	Physical Activity	**Diet**	**Physical Activity**	**Diet**
Frequency	• To be effective, activity must be regular, preferably daily, though fat can be lost over the long term with almost any frequency that results in increased caloric expenditure.	• It is best to reduce caloric intake consistently and daily. To restrict calories only on certain days is *not* best, though fat can be lost over a period of time by reducing caloric intake at any time.	• Daily moderate activity is recommended. For people who do regular vigorous activity, 3 to 6 days per week may be best.	• It is best to diet consistently and daily.
Intensity	• To lose 1 pound of fat, you must expend 3,500 calories more than you normally expend.	• To lose 1 pound of fat, you must eat 3,500 calories fewer than you normally eat.	• Slow, low-intensity aerobic exercise that results in no more than 1–2 pounds of fat loss per week is best.	• Modest caloric restriction resulting in no more than 1–2 pounds of fat loss per week is best.
Time	• To be effective, exercise must be sustained long enough to expend a considerable number of calories. At least 15 minutes per exercise bout are necessary to result in consistent fat loss.	• Eating moderate meals is best. Do not skip meals.	• Exercise durations similar to those for achieving aerobic cardiovascular fitness seem best. An exercise duration of 30–60 minutes is recommended.	• Eating moderate meals is best. Skipping meals or fasting is *not* most effective.

Note: It is best to combine exercise and diet to achieve the 3,500 caloric imbalance necessary to lose a pound of fat. Using both exercise and diet in the target zone is most effective.

Inactivity is more often the cause of childhood obesity than overeating. Many fat children eat less but are considerably less active than their nonfat peers. Excessive television watching may be one reason for inactivity among children if the television viewing is done during daytime hours when children have the opportunity to be active. Studies show that adults who watch more than three hours of television per day are twice as likely to be obese as those who view television for less than one hour per day.

If you exercise moderately for an extra 15 minutes a day, you will lose up to 10 pounds in a year's time. Regular walking, jogging, swimming, or any type of sustained exercise can be effective in producing losses in body fat.

> Physical activity that can be sustained for relatively long periods is considered the most effective for losing body fat.

Physical activities from virtually any level of the physical activity pyramid (see Figure 6) can be effective in controlling body fatness because all physical activities expend calories. Among the most effective activities are those in the aerobic activity section of the pyramid because they can be done for relatively long periods of time. Lifestyle activities are also effective, if performed regularly for extended periods of time. Table 4 shows the caloric expenditures for one hour of involvement in various physical activities. Heavier people expend more **calories** than lighter people because more work is required to move larger bodies.

Popular books have recently claimed that vigorous activities are not effective in helping with body fat loss because they say vigorous activities burn less fat than less intense activities. While this is true in theory, it has little practical meaning for most people. It is the total calories expended in your activity that counts. If you run for the same period of time that you walk, you will expend more calories in running.

Even though vigorous activity can be effective, it will not work if you do not do it regularly. For this reason, more vigorous activity may not be as effective as some less vigorous activities for certain people. For example, running at 10 miles per hour (a 6-minute mile) will cause a 150-pound person to expend 900 calories in one hour. Jogging about half as fast, or at 5 1/2 miles per hour (approximately an 11-minute mile), will result in an expenditure of about 650 calories in the same amount of time. At first glance, the more vigorous exercise seems to be a better choice. But how many people can continue to run at a 10-mile-per-hour pace for a full hour? Each mile run at 10 miles per hour results in an expenditure of 90 calories, while each mile run at 5 1/2 miles per hour results in an expenditure of 118 calories. Per mile, you expend more calories in slow running. It takes longer to run a mile, but by the same token, you can also persist longer. The key is to expend as many calories as possible during each regular exercise period. Doing less vigorous activity for longer periods is better for fat control than doing very vigorous activities that

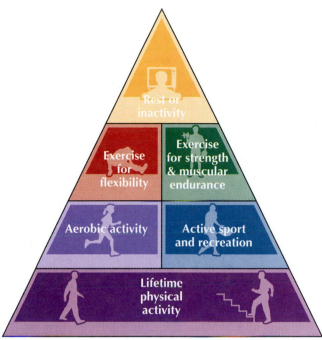

Figure 6

Activities from the lower three levels of the pyramid expend calories, but those from level 1 are especially effective in fat loss.

can be done only for short periods. Nevertheless, vigorous activity can be very effective for some people.

Strength training can be effective in maintaining a desirable body composition.

Performing exercises from the strength and muscular endurance level of the physical activity pyramid can be effective in maintaining desirable body fat levels. People who do strength training increase their muscle mass (lean body mass). This extra muscle mass expends extra calories at rest resulting

Diet The usual food and drink for a person or animal.

Caloric Balance Consuming calories in amounts equal to the number of calories expended.

MET METs are multiples of the amount of energy expended at rest, or approximately 1 calorie per kilogram (2.2 pounds) per hour.

Calorie A unit of energy supplied by food; the quantity of heat necessary to raise the temperature of a kilogram of water 1° C (actually a kilocalorie, but usually called a calorie for weight-control purposes).

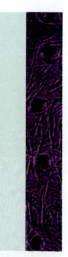

Table 4 Calories Expended per Hour in Various Physical Activities (Performed at a Recreational Level)*

Activity	Calories Used per Hour				
	100 lbs (146 kgs)	120 lbs (55 kgs)	150 lbs (68 kgs)	180 lbs (82 kgs)	200 lbs (91 kgs)
Archery	180	204	240	276	300
Backpacking (40-lb. pack)	307	348	410	472	513
Badminton	255	289	340	391	425
Baseball	210	238	280	322	350
Basketball (half-court)	225	255	300	345	375
Bicycling (normal speed)	157	178	210	242	263
Bowling	155	176	208	240	261
Canoeing (4 mph)	276	344	414	504	558
Circuit training	247	280	330	380	413
Dance, aerobics	315	357	420	483	525
Dance, ballet (choreographed)	240	300	360	432	480
Dance, modern (choreographed)	240	300	360	432	480
Dance, social	174	222	264	318	348
Fencing	225	255	300	345	375
Fitness calisthenics	232	263	310	357	388
Football	225	255	300	345	375
Golf (walking)	187	212	250	288	313
Gymnastics	232	263	310	357	388
Handball	450	510	600	690	750
Hiking	225	255	300	345	375
Horseback riding	180	204	240	276	300
Interval training	487	552	650	748	833
Jogging (5 1/2 mph)	487	552	650	748	833
Judo/karate	232	263	310	357	388
Mountain climbing	450	510	600	690	750
Pool; billiards	97	110	130	150	163
Racquetball; paddleball	450	510	600	690	750
Rope jumping (continuous)	525	595	700	805	875
Rowing, crew	615	697	820	943	1025
Running (10 mph)	625	765	900	1035	1125
Sailing (pleasure)	135	153	180	207	225
Skating, ice	262	297	350	403	438
Skating, roller/inline	262	297	350	403	438
Skiing, cross-country	525	595	700	805	875
Skiing, downhill	450	510	600	690	750
Soccer	405	459	540	621	775
Softball (fast pitch)	210	238	280	322	350
Softball (slow pitch)	217	246	290	334	363
Surfing	416	467	550	633	684
Swimming (fast laps)	420	530	630	768	846
Swimming (slow laps)	240	272	320	368	400
Table tennis	180	204	240	276	300
Tennis	315	357	420	483	525
Volleyball	262	297	350	403	483
Walking	204	258	318	372	426
Waterskiing	306	390	468	564	636
Weight training	352	399	470	541	558

*Note: Locate your weight to determine the calories expended per hour in each of the activities shown in the table based on recreational involvement. More vigorous activity, as occurs in competitive athletics, may result in greater caloric expenditures.

From *Fitness for Life*, 4th edition by Charles B. Corbin and Ruth Lindsey. Copyright © 1997 by Scott Foresman and Company. Reprinted by permission.

in a higher metabolic rate. Also, people with more muscle mass expend more calories when doing physical activity.

Appetite is not necessarily increased through exercise.

The human animal was intended to be an active animal. For this reason, the human "appetite thermostat" (called the "appestat" by some) is set as if all people are active. Those who are inactive do not have a decreased appetite. Likewise, if a person is sedentary and then begins regular exercise, the appetite does not necessarily increase because this appetite thermostat expects activity. Very vigorous activity does not necessarily cause an appetite increase that is proportional to the calories expended in the vigorous exercise.

Strategies for Action: The Facts

Making a variety of self-assessments can help you make informed decisions about body composition.

www.mhhe.com/hper/physed/clw/student/
In Lab 15A you will take a variety of body composition self-assessments. It is important that you take all of the measurements and consider all of the information before making final decisions about your body composition. Each of the self-assessment techniques has its strengths and weaknesses, and you should be aware of these when making personal decisions. The importance you place on one particular measure may be different than the importance another person places on that measure because you are a unique individual and should use information that is more relevant for you personally.

Estimating your basal metabolic rate (BMR) can help you determine the number of calories you expend each day.

In Lab 15C, you can estimate your basal metabolic rate. This will give you an idea of how much energy you expend when you are resting. You can use this information together with the information about the energy you expend to help you balance the calories you consume with the calories you expend each day.

Logging your daily activities can help you determine the number of calories you expend each day.

www.mhhe.com/hper/physed/clw/student/
In Lab 15C, you will also log the activities you perform in a day. You can then determine your energy expenditure in these activities. You can combine this information with the information about your basal metabolism to determine your total daily energy expenditure.

Counting the calories you consume each day can help you balance the calories you expend with the calories you consume.

In the concept on nutrition, you will learn how to count the number of calories you consume each day. You can use this information with the information in Lab 15A to determine if there is a balance in calories consumed and calories expended.

Self-assessment information—especially body composition information—is personal and confidential.

www.mhhe.com/hper/physed/clw/student/
Body composition self-assessment information is personal and should be confidential. When performing the self-assessments in Lab 15A be aware of the following:

1. If doing a self-assessment around other people makes you self-conscious, do the measurement in private.
2. If the measurement requires the assistance of another person, choose a person you trust and feel comfortable with. If you have someone help you make measurements, try to identify a person who will be available over time. This will allow the same person to make the measurements each time you make assessments. For Lab 15A, get the assistance of an expert and/or a partner to do skinfold measures. Of course, doing your own measurements when possible is the best way to make sure that the same person does the measures each time you do them. Recent studies show that self-measurements can be relatively accurate if done consistently with the same caliper and you practice to become skilled.
3. The formulae used to determine body fatness from skinfolds and other procedures were based on normal distributions of people. The more a person differs from normal, the less accurate the measurements will be. For this

reason, most measurements are less accurate for the very lean and people with higher than normal levels of fat. Special procedures are available for athletes, and techniques such as underwater weighing, the BodPod, or bioelectrical impedance are best for those with exceptionally high levels of body fatness.

4. Some measurements, such as the thigh skinfold, are hard to make on some people. This is one reason why two different skinfolding procedures are presented in Lab 15A.

5. Self-assessments require skill. With practice, you can become skillful in making measurements. Your first few attempts will no doubt lack accuracy.

6. Use the same measuring device each time you measure (scale, caliper, measuring tape, etc.). This will assure that any measurement error is constant and will allow you to track your progress over time. For example, your scale may be off by 2 pounds, but if you use the same scale every time you always know the amount of the error and you can correct for it. If you use a different scale each time you weigh, the error is variable. It is difficult to correct for variable errors.

7. Once you have tried all of the self-assessments in Lab 15A, choose the ones you want to continue to do and use the same measurement techniques each time you do the measurements.

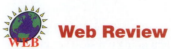

Web Review

Web review materials for Concept 15 are available are at *www.mhhe.com/hper/physed/clw/student/*.

American Anorexia/Bulimia Association
http://www.abainc.org

Morbidity and Mortality Weekly Reports
www.cdc.gov/epo/mmwr/mmwr.html

Shape up America
www.shapeup.org

Suggested Readings

Lee, C. D., Jackson, A. S., and Blair, S. N. US Weight Guidelines: It Is Also Important to Consider Cardiorespiratory Fitness. *International Journal of Obesity.* 22(supplement 2)(1998):S2.

Lohman, T. G., Houtkooper, L. H., and Going, S. B. Body Fat Measurement Goes Hi Tech. *ACSM's Health and Fitness Journal.* 1(1)(1998).

Loy, S. F. et al. Easy Grip on Body Composition Measurements. *ACSM's Health and Fitness.* 2(5)(1998):16.

Otis, C. L. The Female Athlete Triad. *ACSM's Health and Fitness.* 2(1)(1998):20.

Otis, C. L., Drinkwater, B., Johnson, M., Loucks, A., and Wilmore, J. ACSM Position Stand on the Female Athlete Triad. *Medicine and Science in Sports and Exercise.* 29(5)(1997):i.

Roche, A. F., Hyemsfield, S. B., and Lohman, T. G. *Human Body Composition.* Champaign, IL: Human Kinetics, 1996.

Schneider, K. S., et al. Mission Impossible: Too Fat? Too Thin? *People.* 45(22)(1996):65.

Lab Resource Materials: Evaluating Body Fatness

General Information about Skinfold Measurements

It is important to use a consistent procedure for "drawing up" or "pinching up" a skinfold and making the measurement with the caliper. The following procedures should be used for each skinfold site.

1. Lay the caliper down on a nearby table. Use the thumbs and index fingers of both hands to draw up a skinfold or layer of skin and fat. The fingers and thumbs of the two hands should be about 1 inch apart, or half an inch on either side of the location where the measurement is to be made.
2. The skinfolds are normally drawn up in a vertical line rather than a horizontal line. However, if the natural tendency of the skin aligns itself less than vertical, the measurement should be done on the natural line of the skinfold, rather than on the vertical.
3. Do not pinch the skinfold too hard. Draw it up so that your thumbs and fingers are not compressing the skinfold.
4. Once the skinfold is drawn up, let go with your right hand and pick up the caliper. Open the jaws of the caliper and place it over the location of the skinfold to be measured and one-half inch from your left index finger and thumb. Allow the tips, or jaw faces, of the caliper to close on the skinfold at a level about where the skin would be normally.
5. Let the reading on the caliper settle for 2 or 3 seconds, then note the thickness of the skinfold in millimeters.
6. Three measurements should be taken at each location. Use the middle of the three values to determine your measurement. For example, if you had values of 10, 11, and 9, your measurement for that location would be 10. If the three measures vary by more than 3 millimeters from the lowest to the highest, you may want to take additional measurements.

Skinfold Locations for Women

Triceps skinfold— Make a mark on the back of the right arm, one-half the distance between the tip of the shoulder and the tip of the elbow. Make the measurement at this location.

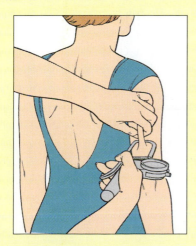

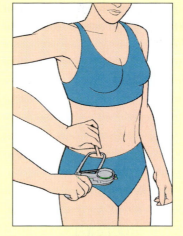

Iliac crest skinfold— Make a mark at the top front of the iliac crest. This skinfold is taken slightly diagonally because of the natural line of the skin.

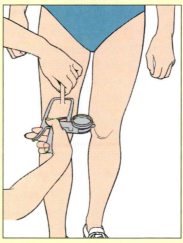

Thigh skinfold— Make a mark on the front of the thigh midway between the hip and the knee. Make the measurement vertically at this location.

Abdominal Skinfold—Make a mark on the skin approximately one inch to the right of the navel. Make a horizontal measurement at this location for the Fitnessgram Method and a vertical measure for the Jackson-Pollock Method. (See page 290.)

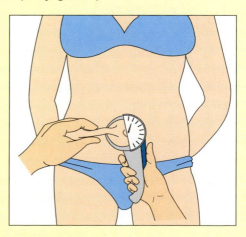

Calf skinfold—Same as for men.

Skinfold Locations for Men

Chest skinfold—Make a mark above and to the right of the right nipple (one-half the distance from the midline of the side and the nipple). The measurement at this location is often done on the diagonal because of the natural line of the skin.

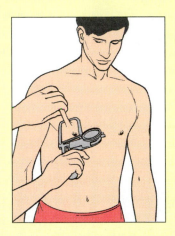

Abdominal skinfold—Make a mark on the skin approximately 1 inch to the right of the naval. Make a vertical measurement at that location for the Jackson-Pollock Method and horizontally for the Fitnessgram Method. (See page 289.)

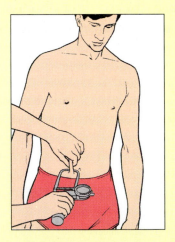

Thigh skinfold—Same as for women (see previous page).

Calf skinfold—Make a mark on the inside of the calf of the right leg at the level of the largest calf size (girth). Place the foot on a chair or other elevation so that the knee is kept at approximately 90 degrees. Make a vertical measurement at the mark.

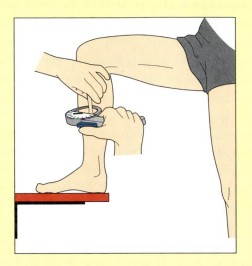

Self-Measured Tricep Skinfold for Both Men and Women

This measurement is made on the left arm so that the caliper can easily be read. Hold the arm straight at shoulder height. Make a fist with the thumb faced upward. Place the fist against a wall. With the right hand place the caliper over the skinfold at it "hangs freely" on the back of the tricep (half way from the tip of the shoulder to the elbow).

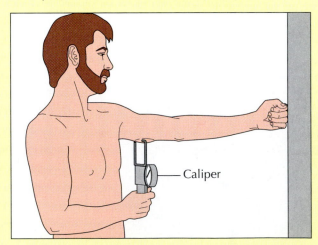

Caliper

Calculating Fatness from Skinfolds (Jackson-Pollock Method)

1. Sum three skinfolds (triceps, iliac crest, and thigh for women; chest, abdominal (vertical), and thigh for men).
2. Use the skinfold sum and your age to determine your percent fat using chart 1 for men and chart 2 for women. Locate your sum of skinfold in the left column and your age at the top of the chart. Your estimated body fat percentage is located where the values intersect.
3. Use the Standards for Body Fatness (chart 4) to determine your fatness rating.

Chart 1 Percent Fat Estimates for Men (Sum of Thigh, Chest, and Abdominal Skinfolds)

Sum of Skinfolds (mm)	Age to the Last Year								
	22 and Under	23 to 27	28 to 32	33 to 37	38 to 42	43 to 47	48 to 52	53 to 57	Over 58
8–10	1.3	1.8	2.3	2.9	3.4	3.9	4.5	5.0	5.5
11–13	2.2	2.8	3.3	3.9	4.4	4.9	5.5	6.0	6.5
14–16	3.2	3.8	4.3	4.8	5.4	5.9	6.4	7.0	7.5
17–19	4.2	4.7	5.3	5.8	6.3	6.9	7.4	8.0	8.5
20–22	5.1	5.7	6.2	6.8	7.3	7.9	8.4	8.9	9.5
23–25	6.1	6.6	7.2	7.7	8.3	8.8	9.4	9.9	10.5
26–28	7.0	7.6	8.1	8.7	9.2	9.8	10.3	10.9	11.4
29–31	8.0	8.5	9.1	9.6	10.2	10.7	11.3	11.8	12.4
32–34	8.9	9.4	10.0	10.5	11.1	11.6	12.2	12.8	13.3
35–37	9.8	10.4	10.9	11.5	12.0	12.6	13.1	13.7	14.3
38–40	10.7	11.3	11.8	12.4	12.9	13.5	14.1	14.6	15.2
41–43	11.6	12.2	12.7	13.3	13.8	14.4	15.0	15.5	16.1
44–46	12.5	13.1	13.6	14.2	14.7	15.3	15.9	16.4	17.0
47–49	13.4	13.9	14.5	15.1	15.6	16.2	16.8	17.3	17.9
50–52	14.3	14.8	15.4	15.9	16.5	17.1	17.6	18.1	18.8
53–55	15.1	15.7	16.2	16.8	17.4	17.9	18.5	18.2	19.7
56–58	16.0	16.5	17.1	17.7	18.2	18.8	19.4	20.0	20.5
59–61	16.9	17.4	17.9	18.5	19.1	19.7	20.2	20.8	21.4
62–64	17.6	18.2	18.8	19.4	19.9	20.5	21.1	21.7	22.2
65–67	18.5	19.0	19.6	20.2	20.8	21.3	21.9	22.5	23.1
68–70	19.3	19.9	20.4	21.0	21.6	22.2	22.7	23.3	23.9
71–73	20.1	20.7	21.2	21.8	22.4	23.0	23.6	24.1	24.7
74–76	20.9	21.5	22.0	22.6	23.2	23.8	24.4	25.0	25.5
77–79	21.7	22.2	22.8	23.4	24.0	24.6	25.2	25.8	26.3
80–82	22.4	23.0	23.6	24.2	24.8	25.4	25.9	26.5	27.1
83–85	23.2	23.8	24.4	25.0	25.5	26.1	26.7	27.3	27.9
86–88	24.0	24.5	25.1	25.5	26.3	26.9	27.5	28.1	28.7
89–91	24.7	25.3	25.9	25.7	27.1	27.6	28.2	28.8	29.4
92–94	25.4	26.0	26.6	27.2	27.8	28.4	29.0	29.6	30.2
95–97	26.1	26.7	27.3	27.9	28.5	29.1	29.7	30.3	30.9
98–100	26.9	27.4	28.0	28.6	29.2	29.8	30.4	31.0	31.6
101–103	27.5	28.1	28.7	29.3	29.9	30.5	31.1	31.7	32.3
104–106	28.2	28.8	29.4	30.0	30.6	31.2	31.8	32.4	33.0
107–109	28.9	29.5	30.1	30.7	31.3	31.9	32.5	33.1	33.7
110–112	29.6	30.2	30.8	31.4	32.0	32.6	33.2	33.8	34.4
113–115	30.2	30.8	31.4	32.0	32.6	33.2	33.8	34.5	35.1
116–118	30.9	31.5	32.1	32.7	33.3	33.9	34.5	35.1	35.7
119–121	31.5	32.1	32.7	33.3	33.9	34.5	35.1	35.7	36.4
122–124	32.1	32.7	33.3	33.9	34.5	35.1	35.8	36.4	37.0
125–127	32.7	33.3	33.9	34.5	35.1	35.8	36.4	37.0	37.6

From Ted A. Baumgartner and Andrew S. Jackson, *Measurement for Evaluation*, 5th edition. Copyright © 1995 Times Mirror Higher Education Group, Inc. Dubuque, Iowa. All rights reserved. Reprinted by permission.

*Percent fat calculated by the formula by Siri. Percent fat = $[(4.95/BD) - 4.5] \times 100$, where BD = body density.

Chart 2 Percent Fat Estimates for Women (Sum of Triceps, Iliac Crest, and Thigh Skinfolds)

	Age to the Last Year								
Sum of Skinfolds (mm)	22 and Under	23 to 27	28 to 32	33 to 37	38 to 42	43 to 47	48 to 52	53 to 57	Over 58
23–25	9.7	9.9	10.2	10.4	10.7	10.9	11.2	11.4	11.7
26–28	11.0	11.2	11.5	11.7	12.0	12.3	12.5	12.7	13.0
29–31	12.3	12.5	12.8	13.0	13.3	13.5	13.8	14.0	14.3
32–34	13.6	13.8	14.0	14.3	14.5	14.8	15.0	15.3	15.5
35–37	14.8	15.0	15.3	15.5	15.8	16.0	16.3	16.5	16.8
38–40	16.0	16.3	16.5	16.7	17.0	17.2	17.5	17.7	18.0
41–43	17.2	17.4	17.7	17.9	18.2	18.4	18.7	18.9	19.2
44–46	18.3	18.6	18.8	19.1	19.3	19.6	19.8	20.1	20.3
47–49	19.5	19.7	20.0	20.2	20.5	20.7	21.0	21.2	21.5
50–52	20.6	20.8	21.1	21.3	21.6	21.8	22.1	22.3	22.6
53–55	21.7	21.9	22.1	22.4	22.6	22.9	23.1	23.4	23.6
56–58	22.7	23.0	23.2	23.4	23.7	23.9	24.2	24.4	24.7
59–61	23.7	24.0	24.2	24.5	24.7	25.0	25.2	25.5	25.7
62–64	24.7	25.0	25.2	25.5	25.7	26.0	26.2	26.4	26.7
65–67	25.7	25.9	26.2	26.4	26.7	26.9	27.2	27.4	27.7
68–70	26.6	26.9	27.1	27.4	27.6	27.9	28.1	28.4	28.6
71–73	27.5	27.8	28.0	28.3	28.5	28.8	28.0	29.3	29.5
74–76	28.4	28.7	28.9	29.2	29.4	29.7	29.9	30.2	30.4
77–79	29.3	29.5	29.8	30.0	30.3	30.5	30.8	31.0	31.3
80–82	30.1	30.4	30.6	30.9	31.1	31.4	31.6	31.9	32.1
83–85	30.9	31.2	31.4	31.7	31.9	32.2	32.4	32.7	32.9
86–88	31.7	32.0	32.2	32.5	32.7	32.9	33.2	33.4	33.7
89–91	32.5	32.7	33.0	33.2	33.5	33.7	33.9	34.2	34.4
92–94	33.2	33.4	33.7	33.9	34.2	34.4	34.7	34.9	35.2
95–97	33.9	34.1	34.4	34.6	34.9	35.1	35.4	35.6	35.9
98–100	34.6	34.8	35.21	35.3	35.5	35.8	36.0	36.3	36.5
101–103	35.3	35.4	35.7	35.9	36.2	36.4	36.7	36.9	37.2
104–106	35.8	36.1	36.3	36.6	36.8	37.1	37.3	37.5	37.8
107–109	36.4	36.7	36.9	37.1	37.4	37.6	37.9	38.1	38.4
110–112	37.0	37.2	37.5	37.7	38.0	38.2	38.5	38.7	38.9
113–115	37.5	37.8	38.0	38.2	38.5	38.7	39.0	39.2	39.5
116–118	38.0	38.3	38.5	38.8	39.0	39.3	39.5	39.7	40.0
119–121	38.5	38.7	39.0	39.2	39.5	39.7	40.0	40.2	40.5
122–124	39.0	39.2	39.4	39.7	39.9	40.2	40.4	40.7	40.9
125–127	39.4	39.6	39.9	40.1	40.4	40.6	40.9	41.1	41.4
128–130	39.8	40.0	40.3	40.5	40.8	41.0	41.3	41.5	41.8

From Ted A. Baumgartner and Andrew S. Jackson, *Measurement for Evaluation*, 5th edition. Copyright © 1995 Times Mirror Higher Education Group, Inc. Dubuque, Iowa. All rights reserved. Reprinted by permission.

*Percent fat calculated by the formula by Siri. Percent fat = $[(4.95/BD) - 4.5] \times 100$, where BD = body density.

Chart 3 Percent Fat Estimates for Sum of Triceps, Abdominal, and Calf Skinfolds

Men		Women	
Sum of Skinfolds	Percent Fat	Sum of Skinfolds	Percent Fat
8–10	3.2	23–25	16.8
11–13	4.1	26–28	17.7
14–46	5.0	29–31	18.5
17–19	6.0	32–34	19.4
20–22	6.0	35–37	20.2
23–25	7.8	38–40	21.0
26–28	8.7	41–43	21.9
29–31	9.7	44–46	22.7
32–34	10.6	47–49	23.5
35–37	11.5	50–52	24.4
38–40	12.5	53–55	25.2
41–43	13.4	56–58	26.1
44–46	14.3	59–61	26.9
47–49	15.2	62–64	27.7
50–52	16.2	65–67	28.6
53–55	17.1	68–70	29.4
56–58	18.0	71–73	30.2
59–61	18.9	74–76	31.1
62–64	19.9	77–79	31.9
65–67	20.8	80–82	32.7
68–70	21.7	83–85	33.6
71–73	22.6	86–88	34.4
74–76	23.6	89–91	35.5
77–79	24.5	92–94	36.1
80–82	25.4	95–97	36.9
83–85	26.4	98–100	37.8
86–88	27.3	101–103	38.6
89–91	28.2	104–106	39.4
92–94	29.1	107–109	40.3
95–97	30.1	110–112	41.1
98–100	31.0	113–115	42.0
101–103	31.9	116–118	42.8
104–106	32.8	119–121	43.6
107–109	33.8	122–124	44.5
110–112	34.7	125–127	45.3
113–115	35.6	128–130	46.1
116–118	36.6	131–133	47.0
119–121	37.5	134–136	47.8
122–124	38.4	137–139	48.7
125–127	39.3	140–142	49.5

Calculating Fatness from Skinfolds (Fitnessgram Method)

1. Sum the three skinfolds (triceps, abdominal, and calf) for both men and women. Use horizontal abdominal measure.
2. Use the skinfold sum and your age to determine your percent fat using chart 3. Locate your sum of skinfold in the left column and your age at the top of the chart. Your estimated body fat percentage is located where the values intersect.
3. Use the Standards for Body Fatness (chart 4) to determine your fatness rating.

Calculating Fatness from Self-Measured Skinfolds

1. Use either the Jackson-Pollock or Fitnessgram method but make the measures on yourself rather than have a partner do the measures. When doing the tricep measure use the self-measurement technique for both men and women. (See page 290.)
2. Calculate fatness using the methods described previously.
3. Use chart 4 to determine ratings.

Chart 4 Standards for Body Fatness (Percent Body Fat)

Classification	Males	Females
Essential fat	No less than 5%	No less than 10%
Borderline	5%–9%	10%–16%
High performance	5%–15%	10%–23%
Good fitness (healthy)	10%–20%	17%–28%
Marginal	21%–25%	29%–35%
Overfat	25%+	35%+

Height-Weight Measurements

1. *Height*—Measure your height in inches or centimeters. Take the measurement without shoes, but add 2.5 centimeters or 1 inch to measurements, as the charts include heel height.

2. *Weight*—Measure your weight in pounds or kilograms without clothes. Add 3 pounds or 1.4 kilograms because the charts include weight of clothes. If weight must be taken with clothes on, wear indoor clothing that weigh 3 pounds or 1.4 kilograms.

3. Determine your frame size using the elbow breadth. The measurement is most accurate when done with a broad-based sliding caliper. However, it can be done using a skinfold caliper or can be estimated with a metric ruler. The right arm is measured when it is elevated with the elbow bent at 90 degrees and the upper arm horizontal. The back of the hand should face the person making the measurement. Using the caliper, measure the distance between the epicondyles of the humerus (inside and outside bony points of the elbow). Measure to the nearest millimeter (1/10 of a centimeter). If a caliper is not available, place the thumb and the index finger of the left hand on the epicondyles of the humerus and measure the distance between the fingers with a metric ruler. Use your height and elbow breadth in centimeters to determine your frame size (Chart 5), you need not repeat this procedure each time you use a height-weight chart.

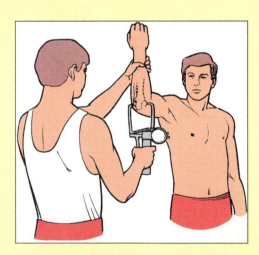

4. Use chart 6 to determine your healthy weight range. The new healthy weight range charts do not account for frame size. However, you may want to consider frame size when determining a personal weight within the health weight range. People with a larger frame size typically can carry more weight within the range than those with a smaller frame size.

Chart 5 Frame Size Determined from Elbow Breadth (mm)

Height	Elbow Breadth (mm).		
	Small Frame	Medium Frame	Large Frame
Males			
5'2" or less	<64	64–72	>72
5'3"–5'6 1/2"	<67	67–74	>74
5'7"–5'10 1/2"	<69	69–76	>76
5'11"–6'2 1/2"	<71	71–78	>78
6'3" or less	<74	74–81	>81
Females			
4'10 1/2" or less	<56	56–64	>64
4'11"–5'2 1/2"	<58	58–65	>65
5'3"–5'6 1/2"	<59	59–66	>66
5'7"–5'10 1/2"	<61	61–68	>69
5'11" or less	<62	62–69	>69

Courtesy of the Metropolitan Life Insurance Company.

Height is given including 1-inch heels.

Chart 6 Healthy Weight Ranges for Adult Women and Men

	Women			Men	
Feet	Height Inches	Pounds	Feet	Height Inches	Pounds
4	10	91–119	5	9	129–169
4	11	94–124	5	10	132–174
5	0	97–128	5	11	136–179
5	1	101–132	6	0	140–184
5	2	104–137	6	1	144–189
5	3	107–141	6	2	148–195
5	4	111–146	6	3	152–200
5	5	114–150	6	4	156–205
5	6	118–155	6	5	160–211
5	7	121–160	6	6	164–216
5	8	125–164			

SOURCE: Data from 1995 Dietary Guidelines U.S. Department of Agriculture and Department of Health and Human Services.

Chart 7 Body Mass Index

Height	100	105	110	115	120	125	130	135	140	145	150	155	160	165	170	175	180	185	190	195	200	205	210	215	220	225	230	235	240	245	250
5'0"	20	21	21	22	23	24	25	26	27	28	29	30	31	32	33	34	35	36	37	38	39	40	41	42	43	44	45	46	47	48	49
5'1"	19	20	21	22	23	24	25	26	26	27	28	29	30	31	32	33	34	35	36	37	38	39	40	41	42	43	43	44	45	46	47
5'2"	18	19	20	21	22	23	24	25	26	27	27	28	29	30	31	32	33	34	35	36	37	37	38	39	40	41	42	43	44	45	46
5'3"	18	19	19	20	21	22	23	24	25	26	27	27	28	29	30	31	32	33	34	35	35	36	37	38	39	40	41	42	43	43	44
5'4"	17	18	19	20	21	21	22	23	24	25	26	27	27	28	29	30	31	32	33	33	34	35	36	37	38	39	39	40	41	42	43
5'5"	17	17	18	19	20	21	22	22	23	24	25	26	27	27	28	29	30	31	32	32	33	34	35	36	37	37	38	39	40	41	42
5'6"	16	17	18	19	19	20	21	22	23	23	24	25	26	27	27	28	29	30	31	31	32	33	34	35	36	36	37	38	39	40	40
5'7"	16	16	17	18	19	20	20	21	22	23	23	24	25	26	27	27	28	29	30	31	31	32	33	34	34	35	36	37	38	38	39
5'8"	15	16	17	17	18	19	20	21	21	22	23	24	24	25	26	27	27	28	29	30	30	31	32	33	33	34	35	36	36	37	38
5'9"	15	16	16	17	18	18	19	20	21	22	23	24	24	25	26	27	27	28	29	30	30	31	32	32	33	34	35	35	36	37	37
5'10"	14	15	16	17	17	18	19	19	20	21	22	22	23	24	24	25	26	27	27	28	29	29	30	31	32	32	33	34	34	35	36
5'11"	14	15	15	16	17	17	18	19	20	20	21	22	22	23	24	24	25	26	26	27	28	29	29	30	31	31	32	33	33	34	35
6'0"	14	14	15	16	16	17	18	18	19	20	20	21	22	22	23	24	24	25	26	26	27	28	28	29	30	31	31	32	33	33	34
6'1"	13	14	15	15	16	16	17	18	18	19	20	20	21	22	22	23	24	24	25	26	26	27	28	28	29	30	30	31	32	32	33
6'2"	13	13	14	15	15	16	17	17	18	19	19	20	21	21	22	22	23	24	24	25	26	26	27	28	28	29	30	30	31	31	32
6'3"	12	13	14	14	15	16	16	17	17	18	19	19	20	21	21	22	22	23	24	24	25	26	26	27	27	28	29	29	30	31	31
6'4"	12	13	13	14	15	15	16	16	17	18	18	19	19	20	21	21	22	23	23	24	24	25	26	26	27	27	28	29	29	30	30

Weight

■ Low   ■ Good fitness zone   ■ Marginal   ■ Obese

Body Mass Index (BMI)

Use the steps listed below or use chart 7 to calculate your BMI.
1. Divide your weight in pounds by 2.2 to determine your weight in kilograms.
2. Multiply your height in inches by 0.0254 to determine your height in meters.
3. Square your height in meters (multiply your height in meters by your height in meters).
4. Divide the value you obtain in step 3 (square of height in meters) into the value you obtain in step 1 (weight in kilograms).
5. If you use these steps to determine your BMI, use the Rating Scale for Body Mass Index (chart 8) to obtain a rating for your BMI.

Chart 8 Rating Scale for Body Mass Index

Classification	BMI
Obese (high risk)	Over 30
Marginal	25–30
Good fitness zone	17–24.9
Low	Less than 17

NOTE: An excessively low BMI is not desirable. Low BMI values can be indicative of eating disorders and other health problems. The government rating for marginal is "overweight."

Determining the Waist-to-Hip Circumference Ratio

The waist-to-hip circumference ratio is recommended as the best available index for determining risk and disease associated with fat and weight distribution. Disease and death risk are associated with abdominal and upper body fatness. When a person has both high fatness and a high waist-to-hip ratio, additional risks exist. The following steps should be taken in making measurements and calculating the waist-to-hip ratio.

1. Both measurements should be done with a nonelastic tape. Make the measurements while standing with the feet together and the arms at the sides, elevated only high enough to allow the measurements. Be sure that the tape is horizontal and around the entire circumference. Record scores to the nearest millimeter or 1/16th of an inch. Use the same units of measure for both circumferences (millimeters or 1/16th of an inch). The tape should be pulled snugly but not to the point of causing an indentation in the skin.

2. *Waist measurement*—Measure at the natural waist (smallest waist circumference). If there is no natural waist, the measurement should be made at the level of the umbilicus. Measure at the end of a normal inspiration.

3. *Hip measurement*—Measure at the maximum circumference of the buttocks. It is recommended that you wear thin-layered clothing (such as a swimming suit or underwear) that won't add significantly to the measurement.

4. Divide the hip measurement into the waist measurement or use the waist-to-hip nomogram (chart 9) to determine your waist-to-hip ratio.

5. Use the Waist-to-Hip Ratio Rating Scale (chart 10) to determine your rating for the waist-to-hip ratio.

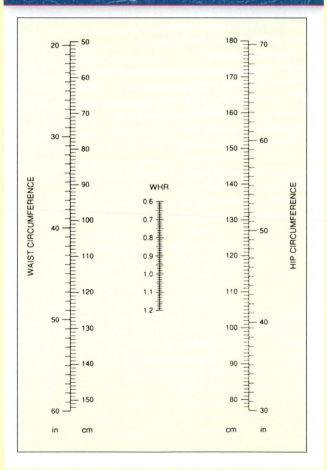

Chart 9 Waist-to-Hip Ratio Nomogram

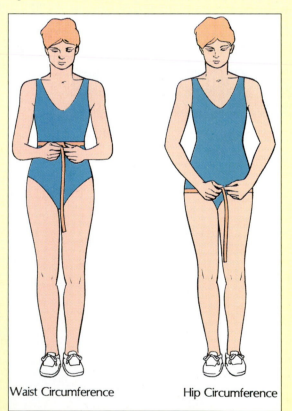

Waist Circumference   Hip Circumference

Note: Using a partner or a mirror will aid you in keeping the tape horizontal.

Chart 10 Waist-to-Hip Ratio Rating Scale

Classification	Men	Women
High risk	>1.0	>0.85
Moderately high risk	0.90–1.0	0.80–0.85
Lower risk	<0.90	<0.80

Lab 15A: Evaluating Body Composition: Skinfold Measures

Name	**Section**	**Date**

Purpose: To estimate body fatness using two different skinfold procedures; to compare measures made by an expert, by a partner, and by self-measurements; to learn the strengths and weaknesses of each technique; and to use the results to establish personal standards for evaluating body composition.

General Procedures: Follow the specific procedures for the two different self-assessment techniques. If possible, have one set of measurements made by an expert (instructor) for each of the two techniques. Next, work with a partner you trust. Have the partner make measurements at each site for both techniques. Finally, make self-measurements for each of the sites. If you are just learning a measurement technique, it is important to practice the skills of making the measurement. If you do measurements over time, use the same instrument (if possible) each time you measure. If your measurements vary widely, take more than one set until you get more consistent results.

If you have had an underwater weighing, an electric impedance measurement, a near-infrared interactance measure, or some other body fatness measurement done recently, record your results below.

Measurement Technique	**% Body Fat**	**Rating**
1.		
2.		

Skinfold Measurements (Jackson-Pollock Method)

Procedures:

1. Read the directions for the Jackson-Pollock Method measurements in the lab resource materials.
2. If possible, observe a demonstration of the proper procedures for measuring skinfolds at each of the different locations before doing partner or self-measurements.
3. Make expert, partner, and self-measurements (see lab resource materials). When doing the self-measure of the triceps use the self-measurement technique described on page 290 (women only).
4. Record each of the measurements in the Results section.
5. Calculate your body fatness from skinfolds by summing the appropriate skinfold values (chest, thigh, and abdominal for men; triceps, iliac crest, and thigh for women). Using your age and the sum of the appropriate skinfolds, determine your body fatness using charts 1 and 2 in the lab resource materials.
6. Rate your fatness using chart 4 in the lab resource materials.

Skinfolds by an expert (if possible)		Skinfolds by Partner		Self-Measurements	
Male		*Male*		*Male*	
Chest		Chest		Chest	
Thigh		Thigh		Thigh	
Abdominal		Abdominal		Abdominal	
Sum		Sum		Sum	
% body fat		% body fat		% body fat	
Rating		Rating		Rating	
Female		*Female*		*Female*	
Triceps		Triceps		Triceps	
Iliac crest		Iliac crest		Iliac crest	
Thigh		Thigh		Thigh	
Sum		Sum		Sum	
% body fat		% body fat		% body fat	
Rating		Rating		Rating	

Make a check by the statements that are true about your measurements.

☐   Person doing measurements has experience with these three skinfold measurements.

☐   Self-measurements were practiced until measurements became consistent.

☐   Results of several trials for each measure are consistent (do not vary more than 2–3 mm).

☐   You are not exceptionally low or exceptionally high in body fat.

The more checks you have, the more likely your measurements are accurate.

Skinfold Measurements (Fitnessgram Method)

Procedures:
1. Read the directions for the Fitnessgram measurements in the lab resource materials.
2. Use the procedures as for the Fitnessgram Method using the triceps, abdominal, and calf sites described in the lab resource materials. When doing the self-measure of the triceps use the self-measurement technique on page 290.
3. Calculate your body fatness from skinfolds by summing the appropriate skinfold values (same for both men and women). Using the sum of the appropriate skinfolds, determine your body fatness using chart 3 in the lab resource materials.
4. Rate your fatness using chart 4 in the lab resource materials.

Results:

Skinfolds by an expert (if possible)

Triceps [ ]

Abdominal [ ]

Calf [ ]

Sum [ ]

% body fat [ ]

Rating [ ]

Skinfolds by Partner

Triceps [ ]

Abdominal [ ]

Calf [ ]

Sum [ ]

% body fat [ ]

Rating [ ]

Self-Measurements

Triceps [ ]

Abdominal [ ]

Calf [ ]

Sum [ ]

% body fat [ ]

Rating [ ]

Make a check by the statements that are true about your measurements.

[ ] Person doing measurements has experience with these three skinfold measurements.

[ ] Self-measurements were practiced until measurements became consistent.

[ ] Results of several trials for each measure are consistent (do not vary more than 2–3 mm).

[ ] You are not exceptionally low or exceptionally high in body fat.

The more checks you have, the more likely your measurements are accurate.

Conclusion and Implications:

In the space provided below, discuss your current body composition based on the two different skinfold procedures and any other measures of body fatness you may have done. Note any discrepancies in the measurements and discuss which of the measurements you think provide the most useful information. To what extent do you think you need to alter your level of body fatness?

Lab 15B: Evaluating Body Composition: Height/Weight and Circumference Measures

Name	**Section**	**Date**

Purpose: To assess body composition using a variety of procedures, to learn the strengths and weaknesses of each technique, and to use the results to establish personal standards for evaluating body composition.

General Procedures: Follow the specific procedures for the three different self-assessment techniques. If possible, work with a partner you trust to help with measurements that you have difficulty making on yourself. If you are just learning a measurement technique, it is important to practice the skills of making the measurement. If you do measurements over time, use the same instrument (if possible) each time you measure. If your measurements vary widely, take more than one set until you get more consistent results. If possible, have an expert make measurements on you using the two procedures.

Height and Weight Measurements

Procedures:
1. Read the directions for height and weight measurements in the lab resource materials.
2. Determine your healthy weight range using chart 6 in the lab resource materials. You may want to use your elbow breadth (chart 5). People with smaller frame sizes should typically weigh less than those with a larger frame size within the healthy weight range. You may need the assistance of a partner to make the elbow breadth measurement.
3. Record your scores in the Results section.

Results:

Weight [ ]   Healthy weight range [ ]

Height [ ]

Make a check by the statements that are true about your measurements.

[ ]   You are confident in the accuracy of the scale you used.

[ ]   You are confident that the height technique is accurate.

The more checks you have, the more likely your measurements are accurate.
If you are a very active person with a high amount of muscle, use this method with caution.

The Body Mass Index

Procedures:
1. Use the height and weight measures from Part 1 above.
2. Determine your BMI score by using chart 7 or the directions in the lab resource materials. Determine your rating using chart 8.
3. Record your scores and rating in the Results section.

Results:

Body mass index [ ]   Rating [ ]

If you are a very active person with a high amount of muscle, use this method with caution.

Waist to Hip Ratio

Procedures:

1. Measure your waist and hip circumferences using the procedures in the lab resource materials.
2. Divide your hip circumference into your waist circumference or use chart 9 in the lab resource materials to calculate your waist-to-hip ratio.
3. Determine your rating using chart 10 in the lab resource materials.
4. Record your scores in the Results section.

Results:

Waist circumference

Hip circumference

Waist-to-hip ratio   Rating

Make a check by the statements that are true about your measurements.

☐ You are confident in the accuracy of the waist and hip measurement.

Make a check by the statements that are true about you.

☐ I am a male 5′9″ or less and have a waist girth of 34 or more.

☐ I am a male 5′10″ to 6′4″ and have a waist girth of 36 or more.

☐ I am a male 6′5″ or more and have a waist girth of 38 or more.

☐ I am a female 5′2″ or less and have a waist girth of 29 or more.

☐ I am a female 5′3″ to 5′10″ and have a waist girth of 31 or more.

☐ I am a female 5′11″ or more and have a waist girth of 33 or more.

If you checked one of the boxes above, the waist-to-hip ratio is especially relevant for you.

Conclusions and Implications:

In the space provided below, discuss your results for the three height, weight, and circumference procedures. Note any discrepancies in the measurements. Indicate the strengths and weaknesses of the various methods. Which of the measures do you think provided you with the most useful information? If you also did the skinfold measures (Lab 15A), discuss your body composition based on all of the information you have collected (skinfolds and height, weight, and circumference measures).

Lab 15C: Determining Your Daily Energy Expenditure

Name	**Section**	**Date**

Purpose: To learn how many calories you expend in a day.

Procedures:

1. Estimate your basal metabolism using step 1 in the Results section. First determine the number of minutes you sleep.
2. Monitor your activity expenditure for one day using Chart 1. Record the number of 5-, 15-, and 30-minute blocks of time that you perform each of the different types of physical activities (e.g., if an activity lasted 20 minutes, you would use one 15-minute block and one 5-minute block). Be sure to distinguish between moderate (Mod) or vigorous (Vig) intensity in your logging. If you perform an activity that is not listed, specify the activity on the line labeled "Other" and estimate if it is moderate or vigorous. You may want to keep copies of Chart 1 for future use. One extra copy is provided.
3. Sum the total number of minutes of moderate and vigorous activity. Determine your calories expended during moderate and vigorous activity using steps 2 and 3.
4. Determine your nonactive minutes using step 4. This is all time that is not spent sleeping or being active.
5. Determine your calories expended in nonactive minutes using step 5.
6. Determine your calories expended in a day using step 6.

Results:

Daily Caloric Expenditure Estimates

Step 1:

Basal calories = .0076 × [Body wt (lbs)] × [Minutes of sleep] = [Basal calories] (A)

Step 2:

Calories (moderate activity) = .036 × [Body wt (lbs)] × [Minutes of moderate activity] = [Calories in moderate activity] (B)

Step 3:

Calories (vigorous activity) = .053 × [Body wt (lbs)] × [Minutes of vigorous activity] = [Calories in vigorous activity] (C)

Step 4:

Minutes (nonactive) = 1,440 min. − [Minutes of sleep] − [Minutes of moderate activity] − [Minutes of vigorous activity] = [Nonactive minutes]

Step 5:

Calories (rest and light activity) = .011 × [Body wt (lbs)] × [Nonactive minutes] = [Calories in other activities] (D)

Step 6:

Calories expended (per day) = [(A)] + [(B)] + [(C)] + [(D)] = [Daily calories]

Answer these questions about your daily calorie expenditure estimate.

Yes	No	
☐	☐	Were the activities you performed similar to what you normally perform each day?
☐	☐	Do you think your daily estimated calorie expenditure is an accurate estimate?
☐	☐	Do you think you expend the correct amount of calories in a typical day to maintain the body composition (body fat level) that is desirable for you?

Conclusions and Interpretations: In several paragraphs, discuss your daily calorie expenditure. Comment on your answers to the questions listed above. In addition, comment on whether you think you should modify your daily calorie expenditure for any reason.

Chart 1   Daily Activity Log

Day of Monitoring:

Physical Activity Category		5 Minutes	15 Minutes	30 Minutes	Minutes
Lifestyle Activity		1 2 3 4 5 6	1 2 3 4 5 6	1 2 3	
Dancing (general)	Mod				
Gardening	Mod				
Home repair/maintenance	Mod				
Occupation	Mod				
Walking/hiking	Mod				
Other:	Mod				
Aerobic Activity		1 2 3 4 5 6	1 2 3 4 5 6	1 2 3	
Aerobic dance (low impact)	Mod				
	Vig				
Aerobic eq. (rowing, stair, ski)	Mod				
	Vig				
Bicycling	Mod				
	Vig				
Running	Mod				
	Vig				
Skating (roller/ice)	Mod				
	Vig				
Swimming (laps)	Mod				
	Vig				
Other:	Mod				
	Vig				
Sport/Recreation Activity		1 2 3 4 5 6	1 2 3 4 5 6	1 2 3	
Basketball	Mod				
	Vig				
Bowling/billards	Mod				
Golf	Mod				
Martial arts (judo, karate)	Mod				
	Vig				
Racquetball/tennis	Mod				
	Vig				
Soccer/hockey	Mod				
	Vig				
Softball/baseball	Mod				
Volleyball	Mod				
	Vig				
Other:	Mod				
Flexibility Activity		1 2 3 4 5 6	1 2 3 4 5 6	1 2 3	
Stretching	Mod				
Other:	Mod				
Strengthening Activity		1 2 3 4 5 6	1 2 3 4 5 6	1 2 3	
Calisthenics (push-ups/sit-ups)	Mod				
Resistance Exercise	Mod				
Other:	Mod				

Minutes of moderate activity

Minutes of vigorous activity

Total minutes of activity

Chart 2   Daily Activity Log

Day of Monitoring:

Physical Activity Category		5 Minutes	15 Minutes	30 Minutes	Minutes
Lifestyle Activity		1 2 3 4 5 6	1 2 3 4 5 6	1 2 3	
Dancing (general)	Mod				
Gardening	Mod				
Home repair/maintenance	Mod				
Occupation	Mod				
Walking/hiking	Mod				
Other:	Mod				
Aerobic Activity		1 2 3 4 5 6	1 2 3 4 5 6	1 2 3	
Aerobic dance (low impact)	Mod				
	Vig				
Aerobic eq. (rowing, stair, ski)	Mod				
	Vig				
Bicycling	Mod				
	Vig				
Running	Mod				
	Vig				
Skating (roller/ice)	Mod				
	Vig				
Swimming (laps)	Mod				
	Vig				
Other:	Mod				
	Vig				
Sport/Recreation Activity		1 2 3 4 5 6	1 2 3 4 5 6	1 2 3	
Basketball	Mod				
	Vig				
Bowling/billards	Mod				
Golf	Mod				
Martial arts (judo, karate)	Mod				
	Vig				
Racquetball/tennis	Mod				
	Vig				
Soccer/hockey	Mod				
	Vig				
Softball/baseball	Mod				
Volleyball	Mod				
	Vig				
Other:	Mod				
Flexibility Activity		1 2 3 4 5 6	1 2 3 4 5 6	1 2 3	
Stretching	Mod				
Other:	Mod				
Strengthening Activity		1 2 3 4 5 6	1 2 3 4 5 6	1 2 3	
Calisthenics (push-ups/sit-ups)	Mod				
Resistance Exercise	Mod				
Other:	Mod				

Minutes of moderate activity

Minutes of vigorous activity

Total minutes of activity

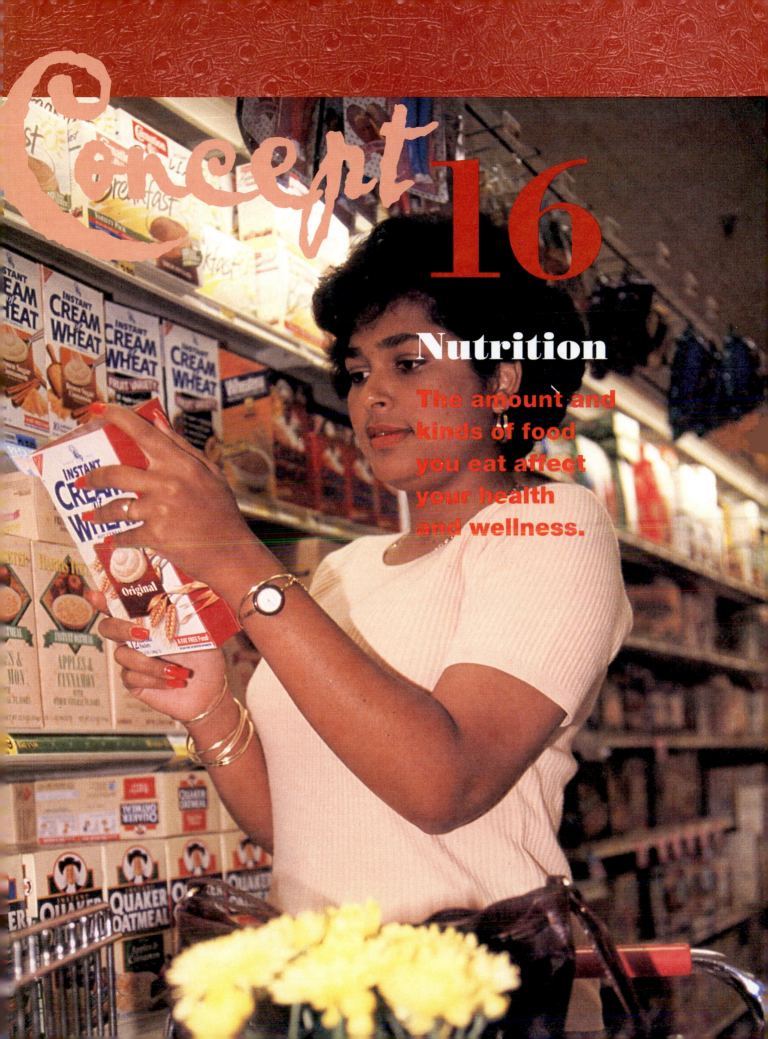

Concept 16

Nutrition

The amount and kinds of food you eat affect your health and wellness.

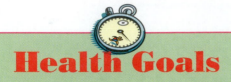

Health Goals

for year 2010

Promote health by improving dietary factors and nutritional status.

Reduce chronic disease risk, disease progression, debilitation, and premature death associated with dietary factors and nutritional status.

Increase proportion of people who meet national dietary guidelines.

Increase proportion of people who eat no more than 30 percent of calories as fat.

Increase proportion of people who eat no more than 10 percent of calories as saturated fat.

Increase proportion of people who eat at least five servings of vegetables and fruits daily.

Increase proportion of people who eat at least six servings of grain products daily.

Increase proportion of people who meet dietary recommendation for calcium.

Reduce proportion of people who consume excess sodium.

Reduce incidence of iron deficiency and anemia (especially children and women).

Increase teaching about nutrition (school, work-site and health care agencies).

Introduction

The importance of good nutrition for optimal health is well established. Most people believe that nutrition is important but still find it difficult to maintain a healthy diet. One reason is that foods are usually developed, marketed and advertised for convenience and taste rather than for health or nutritional quality. Another reason is that many individuals have misconceptions about what constitutes a healthy diet. Some of these misconceptions are propagated by so called "experts" with less than impressive credentials and those with commercial interests. Others are created by the confusing, and often contradictory, news reports about new nutrition research. In spite of the fact that nutrition is an advanced science, there are still many unanswered questions.

In this concept some basic nutrition guidelines are presented to inform the reader and dispel various nutrition myths. A special section is presented on nutrition and physical performance to assist those interested in sports and high-level performance. If you are interested in learning more about nutrition than is covered here you are encouraged to seek the advice of a registered dietitian or to study reliable books, journals, or government documents (see Suggested Readings and Web Review).

The Facts about Basic Nutrition and Health

The amount and kinds of food you eat affect your health and well-being.

There are about 45 to 50 nutrients in food that are believed to be essential for the body's growth, maintenance, and repair. These are classified into six categories: carbohydrates (and fiber), fats, proteins, vitamins, minerals, and water. The first three provide energy, which is measured in calories. Specific dietary recommendations for each of the six nutrients are presented later in this concept.

www.mhhe.com/hper/physed/clw/student/
Recommended Daily Allowances (RDA) values published by the Food and Nutrition Board of the National Academy of Sciences have served as the standard for nutritional adequacy for the past two decades. Recently the Academy, in partnership with Health Canada, has recognized the need for additional nutrition standards resulting in the establishment of four types of values all classified under the heading of **Dietary Reference Intakes** (DRI). RDA values are established when adequate scientific information is available for most foods (Recommended Nutrient Intake—RNI values—in Canada). They are based on **Estimated Average Requirements** (EAR) values when they are available. **Adequate Intake** (AI) is an alternative term used to describe the amount of a nutrient people should consume when scientific data is not adequate to establish RDA values. **Tolerable Upper Intake Level** (UL) is a new type of dietary reference. To date values have been established for only a few nutrients. The goal is to establish UL values for all, or at least most nutrients, in the next few years. The establishment of UL values makes it clear that while too little of a nutrient can be harmful to health, so can too much. For now, RDA values are the most relevant reference term, though UL values will become more meaningful when they are established for most nutrients. In many ways the RDAs are threshold values similar to the threshold of training values for physical activity. The target zone for healthy eating would range from the RDA values to the UL values.

The quantity of nutrients recommended varies with age and other considerations; for example, young children need

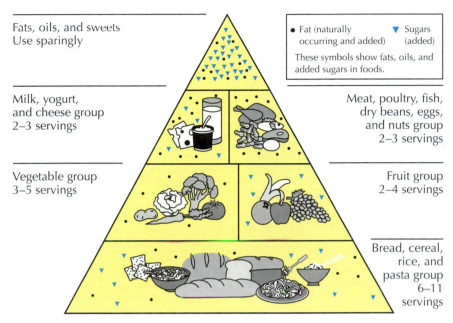

Fats, oils, and sweets
Use sparingly

● Fat (naturally ▼ Sugars
occurring and added) (added)
These symbols show fats, oils, and
added sugars in foods.

Milk, yogurt,
and cheese group
2–3 servings

Meat, poultry, fish,
dry beans, eggs,
and nuts group
2–3 servings

Vegetable group
3–5 servings

Fruit group
2–4 servings

Bread, cereal,
rice, and
pasta group
6–11
servings

Figure 1
The food guide pyramid.
SOURCE: Data from the U.S. Department of Agriculture.

more calcium than adults and pregnant women or post-menopausal women need more calcium than other women. Accordingly dietary reference intakes, including RDAs, have been established for several age/gender groups. In this book, the values used are those that are appropriate for most adult men and women.

Some foods contain some of all six classes of nutrients (e.g., whole wheat bread) whereas others contain only one (e.g., sugar). No food is a "complete" food because none contains all of the specific essential nutrients.

> Eating the recommended servings of food from the food guide pyramid will provide key nutrients and enable a person to meet dietary recommendations.

The food guide pyramid (Figure 1) was designed to guide people in the selection of nutritious food. Selecting the appropriate number of servings from each portion of the pyramid will assure inclusion of necessary nutrients in the diet. A greater number of servings is recommended from the foods near the base of the pyramid (complex carbohydrates) with fewer servings from the upper levels. Foods from the lower level of the pyramid are "nutritionally dense," meaning that they have more nutrients per calorie than low-density foods. For example, a 200-calorie piece of Boston cream pie (from tip of pyramid) has very few vitamins and minerals and is high in fat and refined carbohydrates. On the other hand, 200 calories of tuna has very little

fat; 100 percent of the RDA for protein, niacin, and vitamin B_{12}; and substantial B_6 and phosphorus. Eating nutritionally dense food is particularly important for someone on a low-

Recommended Daily Allowance (RDA) The minimum amount of a specific nutrient that should be included in the daily diet to meet the health needs of nearly all people in a specific age/gender group.

Dietary Reference Intakes (DRI) A generic term used to describe four types of values used to describe appropriate amounts of nutrients in the diet (AI, EAR, RDA, and UL).

Estimated Average Requirement (EAR) A term that described the amount of a nutrient that meets the needs of at least 50 percent of the people in a specific age/gender group.

Adequate Intakes (AI) A term used instead of recommended dietary allowance (RDA) when sufficient data are not available to establish RDA values for a specific nutrient.

Tolerable Upper Intake Level (UL) A term used to describe the maximum level of a daily nutrient that will not pose a risk of adverse health effects for most people.

Food Groups

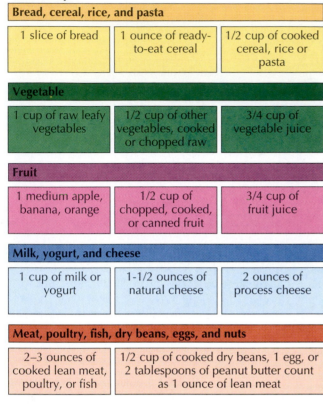

Bread, cereal, rice, and pasta		
1 slice of bread	1 ounce of ready-to-eat cereal	1/2 cup of cooked cereal, rice or pasta

Vegetable		
1 cup of raw leafy vegetables	1/2 cup of other vegetables, cooked or chopped raw	3/4 cup of vegetable juice

Fruit		
1 medium apple, banana, orange	1/2 cup of chopped, cooked, or canned fruit	3/4 cup of fruit juice

Milk, yogurt, and cheese		
1 cup of milk or yogurt	1-1/2 ounces of natural cheese	2 ounces of process cheese

Meat, poultry, fish, dry beans, eggs, and nuts	
2–3 ounces of cooked lean meat, poultry, or fish	1/2 cup of cooked dry beans, 1 egg, or 2 tablespoons of peanut butter count as 1 ounce of lean meat

Figure 2

What counts as a serving?

SOURCE: Data from the U.S. Department of Agriculture.

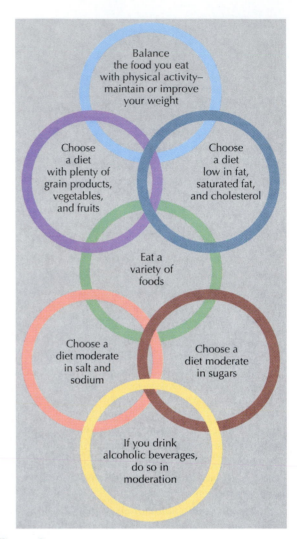

Figure 3

Dietary guidelines for Americans.

SOURCE: Data from *Home and Garden Bulletin No. 232*, 4th edition, December 1995, U.S. Department of Agriculture, U.S. Department of Health and Human Services, Washington, DC.

calorie diet because it is especially hard to get all the essential nutrients when you do not eat very much food.

There are other models used to describe methods for helping people eat healthy nutritious diets. For example, the American Heart Association has adapted the pyramid to aid in selection of foods for heart disease prevention, a pyramid for older adults is now available, and in Canada the Food Guide is used to help people choose nutritious foods (see Appendix E).

Counting food servings is important to assuring that adequate choices are made from the pyramid.

Figure 2 provides you with examples of what constitutes a serving for each food group. Use this information to help you see if you have made the appropriate number of choices from the pyramid. National health goals for nutrition specifically target fruits, vegetables, and grains.

Though many people in western society do not eat adequate portions of nutritionally dense foods even when they are readily available, there is evidence that the diets of Americans have improved in recent years. Over the past two to three

decades, the percentage of calories from fat has decreased and the intake of fruits (up 19 percent), vegetables (up 22 percent), and grains (up 47 percent) has increased. Still the number of servings of fruit now averages 1.5 per day, an amount lower than the dietary recommendation of two servings per day. It is encouraging that vegetable intake (3.6 per day) is above the recommended amount of three servings per day. Discouraging is the fact that nearly half of the vegetable intake is from potatoes, and half of the potato intake is from French fries.

New dietary guidelines are available to help you plan for sound nutrition.

Federal law requires the publication of national dietary guidelines every five years. The most recent guidelines are illustrated in Figure 3. These guidelines are intended to sup-

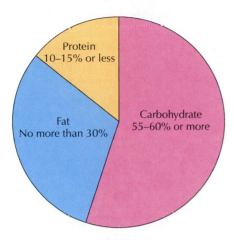

Figure 4
Recommended dietary intake.

plement previous guidelines and the food guide pyramid in helping Americans select a nutritious diet. Among the major differences in these guidelines and previous ones are an emphasis on selecting a variety of foods in the diet, an emphasis on foods from the base of the pyramid, an emphasis on physical activity as part of balancing calories, a recognition that vegetarian diets can be sound when properly selected, and a change in weight standards (age-neutral standards) so as not to allow weight gain as people grow older.

> The number of calories needed per day depends upon the body's metabolic rate (MR), which, in turn, depends upon such factors as age, sex, size, muscle mass, glandular function, emotional state, climate, and exercise.

www.mhhe.com/hper/physed/clw/student/
Your **basal metabolic rate (BMR)** is the basis for your caloric needs. The higher the BMR, the more calories you burn at rest. Your **metabolic rate (MR)** is a combination of your BMR and calories expended in normal daily activities. The MR is usually higher in males, young people, large people, lean and muscular people, and in nervous people; in cold and hot weather; and during exercise.

A moderately active college-age woman needs about 2,000 calories per day, whereas a moderately active man of the same age needs about 2,800 calories. A female athlete in training might burn 2,600 to 4,500 calories; a male athlete in training might expend 3,500 to 6,000. If your weight remains at the optimum, the caloric content of your diet is correct. If weight varies from optimal, the caloric content of the diet may need to be altered.

The three primary sources of calories in the diet are fat, protein, and carbohydrates. The typical adult consumes too much fat and too little carbohydrate, especially complex carbohydrates. Health goals want Americans to reduce the amount of dietary fat and increase the amount of complex carbohydrates in the diet (see Figure 4). Currently, only 33 percent of people aged 2 and above meet the goal of eating no more than 30 percent of the diet as fat, and 35 percent consume more than 10 percent saturated fat. For fruits and vegetables, the proportion of the population eating adequate servings is 40 percent and for grains 52 percent.

> Eating well can reduce risk of various health problems and increase quality of life.

As will be more clearly described in the sections that follow, the risk of many diseases is reduced by proper nutrition. Among the conditions especially affected by eating patterns are heart disease, stroke, diabetes, colon cancer, high blood pressure, and osteoporosis. Proper nutrition can also enhance the quality of life by improving the ability to carry out work and leisure-time activities without fatigue.

Dietary Recommendations for Fat: The Facts

> Excess fat in the diet, particularly saturated fat, is associated with an increased risk of disease and is inversely related to optimal health.

www.mhhe.com/hper/physed/clw/student/
Humans need some fat in their diet because fats are carriers of vitamins A, D, E, and K. They are a source of essential linoleic acid, make food taste better, and provide a concentrated form of calories, which serve as an important source of energy during moderate to

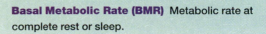
Metabolic Rate (MR) The rate at which the body produces heat that is measured in calories; an indication of the body's activities, including exercise and normal body functions.

Basal Metabolic Rate (BMR) Metabolic rate at complete rest or sleep.

vigorous exercise. Fats have more than twice the calories per gram as carbohydrates.

There is evidence that excessive total fat in the diet is associated with atherosclerotic cardiovascular disease and breast, prostate, and colon cancer, as well as obesity. **Saturated fats** come primarily from animal sources such as red meat, dairy products, and eggs, but they are also found in some vegetable sources such as coconut and palm oils. They are considered most likely to contribute to the health problems mentioned above. In addition, excess saturated fat in the diet contributes to increased cholesterol, and increased LDL (low-density lipoprotein) cholesterol in the blood. It is for this reason that no more than 10 percent of your total calories should come from saturated fats.

Unsaturated fats, also a part of a normal diet, are of two basic types: polyunsaturated and monounsaturated. Polyunsaturated fats are derived principally from vegetable sources such as safflower, cottonseed, soybean, sunflower, and corn oils (Omega-6 fats), and cold-water fish sources such as salmon and mackerel (Omega-3 fats). Monounsaturated fats are derived primarily from vegetable sources including olive, peanut, and canola oil.

Unsaturated fats are generally considered to be less likely to contribute to cardiovascular disease, cancer, and obesity than saturated fats. When polyunsaturated fats (Omega-6) are substituted for saturated fats, there is a reduction in total cholesterol and LDL cholesterol in the blood, but there may be a decrease in HDL (high-density lipoprotein) cholesterol as well. However, when monounsaturated fats are substituted for saturated fats, total cholesterol and LDL cholesterol are thought to decrease without an accompanying decrease in the desirable HDL. There is limited evidence that Omega-3 unsaturated fats may inhibit cancers, but Omega-6 fats may not have the same effect. Fish oils have been shown to reduce triglycerides, but there is no conclusive evidence that they are especially successful in reducing blood cholesterol.

Humans produce their own cholesterol even when dietary cholesterol is limited. Still, there is evidence that high dietary cholesterol can increase the risk of atherosclerosis and coronary heart disease. Principal sources of dietary cholesterol are organ meats, some shellfish, and egg yolks.

It is interesting that the new dietary guidelines have changed the wording concerning fat in the diet (see Figure 4). Formerly, it was recommended that "30 percent or less" of the diet should consist of fat. The new wording states that "no more than 30 percent" of the diet should be from fat. This change was made to downplay the notion that "the lower the fat the better." While the experts want to encourage lower fat in the diet, they also want to emphasize that some fat is necessary in a healthy diet. Recent research has challenged the idea that exceptionally low fat diets (15 percent or lower) are beneficial for most people. While they may be appropriate for small segments of the population who are at high risk of heart disease and other medical condition, exceptionally low-fat diets may have harmful effects to most people, especially without expert supervision. For example, the evidence suggests that very low-fat diets may not provide adequate nutrients, may reduce HDL (the good cholesterol), and may increase some of the less desirable blood fats. Exceptionally low-fat diets may pose special problems for pregnant women and children.

Modified fats and fat substitutes in the diet can have varying health consequences.

For decades, the public has been cautioned to avoid saturated fat. As a result, many people changed from eating butter—a product high in saturated fat—to margarine, a product typically made from vegetable products that are primarily unsaturated fat. Recent studies show that foods, such as margarine and shortening containing hydrogenated fats or **trans fatty acids,** can result in greater total blood cholesterol levels and higher LDL levels. This suggests that food containing trans fatty acids should be limited in the diet. Also, experts have recommended that future food labels stipulate the amounts of trans fatty acids included in processed foods. It is not surprising that some people who changed from butter to margarine felt betrayed because they modified their habits only to find that their behavior modification was not effective. This only points out the fact that it takes time to discover the health consequences of dietary changes. People who follow general guidelines for good eat-

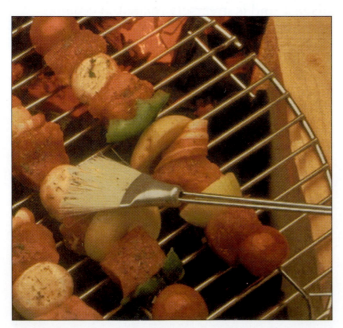

Broiled foods have less fat than fried foods.

ing will benefit, even if some specific recommendations are modified in the future.

While trans fatty acids have been found to have more risk to health than expected, a fat substitute now commonly used in snack foods has been found to be safer than previously thought. Olestra is a product approved several years ago by the FDA that is sometimes referred to as fake fat. It is a synthetic fat substitute in foods that passes through the gastrointestinal system without being digested. Thus, foods cooked with Olestra have fewer calories. For example, a chocolate chip cookie cooked in a normal way would have 138 calories while an Olestra cookie would have 63. One ounce of normal potato chips contains 160 calories while the same amount prepared using Olestra has 70. Many consumer groups opposed the approval of Olestra because it has possible side effects. A warning label must be included on this product noting these possible effects. The label reads: *"This product contains Olestra. Olestra may cause abdominal cramping and loose stools. Olestra inhibits the absorption of some vitamins and other nutrients. Vitamins A, D, E, and K have been added."* Research conducted after several years of product use led to a recent decision by the FDA that there is a "reasonable certainty of no harm" from Olestra use. Fears of significant gastrointestinal problems among large numbers of users did not materialize. Currently, there is discussion concerning possible modification of the warning label for this product. Some consumer groups are still concerned that consumers may not eat less fat even when they eat foods with Olestra, but rather will feel that they can eat more foods not especially dense in nutrients. One thing is certain—Olestra does not add significantly to the nutritional value of food. Its only value is to reduce calories and fat in the diet. If it does not do this, as many experts expect it won't, it will not enhance your diet. Though all people do not experience side effects, some do.

There are several new products that will probably be widely distributed in the years ahead. The first is a product used in a special kind of margarine that has been used in Finland for a number of years. Benecol margarine is a butter substitute that contains an active ingredient called sitostanol. There is some evidence that this product is less of a health risk than butter or margarine containing trans fatty acids. The active ingredient, which comes from pine trees, is purported to be effective in reducing cholesterol levels in the blood. The product was introduced to American markets. Foods such as Benecol margarine are often referred to as "neutraceuticals" or "functional foods" because they are a combination of pharmaceuticals and food. Debate continues as to whether this type of product will be regulated by the FDA as a food or will be classified as a food supplement and not be regulated by FDA. Decisions on these products will, no doubt, influence the way similar "neutraceuticals" will be regulated in the future. If and when these products are widely used in the United States, nutrition experts will be interested to see if these products have health benefits for Americans and whether it will satisfy their tastes.

The second product that will soon appear is another fake fat. This product will be sold under the name Nu-Trim. It is made exclusively from oats, a grain that has been shown to reduce cholesterol in many people. This product has also been shown to reduce cholesterol—particularly LDL cholesterol (the bad cholesterol). Unlike other products that are marketed by large food or pharmaceutical companies, all proceeds from Nu-Trim will go to the federal government because it was developed by the Department of Agriculture. It is expected that this product will appear in foods such as cookies, cakes, and other baked items.

There are some recommendations that can be followed to assure healthy amounts of fat in the diet.

 www.mhhe.com/hper/physed/clw/student/ The following list includes basic recommendations for fat content in the diet.

- Total fat in the diet should consist of no more than 30 percent of the total calories consumed.
- Saturated fat in the diet should be no more than 10 percent of total calories consumed.
- Polyunsaturated and monounsaturated fats should be substituted for saturated fat in the diet.
- Dietary cholesterol should be limited to 300 milligrams per day.

The following guidelines will help you implement the recommendations above.

- Substitute lean meat, fish, poultry, nonfat milk, and other low-fat dairy products for high-fat foods.
- Reduce intake of fried foods, especially those cooked in saturated fats (often true of fast-food restaurants), desserts with high levels of fat (many cookies and cakes), and dressings with high-fat ingredients.
- Limit dietary intake of foods high in cholesterol such as egg yolks, organ meats, and shellfish.

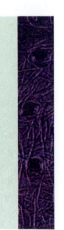

Saturated Fat Dietary fat that is usually solid at room temperature and comes primarily from animal sources.

Unsaturated Fat Monounsaturated or polyunsaturated fat that is usually liquid at room temperature and comes primarily from vegetable sources.

Trans Fatty Acids Fats that result when liquid oil has hydrogen added to it to make it more solid. Hydrogenation transforms unsaturated fats so that they take on characteristics of saturated fats, as is the case for margarine and shortening.

- Use monounsaturated or polyunsaturated fats for cooking.
- Limit the amount of trans fatty acids in the diet and in cooking.
- Though two or three servings of fish per week may be prudent because of its content of Omega-3 polyunsaturated oils, there is not sufficient evidence to endorse a fish-oil dietary supplement.
- Be careful of the total elimination of a single food source from the diet. For example, the elimination of meat and dairy products could result in iron or calcium deficiencies, especially among women and children.

Dietary Recommendations for Carbohydrates: The Facts

For optimal health, carbohydrates, especially complex carbohydrates, should be the principal source of calories in the diet.

Complex carbohydrates are known as starches and include fruits, vegetables, whole-grain breads, and cereals. These foods are nutritionally dense and also contain **cellulose** (a type of dietary **fiber**). Cellulose does not provide nutrition and is not digested, but is considered essential for the bulk it provides for efficient digestion.

Research evidence shows that diets high in complex carbohydrates such as whole-grain cereals, legumes, vegetables, and fruits are associated with a low incidence of lung, colon, esophagus, and stomach cancer as well as coronary heart disease. Some of this benefit may be due to the fact that complex carbohydrate diets are likely to be low in saturated fat. Water-soluble fiber, such as pectin and oat bran, has recently been shown to produce small reductions in total blood cholesterol, independent of the effects of reduced dietary fat. Long-term studies indicate that high-fiber diets may also be associated with a lower risk of diabetes mellitus, diverticulosis, hypertension, and gallstone formation. It is not known whether these health benefits are directly attributable to high dietary fiber or other effects associated with the ingestion of vegetables, fruits, and cereals in the diet. Complex carbohydrates may also be beneficial to health because they provide rich sources of vitamins and minerals. The possible benefits of consuming a diet high in complex carbohydrates and certain vitamins are discussed in the section on vitamins. For the reasons mentioned above, the new dietary guidelines for Americans place a special emphasis on complex carbohydrates (see Figure 3). Since 1991, the amount of fiber in the diet has increased from 11 to 16 grams per day. This is still short of the 20 to 30 grams per day recommended by the National Cancer Institute.

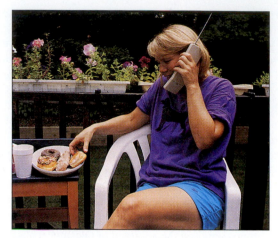

Candy, soft drinks, potato chips and other foods with empty calories have little nutritional value.

www.mhhe.com/hper/physed/clw/student/

Simple carbohydrates are sugars such as sucrose, lactose, maltose, glucose, and fructose. They are low in nutritional density and are commonly found in foods considered to possess "empty calories" such as candy and soft drinks. The national dietary guidelines note that "the body cannot tell the difference between naturally occurring and added sugars because they are identical chemically." This statement was added to counter the public perception that some types of sugars are better than others. Foods high in simple carbohydrates do not, however, have the same benefits to health as do foods high in complex carbohydrates. Foods high in simple carbohydrates are often high in fat as well. Simple carbohydrates, especially sucrose, a sugar often found in candy and soft drinks, have also been shown to increase the incidence of dental caries. Sugar consumption, among people who have an adequate diet, is not a risk factor for diseases such as cancer and heart disease. It should be noted that athletes and other active people who need supplemental calorie intake to maintain body weight may need to consume more carbohydrates, including simple carbohydrates, than people who are sedentary. Increasing carbohydrates in the diet is more desirable than supplementing proteins or consuming higher amounts of fat.

There are some recommendations that can be followed to assure healthy amounts of carbohydrates in the diet.

The following list includes basic recommendations for carbohydrate content in the diet.

- Total carbohydrates in the diet should account for 55 percent or more of total calories consumed.

- Simple carbohydrates should be limited to 15 percent or less of total calories consumed, except for very active people.
- High-fiber foods should be included in the daily diet.

The following guidelines will help you implement these recommendations.

- Consume at least five servings of vegetables and/or fruits each day. Servings of green and yellow vegetables as well as citrus fruits are recommended. A serving of vegetables equals approximately one-half cup. A serving of fruit equals one medium-size piece.
- Consume at least six servings a day of complex carbohydrates such as breads, cereals, and/or legumes. A serving of legumes or cereal equals approximately one-half cup. A serving of bread is one slice, or one roll or muffin.
- Limit intake of desserts, baked goods, and other foods high in simple sugars or empty calories.
- Dietary fiber supplements other than in the form of food (such as oat bran) are not recommended unless prescribed for medical reasons.

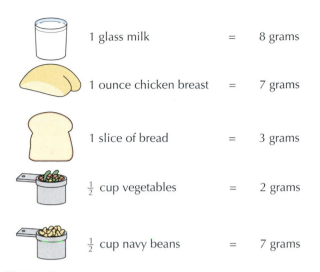

1 glass milk	=	8 grams
1 ounce chicken breast	=	7 grams
1 slice of bread	=	3 grams
½ cup vegetables	=	2 grams
½ cup navy beans	=	7 grams

Figure 5

Protein content of various foods.

Adapted from Williams, M. *Nutrition for Fitness and Sport* 4th ed. St. Louis: McGraw-Hill, 1995.

Dietary Recommendations for Proteins: The Facts

> Protein is the basic building block for the body, but dietary protein constitutes a relatively small amount of daily calorie intake.

Proteins are often referred to as the building blocks of your body because all body cells are made of protein. Proteins are formed from 20 different **amino acids**. More than 100 proteins are made of these amino acids. Eleven of these amino acids are made in your own body, but nine **essential amino acids** are not. You must consume foods that contain the essential amino acids if your body is to function properly. Certain foods, called complete proteins, contain all of the essential amino acids. Examples of complete proteins are meat, dairy products, and fish. Incomplete proteins contain some, but not all, of the essential amino acids. Examples of incomplete proteins are beans, nuts, and rice.

One way to identify amino acids is the *-ine* at the end of their name. For example, arginine and lysine are two of the amino acids that have received recent attention in the press. Only three of the 20 amino acids do not have the *-ine* suffix. They are aspartic acid, glutamic acid, and tryptophan.

All of the amino acids can be obtained from food, and recommended amounts are essential to good health (see Figure 5). Experts agree that there are no known benefits and some possible risks to consuming diets exceptionally high in animal protein. Certain cancers and coronary heart disease risk have been associated with high dietary intake of animal protein. Researchers are not certain whether the increased risk of contracting these diseases is because of the protein itself or the fact that diets high in animal protein are also high in fat. Excessive protein intake can lead to urinary calcium loss, which can weaken bones and lead to osteoporosis.

Some scientists are concerned that restriction of animal protein might result in lower than necessary dietary intake of essential nutrients such as iron, especially for women and children. If the recommendations suggested in this section are followed, this should not be a problem. It is not our intent to suggest that animal protein should not be part of the normal diet, but rather consumption of animal protein be restricted somewhat, especially when the fat content is high. In fact, the most recent national dietary guidelines for the first time include a statement indicating that "vegetarian diets are consistent with the Dietary Guidelines for Americans and can meet Recommended Dietary Allowances for nutrients.

Cellulose Indigestible fiber (bulk) in foods.

Fiber Indigestible bulk in foods that can be either soluble or insoluble in body fluids.

Amino Acids Twenty basic building blocks of the body that make up proteins.

Essential Amino Acids Nine basic amino acids that the human body cannot produce and that must be obtained from food sources.

You can get enough protein as long as the variety and amounts of foods consumed are adequate." It is noted that **vegans** must supplement the diet with vitamin B_{12} because this vitamin's only source is animal foods. **Lacto-ovo vegetarians** do not have the same concerns. The guidelines also emphasize the need for vegans to take care that, especially for children, adequate vitamin D and calcium are contained in the diet because most people get these nutrients from milk products.

People who eat a variety of foods including meat, dairy products, eggs, and plants rich in protein virtually always eat more protein than the body needs. Eating a variety of foods assures that all essential amino acids are consumed. Because of problems associated with excessive protein intake and health problems encountered by people who have used protein supplements, the latter are not recommended. In fact, many of the more serious health problems resulting from the consumption of dietary supplements are associated with excessive protein intake. More information concerning high-protein diets and protein supplements is included later in this concept and in the concept on managing diet and activity.

There are some recommendations that can be followed to assure healthy amounts of protein in the diet.

The following list includes basic recommendations for protein content in the diet.

- Protein in the diet should account for 10 to 15 percent of the total calories consumed.
- Protein in the diet should meet the RDA of 0.8 grams per kilogram (2.2 pounds) of a person's desirable weight. This is about 36 grams for a 100-pound person.
- Protein in the diet should not exceed twice the RDA (1.6 grams per kilogram of a person's desirable weight).
- Vegetarians (people who severely limit the intake of animal products) must be especially careful to eat combinations of foods that assure adequate intake of essential amino acids, and vegans should supplement their diets with vitamin B_{12}.

The following guidelines will help you implement these recommendations.

- Consume at least two servings a day of lean meat, fish, poultry, and dairy products (especially those low in fat content) or adequate combinations of foods such as beans, nuts, grains, and rice in the diet.
- Dietary supplements of protein such as tablets and powders are not recommended (see section later in this concept and the concept of managing diet.

Dietary Recommendations for Vitamins: The Facts

Adequate vitamin intake is necessary to good health and wellness, but excessive vitamin intake is not necessary and can be harmful.

Consuming foods containing the minimum RDA of each of the vitamins is essential to the prevention of disease and maintenance of good health. Consuming foods high in carotinoid and retinoid is recommended because these foods are associated with the reduced risk of some forms of cancer. Carotinoid- and retinoid-rich foods such as green and yellow vegetables, (carrots, and sweet potatoes) contain high amounts of vitamin A. Diets high in vitamin C (citrus fruits and vegetables) and vitamin E (green leafy vegetables) are also associated with reduced risk of cancer. One recent study indicated that diets high in vitamin E are associated with reduced risk of heart disease. It has been hypothesized that vitamins C, E, and carotinoid-rich foods act as **antioxidants**, which help prevent cancer and other forms of disease. Most experts point out that selecting more servings from the second level of the food pyramid is wise, but they express caution concerning the use of vitamin supplements.

Nevertheless, a number of respected health and wellness publications and popular books have advocated antioxidant supplements, including beta-carotene (a plant product that is converted to vitamin A in the body) and vitamins C and E, to protect the body from cell-damaging free radicals resulting from environmental pollution. These publications also assumed that supplements of these vitamins had the same health effect as consuming good food high in vitamin content. Several very recent large-scale studies have shown either no benefit from beta-carotene supplements or have shown that the supplements may have negative effects. One study was discontinued early because of higher heart disease and lung cancer rates among the supplement group. While some advocates of antioxidants still recommend supplements of vitamins C and E, most have backed off recommendations for beta-carotene based on the results of the studies cited above.

Just as some have advocated antioxidant supplements, others have not. For example, the National Council for Reliable Health Information suggests the value of antioxidants has been more an "illusion created by the vitamin hucksters than scientific reality." Also, the committee that developed the dietary guidelines for Americans chose to emphasize good food rather than food supplements. Most experts agree. Some foods that are especially rich in vitamins and minerals are considered nutrition "all-stars" and make good dietary choices (see Table 1).

While one type of supplement for all people is not deemed wise, there is little doubt that certain segments of the population do not eat a balanced diet, and as a matter of

Table 1 Top Ten Antioxidant All-Stars

	C (mg)	Beta Carotine (mg)	E (mg)	Folacin (mg)
Broccoli (1/2 cup cooked)	49	0.7	0.9	53
Cantaloupe (1 cup cubed)	68	3.1	0.3	17
Carrot (1 medium)	7	12.2	0.3	10
Kale (1/2 cup cooked)	27	2.9	3.7	9
Mango (1 medium)	57	4.8	2.3	31
Pumpkin (1/2 cup canned)	5	10.5	1.1	15
Red bell pepper (1/2 cup raw)	95	1.7	0.3	8
Spinach (1/2 cup cooked)	9	4.4	2.0	131
Strawberries (1 cup)	86	—	0.3	26
Sweet potato (1 medium, cooked)	28	14.9	5.5	26
Adult RDA or suggested intake	60	5–6	8–10	180–200

Runners-up: Brussels sprouts, all citrus fruits, tomatoes, potatoes, other berries, other leafy greens (dandelion, turnip, and mustard greens, swiss chard, arugula), cauliflower, green pepper, asparagus, peas, beets, and winter squash.
SOURCE: Reprinted with permission from the *University of California at Berkeley Wellness Letter,* © Health Letter Associates, 1994.

national policy, many foods have been fortified. National policy dictates that milk be fortified with vitamin D, low-fat milk with vitamins A and D, and margarine with vitamin A. These foods were selected because they are common food sources for growing children. Recently the FDA announced that breads, flours, rice, grits and other grain products would be fortified with folic acid because of the evidence that such fortification would help reduce birth defects. In fact, less than half of young women get sufficient folic acid (a B vitamin), adding to the concern about birth defects. Also, there is some evidence that this vitamin can help reduce risk of heart disease. The public policy of food fortification continues to emphasize consuming a variety of healthy foods (in this case fortified foods) rather than using supplements.

Sometimes supplements are needed to meet specific nutrient requirements for specific groups. For example, older people may need a vitamin D supplement if they get little exposure to sunlight, and iron supplements are often recommended for pregnant women. Daily vitamin supplements at or below the RDA are considered safe, but are rarely needed by people who eat a variety of foods as recommended by the food guide pyramid. However, excess doses of vitamins have been shown to cause health problems. For example, excessively high amounts of vitamin C are dangerous for the 10 percent of the population who inherit a special gene related to health problems. Excessively high amounts of vitamin D are toxic, and mothers who take too much vitamin A risk birth defects to unborn children.

There are some recommendations that can be followed to assure healthy amounts of vitamins in the diet.

The following list includes basic recommendations for vitamin content in the diet.

- Vitamins in the amounts equal to the RDAs should be included in the diet each day.

Vegan A strict vegetarian who not only excludes all forms of meat from the diet, but also excludes dairy products and eggs.

Lacto-ovo Vegetarians A vegetarian who includes dairy and eggs in the diet.

Antioxidants Vitamins (C, E, and plant forms of A or beta carotene) that are thought to inactivate "activated oxygen molecules," sometimes called free radicals. Free radicals are naturally created by human cells but are also caused by environmental factors such as smoke and radiation. Free radicals may cause cell damage that leads to diseases of various kinds. Antioxidants may inactivate the free radicals before they do their damage.

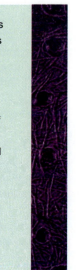

The following guidelines will help you implement these recommendations.

- A diet containing the food servings recommended for carbohydrates, proteins, and fats will more than meet the RDA standards.
- Extra servings of green and yellow vegetables, citrus and other fruits, and other non-animal food sources high in fiber, vitamins, and minerals are wise (especially foods from the nutrition all-stars).
- People who eat a sound diet as described in this concept do not need a vitamin supplement. When UL (upper level) values are established for all vitamins it will be easier to determine how much is too much for any and all vitamins. Daily vitamin supplements may be appropriate for those who restrict calories. In the meantime, those who choose to take a supplement are advised not to take daily amounts larger than the RDA. The guidelines suggested later in this concept should be considered before taking any supplement.
- People with special needs should seek medical advice before selecting supplements and should inform medical personnel as to amounts and content of all supplements (vitamin or other).

Dietary Recommendations for Minerals: The Facts

> Adequate mineral intake is necessary for good health and wellness, but excessive mineral intake is not necessary and can be harmful.

Like vitamins, minerals have no calories and provide no energy for the body. They are important in regulating various bodily functions. Two particularly important minerals are calcium and iron. Calcium is important to bone, muscle, nerve, blood development and function, and has been associated with reduced risk of heart disease. Iron is necessary for the blood to carry adequate oxygen. Other important minerals are phosphorus, which builds teeth and bones; sodium, which regulates water in the body; zinc, which aids in the healing process; and potassium, which is necessary for proper muscle function.

RDAs for minerals are established to determine the amounts of each necessary for healthy day-to-day functioning. A sound diet provides all of the RDA for minerals. Evidence indicating that some segments of the population may be mineral-deficient have led to the establishment of health goals identifying a need to increase mineral intake for some segments of the population.

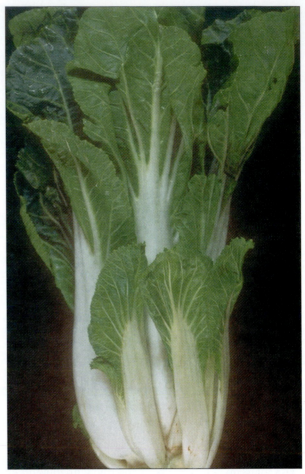

Green leafy vegetables and low fat milk are good sources of calcium.

A recent National Institutes of Health (NIH) consensus statement indicates that a large percentage of Americans fail to get enough calcium in their diet and emphasizes the need for increased calcium—particularly for women who are pregnant, postmenopausal women, and people over 65 who need 1,500 mg/day, which is higher than previous RDA amounts. Recent research suggests that a calcium supplement may help relieve PMS symptoms among postmenopausal women. The NIH has indicated that a total intake of 2,000 mg/day of calcium is safe and that adequate vitamin D in the diet is necessary for optimal calcium absorption to take place. Though getting these amounts in a calcium-rich diet is best, calcium supplementation for those not eating properly seems wise. Check with your physician or a dietitian before you consider a supplement because individual needs vary. Several of the suggested readings at the end of this concept provide information on the topic.

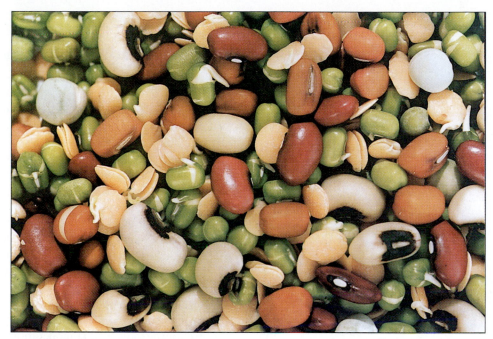

Cooked dried beans are a good low fat source of protein and iron.

One national health goal is to reduce the proportion of people who consume more than recommended amounts of sodium (2,400 mg per day) and sodium chloride or table salt (6 grams a day). Some researchers have questioned the relationship between sodium intake and health especially among apparently healthy adults. The conventional wisdom is that excessive sodium intake is especially problematic among people with high blood pressure. Salt intake up to recommended amounts is necessary for good health. Beyond those amounts, there is no apparent benefit, so restriction of salt consistent with national goals seems wise. Because many fast foods have a high salt, many people in our culture consume amounts well above the recommended levels. Currently, 79 percent of the population exceeds these amounts.

Another concern is iron deficiency among very young children and women of child-bearing age. Low iron may be a special problem for women taking birth control pills because the combination of low iron levels and birth control pills has been associated with depression and generalized fatigue. Also, a decrease in salt and sodium intake is a health goal established for people of all ages because of the association of dietary salt and sodium with elevated blood pressure. Eating the appropriate number of servings from the food pyramid provides all the minerals necessary for meeting the RDA for minerals. Nutrition goals for the nation emphasize the importance of adequate servings of foods rich in calcium, such as green leafy vegetables and milk products; adequate servings of foods rich in iron, such as beans, peas, spinach, or meat; and reduced salt in the diet.

There are some recommendations that can be followed to assure healthy amounts of minerals in the diet.

The following list includes basic recommendations for mineral content in the diet.

- Minerals in amounts equal to the RDAs should be consumed in the diet each day.
- In general, a calcium dietary supplement is not recommended for the general population; however, supplements may be appropriate for adults who do not eat well (up to 1,000 mg/day). For postmenopausal women, a calcium supplement is recommended (up to 1,500 mg/day for those who do not eat well). A supplement may also be appropriate for people who restrict calories but RDA values should not be exceeded unless the person consults with a registered dietitian or a physician regarding amounts and types of supplements and considers the guidelines for food supplements suggested later in this concept.
- Salt should be limited in the diet to no more than 4–6 grams per day, and even less would be desirable (3 grams). Three grams equals one teaspoon of table salt.

The following guidelines will help you implement these recommendations.

- A diet containing the food servings recommended for carbohydrates, proteins, and fats will more than meet the RDA standards.

- Extra servings of green and yellow vegetables, citrus and other fruits, and other non-animal sources of foods high in fiber, vitamins, and minerals are recommended as a substitute for high-fat foods.

Dietary Recommendations for Water and Other Fluids: The Facts

Water is a critical component in the healthy diet.

Though water is not in the food pyramid because it contains no calories, provides no energy, and provides no key nutrients, it is very important to health and survival. Water is a major component of most of the foods you eat, and more than half of all body tissues are composed of it. Regular water intake maintains water balance and is critical to many important bodily functions.

Beverages other than water are a part of many diets. Some beverages can have an adverse effect on good health.

Coffee, tea, soft drinks, and alcoholic beverages are often substituted for water in the diet. Too much caffeine consumption has been shown to cause symptoms such as irregular heartbeat in some people. Tea has not been shown to have similar effects, though this may be because tea drinkers typically consume less volume than coffee drinkers, and tea has less caffeine per cup than coffee. Both beverages contain caffeine, as do many soft drinks, though drip coffee typically contains two to three times the caffeine of a typical cola drink.

Excessive consumption of alcoholic beverages can have negative health implications because the alcohol often replaces nutrients. Excessive alcohol consumption is associated with the increased risk of heart disease, high blood pressure, stroke, and osteoporosis. Long-term excessive alcoholic beverage consumption leads to cirrhosis of the liver and to the increased risk of hepatitis and cancer. Alcohol consumption during pregnancy can result in low birth weight, fetal alcoholism, and other damage to the fetus. The National Dietary Guidelines indicate that alcohol used in moderation can "enhance the enjoyment of meals" and is associated with a lower risk of coronary heart disease for some individuals.

There are some recommendations that can be followed to assure healthy amounts of water and other fluids in the diet.

The following list includes basic recommendations for water and other fluids in the diet.

- In addition to foods containing water, the average adult needs about eight glasses (8 ounces each) of water every day. Water intake must be increased even more for active people and those in hot environments.
- Coffee, tea, and soft drinks should not be substituted for water and/or other beverages or foods such as low-fat milk, fruit juices, or foods rich in calcium, which provide sources of key nutrients.
- Limit daily servings of beverages containing caffeine to no more than three.
- If you are an adult and you choose to drink alcohol, do so in moderation. The latest dietary guidelines for Americans indicate that moderation includes no more than one drink per day for women and no more than two drinks per day for men (one drink equals 12 ounces of regular beer, 5 ounces of wine—small glass, or one average-size cocktail—1.5 ounces of 80 proof alcohol).

The Facts about Sound Eating Practices

Healthy snacks can be an important part of good nutrition.

Snacking is not necessarily bad. For people interested in losing or maintaining their current weight, small snacks of appropriate foods can help fool the appetite. For people interested in gaining weight, snacks can provide additional calories. For people trying to maintain or lose weight, the calories consumed in snacks will probably necessitate limiting the calories consumed at meals. The key is proper selection of the foods for snacking.

As with your total diet, the best snacks are those that are nutritionally dense. Too often, snacks are high in calories, fats, simple sugar, and salt. Check the content of snacks. Even foods sold as "healthy snacks," such as granola bars, are often high in fat and simple sugar. Some common snacks such as chips, pretzels, and even popcorn may be high in salt and may be cooked in fat.

Some suggestions for healthy snacks include ice milk (instead of ice cream), fresh fruits, vegetable sticks, popcorn not cooked in fat and with little or no salt, crackers, and nuts with little or no salt.

Consistency (with variety) is a good general rule of nutrition.

Eating regular meals every day, including a good breakfast, is wise. Many studies have shown breakfast to be an important meal. One-fourth of the day's calories should be consumed at breakfast. Skipping breakfast impairs performance because blood sugar levels drop in the long period between dinner the night before and lunch the following day. Eating every four to six hours is wise.

Moderation is a good general rule of nutrition.

Just as too little food can cause problems, excessive intake of various nutrients can cause problems. More is not always better. Moderation (neither too much nor too little) in choices of foods is advised.

It is not necessary to permanently eliminate foods that you really enjoy, but some of your favorite foods may not be among the best of choices. Enjoying special foods on occasion is part of moderation. The key is to limit choices that are not consistent with the recommendations made in this concept.

Careful selection of food choices is important for people who rely on fast foods as a significant part of their diet.

More and more Americans rely on fast foods as part of their normal diet. Unfortunately, many fast foods are poor nutritional choices. Many hamburgers are high in fat. French fries are high in fat because they are usually cooked in saturated fat. Even choices deemed to be more nutritious, such as chicken or fish sandwiches, are often high in fat and calories because they are cooked in fat and covered with special high-fat/high-calorie sauces. Become informed about the content of fast foods before you make your selection. Some guidelines for selection of foods are provided in the concept on managing diet.

The Facts about Nutrition and Physical Performance

There are some basic dietary guidelines for active people.

In general, the nutrition rules described in this concept apply to all people, whether active or sedentary, but there are some additional nutrition facts that are important for

Table 2 Dietary Recommendations for Athletes and Active People	
Fat	Active people, like everyone else, should restrict fat to no more than 30 percent, especially saturated fat (no more than 10 percent).
Protein	The American Dietetics Association (ADA) recommends 1.0 gram per kg of body weight for active people such as athletes. This is higher than the 0.8 per kg recommended for normal adults. A normal healthy diet easily meets this need, so protein above 15 percent of the diet is not recommended, nor are protein supplements (including amino acids).
Carbohydrates	Because active people often expend calories in amounts considerably above normal, extra calories are necessary in the diet. Carbohydrates are the best source. To avoid excess fat and protein intake, carbohydrates (especially complex carbohydrates) may constitute as much as 70 percent of total calorie intake.
Vitamins and Minerals	People in activities for which caloric restriction may be encouraged, such as wrestling, must be especially careful in the food choices they make. Also, female athletes should consider a calcium supplement after consultation with an expert. This is especially true for those who are amenorrheic and/or are involved in extensive training.

exercisers and athletes. This information is outlined in Table 2.

Carbohydrate loading and carbohydrate replacement during exercise can enhance sustained aerobic performances exceeding one hour in length.

www.mhhe.com/hper/physed/clw/student/
Athletes and vigorously active people must maintain a high level of readily available fuel, especially in the muscles. Adequate complex carbohydrate consumption is the best way to assure this.

Prior to an activity that will require extended duration of physical performance (more than one hour in length, such as a marathon), **carbohydrate loading** can be useful. Carbohydrate loading is accomplished by resting one or two days before the event and eating a higher than normal amount of complex carbohydrates. This procedure helps prevent the depletion of muscle **glycogen**, which is necessary for sustained performance. However, this procedure could cause problems for people with diabetes, hypertriglycemia, and kidney disorders.

Ingesting carbohydrate solutions during long, sustained exercise can also aid performance by preventing or forestalling muscle glycogen depletion. Drinking fluids that have no more than 6–8 percent sugar helps prevent dehydration and replenishes energy stores. These solutions should be taken regularly in long, sustained performances. After the long, sustained activity is over, consuming carbohydrates within fifteen to thirty minutes can aid in rapid replenishment of muscle glycogen, which may be important to future performances. Carbohydrate drinks are not helpful for short (less than an hour) endurance activity.

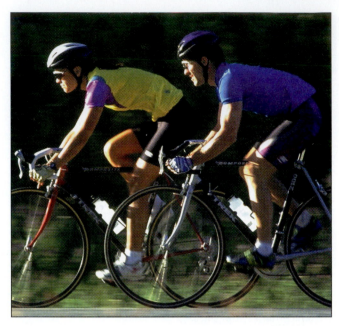

Good nutrition is essential for active people.

The timing may be more important than the makeup of the pre-event meal.

It is probably best to eat about three hours before competition or heavy exercise to allow time for digestion. Generally, the athlete can make his or her food selection on the basis of past experience. Tension, anxiety, and excitement are more likely to cause gastric distress than is food selection. It is generally accepted that fat intake should be minimal because it digests more slowly; "gas formers" should probably be avoided; and proteins and high-cellulose foods should be kept to a moderate amount prior to prolonged events to avoid urinary and bowel excretion. Drinking 2 or 3 cups of liquid will ensure adequate hydration.

Consuming simple carbohydrates (sugar, candy) within an hour or two of an event is not recommended because it may cause an insulin response that results in weakness and fatigue, or may cause stomach distress, cramps, or nausea.

It should be noted that the excitement associated with competition is probably the main reason for having a special diet before participation. Because many people who exercise regularly usually are not competing, there is little reason to alter normal diet before regular exercise. Likewise, there is no need to delay exercise for long periods after the meal if exercise is moderate and noncompetitive.

High-protein diets for active people and athletes have been questioned by leading organizations in the areas of health, physical activity, and nutrition.

In recent years, several books have recommended high-protein/low-carbohydrate diets for active people and for those interested in improving athletic performance. A com-

mon high-protein diet is often referred to as the 40/30/30 diet because it recommends 40 percent carbohydrates, 30 percent proteins, and 30 percent fat. The 40/30/30 plan is well above the national recommendation for protein of 10 to 15 percent and well below the 55 to 60 percent recommendation for carbohydrates.

The American College of Sports Medicine, the American Dietetic Association, and several other groups (see Suggested Readings) have challenged the soundness of the 40/30/30 diet. They note that claims of books promoting high-protein diets are often based on unfounded ideas and oversimplification of the facts. Some false claims and correct facts about high-protein diets are described in greater detail in the concept on managing diet. Most athletes need more carbohydrates in the diet, not less. As noted earlier, athletes get the extra protein they need by consuming extra calories; thus, 10 to 15 percent of the diet as protein is adequate to meet their needs. Contrary to popular opinion, extra protein (more than 15 percent) does not result in extra muscle development.

People who are interested in enhancing physical performance are especially subject to nutrition quackery.

A food or nutrition product thought to enhance performance is considered to be an **ergogenic aid**. Many so-called ergogenic aids can be classified as quack products because they do not enhance performance as promised and are often exceptionally expensive. In some cases, so-called performance-enhancing supplements are dangerous to health and wellness. Examples of products that are misrepresented in terms of potential

Table 3 Some Commonly Misrepresented Dietary Supplements Alleged to Enhance Performance

Product	Claim	The Facts
Plant steroids	• Alleged to promote muscle development similar to animal steroids.	• Plant steroids do not promote muscle mass gains in humans. One plant product is a steroid precursor (androstendione*).
Trace elements (e.g., chromium picolinate)	• Alleged to promote muscle development.	• No evidence of effectiveness. It could lead to anemia if taken in excess. One recent study indicates possible link to cancer and chromosome damage.
Amino acids (e.g., arginine, lysine)	• Alleged to promote increases in human growth hormone that lead to increased muscle mass.	• Some evidence that increased HGH* results from intake of amino acids, but little evidence of resulting muscle mass increases. There is risk in taking the high doses recommended by sellers. Banned in Canada.
Protein supplements	• Alleged muscle mass gains.	• No evidence of effectiveness; some are not digestible. Not superior to dietary protein as some claim, and far more costly. Overuse can lead to excess loss of body water, diarrhea, abdominal cramps, and altered kidney function.
Caffeine	• Alleged to enhance endurance performance.	• Inconsistent results. Banned by Olympic rules. Some negative health consequences. Can cause dehydration.
Vitamin supplements (e.g., B complex, B_{15})	• Alleged stress reduction and performance enhancement.	• No evidence of benefits to those who are not vitamin deficient. B_{15} (pangamic acid) is not a vitamin and can be harmful. No evidence of stress-reducing effects.
Minerals (e.g., iron)	• Alleged that athletes and active people need more than other people.	• Some evidence that active people have increased need, but the consensus is that a sound diet provides for those needs.
Hormones (e.g., melatonin)	• Claims to enhance sex life, combat aging, and reduce disease risk.	• Effects not known, especially long term. All sales banned in some European countries; a prescription is required in Canada. Hormones are powerful substances that can produce unexpected results. Actual content of product is not regulated, so there is no certainty of content. Users are considered to be "human guinea pigs" by some experts.

Note: FDA standards have not been set for many advertised products. For this reason, the consumer cannot be assured of the exact content of products, and product safety cannot be assured. This is illustrated by the recall of products containing the amino acid L-tryptophan after the deaths of 32 people were linked to its use.

*For more information on these supplements, see the concept on muscle fitness.

performance-enhancing benefits are dietary supplements such as vitamins, minerals, proteins and amino acids, and plant steroids. Among the most-often misrepresented products are protein and amino acid supplements, sometimes referred to as "steroid alternatives." Table 3 lists some of these.

The Facts: Nutrition Quackery

The Food and Drug Administration has labeled the "health-food" racket as the most widespread quackery in the United States.

Whether athletic or sedentary, the individual on a well-balanced diet does not benefit from special foods, phosphate, alkaline salts, choline, lecithin, wheat germ, honey, gelatin,

Carbohydrate Loading Extra consumption of complex carbohydrates in the days prior to a long, sustained performance.

Glycogen A source of energy stored in the muscles and liver that is necessary for sustained physical activity.

Ergogenic Aid In this concept, this term will refer to a nutritional supplement claimed by its promoters to improve performance.

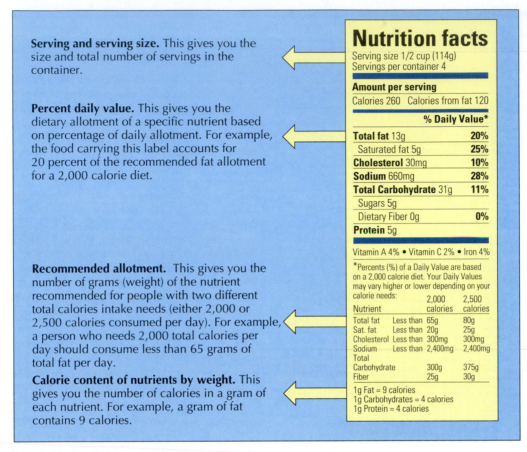

Serving and serving size. This gives you the size and total number of servings in the container.

Percent daily value. This gives you the dietary allotment of a specific nutrient based on percentage of daily allotment. For example, the food carrying this label accounts for 20 percent of the recommended fat allotment for a 2,000 calorie diet.

Recommended allotment. This gives you the number of grams (weight) of the nutrient recommended for people with two different total calories intake needs (either 2,000 or 2,500 calories consumed per day). For example, a person who needs 2,000 total calories per day should consume less than 65 grams of total fat per day.

Calorie content of nutrients by weight. This gives you the number of calories in a gram of each nutrient. For example, a gram of fat contains 9 calories.

Figure 6
Using food labels.
SOURCE: Data from the U.S. Food and Drug Administration.

aspartates, brewer's yeast, or royal jelly unless prescribed for medical purposes by a physician. Because these products do not produce the special benefits claimed for them, their use and/or sale can be considered nutritional quackery. A complete discussion of nutrition quackery is provided in the concept on quackery.

Recent legislation designed to regulate food supplements has not been effective in protecting the consumer.

The Dietary Supplements Health and Education Act was passed in 1994. It was considered by many experts to be a compromise between health-food manufacturers who wanted no regulation of dietary supplements (such as vita-mins, minerals, proteins, and herbs) and those who wanted strict control of these substances. Many nutrition experts now feel that the Act is responsible for an explosion in sales of products that have not been proven to be effective. A more detailed discussion of nutrition supplements is included in the concept on quackery.

Claims for foods in advertisements may not provide accurate information about the nutritional value of the foods.

Until recently, food labels have failed to provide useful information concerning the nutritional values of foods. Recently, Congress enacted laws to make food labels more uniform and to protect consumers. Now products sold in stores must meet specified standards to be able to use words such as "fat-free" on the label. For example, a food must have less than one-half of a gram of fat per serving (50 grams) to be labeled "fat-free," and it must have less than 3 grams per serving to be labeled "low-fat." To be labeled "low in saturated fat," a food must have less than 15 percent of its calories from saturated fat.

The labels required on foods sold in stores (see Figure 6) provide information based on diets of 2,000 calories per day. As noted earlier in this concept, the number of calories you consume depends on your age, body size, gender, metabolic rate, and activity level. The 2,000-calorie value is better suited for children and women than for men, who typically consume more calories in a day. Values must be adjusted for people whose daily calorie intake is above 2,000 calories.

In spite of recent improvements in food labeling, consumers must continue to be wary of deceptive advertising. While the use of words such as "light" or "low-fat" has been regulated to some extent, consumers should be sure that products live up to claims made for them. It is wise to read food labels, to ask for information about food content in restaurants, and to be wary of claims about supplements advertised for health or fitness improvement.

Strategies for Action: The Facts

> An analysis of your current diet is a good first step in making future decisions about what you eat.

In Lab 16A, you will have an opportunity to analyze your current diet. Many experts recommend keeping a log of what you eat for at least a week if you are to get a good picture of your typical eating patterns. You will be given the opportunity to analyze your diet for one or two days. You may want to do a longer assessment in the future. In Lab 16B, you will be given the opportunity to compare a "nutritious diet" to a "favorite diet." Doing the analyses of two different daily meal plans will help you get a more accurate picture as to whether foods you think are nutritious actually meet current healthy lifestyle goals.

Web Review

Web review materials for Concept 16 are available are at *www.mhhe.com/hper/physed/clw/student/*.

American Dietetic Association
  www.eatright.org

Berkeley Nutrition Services
  www.nutritionquest.com

Center for Science in the Public Interest
  www/cspinet.org

Food and Drug Administration (FDA)
  www.fda.gov

National Academy of Sciences
  www.nas.edu

Office of Dietary Supplements
  http://odp.od.nih.gov/ods/default.html

U.S. Department of Agriculture (USDA)
  www.usda.gov

USDA Food and Nutrition Information Center
  http://www.nalusda.gov/fnic/

Suggested Readings

ACSM's Health and Fitness Journal 2(July–August) (1998):18.

The Antioxidant Scare. *National Council for Reliable Health Information* 17(May–June) (1994):1.

Armsey, T. D., and Green, G. A. Nutrition Supplements: Science vs Hype. *Physician and Sportsmedicine*. 25(6)(1997):76.

Beta Carotine Pills: Should You Take Them? *University of California at Berkeley Wellness Letter* 12(April 1996):1.

Calcium: Vital for Women and Men. *Consumer Reports on Health* 6(1994):13.

Clark, K. Water, Sports Drinks, Juice, or Soda? *ACSM's Health and Fitness Journal*. 2(5)(1998):41.

Clarkson, P. M. "The Skinny On Weight Loss Supplements and Drugs." *ACSM's Health and Fitness Journal*. 2 (4) (1988):18.

Coleman, E. Carbohydrate Unloading. *Physician and Sports Medicine*. 25(2)(1997):97.

Farley, D. Making Sure Hype Doesn't Overwhelm Science. *FDA Consumer* 56(1996):1.

Lemonick, M.D. Is America Ready for Fat-Free Fat? *Time* 147(1996):53.

National Institute of Health. Optimal Calcium Intake. *Consensus Development Conference Statement, June 1994.* Available from NIH Office of Medical Applications Research.

Public Health Service. *The Surgeon General's Report on Nutrition and Health.* Washington, D.C.: Department of Health and Human Services, 1988, Pub. No. 88–50210.

Questioning 40/30/30: A Guide to Understanding Sports Nutrition Advice. A 22 page booklet published jointly by the American College of Sport Medicine, The American Dietetics Association, The Women's Sports Foundation and the Cooper Institute for Aerobics Research, 1997.

The Supplement Story: Can Vitamins Help? *Consumer Reports* 57(1992):12.

U.S. Department of Health and Human Services. *Healthy People 2010 Objectives:* Draft for Comment. Washington, D.C.: U.S. Department of Health and Human Services, 1998, Objectives Chapter 2: Nutrition.

U.S. Department of Agriculture and U.S. Department of Health and Human Services. *Nutrition and Your Health: Dietary Guidelines for Americans,* 4th ed. Washington, D.C.: U.S. Department of Agriculture and U.S. Department of Health and Human Services, 1995.

U.S. Department of Agriculture and U.S. Department of Health and Human Services. *Report of the Dietary Guidelines Advisory Committee.* Washington, D.C.: U.S. Department of Agriculture and U.S. Department of Health and Human Services, 1995.

Williams, M. H. *Nutrition for Sport and Fitness* 4th ed. St. Louis: WCB/McGraw-Hill, 1995.

Lab 16A: Nutrition Analysis

Name **Section** **Date**

Purpose: To learn to keep a dietary log, to determine the nutritional quality of your diet, to determine your average daily caloric intake, and to determine necessary changes in eating habits.

Procedure:
1. Record your dietary intake for two days using the Daily Diet Record sheets. Record intake for one weekday and one weekend day. You may wish to make copies of the Record sheet for future use.
2. Include the actual foods eaten, the amount (size of portion in teaspoons, tablespoons, cups, ounces, or other standard units of measurement). Be sure to include all drinks (coffee, tea, soft drinks, etc.) Include *all* foods eaten, including sauces, gravies, dressings, toppings, spreads, etc. Determine your calorie consumption for each of the two days. Use the Calorie Guide to Common Foods in the appendix or the Guides to Food available on the Web.
3. List the number of servings from each food group by each food choice.
4. Estimate the proportion of complex carbohydrate, simple carbohydrate, protein, and fat in each meal and in snacks, as well as for the total day.
5. Answer the questions in chart 1 using information for a typical day based on the dietary record sheets. Score one point for each "yes" answer on chart 1. Use chart 2 to rate your dietary habits. Circle the appropriate rating.

Results:
Record the number of calories consumed for each of the two days.

Weekday [ ] calories   Weekend [ ] calories

Conclusions and Implications: In several sentences, discuss your diet as recorded in this lab. Explain any changes in your eating habits that may be necessary. Comment on whether the days you surveyed are typical of your normal diet.

Chart 1 Dietary Habits Questionnaire

Yes   **No**   Answer questions based on a typical day (use your Daily Records to help).

○   ○   1. Do you eat 3 normal-size meals?

○   ○   2. Do you eat a healthy breakfast?

○   ○   3. Do you eat lunch regularly?

○   ○   4. Does your diet contain about 55 to 60 percent carbohydrates with a high concentration of fiber?

○   ○   5. Are less than one-fourth of the carbohydrates you eat simple carbohydrates?

○   ○   6. Does your diet contain 10 to 15 percent protein?

○   ○   7. Does your diet contain no more than 30 percent fat?

○   ○   8. Do you limit the amount of saturated fat in your diet (no more than 10 percent)?

○   ○   9. Do you limit salt intake to acceptable amounts?

○   ○   10. Do you get adequate amounts of vitamins in your diet without a supplement?

○   ○   11. Do you typically eat 6–11 servings from the bread, cereal, rice, and pasta group of foods?

○   ○   12. Do you typically eat 3–5 servings of vegetables?

○   ○   13. Do you typically eat 2–4 servings of fruits?

○   ○   14. Do you typically eat 2–3 servings from the milk, yogurt, and cheese group of foods?

○   ○   15. Do you typically eat 2–3 servings from the meat, poultry, fish, beans, eggs, and nuts group of foods?

○   ○   16. Do you drink adequate amounts of water?

○   ○   17. Do you get adequate minerals in your diet without a supplement?

○   ○   18. Do you limit your caffeine and alcohol consumption to acceptable levels?

○   ○   19. Is your average calorie consumption reasonable for your body size and for the amount of calories you normally expend?

[   ]   Total number of "Yes" answers

Chart 2 Dietary Habits Rating Scale

Score	Rating
18–19	Very good
15–17	Good
13–14	Marginal
12 or less	Poor

Daily Diet Record

Day 1

Breakfast Food	Amount (cups, tsp., etc.)	Calories	Food Servings				Estimated Meal Calorie %
			Bread/Cereal	Fruit/Veg.	Milk/Meat	Fat/Sweet	
							☐ % Protein
							☐ % Fat
							☐ % Complex carbohydrate
							☐ % Simple carbohydrate
							100% Total

Lunch Food	Amount (cups, tsp., etc.)	Calories	Food Servings				Estimated Meal Calorie %
			Bread/Cereal	Fruit/Veg.	Milk/Meat	Fat/Sweet	
							☐ % Protein
							☐ % Fat
							☐ % Complex carbohydrate
							☐ % Simple carbohydrate
							100% Total

Dinner Food	Amount (cups, tsp., etc.)	Calories	Food Servings				Estimated Meal Calorie %
			Bread/Cereal	Fruit/Veg.	Milk/Meat	Fat/Sweet	
							☐ % Protein
							☐ % Fat
							☐ % Complex carbohydrate
							☐ % Simple carbohydrate
							100% Total

Snack Food	Amount (cups, tsp., etc.)	Calories	Food Servings				Estimated Snack Calorie %
			Bread/Cereal	Fruit/Veg.	Milk/Meat	Fat/Sweet	
							☐ % Protein
							☐ % Fat
							☐ % Complex carbohydrate
							☐ % Simple carbohydrate
							100% Total
Daily Totals							**Estimated Daily Total Calorie %**
		Calories	Servings	Servings	Servings	Servings	☐ % Protein
							☐ % Fat
							☐ % Complex carbohydrate
							☐ % Simple carbohydrate
							100% Total

Daily Diet Record

Day 2

Breakfast Food	Amount (cups, tsp., etc.)	Calories	Food Servings				Estimated Meal Calorie %
			Bread/Cereal	Fruit/Veg.	Milk/Meat	Fat/Sweet	
							☐ % Protein
							☐ % Fat
							☐ % Complex carbohydrate
							☐ % Simple carbohydrate
							100% Total

Lunch Food	Amount (cups, tsp., etc.)	Calories	Food Servings				Estimated Meal Calorie %
			Bread/Cereal	Fruit/Veg.	Milk/Meat	Fat/Sweet	
							☐ % Protein
							☐ % Fat
							☐ % Complex carbohydrate
							☐ % Simple carbohydrate
							100% Total

Dinner Food	Amount (cups, tsp., etc.)	Calories	Food Servings				Estimated Meal Calorie %
			Bread/Cereal	Fruit/Veg.	Milk/Meat	Fat/Sweet	
							☐ % Protein
							☐ % Fat
							☐ % Complex carbohydrate
							☐ % Simple carbohydrate
							100% Total

Snack Food	Amount (cups, tsp., etc.)	Calories	Food Servings				Estimated Snack Calorie %
			Bread/Cereal	Fruit/Veg.	Milk/Meat	Fat/Sweet	
							☐ % Protein
							☐ % Fat
							☐ % Complex carbohydrate
							☐ % Simple carbohydrate
							100% Total

Estimated Daily Total Calorie %

☐ % Protein
☐ % Fat
☐ % Complex carbohydrate
☐ % Simple carbohydrate
100% Total

Daily Totals	✕	Calories	Servings	Servings	Servings	Servings

Lab 16B: Selecting Nutritious Foods

Name	Section	Date

Purpose: To learn to select a nutritious diet, to determine the nutritive value of favorite foods, and to compare a nutritious foods values to a favorite foods values.

Procedure:
1.   Select a breakfast, lunch, and dinner from the foods list in Appendix D. Include between-meal snacks with the nearest meal. If you cannot find foods you would normally choose, select those most similar to choices you might make.
2.   Select a breakfast, lunch, and dinner from foods you feel would make the most nutritious meals. Include between-meal snacks with nearest meal.
3.   Record your "favorite foods" and "nutritious foods" on the log on the back of this sheet. Record the calories for proteins, carbohydrates, and fats for each of the foods you choose.
4.   Total each column for the "favorite" and the "nutritious" meal.
5.   Determine the percentages of your total calories that are protein, carbohydrate, and fat by dividing each column total by the total number of calories consumed.
6.   Answer the questions in the Conclusions and Implications section.

Results: Record your results below. Calculate percent of calories from each source by dividing total calories into calories from each food source (protein, fat, or carbohydrate).

	Favorite Foods		Nutritious Foods	
Source	**Calories**	**% of Total Calories**	**Calories**	**% of Total Calories**
Protein				
Fat				
Carbohydrates				
Total		100%		100%

Conclusion and Implications: In several sentences, discuss differences you found between your nutritious diet and your favorite diet. Discuss the quality of your nutritious diet as well as other things you learned from doing this lab.

"Favorite" versus "Nutritious" Food Choices for Three Daily Meals

Breakfast Favorite — Food Choices

Food No.	Cal.	Pro. Cal.	Car. Cal.	Fat Cal.
Totals				

Breakfast Nutritious — Food Choices

Food No.	Cal.	Pro. Cal.	Car. Cal.	Fat Cal.
Totals				

Lunch Favorite — Food Choices

Food No.	Cal.	Pro. Cal.	Car. Cal.	Fat Cal.
Totals				

Lunch Nutritious — Food Choices

Food No.	Cal.	Pro. Cal.	Car. Cal.	Fat Cal.
Totals				

Dinner Favorite — Food Choices

Food No.	Cal.	Pro. Cal.	Car. Cal.	Fat Cal.
Totals				
Daily Totals (Calories)				
Daily % of Total Calories				

Dinner Nutritious — Food Choices

Food No.	Cal.	Pro. Cal.	Car. Cal.	Fat Cal.
Totals				
Daily Totals (Calories)				
Daily % of Total Calories				

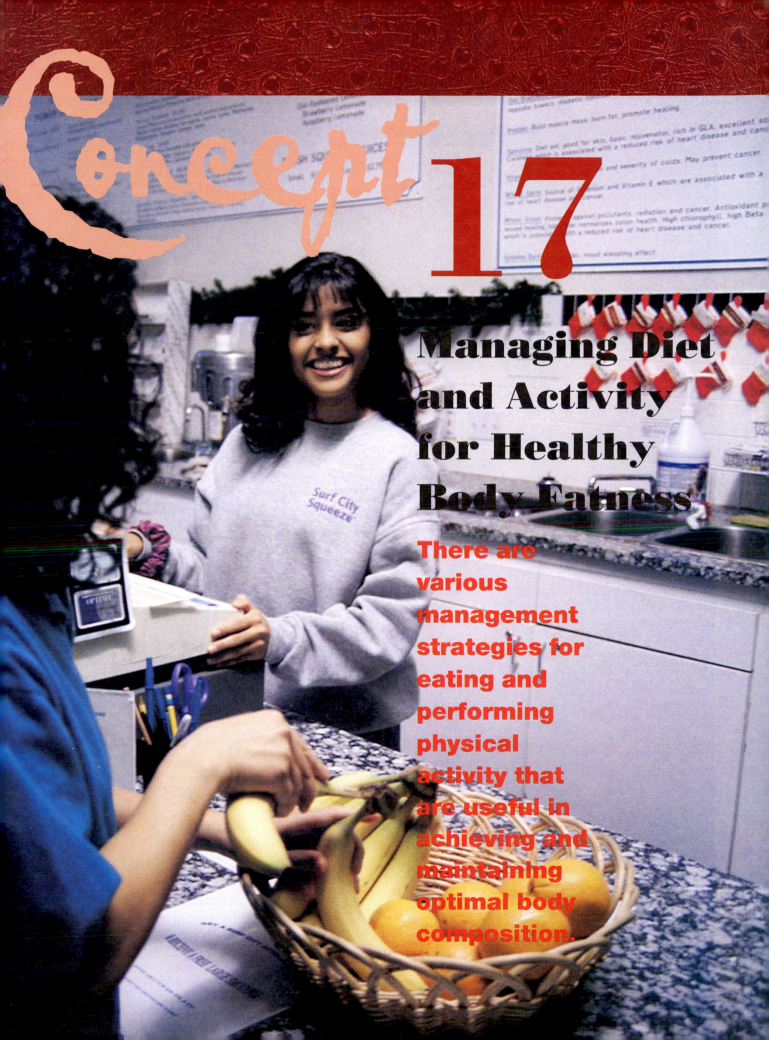

Concept 17

Managing Diet and Activity for Healthy Body Fatness

There are various management strategies for eating and performing physical activity that are useful in achieving and maintaining optimal body composition.

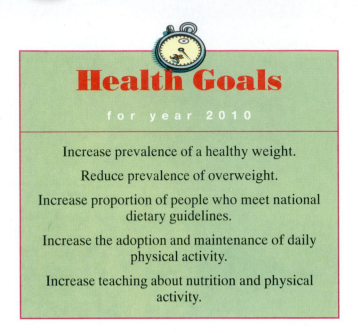

Health Goals

for year 2010

Increase prevalence of a healthy weight.

Reduce prevalence of overweight.

Increase proportion of people who meet national dietary guidelines.

Increase the adoption and maintenance of daily physical activity.

Increase teaching about nutrition and physical activity.

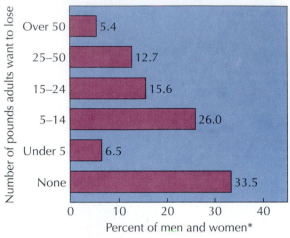

* Note: does not equal 100% due to rounding

Figure 1

Pounds of weight Americans want to lose.

Introduction

A recent poll indicated that 96 percent of all adult males and 99 percent of all adult females would change something about their physical appearance. The leading concern was weight loss. In fact, 66.5 percent of all Americans want to lose weight in the upcoming year (see Figure 1). Experts suggest that movies, television, and magazines have created an obsession with weight loss among many teens and adults. In many cases, the concern is with losing weight rather than fat, and with appearance rather than good health. Caution is necessary so that we do not create more problems than we solve.

Because of the misplaced concern with weight loss among large numbers of people, the emphasis of this concept will be on fat loss for good health. When properly done, fat control can be safe and effective. This concept will make suggestions for losing, maintaining, and gaining body fat.

The Facts about Goal Setting for Fat Control

The first step in fat control is establishing realistic goals.

Too many teens and adults, both men and women, establish unrealistic goals for their physical appearance. Fat, weight, and body proportions are all factors that can be changed, but people often set standards for themselves that are difficult, if not impossible, to achieve. Figure 1 illustrates the fact that large segments of the population would like to lose weight, and many want to lose very large amounts of weight. Start-

ing with small goals is preferable to establishing goals that seem impossible to accomplish. This necessitates developing an understanding of your own body proportions as well as your body fatness. Unrealistic goals may result in eating disorders, failure to meet goals, or failure to maintain fat loss over time.

Goals that emphasize the behavior of eating less and exercising more are more effective than those emphasizing a specific outcome such as weight or fat lost (or gained).

Researchers have shown that setting **outcome goals,** or goals that set a specific amount of weight or fat loss (gain), can be discouraging. If a **behavioral goal** of eating a reasonable number of calories per day and expending a reasonable number of calories in exercise is met, outcome goals will be achieved. Most experts believe that behavioral goals work better than weight or fat loss goals, especially in the short term.

People who have a large amount of fat to lose may do better setting short-term rather than long-term goals.

Losing 50 pounds (22.7 kilograms) may seem impossible and for this reason is not a good **short-term goal.** Losing 2 pounds (1 kilogram) in a week may seem more achievable. Because your weight can fluctuate with the amount of water lost or retained, daily monitoring of weight can also be discouraging. Weight may drop dramatically one day because of water loss and increase the next. Care must be taken not to worry too much about daily weight or fat losses or gains in the early stages of a program. **Long-term goals** are best established after a series of short-term goals have been met.

Record keeping is important to meeting fat-control goals and making moderation a part of your normal lifestyle.

---

www.mhhe.com/hper/physed/clw/student/

Studies have shown that it is easy to fool yourself when determining the amount of food you have eaten or the amount of exercise you have done. Once fat-control goals have been set, whether for weight loss, maintenance, or gain, it is important to keep records of your behavior. People often underestimate the amount of food they have eaten, particularly the number of calories consumed. They also tend to overestimate the amount of exercise they do. Keeping a diet log and an exercise log can help you monitor your behavior and maintain the lifestyle necessary to meet your goals. A log can also help you monitor changes in weight and body fatness. But remember, care should be taken to avoid too much emphasis on short-term weight changes. A log can be used for record keeping. In Lab 17B you will have the opportunity to keep records to monitor your calorie intake and energy expenditure.

Be aware of changes in body water when monitoring body weight.

As noted in the concept on body composition, much of our body weight is water. Large short-term changes in body weight from day to day most likely result from changes in water rather than changes in body fat. To get accurate assessments of true changes in body fatness, weight and body fatness assessments should not be done too frequently. Drinking adequate amounts of water is important to people who are restricting calories and will reduce the risk of false changes in body fat. Measuring weight is best done early in the morning before you have eaten breakfast.

Crash diets that bring about weight loss by dehydration of only 5 percent in 48 hours have been shown to reduce the individual's working capacity by as much as 40 percent. The practice of "making weight" in athletics, whether by dehydration, induced vomiting, or starvation diets, is dangerous to health and should be condemned. Much of the weight loss from fad diets is loss of valuable lean muscle mass.

The best way to control body fatness is to establish a healthy lifestyle.

One way to ascertain whether fat control goals are realistic is to determine if they can be maintained for a lifetime. Diets that require severe caloric restriction or exercise programs that require exceptionally large caloric expenditure can be

effective in fat loss over a short period, but are seldom maintained for a lifetime. Studies show that extreme programs for fat and weight control, designed to "take it off fast," result in long-term success rates of less than 5 percent. Research shows that one reason extremely low-calorie diets are ineffective is that they may promote "calorie sparing." When calorie intake is 800–1,000 or less, the body protects itself by reducing basal and resting metabolism levels (sparing calories). This results in less fat loss, even though the calorie intake is very low.

A healthy lifestyle includes a healthy diet and regular exercise. For some people, it may be necessary to develop a daily habit of eating several hundred calories less than other people or maintaining an exercise schedule that expends more calories than the normal person if desirable body fat levels are to be maintained. These habits of moderation can realistically become part of your normal lifestyle.

Some Facts about Eating and Fat Control

There are some general guidelines for eating that can help people interested in losing body fat.

---

www.mhhe.com/hper/physed/clw/student/

- Restrict calories in moderate amounts per day rather than make large reductions in daily caloric intake.

Outcome Goal   A statement of intent to achieve a specific test score or a specific standard associated with good health or wellness. An example would be, "I will lower my body fat level by three percent."

Behavioral Goal   A statement of intent to perform a specific behavior (changing a lifestyle) for a specific period of time. An example would be, "I will reduce the fat in my diet to 30 percent or less of my total calories."

Short-Term Goal   A statement of intent to change a behavior or outcome in a period of days or weeks.

Long-Term Goal   A statement of intent to change behavior or achieve a specific outcome in a period of months or years.

- Eat less fat. Research shows that reduction of the fat in the diet not only results in fewer calories consumed (fats have more than twice the calories per gram as carbohydrates or proteins), but in greater body fat loss as well!
- Severely restrict **empty calories** which provide little nutrition and can account for an excessive amount of your daily caloric intake. Examples of these foods are candy (often high in simple sugar) and potato chips (often fried in saturated fat).
- Increase complex carbohydrates. Foods high in fiber, such as fresh fruits and vegetables, contain few calories for their volume. They are nutritious and filling, and are especially good foods for a fat loss program.
- Learn the difference between craving and hunger. Hunger is a physiological phenomenon that is a result of the body's need to supply energy to sustain life. A craving is simply a desire to eat something, sometimes even a food that is not particularly liked. When you feel the urge to eat, you may want to ask yourself: Is this real hunger or a craving? Hunger is accompanied by growling of the stomach and is most likely to occur after long periods without food. If you have the urge to eat soon after a meal, it is probably from craving, not hunger.

There are some guidelines for shopping that can help people interested in fat control.

- Shop from a list. This helps you avoid buying foods that contain empty calories and other foods that will tempt you to overeat.
- Shop with a friend. This is another way to help you avoid the purchase of unneeded foods. For this technique to work, the other person must be sensitive to your goals. In some cases, a friend can have a bad, rather than a good, influence.
- Shop on a full stomach to avoid the temptations of buying junk food.
- Check the label for contents of foods. If the calories are not listed, be wary of buying them. Many so-called weight-reduction foods have caloric contents equal to or in excess of normal foods.
- Consider foods that take some preparation time. If it takes time to prepare food, you may be less likely to eat it on the spur of the moment. It is acceptable to purchase foods prepackaged in small portions and that contain low caloric content, even if they require little preparation.

There are some guidelines about the way you eat that can be useful in fat loss.

- When you eat, do nothing else but eat. If you watch television, read, or do some other activity while you eat, you may be unaware of what you have eaten. Also, you

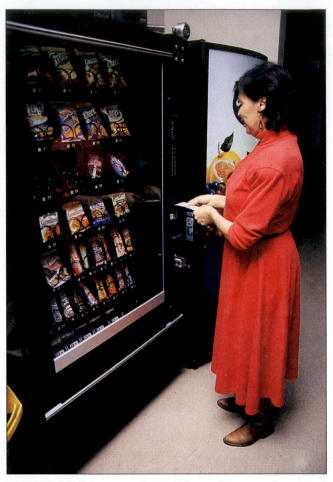

Foods with "empty calories" have few nutrients and often are relatively high in calorie content.

should enjoy your eating, not share it with some other activity.
- Eat slowly. Taste your food. Pause between bites. Chew slowly. Don't take the next bite until you have swallowed what you have in your mouth. Periodically take a longer pause. Be the last one finished eating.
- Do not eat food you do not want. Some people do not want to waste food so they clean their plate even when they feel full.
- Follow an eating schedule. Eating at regular meal times can help you avoid snacking. If meals are spaced equally throughout the day, it can help reduce appetite.
- Eat in designated areas only. Designate areas such as the kitchen and dining room as eating areas.
- Eat meals of equal size. Some people try to restrict calories at one or two meals to save up for a big meal. Eating several *small* meals helps you avoid hunger (fools the appetite) and helps you keep from losing control at one meal.
- Leave the table after eating and clear dishes early, which help prevent you from taking extra unwanted bites and servings.

- Avoid second servings. Limit your intake to one moderate serving. If second servings are taken, make them one-half the size of first servings.
- Limit servings of salad dressings and condiments (catsup, etc.). These are often high in fat and calories, and can sometimes amount to greater calorie consumption than the food on which you put them.
- Limit servings of nonbasic parts of the meal. It is easy to consume large numbers of calories on alcohol, soft drinks, breads, and desserts. Limit these items.

There are some guidelines that are useful for controlling the home environment to aid in fat loss.

- Keep busy, especially at high-risk times when you are most likely to eat when you are not hungry. If you have an urge to eat, exercise, talk to someone, go shopping, drink a glass of water, or find something active to do.
- Store food out of sight. Avoid containers that allow you to see the food. It is especially important to limit the accessibility of foods that tempt you and foods with empty calories. "Foods that are out of sight, are out of mouth."
- Avoid serving food to other people, especially between meals. Let them prepare their own snacks.
- If you snack, eat foods high in complex carbohydrates and low in fats, such as fresh fruits and carrot sticks.
- Freeze leftovers, which are often tempting to eat. Freezing them so that it takes time to eat them will help you avoid temptation.

There are some guidelines for controlling the work environment to aid in fat loss.

- Take food from home rather than eating from vending machines or catering trucks. Even snacks should be brought from home, where they can be prepared based on guidelines listed above.
- Avoid snack machines. Most snacks from machines are high in calories and low in nutritional value. Fresh fruit from machines is an exception.
- If you eat out, plan your meal selection ahead of time. Write it down and know its calorie content. Be aware that many fast foods are high in caloric content and fat.
- Do not eat while working.
- Avoid sources of food provided by co-workers (for example, food in work rooms, such as birthday cakes, or candy in jars).
- Do something active during breaks. For example, take a walk.
- Have drinking water or low-calorie drinks available to substitute for snacks.

There are some guidelines for eating on special occasions that can be useful in fat loss.

- Practice ways to refuse food. Practice in front of a mirror or with friends. Know exactly what to say when you refuse food. Do not let yourself be intimidated into eating something you do not want. For example, you might say something as simple as "No thank you." Be wary of persistent hosts. Do not let them make you feel guilty for not eating. Be polite but emphatic; give no indication that you might change your mind.
- In extreme cases, you may wish to avoid situations that create a high risk of overeating.
- Eat before you go out.
- Do not stand near food sources.
- If you feel the urge to eat, talk to someone or find something else to occupy your thoughts.

There are some guidelines for eating out that can be useful in fat loss.

In recent years, more and more people eat meals away from home with greater frequency. To save time and money, fast foods are often the foods of choice. The following guidelines are designed to aid in making good choices about foods when eating out.

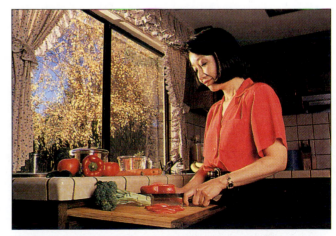

If you snack, consider foods high in complex carbohydrates.

Empty Calories Calories in foods considered to have little nutritional value.

- Limit deep-fat–fried foods.
- Ask establishments for information about food content before ordering.
- Limit use of sauces and condiments such as butter, margarine, catsup, and mayonnaise.
- Limit use of salad dressings. Salads are healthy and low in calories until large amounts of dressing are added.
- Choose low-fat products such as skim (not whole) milk, and ask for information about any food considered to be low-fat or reduced-fat.
- Choose chicken without skin, fish, or lean (well-trimmed) cuts of meat that are grilled or broiled rather than fried.
- Do not eat everything on your plate if very large portions are served.
- Order à la carte rather than full meals that come with several courses.
- If you eat dessert, avoid those high in fat or those covered with sauces or toppings.

Fad diets are not a satisfactory means of long-term weight reduction and may adversely affect your health.

www.mhhe.com/hper/physed/clw/student/

There are hundreds of fad diets and diet books, but dietitians warn that there is no scientific basis for drastic juggling of food constituents. Such diets are usually unbalanced and may result in serious illness or even death, especially for the obese person who is already apt to be suffering from a number of health disorders. Fad diets cannot be maintained for long periods; therefore, the individual usually regains any lost weight. Less than 5 percent of people who lose weight maintain the loss for more than a year. Constant losing and gaining, known as the "yo-yo syndrome," may be as harmful as the original obese condition.

Total fasting is dangerous, as are crash (fast) diets. Pill popping, hormone injections, and powder and liquid diets have little value in long-term weight-control programs and present many health hazards. When in doubt, avoid diets that:

- Promise fast, easy solutions.
- Promise to help you achieve ideal weight without mental inspiration and perspiration.
- Favor one food as the answer to weight problems.
- Promise that your fat will melt away.

Artificial sweeteners and fat substitutes may help, but are not a "sure cure" for body fatness problems.

www.mhhe.com/hper/physed/clw/student/

Artificial sweeteners have dramatically reduced the calories in some soft drinks and foods. However, since they were introduced, the general

public has not eaten fewer calories, and more people are now overweight than before they were introduced. Also, new products often referred to as "fake fat" are used as a fat substitute in baking and cooking. Potato chips and other fried foods cooked in these products as well as baked goods using these products have less fat and fewer calories. If you eat no more food than usual and substitute foods made with these products, you will consume fewer calories and less fat. Experts worry that consumers will not eat the same amount of foods with these fake fats but will feel that they can eat more because these foods contain fewer calories and less fat.

Diets that emphasize one specific nutrient are typically ineffective and can be dangerous.

In recent years, diets that emphasize one nutrient at the expense of others have been widely advocated by authors of books and sellers of nutritional supplements. Among these are high-fat or low-fat diets, high- or low-carbohydrate diets, and the commonly advocated high-protein diet. There are many obvious reasons for avoiding high-fat diets. First, each fat gram contains more than twice the calories of protein or carbohydrate. Second, the health risks of high-fat diets are well-documented. Recent research suggests that for most people, diets excessively low in fat are also not advised without advice from a physician or registered dietitian.

If a person increases carbohydrates, it means cutting protein or fat in the diet. As long as there is adequate protein (10 to 15 percent) and fat amounts are not excessively low, high-carbohydrate diets can be appropriate. For higher than normal carbohydrate diets, it is important to distribute protein and fat intake across the day. Meals consisting entirely of carbohydrate are not recommended.

High-protein diets are the most common advocated diets that emphasize one nutrient. High-protein diets are basically the same as low-carbohydrate diets because the increase in proteins is typically at the expense of carbohydrates. The recent claims in several best-selling nutrition books about high-protein diets prompted the American College of Sports Medicine, The American Dietetics Association, and several other organizations to prepare a guide to make consumers aware of the false claims about high-protein/low-carbohydrate diets. These diets are sometimes referred to as 40/30/30 diets because they recommend low carbohydrate (40 percent rather than 55 or 60 percent) and high protein (30 percent rather than 10 to 15 percent). Table 1 provides some information about high-protein diets such as 40/30/30.

In the final analysis, the percentages of calories recommended as national health goals are most likely to be effec-

Table 1 Claims and Facts about High Protein/Low Carbohydrate Diets

Claim	Fact
A high-protein/low-carbohydrate (HP/LC) diet will decrease "bad" eicosanoids and produce "good" eicosanoids. Eicosanoids are derivatives of fatty acids formed by oxidization that may have hormonelike properties.	No published findings have shown eicosanoids to affect health.
A HP/LC diet will reduce substances in the body (Profactor-H) that produce a deadly imbalance that comes from having too much insulin in the blood.	No published findings have shown Profactor-H to affect health.
A high-carbohydrate diet promotes insulin resistance thus causing the body to store extra fat.	Insulin resistance (inability of the cells to use insulin effectively) occurs most commonly in overweight and sedentary people. Loss of weight and moderate exercise can often reduce these symptoms. Loading carbohydrates before activity can increase insulin in the blood, but this increase has not been found to decrease performance.
A HP/LC diet enhances health and performance.	Evidence suggests that 10 to 15 percent protein and 55 to 60 percent carbohydrate are best for health and wellness, even for active people.
A HP/LC diet is effective in improving performance and health and can be used safely for long periods of time.	Short-term effects may include dizziness, diarrhea, insomnia, fatigue, and aching legs. Long-term effects can include kidney damage (especially for people with renal decrease) and other conditions associated with lack of adequate balance of nutrients. Much of the research cited by HP/LC advocates was done with subjects who have insulin resistance problems, and it is not reasonable to apply these results to people without pathology.
A 40/30 carbohydrate-to-protein ratio will help the body burn calories more effectively and result in achieving and maintaining a healthy weight.	The main reason high-protein/low-carbohydrate diets result in weight loss is the low total calorie count. Low-calorie diets may result in deficiencies of various nutrients and are unlikely to be adhered to over the long haul. The excessively high protein and fat content can lead to health problems.
Advocates of HP/LC diets suggest that fat is the primary source of energy for muscles.	Fat can be a source of energy for muscles, but during intense activity, carbohydrates stored in muscles are the primary source. Carbohydrates are essential to the body's ability to supply energy, and for competitive athletes, the 40/30/30 plan does not provide enough to reach peak performance. Eating more fat does not help you burn fat better, and excess fat in the diet will likely be stored in the body as fat.

Adapted from Questioning 40/30/30, see suggested readings.

tive for those interested in achieving and maintaining healthy body fat levels and achieving optimal performance.

Many of the eating guidelines that are useful for fat loss are also valuable in maintaining desirable levels of body fat.

Once a person has achieved a desirable level of body fatness, it is important that this level be maintained throughout life. Many of the eating strategies for losing body fatness listed in the previous sections are also appropriate for maintaining body fat levels at desirable levels. If you follow them, you will develop new and healthier eating patterns that you will retain for the rest of your life.

Some people need to gain weight and can benefit from a change in their eating patterns.

Most people who want to gain weight want to gain lean body tissue. Only those who have body fat percentages less than what is considered to be essential for good health need to gain body fat. Some eating guidelines for people interested in gaining weight are listed here:

- Increase the calories consumed. Increasing caloric intake by amounts of 500–1,000 calories a day will help most people gain weight over time.

- The majority of extra calories should come from complex carbohydrates: breads, pasta, rice, fruits such as bananas, and potatoes are good sources. High-protein diets or diet supplements are not particularly effective if you maintain a normal diet. High-fat diets can result in weight gain but may not be best for good health, especially if they are high in saturated fat.

- If extra exercise results in extra calories expended, caloric intake will need to be adjusted to compensate. It may be difficult to eat when you are not hungry. Eating more than three meals per day may help.

- Drink lots of juice and milk. Grape and cranberry juices are good because they are high in calories.

- Eat snacks. Bananas, granola, and nuts are high-calorie, healthy snacks.

- If weight gain does not occur over a period of weeks and months with extra caloric consumption, medical assistance may be necessary.

> **More calories are required to maintain weight during the growing years than during adulthood.**

Typically, the people most likely to have difficulty in gaining weight are age 10 to 20. They have probably been told more than once that they will not have trouble gaining weight when they grow older. This is true for most people, but it is of little consolation if they want to gain weight now. During adolescence, most people begin to gain weight, including muscle mass that can be enhanced with regular exercise. If they follow the guidelines just listed, they may have success in gaining weight. Excessive eating to gain weight (especially during adolescence) is not without its problems. The body requires more caloric intake during the teen years because the body is growing. A person who develops a habit of high caloric intake during this time may have a difficult time controlling fatness when the demands on the body are less.

Some Facts about Physical Activity and Fat Control

> **There are some guidelines for physical activity that can be of value in losing or maintaining desirable body-fat levels.**

www.mhhe.com/hper/physed/clw/student/

- Perform regular aerobic exercise. Since aerobic exercise can be maintained for a long period, it allows you to expend large numbers of calories. For this reason, it is the best type of physical activity for fat loss and maintenance.

- Find a time, a place, and a type of physical activity that will permit you to work out regularly. Regularity is the key to exercise being of value.

- Strength training can increase muscle mass and result in fat loss without loss in weight. If you follow the guidelines for strength training, you can increase your muscle mass provided calorie intake is constant.

> **Two principal guidelines for physical activity are of value in gaining weight, including muscle mass.**

- Strength training is the best form of exercise for people interested in gaining weight. Of course, strength training is most effective in weight gain when accompanied by an increase in calorie intake.

- Excessive aerobic exercise may make it difficult to gain weight. Although some regular aerobic exercise is necessary for health and cardiovascular fitness, it may be necessary to limit aerobic exercise if weight gain is the goal. Studies have shown that extensive aerobic training can even cause a reduction in muscle mass. When training to gain weight, limiting aerobic exercise to 3 or 4 days a week can be beneficial.

Strategies for Action: The Facts

> **Knowing about guidelines for controlling body fatness is not as important as following them.**

The guidelines presented in this concept are only of value if you use them. In Lab 17A, you will have the opportunity to identify some of the guidelines that you feel will help you the most in the future.

> **The support of family and friends can be of great importance in balancing calorie intake and calorie expenditure.**

The importance of family and friends to successful adherence to a regular physical activity program can't be overemphasized. Family and friends can also help you in changing and adhering to healthy eating practices. It is known that parents who overeat often have children who eat more than normal. In these cases, it is important for the entire family to participate in a program to control fatness. Family and friends should provide support for the person trying to gain or lose fat by helping them follow the guidelines presented in this concept, rather than tempting the person to eat improperly. Unfortunately, sometimes friends and family members can put too much emphasis on the person's fat loss. This can have the opposite effect of that intended if it is perceived as an attempt to control one's behavior. Studies have shown that the use of extrinsic rewards such as money or special gifts for achieving goals may be effective in the short-term, but may result in resentment rather than adherence over the long-term. Encouragement and support rather than control of behavior is the key!

Group support can be one of the best reinforcers of proper eating and exercise behavior.

Group support has been found to be beneficial to many individuals who are attempting to change their behavior. Alcoholics have found that the support of others is critical to their rehabilitation. (Alcoholics Anonymous grew as a result of this need.) If you want to alter your body composition, especially to lose body fat, group support is important if you are to make permanent lifestyle changes in diet and exercise. Groups such as Overeaters Anonymous and Weight Watchers have been organized to help those who need the support of peers in attaining and maintaining desirable fat levels for a lifetime.

There are some psychological strategies that can be of assistance in eating and exercising to attain and maintain a desirable level of body fatness.

- Avoid food fantasies. Sometimes the thought of food is what causes overeating. Practice restructuring your thought process to something other than food fantasies. Use mental imagery to create a mind's-eye view of something you enjoy other than food. When food fantasies occur, you may want to exercise or engage in some activity that refocuses your attention.
- Avoid weight fantasies. Sometimes the thought of being excessively thin or muscular occurs. By itself, this may not be bad. If, however, it causes you to become discouraged and makes your goals seem unattainable, it is bad. When weight fantasies occur, do some other activity to redirect your focus of attention or imagine something other than the weight fantasy. Altering mental fantasies takes practice.
- Avoid **negative self-talk.** One type of negative self-talk occurs when a person starts self-criticism for not meeting a goal. For example, if a person is determined not to

eat more than one serving of food at a party, but fails to meet this goal, he or she might say, "It's no use stopping now; I've already blown it." It is not too late. Failing to meet goals can happen to anyone. Negative self-talk makes it easy to fail in the future. A more appropriate response would involve **positive self-talk** such as, "I'm not going to eat anything else tonight; I can do it."

Keeping records of calories consumed and calories expended can be an effective tool in maintaining a healthy body composition throughout life.

Moderate changes in the number of calories you consume or the number of calories you expend in physical activity can have meaningful long-term effects on body fatness. In Lab 17B, you will have the opportunity to keep records to help you monitor your calorie intake and calorie expenditure.

Web Review

Web review materials for Concept 17 are available are at *www.mhhe.com/hper/physed/clw/student/*.

American Dietetic Association
   www.eatright.org
Berkeley Nutrition Sciences
   www.nutritionquest.com
Center for Science in the Public Interest
   http://www.cspinet.org/
Fast Food Facts: Interactive Food Finder
   www.olen.com/food
Meals Online
   www.meals.com
Office of Dietary Supplements
   http://www.odp.od.nih.gov/ods/default.html
USDA Food and Nutrition Information Center
   http://www.nalusda.gov/fnic/

Negative Self-Talk Self-defeating discussions with yourself focusing on your failures rather than your successes.

Positive Self-Talk Telling yourself positive, encouraging things that help you succeed in accomplishing your goals.

Suggested Readings

Brownell, K., et al. "Matching Weight Control Programs to Individuals." *The Weight Control Digest* 1(1991):65.

Brownell, K., Rodin, J., and Wilmore, J., eds. *Eating, Body Weight, and Performance in Athletes: Disorders of Modern Society.* Philadelphia: Lea & Febiger, 1992.

Clarkson, P. M. "The Skinny on Weight Loss Supplements and Drugs: Winning the War Against Fat." *ACSM's Health and Fitness Journal* 2(4)(1998):18.

Hawley, J. A. "Fat Burning During Exercise: Can Ergogenics Change the Balance?" *Physician and Sportsmedicine.* 26(9)(1998):56.

Lemonick, M. D. "Are We Ready for Fat Free Fat?" *Time* 4(January 22, 1996), 40.

Peterson, J. A., Bryant, C. X., and Franklin, B. A. "50 Nifty Ways to Reduce Fat in Your Diet." *Fitness Management* 14(11)(1998):40.

Questioning 40/30/30: A Guide to Understanding Sports Nutrition Advice." A 22-page booklet published jointly by The American College of Sports Medicine, The American Dietetics Association, The Women's Sports Foundation, and The Cooper Institute for Aerobics Research, 1997.

U.S. Department of Health and Human Services. *Healthy People 2010 Objectives: Draft for Comment.* Washington, DC: U.S. Department of Health and Human Services, 1998, Objectives Chapters 1: Physical Activity and 2: Nutrition.

Wardlaw, G. M., Insel, P. M., and Seyler, M. F. *Contemporary Nutrition (2nd ed.).* St. Louis: Mosby, 1994.

Wilmore, J. H. "Exercise, Obesity and Weight Control." In Corbin, C. B. and Pangrazi, R. P. (ed.). *Towards a Better Understanding of Physical Fitness and Activity.* Scottsdale, AZ: Holcomb-Hathaway, 1999, Chapter 16.

Lab 17A: Selecting Strategies
for Managing Eating

Name	**Section**	**Date**

Purpose: To help you select strategies for managing eating to control body fatness.

Procedures:
1.   Read the strategies listed in chart 1.
2.   Make a check in the box beside five to ten of the strategies that you think will be most useful to you.
3.   Answer the questions in the Conclusions and Implications section.

Chart 1 Strategies for Managing Eating to Control Body Fatness

✔	Check 5 to 10 strategies that you might use in the future.
	Shopping Strategies
	Shop from a list.
	Shop with a friend.
	Shop on a full stomach.
	Check food labels.
	Consider foods that take some time to prepare.
	Methods of Eating
	When you eat, do nothing but eat. Don't watch television or read.
	Eat slowly.
	Do not eat food you do not want.
	Follow an eating schedule.
	Do your eating in designated areas such as kitchen or dining room only.
	Leave the table after eating.
	Avoid second servings.
	Limit servings of condiments.
	Limit servings of nonbasics such as dessert, breads, and soft drinks.
	Eat several meals of equal size rather than one big meal and two small ones.
	Eating in the Work Environment
	Take your own food to work.
	Avoid snack machines.
	If you eat out, plan your meal ahead of time.
	Do not eat while working.
	Avoid sharing foods from coworkers including birthday cakes, etc.
	Have activity breaks during the day.
	Have water available to substitute for soft drinks.
	Have low-calorie snacks to substitute for office snacks.

✔	Check 5 to 10 strategies that you might use in the future.
	Eating on Special Occasions
	Practice ways to refuse food.
	Avoid tempting situations.
	Eat before you go out.
	Don't stand near food sources.
	If you feel the urge to eat, find someone to talk to.
	Strategies for Eating Out
	Limit deep-fat fried foods.
	Ask for information about food content.
	Limit use of condiments.
	Choose low-fat foods (e.g., skim milk, low-fat yogurt).
	Choose chicken, fish or lean meat.
	Order á la carte.
	If you eat desserts, avoid those with sauces or toppings.
	Eating at Home
	Keep busy at times when you are at risk of overeating.
	Store food out of sight.
	Avoid serving food to others between meals.
	If you snack, choose snacks with complex carbohydrates such as carrot sticks or apple slices.
	Freeze leftovers to avoid temptation of eating them between meals.

Conclusions and Implications:

1. In several sentences, discuss your need to use strategies for effective eating. Do you need to use them? Why or why not?

2. In several sentences, discuss the effectiveness of the strategies contained in Chart 1. Do you think they can be effective for people who have a problem controlling their body fatness?

Lab 17B: Keeping Records for Fat Control

Name	Section	Date

Purpose: To allow you to keep records of calories taken in and calories expended to help you maintain a healthy level of body fat.

Procedures:
1. Establish a calorie intake goal for one day.
2. Determine the calories you consumed in one day using information from the dietary records you kept previously (Lab 16A Nutrition). If you did not perform that lab, perform it to provide information for this activity.
3. Record your daily calories consumed in the Results section.
4. Determine the calories you expended in one day using information from the calorie expenditure records you kept previously (Lab 15B Body Composition). If you did not perform that lab, perform it to provide information for this activity.
5. Record your daily calories expended in the Results section.
6. Determine your daily calorie imbalance by subtracting your calories consumed from calories expended.
7. Provide the additional information requested in the Results section.
8. Answer the questions in the Conclusions and Implications section.

Results:

Subtract calories expended from those consumed for the day to determine your calorie imbalance.

Daily calories
actually consumed

−

Daily calories
actually expended

=

Calorie
imbalance

+

−

Divide the calories imbalance into 3,500 calories to determine how many days it would take your daily calorie imbalance to cause a gain or loss of one pound.

$$\frac{3,500}{\text{Calorie imbalance}} = \boxed{} \text{ Days to gain or lose one pound of fat.}$$

Conclusions and Implications:

1. In several sentences, discuss the calorie imbalance (or lack of one) that existed for the one day described in this lab. Are the daily intake and expenditure values recorded for this lab typical of a normal day for you? If not, what do you think would be more typical? Would you like to continue a plan of eating and activity that would result in a calorie intake/expenditure similar to what you experienced in this lab?

Stress Management

Concept

18

Stress and Health

Mental and physical health are affected by an individual's ability to avoid or adapt to stress.

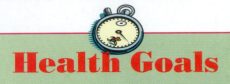

Health Goals

for year 2010

Reduce incidence of depression and resulting loss of quality of life.

Reduce suicide and suicide attempts especially among young people.

Increase mental health screening.

Increase availability of health care and counseling for mental health problems.

Increase healthy and active days.

Reduce worksite stress.

Introduction

Stress has been linked to between 50 and 70 percent of all illnesses. Some mental and physical conditions that can be psychosomatic (or stress-caused) include high blood pressure and heart disease; psychiatric disorders, such as depression and schizophrenia; indigestion; colitis; poor posture; headaches; insomnia; diarrhea; constipation; increased blood-clotting time; increased cholesterol concentration; diuresis; edema; and low back pain. Other serious diseases, such as cancer, can be influenced by a person's state of mind. In many cases, there is considerable time between a major stressor and the onset of a disease, so we do not always associate the two. Because of this, it is likely that the effect of stress on our body's function is underestimated.

Stress affects nearly everyone to some degree. In fact, approximately 67 percent of adults indicate that they feel "great stress" at least one day a week. Because stress is such a common problem in our society, stress management is viewed as a priority lifestyle similar to physical activity and a healthy diet. This concept will review the cause and consequence of stress. The following concept will provide practical guidelines on how to manage stress more effectively.

The Facts about Stress and Tension

Stress is a normal part of life.

All living creatures are in a continual state of **stress** (some more, some less). It is so pervasive that the body has a built-in mechanism that helps it respond and adapt to stress. When the body experiences a significant **stressor,** it triggers an emotional response that, in turn, evokes the autonomic nervous system to activate the "fight-or-flight" response. This adaptive and protective mechanism stimulates the adrenal glands to secrete hormones (epinephrine and cortisol) that prepare the body for what is perceived as a threat or assault on the whole organism. Almost all body systems are alerted to a heightened state of readiness as a result of this hormonal response. In some instances, this alarm reaction of the body may be essential to survival, but when evoked inappropriately or excessively, it may be more harmful than the effects of the original stressor. For example, a fight-or-flight response may cause a coronary spasm that could lead to a heart attack.

Too little stress is undesirable.

Stress is not always harmful. In fact, a lack of stress, sometimes called "rust out," can lead to boredom, apathy, and less than optimal health. Moderate stress may enhance behavioral adaptation and is necessary for maturation and health. It stimulates psychological growth. It has been said that "freedom from stress is death" and "stress is the spice of life."

Individuals tend to adapt best to moderate stress.

According to Hans Selye, the father of modern stress theory, the physiological and emotional effects of stress are adaptive responses that assist the body in adjusting to the stress. You would expect mild stress to produce mild **adaptations,** and strong stress to produce strong adaptive responses, but this is not so. High levels of threat tend to evoke ineffective, disorganized behavior that impairs the ability to function effectively. Figure 1 shows this relationship between stress and adaptive responses. The amount of stress that you can adapt to comfortably is what Selye called **eustress** and would, in a sense, be the target zone for stress (see Figure 2). The excessive level of stress that compromises our function and well-being is known as **distress.**

Individuals react and adapt differently to stressors.

What one person finds stressful may not be stressful to another person, and stress affects people differently. Stress mobilizes some to greater efficiency, while it confuses and disorganizes others. For example, sky diving or riding a roller coaster would be thrilling for some people, but for others it would be a very stressful and unpleasant experience. An individual's response to stress depends upon the intensity of the threat, the type of situation in which it occurs, and such personal variables as cultural background, tolerance levels, past experience, and personality.

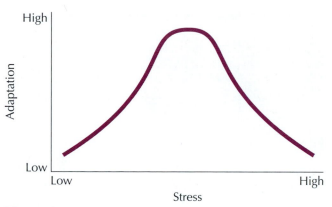

Figure 1
Stress and adaptive responses.

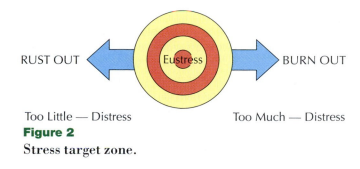

RUST OUT ← Eustress → BURN OUT

Too Little — Distress   Too Much — Distress

Figure 2
Stress target zone.

Many contemporary health psychologists acknowledge the complexity of the stress response and view stress as an interactive process. From this perspective, the nature of the stressor is not as important as the way a person appraises stress and what coping strategies are used to deal with stress. Two people can experience the same stressor but may respond very differently depending on how they appraise it and/or cope with it. These issues will be explored in more detail in this and the following concept.

The Facts about Sources of Stress

Stress can come from a variety of sources.

There are many kinds of stressors. Environmental stressors include heat, noise, overcrowding, climate, and terrain. Physiological stressors may be such things as drugs, caffeine, tobacco, injury, infection or disease, and physical effort.

Emotional stressors are the most frequent and important stressors affecting humans. Some people refer to these as "psychosocial" stressors. These include life-changing events, such as a change in work hours or line of work, family illnesses, problems with superiors, deaths of relatives or friends, and increased responsibilities. In school, pressures such as grades, term papers, and oral presentations may induce stress. A recent national study of daily experiences indicates that more than 60 percent of all stressful experiences fall in 13 areas. These areas are listed in Table 1.

Financial problems are a significant source of stress for college students.

Today, the average age of college students is estimated to be in the upper 20s. This is because many people go back to

Table 1 Leading Sources of Stress	
Source	**%**
1. Arguments or tense moments	8.6
2. Disagreements on issues at work	7.8
3. Concern over physical health of others	7.0
4. Work overload and demands	6.7
5. Worry about other's problems or well-being	6.4
6. Financial issues	4.6
7. Disciplining children	3.5
8. Disagreement over family issues	3.1
9. Being late or missing appointments	3.1
10. Differences of opinions on values	2.7
11. Home overload and demands.	2.7
12. Household and car repairs	2.6
13. Tension over household chores	2.6

SOURCE: National Study of Daily Experiences, with permission of David Almeida.

Stress The nonspecific response (generalized adaptation) of the body to any demand made upon it in order to maintain physiological equilibrium. This positive or negative response results from emotions that are accompanied by biochemical and physiological changes directed at adaptation.

Stressor Anything that places a greater than routine demand on the body or evokes a stress reaction.

Adaptation The body's efforts to restore normalcy.

Eustress Positive stress, or stress that is mentally or physically stimulating.

Distress Negative stress, or stress that contributes to health problems.

school while working or change careers later in life. No matter what your age, financial problems are stressful (see Table 1). However, students who are not self-sufficient or who have to work as well as attend school, are especially likely to experience stress associated with money. Students are often given access to credit cards even though they may have little experience managing money. To avoid financial problems and their associated stresses, all people would be advised to adhere to the following guidelines:

- Prepare a budget and stick to it. A budget should include an itemized list of planned expenditures. The amount budgeted for all expenses should be less than total income.
- Avoid using credit or credit cards. Credit allows you to buy things you cannot afford but it also reduces your buying power by 5 to 25 percent. Saving to buy the things you want and need allows you to get more for your money.
- Communicate with significant others about spending. Lack of communication is associated with many money problems.

Stressors vary in severity.

Because stressors vary in magnitude and duration, many experts categorize them by severity. Major stressors are those that create major emotional turmoil or require tremendous amounts of adjustment. This category includes personal crises (major health problems or death in family, divorce/separation, financial problems, legal problems, etc.), job/school-related pressures or major age-related transitions (college, marriage, career, retirement). Minor stressors are generally viewed as shorter term or less severe. This category includes events or problems such as traffic hassles, peer/work relations, time pressures, or family squabbles, just to name a few. Major stressors can alter our daily patterns of stress and impair our ability to handle the minor stressors or hassles of life. Conversely, minor stressors can accumulate and create more significant problems. It is important to be aware of both types of stressors.

The nature and magnitude of stressors change during the life span.

Depending on your perspective, some periods in life may be more stressful than others, but each phase provides its own challenges and experiences. Some argue that adolescence represents the most stressful time of life. There are drastic changes in a person's body and numerous psychosocial challenges that must be overcome. College provides additional mental challenges as well as financial pressures and the pressures of living independently. During the early adult

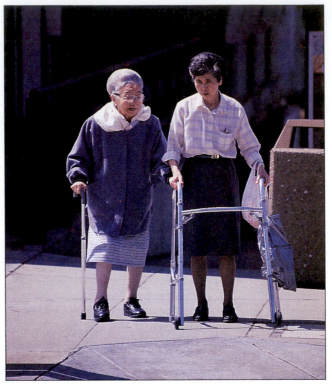

Stress varies with age and stage of life.

years, there are tremendous pressures and responsibilities to juggle career and family obligations. Late adulthood presents still other new challenges such as coping with declining functioning or illness. While the nature of the stressor changes, the presence of stress remains consistent. Learning to manage stress can make it easier to handle the changing stresses in life.

Stress can be self-induced and pleasurable, or unpleasurable.

www.mhhe.com/hper/physed/clw/student/
While many people blame external sources for their stress, much of our stress is self-induced. For example, athletes deliberately place themselves in stressful, competitive situations, lawyers and surgeons attempt the challenge of difficult cases or operations, and pregnant women willingly accept the psychological and physiological stress of bearing children. For some, stress can be addictive. Many **Type A personalities** seek out stressful situations and seemingly thrive on the pressure. Self-induced stress may also be an unpleasant but necessary interlude that cannot be avoided. For example, the risk of falling is necessary in learning to ride a bicycle.

At one time, all people with Type A personalities were thought to be at special risk of health problems, especially heart diseases. More recent studies indicate that many Type A personalities adapt to stress well, while others do not. Those who do not express their anger and have hostility associated with stressful situations are more likely to be at risk. A recent study showed that anger and hostility are as much factors for women as men. The researchers indicate that if you have anger and hostility, it is appropriate to express them in socially acceptable ways. If it is not appropriate, you need to find other ways to cope.

Negative, ambiguous, and uncontrollable events are usually the most stressful.

While stress can come from both positive and negative events, negative ones generally cause more distress. This is because negative stressors usually have harsher consequences and little benefit. Positive stressors on the other hand usually have enough benefit to make them worthwhile. So, while the stress of getting ready for a wedding may be tremendous, it is not as bad as the negative stress associated with losing a job.

Ambiguous stressors are harder to accept than problems that are more clearly defined. In most cases, if the cause of a stressor or problem can be identified, then active measures can be taken to improve the situation. For example, if you are stressed about a project at work or school, you can employ specific strategies to help you complete the task on time. Stress brought on by a relationship with friends or coworkers, on the other hand, may be harder to understand. In some cases, it may not be possible to determine the primary source or cause of the problem. These situations are more problematic because there are fewer clear-cut solutions.

Another factor that makes events stressful is a lack of control. Stress brought on by illness, accidents, or natural disasters often fit into this category. Because little can be done to change the situation, these events leave us feeling powerless. If the stressor is something that can be dealt with more directly, then efforts at minimizing the stress are likely to be effective. This helps us to feel more in control.

Occupations are common sources of stress, and some are more stressful than others.

www.mhhe.com/hper/physed/clw/student/

People spend large amounts of time at their jobs. Challenging tasks, uncertain responsibilities, and uncontrollable situations make occupational stress one of the most common sources of stress. While all jobs can be stressful, one study suggested that the 12 most stressful jobs were laborer, secretary, inspector, clinical lab technician, office manager, foreperson, manager/administrator, waiter/waitress, machine operator, farm owner, miner, and

painter. While not listed, air traffic control is often considered a high-stress occupation. This is because of the tremendous responsibility inherent in guiding planes safely into an airport. Because the prevalence of occupational stress is so high, many businesses hire psychologists to counsel employees about handling stress in the workplace. This can help reduce absenteeism, boredom, and the number of accidents and resignations.

The Facts about the Appraisal of Stress

Your appraisal of a stressful situation influences its severity.

Stressors by themselves generally do not cause problems unless they are perceived or appraised as stressful. Appraisal usually involves a consideration of the consequences of the situation and an evaluation of the resources that are available to help you cope with the situation. Stressors that have major consequences and little hope of resolution pose the greatest threat. By trying to maintain an optimistic view of stressful situations, you can minimize the effect of stress on your lifestyle. Dale Carnegie, a respected lecturer and author, recommended that individuals first accept the worst possible scenario and then take active steps to avoid it. This way you are likely to be positively surprised by the outcome.

Certain personality characteristics have been found to be associated with the ability to deal with stressful situations.

www.mhhe.com/hper/physed/clw/student/

While all people are exposed to stress, some people handle it better than others. Much of the difference lies in how people appraise a stressful situation. Certain characteristics (collectively referred to as **hardiness**) have been found to influence a person's reaction

Type A Personality A personality type characterized by impatience, ambition, and aggression; Type A personalities may be more prone to the effects of stress but may also be more able to cope with stress.

Hardiness A collection of personality traits thought to make a person more resistant to stress.

to stressful situations. Individuals possessing hardiness have been found to appraise and respond to stress in a more favorable ways than people without it. The dimensions of hardiness are:

Commitment: The stressors of everyday life can be overwhelming to many people. While stress cannot be avoided, a sense of commitment to your life and your aspirations can make stress more tolerable. Hardy individuals possess a strong sense of commitment and are willing to put up with adversity to keep pushing toward their desired goals.

Challenge: Many people experience considerable stress from the high-pressure demands of school and work. Much of the stress is caused by concern about being able to meet these new demands and the fear associated with failure. Hardy individuals see new responsibilities and situations as challenges rather than stressors. With this perspective, new situations become opportunities for growth rather than chances for failure.

Control: As previously mentioned, situations tend to be more stressful when they are out of our control. Rather than easily giving up when situations seem out of control, hardy individuals find ways to assume control over their problems. Being proactive rather than reactive is an effective strategy to combating stress. It is important to acknowledge that many stressors may be out of your control. In these situations, it is important to just "go with the flow." In other words, you may not be able "to smooth out the surf, but you can learn to ride the waves." Depending on the degree of control that is available, some coping strategies may be more effective than others. Specific recommendations are provided in the next concept.

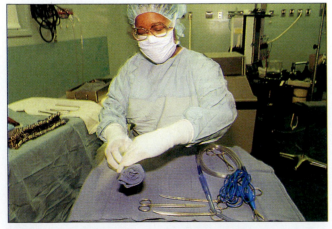

Hardy individuals see new responsibilities as challenges, not as producers of distress.

The Facts about Responses to Stress

Responses to stressors can be short- or long-lived.

Some stress persists only as long as the stressor is present. For example, job-related stress caused by a challenging project would generally subside once that project is completed. Other forms of stress may outlast the experience. For example, getting raped or mugged is an incredibly stressful experience and one that tends to stay with a person long after the crime is over. In these cases, the experiences will have long-term emotional consequences that take a long time to heal.

Stress can have physical effects on the body.

Many of the commonly observed symptoms of stress are physical in nature. Increases in heart rate and blood pressure and sweaty palms are just some of the many physical changes that are commonly observed following acute stress (see Figure 3). Chronic exposure to stress can lead to other physical symptoms such as headaches, indigestion, and stomach cramps.

Muscle tension is another common result of stress. One form of this tension is seen in the unnecessary "bracing" or "splinting" action of muscles—the clinched jaw, hunched shoulders, and white knuckles, or muscles contracting when they are not needed. They may stay contracted for long periods without your being aware of it. This tension can cause muscle spasms and pain that, in turn, becomes an additional stressor.

You can evaluate tension by learning to recognize signs of muscle tension. In Lab 18C, you will have the opportunity to practice evaluating signs of **neuromuscular hypertension.**

Stress can have mental and emotional effects on the body.

The challenges caused by psychosocial stress may lead to a variety of mental and emotional effects. In the short-term, stress can impair concentration and attention span. **Anxiety** is an emotional response to stress that is characterized by both apprehension and compulsion. Because the response usually involves expending a lot of nervous energy, anxiety can lead to fatigue and muscular tension. Unresolved personal stressors can also lead to depression.

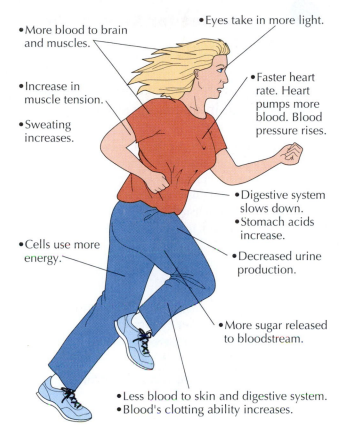

- More blood to brain and muscles.
- Increase in muscle tension.
- Sweating increases.
- Cells use more energy.
- Eyes take in more light.
- Faster heart rate. Heart pumps more blood. Blood pressure rises.
- Digestive system slows down.
- Stomach acids increase.
- Decreased urine production.
- More sugar released to bloodstream.
- Less blood to skin and digestive system.
- Blood's clotting ability increases.

Figure 3
Physical symptoms of stress.

Stress can lead to changes in behavior.

Stress can cause people to adopt nervous habits like biting their nails. It can also cause normally calm people to become irritable and short-tempered. Other behavioral responses to stress include altered eating and sleeping patterns.

The Facts about Stress and Health

Chronic stress can cause or exacerbate a variety of health problems.

Stress is viewed as an important cause of many health problems. It has been linked to chronic health maladies that plague individuals on a daily basis such as headaches, indigestion, and insomnia. It has also been linked to major health problems such as depression and coronary heart disease. While stress can exert direct effects on health, it is generally believed that stress contributes to diseases by interacting with other risk factors and by affecting the body's ability to adapt or cope.

Excessive stress reduces the effectiveness of the immune system.

Research on the immune system indicates that stress compromises the function of your body's immune system. With an inefficient immune system, it is more difficult to fight off bacterial infections and to recover from medical treatments. An altered immune function also increases a person's susceptibility to allergens. Therefore allergies and asthma attacks may be more severe under periods of high stress. Other autoimmune disorders such as rheumatoid arthritis are also made worse from stress.

Chronic fatigue syndrome has been associated with stress.

High levels of stress put a major burden on the mind and body. Fatigue can result from lack of rest or sleep, emotional strain, pain, disease, or combinations thereof. Fatigue can be classified as either **psychological fatigue** or **physiological fatigue**, but both can result in a state of

Neuromuscular Hypertension Unnecessary or exaggerated muscle contractions; excess tension beyond that needed to perform a given task; also called hypertonus.

Anxiety A state of apprehension with a compulsion to do something; excessive anxiety is a tension disorder with physiological characteristics.

Psychological Fatigue A feeling of fatigue usually caused by such things as lack of exercise, boredom, or mental stress that results in a lack of energy and depression; also referred to as "subjective" or "false" fatigue.

Physiological Fatigue A deterioration in the capacity of the neuromuscular system as the result of physical overwork and strain; also referred to as "true" fatigue.

Chronic Fatigue Syndrome A clinical condition characterized by a pronounced fatigue or debilitating tiredness.

exhaustion or **chronic fatigue syndrome** with neuromuscular hypertension.

Headaches and backaches are commonly associated with chronic stress.

Trigger points from excessive muscular tension can lead to myofascial pain syndrome. This syndrome can cause or aggravate backaches and headaches. (See concept on back and neck care.)

Depression is associated with excessive negative stress.

People who are excessively stressed are more likely to be depressed than people who have optimal amounts of stress in their lives. Health care costs for depressed people are 70 percent higher than for those who are not, and costs for people reporting high levels of stress are 50 percent higher than their less-stressed colleagues.

Stress can indirectly influence health.

Chronic levels of stress put a tremendous burden on a person's lifestyle. Many people find it difficult to maintain a healthy lifestyle during periods of high stress. Smoking, drinking, drugs, and unhealthy foods are some of the common vices or escapes that people resort to during periods of stress. Recent research has shown that drugs commonly prescribed to reduce depression can be effective in many cases but that they often do not get to the source of the life stressors that cause depression and often have side effects that are not positive.

In addition to increased tendencies for negative behaviors, stress can result in a reduced tendency toward positive behaviors such as regular physical activity and sufficient sleep. The combination of more negative behaviors and less positive behaviors can lead to additional health problems.

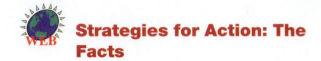

Strategies for Action: The Facts

Self-assessments of stressors in your life can be useful in managing stress.

In Lab 18A you will have the opportunity to evaluate your stress levels using the Life Experience Survey. In Lab 18B you will assess your hardiness, a characteristic associated with effectively coping with stress. If you find that you are high in stress, you can use the techniques described in the next concept to help you reduce your stress levels.

Web Review

Web review materials for Concept 18 are available are at *www.mhhe.com/hper/physed/clw/student/*.

American Institute of Stress
   www.stress.org
American Psychological Association
   www.apa.org
National Institute of Mental Health
   http://www.gopher.nimh.nih.gov/

Suggested Readings

Corbin, D. E. (ed.). *Perspectives: Stress Management.* Boulder, CO: Coursewise Publishing Co., 1999.

Girdano, D. and Everly, G. *Controlling Stress and Tension: A Holistic Approach* (5th ed.). Englewood Cliffs, NJ: Prentice-Hall, 1996.

Landers, D. "The Influence of Exercise on Mental Health." In Corbin, C. B. and Pangrazi, R. P. (ed.). *Towards a Better Understanding of Physical Fitness and Activity.* Scottsdale, AZ: Holcomb-Hathaway, 1999, Chapter 16.

Ortal, M. and Sherman, C. "Exercise Against Depression." *Physician and Sportsmedicine* 26(10)(1998):55.

U.S. Department of Health and Human Services. *Healthy People 2010 Objectives: Draft for Comment.* Washington, DC: U.S. Department of Health and Human Services, 1998, Objectives Chapter 23: Mental Health and Mental Disorders.

Lab 18A: Evaluating Your Stress Level

Name	**Section**	**Date**

Purpose: To evaluate your stress during the past year and determine its implications.

Procedure:
1. Complete the Life Experience Survey based on experiences during the past year. Place an X over the circle of the score representing the impact the experience had on you.
2. Add all of the negative numbers and record your score (distress) in the Results section. Add the positive numbers and record your score (eustress) in the Results section. Use all of the events in the last year.
3. Find your scores on the Rating Scale (Chart 1) and record your ratings.
4. Interpret the results by answering the questions, and discussing the conclusions and implications in the space provided.

Results:

Sum of negative scores [ ] (distress)   Rating on negative scores [ ]

Sun of positive scores [ ] (eustress)   Rating on positive scores [ ]

The higher the negative score, the greater the distress and the more likely you are to:
1. have high anxiety;
2. have some personal maladjustments, psychological problems, and/or neuroticism;
3. be depressed;
4. feel less capable of exerting control over your environment; and
5. have academic problems; lower GPA.
A high positive score (eustress) suggests that your life's experiences are enriching your quality of life.

Chart 1 Rating Scale for Life Experiences and Stress

	Sum of Negative Scores (Distress)	Sum of Positive Scores (Eustress)
May need counseling	14+	
Above-average stress	9–13	
Average	6–9	9–10
Below-average stress	<6	

Scoring the Life Experience Survey:
1. Add all of the negative scores to arrive at your own distress score (negative stress).
2. Add all of the positive scores to arrive at a eustress score (positive stress).

THE LIFE EXPERIENCE SURVEY

Listed below are a number of events that sometimes bring about change in the lives of those who experience them and necessitate social readjustment. Check those events that you have experienced in the past year. For each item, place an X over the circled number that indicates the extent to which you viewed the event as having either a positive or negative impact on your life at the time the event occurred. That is, indicate the type and extent of impact that the event had. A rating of –3 would indicate an extremely negative impact. A rating of 0 suggests neither a positive nor a negative impact. A rating of +3 would indicate an extremely positive impact.

Section I of the test is designed for everyone. It provides three extra blanks (numbers 45, 46, and 47) for you to list any recent experiences that have had an impact on your life but that were not mentioned in the preceding items.

Section II of the test is designed for students only. If there are school-related experiences that have had a noticeable impact on your life but are not listed, you may list them in one or more of the three blanks in Section I.

Note: Some items apply only to males and some apply only to females; these are indicated in the survey.

Section I	Extremely Negative	Moderately Negative	Somewhat Negative	No Impact	Slightly Positive	Moderately Positive	Extremely Positive
1. Marriage	(–3)	(–2)	(–1)	(0)	(+1)	(+2)	(+3)
2. Detention in jail or comparable institution	(–3)	(–2)	(–1)	(0)	(+1)	(+2)	(+3)
3. Death of spouse	(–3)	(–2)	(–1)	(0)	(+1)	(+2)	(+3)
4. Major change in sleeping habits (much more or less sleep)	(–3)	(–2)	(–1)	(0)	(+1)	(+2)	(+3)
5. Death of close family member:							
a. mother	(–3)	(–2)	(–1)	(0)	(+1)	(+2)	(+3)
b. father	(–3)	(–2)	(–1)	(0)	(+1)	(+2)	(+3)
c. brother	(–3)	(–2)	(–1)	(0)	(+1)	(+2)	(+3)
d. sister	(–3)	(–2)	(–1)	(0)	(+1)	(+2)	(+3)
e. child	(–3)	(–2)	(–1)	(0)	(+1)	(+2)	(+3)
f. grandmother	(–3)	(–2)	(–1)	(0)	(+1)	(+2)	(+3)
g. grandfather	(–3)	(–2)	(–1)	(0)	(+1)	(+2)	(+3)
h. other (specify) _____	(–3)	(–2)	(–1)	(0)	(+1)	(+2)	(+3)
6. Major change in eating habits (much more or much less food intake)	(–3)	(–2)	(–1)	(0)	(+1)	(+2)	(+3)
7. Foreclosure on mortgage or loan	(–3)	(–2)	(–1)	(0)	(+1)	(+2)	(+3)
8. Death of a close friend	(–3)	(–2)	(–1)	(0)	(+1)	(+2)	(+3)
9. Outstanding personal achievement	(–3)	(–2)	(–1)	(0)	(+1)	(+2)	(+3)
10. Minor law violations (traffic ticket, disturbing the peace, etc.)	(–3)	(–2)	(–1)	(0)	(+1)	(+2)	(+3)
11. *Male:* Wife's/girlfriend's pregnancy *Female:* Pregnancy	(–3)	(–2)	(–1)	(0)	(+1)	(+2)	(+3)
12. Changed work situation (different working conditions, working hours, etc.)	(–3)	(–2)	(–1)	(0)	(+1)	(+2)	(+3)
13. New job	(–3)	(–2)	(–1)	(0)	(+1)	(+2)	(+3)
14. Serious illness or injury of close family member:							
a. father	(–3)	(–2)	(–1)	(0)	(+1)	(+2)	(+3)
b. mother	(–3)	(–2)	(–1)	(0)	(+1)	(+2)	(+3)
c. sister	(–3)	(–2)	(–1)	(0)	(+1)	(+2)	(+3)
d. brother	(–3)	(–2)	(–1)	(0)	(+1)	(+2)	(+3)
e. grandfather	(–3)	(–2)	(–1)	(0)	(+1)	(+2)	(+3)
f. grandmother	(–3)	(–2)	(–1)	(0)	(+1)	(+2)	(+3)
g. spouse	(–3)	(–2)	(–1)	(0)	(+1)	(+2)	(+3)
h. child	(–3)	(–2)	(–1)	(0)	(+1)	(+2)	(+3)
i. other (specify) _____	(–3)	(–2)	(–1)	(0)	(+1)	(+2)	(+3)
15. Sexual difficulties	(–3)	(–2)	(–1)	(0)	(+1)	(+2)	(+3)
16. Trouble with employer (in danger of losing job, being suspended, demoted, etc.)	(–3)	(–2)	(–1)	(0)	(+1)	(+2)	(+3)

Section I

	Extremely Negative	Moderately Negative	Somewhat Negative	No Impact	Slightly Positive	Moderately Positive	Extremely Positive
17. Trouble with in-laws	−3	−2	−1	0	+1	+2	+3
18. Major change in financial status (a lot better off or a lot worse off)	−3	−2	−1	0	+1	+2	+3
19. Major change in closeness of family members (decreased or increased closeness)	−3	−2	−1	0	+1	+2	+3
20. Gaining a new family member (through birth, adoption, family member moving in, etc.)	−3	−2	−1	0	+1	+2	+3
21. Change of residence	−3	−2	−1	0	+1	+2	+3
22. Marital separation from mate (due to conflict)	−3	−2	−1	0	+1	+2	+3
23. Major change in church activities (increased or decreased attendance)	−3	−2	−1	0	+1	+2	+3
24. Marital reconciliation with mate	−3	−2	−1	0	+1	+2	+3
25. Major change in number of arguments with spouse (a lot more or a lot less arguments)	−3	−2	−1	0	+1	+2	+3
26. *Married Male:* Change in wife's work outside the home (beginning work, ceasing work, changing to a new job) *Married Female:* Change in husband's work (loss of job, beginning new job, retirement, etc.)	−3	−2	−1	0	+1	+2	+3
27. Major change in usual type and/or amount of recreation	−3	−2	−1	0	+1	+2	+3
28. Borrowing more than $10,000 (buying a home, business, etc.)	−3	−2	−1	0	+1	+2	+3
29. Borrowing less than $10,000 (buying car, TV, getting school loan, etc.)	−3	−2	−1	0	+1	+2	+3
30. Being fired from job	−3	−2	−1	0	+1	+2	+3
31. *Male:* Wife/girlfriend having abortion *Female:* Having abortion	−3	−2	−1	0	+1	+2	+3
32. Major personal illness or injury	−3	−2	−1	0	+1	+2	+3
33. Major change in social activities; e.g., parties, movies, visiting (increased or decreased participation)	−3	−2	−1	0	+1	+2	+3
34. Major change in living conditions of family (building new home, remodeling, deterioration of home, neighborhood, etc.)	−3	−2	−1	0	+1	+2	+3
35. Divorce	−3	−2	−1	0	+1	+2	+3
36. Serious injury or illness of close friend	−3	−2	−1	0	+1	+2	+3
37. Retirement from work	−3	−2	−1	0	+1	+2	+3
38. Son or daughter leaving home (due to marriage, college, etc.)	−3	−2	−1	0	+1	+2	+3
39. Ending of formal schooling	−3	−2	−1	0	+1	+2	+3
40. Separation from spouse (due to work, travel, etc.)	−3	−2	−1	0	+1	+2	+3
41. Engagement	−3	−2	−1	0	+1	+2	+3
42. Breaking up with boyfriend/girlfriend	−3	−2	−1	0	+1	+2	+3
43. Leaving home for the first time	−3	−2	−1	0	+1	+2	+3
44. Reconciliation with boyfriend/girlfriend	−3	−2	−1	0	+1	+2	+3
Other recent experiences that have had an impact on your life. List and rate.	−3	−2	−1	0	+1	+2	+3
45. _____	−3	−2	−1	0	+1	+2	+3
46. _____	−3	−2	−1	0	+1	+2	+3
47. _____	−3	−2	−1	0	+1	+2	+3

Section II: For Students Only	Extremely Negative	Moderately Negative	Somewhat Negative	No Impact	Slightly Positive	Moderately Positive	Extremely Positive
48. Beginning new school experience at a higher academic level (college, graduate school, professional school, etc.)	-3	-2	-1	0	+1	+2	+3
49. Changing to a new school at same academic level (undergraduate, graduate, etc.)	-3	-2	-1	0	+1	+2	+3
50. Academic probation	-3	-2	-1	0	+1	+2	+3
51. Being dismissed from dormitory or other residence	-3	-2	-1	0	+1	+2	+3
52. Failing an important exam	-3	-2	-1	0	+1	+2	+3
53. Changing a major	-3	-2	-1	0	+1	+2	+3
54. Failing a course	-3	-2	-1	0	+1	+2	+3
55. Dropping a course	-3	-2	-1	0	+1	+2	+3
56. Joining a fraternity/sorority	-3	-2	-1	0	+1	+2	+3

Adapted from Irwin G. Sarason, James H. Johnson, and Judith M. Siegel, "Assessing the Impact of Life Changes: Development of the Life Experiences Survey," in Journal of Consulting and Clinical Psychology, 46(5):932–46. Copyright © 1978 by the American Psychological Association. Reprinted by permission.

Conclusions and Implications: In several sentences, discuss your current stress level and what, if anything, needs to be done about it. Use your stress rating in your discussion.

Lab 18B: Evaluating Your Hardiness

Name	**Section**	**Date**

Purpose: To evaluate your level of hardiness and to help you identify the ways in which you appraise and respond to stressful situations.

Procedure:
1. Complete the Hardiness Questionnaire. Make an X over the circle that best describes what is true for you personally.
2. Summarize your score using the scoring chart.
3. Evaluate your score using the Hardiness Rating Chart and record your ratings.
4. Interpret the results by answering the questions, and discussing the conclusions and implications in the space provided.

Hardiness Questionnaire

Questions	Not True	Rarely True	Sometimes True	Often True	Score
1. I look forward to school and work on most days.	1	2	3	4	
2. Having too many choices in life makes me nervous.	4	3	2	1	
3. I know where my life is going and look forward to the future.	1	2	3	4	
4. I prefer to not get too involved in relationships.	4	3	2	1	
Commitment Score Sum 1–4					
5. My efforts at school and work will pay off in the long run.	1	2	3	4	
6. You just have to trust your life to fate to be successful.	4	3	2	1	
7. I believe that I can make a difference in the world.	1	2	3	4	
8. Being successful in life takes more luck and good breaks than effort.	4	3	2	1	
Control Score Sum 5–8					
9. I would be willing to work for less money if I could do something really challenging and interesting.	1	2	3	4	
10. I often get frustrated when my daily plans and schedule get altered.	1	2	3	4	
11. Experiencing new situations in life is important to me.	1	2	3	4	
12. I don't mind being bored.	1	2	3	4	
Challenge Score Sum 9–12					

Results:

Commitment score [ ]   Commitment rating [ ]

Control score [ ]   Control rating [ ]

Challenge score [ ]   Challenge rating [ ]

(Sum the three scores)

Hardiness score [ ]   Hardiness rating [ ]

Hardiness Rating Chart:

Rating	Individual Hardiness Scale Scores	Total Hardiness Scores
High hardiness	14–16	40–48
Moderate hardiness	10–13	30–39
Low hardiness	Less than 10	Less than 30

Conclusions and Implications:

1. In several sentences, discuss your three hardiness scores. Commitment scores reflect a dedication toward personal goals and life in general. Control scores reflect a belief that events in your life are within your control. Challenge scores reflect an ability to see stressful situations as opportunities for growth. Do you think these scores have implications for you? Are there changes you can make?

2. In several sentences, discuss your total hardiness score. This collection of traits has been referred to as the "stress-resistant personality" since hardy individuals have been found to respond better to stressful situations. Do you think your score is accurate for you? Do you think the score has implications for you?

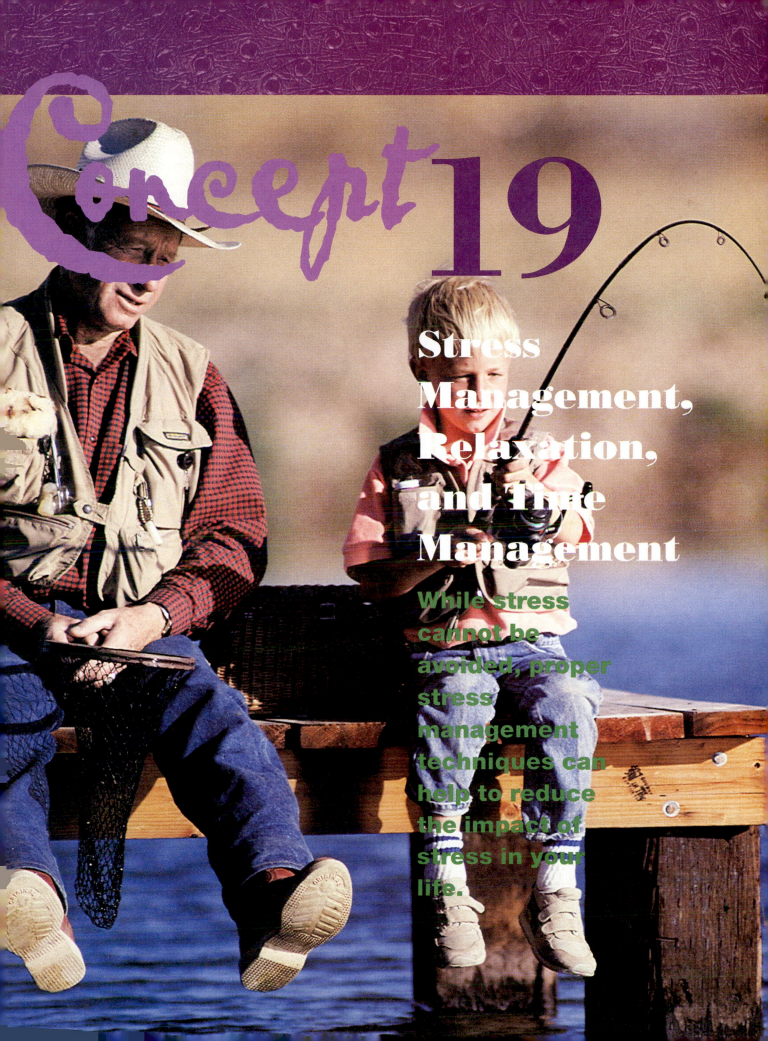

Concept 19

Stress Management, Relaxation, and Time Management

While stress cannot be avoided, proper stress management techniques can help to reduce the impact of stress in your life.

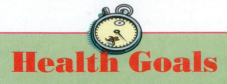

Health Goals

for year 2010

Reduce incidence of depression and resulting loss of quality of life.

Reduce suicide and suicide attempts especially among young people.

Increased mental health screening.

Increase availability of health care and counseling for mental health problems.

Increase healthy and active days.

Reduce worksite stress.

Introduction

When stress gets the best of you, it is important to find ways to cope with stress. **Active coping strategies** (problem solving, social support) are recommended when the stressful situations are largely within your control. **Passive coping strategies** (music, relaxation exercises, exercise) are recommended when the stress is largely out of your control or when you just want some immediate relief from the stress at hand. Most stressors will require both types of strategies. Drugs, alcohol, and food are not good choices for reducing stress since these can lead to more problems than they are intended to solve. This concept will review several approaches for effective stress management.

The Facts about Coping with Stress

Unresolved stress poses the greatest physical and emotional danger.

While some stressors are short lived, many stressors persist over a long period of time. The ability to adapt, or cope with these stressors, largely determines their ultimate effect. If effective coping strategies are used, the effects of a stressful situation can be more tolerable. In many cases, by "staying positive" reasonable solutions or compromises can be found for many problems. On the other hand, if ineffective coping strategies are used, many problems can actually become worse. This can lead to even more stress and more severe outcomes. While stress cannot be avoided, stress can be managed. Effective stress management is a skill that can contribute to both health and quality of life.

Coping strategies can be classified as "active" or "passive" depending on the nature of their influence.

Individuals deal with stress in a variety of ways; however, the methods of **coping** can generally be classified as either active or passive. Active coping strategies are aimed at changing the source or cause of the stress. Passive coping strategies, on the other hand, attempt to regulate the emotions from stress. A description of various coping strategies is provided in Table 1. While some strategies may be more effective for some people than for others, some strategies, like "escaping," are likely to be ineffective for almost everyone.

A key in stress management is to select coping strategies that are appropriate for the type of stress that you are experiencing. If you are confronting a situation that is largely out of your control, then active efforts to change the situation are unlikely to be effective. For these situations, it is more effective to use passive (emotion-based) coping strategies that help to minimize the effects of the stress. On the other hand, if you are experiencing stress from issues or events that you can control, then more active efforts are likely to improve the situation.

Coping with most stress requires a variety of thoughts and actions.

Stress forces our bodies to work under less than optimal conditions; yet, this is the time when we need to function at our best. Effective coping may require some efforts to regulate the emotional aspects of the stress and other efforts directed toward solving the problem. For example, if you are experiencing stress over grades in school, you have to accept your current grades and also take active steps to improve them. It does no good to worry about events that are behind you. Instead, it is important to look ahead for ways to solve the problems at hand.

Table 1 Active and Passive Coping Strategies for Stress Management

Category	Description
Active Coping Strategies	**Strategies that directly seek to solve or minimize the nature of the stressful situation.**
• Accepting	• Realizing that the problem was brought on by you and committing yourself to not let it happen again.
• Re-appraising	• Viewing experience as a learning or growth opportunity.
• Praying	• Looking for spiritual guidance to overcome the problem.
• Problem solving	• Making a plan of action to solve the problem and following the necessary steps to make the situation better.
• Controlling	• Trying to make yourself feel better or looking for ways to get past the situation.
• Seeking active social support	• Getting help or advice from others who can provide specific assistance for your situation.
Passive Coping Strategies	**Strategies that seek to minimize the emotional and physical effects of the stressful situation.**
• Ignoring	• Refusing to think about the situation or trying to move on as if there was no problem.
• Escaping	• Looking for ways to feel better or to stop thinking about the problem.
• Confronting	• Expressing anger over a situation, or challenging authorities to try to change the situation.
• Relaxing	• Using relaxation techniques to reduce the symptoms of stress.
• Exercising	• Using physical activity to reduce the symptoms of stress.
• Seeking passive social support	• Talking with someone about what you are experiencing or accepting sympathy and understanding over your situation.

Coping with this situation may therefore require both passive and active strategies. Passive strategies are needed to stop worrying about your current situation, and active strategies are needed to remove the source of the stress.

Physical Activity and Stress Management: The Facts

Regular activity and a healthy diet can help you adapt to stressful situations

An individual's capacity to adapt is not a static function, but fluctuates with energy, drive, and courage. The better your overall health, the better you can withstand the rigors of tension without becoming susceptible to illness or other disorders. Physical activity is especially important because it conditions your body to function effectively under challenging physiological conditions.

Physical activity can provide effective relief from stress and aid in muscle tension release.

Physical activity has been found to be effective at relieving stress, particularly white-collar job stress. Studies show that regular exercise decreases the likelihood of stress disorders and reduces the intensity of the stress response. It also shortens the time of recovery from an emotional trauma. Its effect tends to be short term, so one must continue to exercise regularly for it to have a continuing effect. Exercise is not like a measles vaccine where one inoculation is good for life. Aerobic exercise is believed to be especially effective in reducing anxiety and relieving

Coping A person's constantly changing cognitive and psychological efforts to manage stressful situations. Coping strategies can be either active or passive.

Active Coping Strategies A method of adapting to stress that is based on changing the source or cause of stress; also called problem-focused coping.

Passive Coping Strategies A method of adapting to stress that is based on regulating the emotions that cause stress; also called emotion-focused coping.

stress (though a wide variety of other activities are also good). Whatever your choice of exercise, it is likely to be more effective as an antidote to stress if it is something you find enjoyable.

Stretching exercises and rhythmical exercises especially aid in relaxation.

People who work long hours at a desk can release tension by getting up frequently and stretching, by taking a brisk walk down the hall, or by performing "office exercises."

Exercising to music or to a rhythmic beat has been found to be relaxing and even "hypnotic." Some exercises designed specifically for relaxation are illustrated in Table 1.

Various mechanisms have been proposed to explain the stress reductions following physical activity.

www.mhhe.com/hper/physed/clw/student/

Numerous studies have examined the anxiety-reducing effects of physical activity. Because physical activity leads to a variety of changes in the mind and body, it has proven difficult to identify the mechanisms through which it exerts its effect. Some of the leading theories are described here:

- *Distraction (**time-out hypothesis**):* Physical activity provides a break from the demands of normal life. This change in focus may allow the brain to process or reinterpret stressful scenarios or to relax. This theory would suggest that participating in other focused activities (e.g., playing the piano) may have similar beneficial effects on stress.
- *Increased endorphins. (**endorphin** hypothesis):* The evidence is equivocal but some research has suggested that exercise causes the release of natural painkilling chemicals known as endorphins that may be related to the affective changes in mood.
- *Neurotransmitter hypothesis:* Regular physical activity reduces the levels of catecholamines (epinephrine and norepinephrine) and cortisol, hormones involved in the stress response. Thus, regular bouts of activity can reduce the end result of stress. Some evidence indicates that physical activity also influences levels of other neurotransmitters, such as dopamine, that are associated with relaxation.

- *Self-esteem hypothesis:* For many people, the completion of a task like exercise boosts confidence and a sense of self-mastery. These perceptions can boost self-esteem and help people feel better about themselves and their situation.
- *Thermogenic hypothesis:* During exercise, the body's core temperature increases as a result of the increased muscular activity. There is some evidence that these elevations may produce therapeutic benefits. Many people report that a sauna or warm shower can promote relaxation—possibly by the same mechanism.

The Facts about Conscious Relaxation Techniques

Conscious relaxation techniques can be an effective way to combat stress.

Conscious relaxation techniques reduce stress and tension by directly altering the symptoms. When you are stressed, heart rate, blood pressure, and muscle tension all increase to help your body deal with the challenge. Conscious relaxation techniques act to reduce these normal effects and bring the body back to a more relaxed state. Most techniques employ the "three Rs" of relaxation to help the body relax: (1) reduce mental activity, (2) recognize tension, and (3) reduce respiration. Because these techniques do not change the nature or impact of a stressor, they are considered to be a passive or emotion-focused coping strategy.

There are a variety of conscious relaxation techniques.

Five examples of these techniques are described here:

- *"The Quick Fix"*—To get relief from a stressful situation during the day, take a timeout for 5 or 10 minutes by finding a quiet place away from the situation with as

Time-Out Hypothesis A possible mechanism for the beneficial effects of exercise on stress.

Endorphins Hormones released by the body during periods of stress or exertion that are thought to suppress pain and promote relaxation.

Table 1
Relaxation Exercises

1. Neck Stretch

Roll the head slowly in a half-circle from 9:00 to 8:00 to 7, 6, 5, 4, and 3, then reverse from 3 to 9. Close your eyes and feel the stretch. Do *not* make a full circle by tipping the head back. Repeat several times.

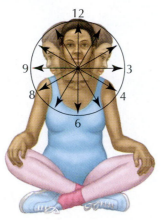

2. Shoulder Lift

Hunch the shoulders as high as possible (contract) and then let them drop (relax). Repeat several times. Inhale on the lift; exhale on the drop.

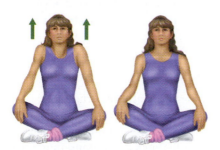

4. Trunk Swings

Following the trunk stretch and drop (see illustration 3), remain in the "drop" position and with a minimum of muscular effort, set the trunk swinging from side to side by shifting the weight from one foot to the other, letting the heels come off the floor alternately. Keep the entire body (especially the neck) limp.

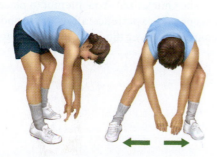

3. Trunk Stretch and Drop

Stand and reach as high as possible; tiptoe and stretch every muscle, then collapse completely, letting knees flex and trunk, head, and arms dangle. Repeat two or three times. Inhale on the stretch and exhale on the collapse.

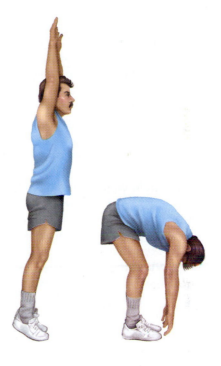

5. Tension Contrast

With arms extended overhead, lie on your side. Tense the body as stiff as a board, then let go and relax, letting the body fall either forward or backward in whatever direction it loses balance. Continue letting go for a few seconds after falling and allow yourself to feel like you are still sinking. Repeat on the other side.

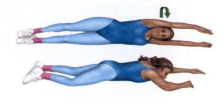

few distractions as possible. Sit, loosen your clothes, take off your shoes, and close your eyes. Then follow these steps: (1) Inhale deeply for about 4 seconds; then exhale, letting the air out slowly for about 8 seconds (twice as long as the inhalation). Do this several times. (2) Mentally visualize a pleasant image, such as a peaceful lake or stream; continue to relax and breathe deeply. (3) When your time is up, breathe deeply and stretch luxuriously; go back to your work refreshed and with a changed attitude. You may need to do this several times a day.

- *Jacobson's Progressive Relaxation Method*—You must be able to recognize how a tense muscle feels before you can voluntarily release the tension. In this technique, contract the muscles strongly, then relax. Each of the large muscles is relaxed first, and later the small ones. The contractions are gradually reduced in intensity until no movement is visible. Always, the emphasis is placed on detecting the feeling of tension as the first step in "letting go," or "going negative." Jacobson, a pioneer in muscle relaxation research, emphasized the importance of relaxing eye and speech muscles, because he believed these muscles trigger reactions of the total organism more than other muscles. A sample contract-relax exercise routine for relaxation is presented in Lab 19B.

- *Autogenic (Self-generated) Relaxation Training*—Several times daily, sit or lie in a quiet room with eyes closed. Block out distracting thoughts by passively concentrating on preselected words or phrases. This technique has been used to focus on heaviness of limbs, warmth of limbs, heart rate regulation, respiratory rate and depth regulation, and coolness in the forehead. It evokes changes opposite to those produced by stress. Research has shown that people who are skilled in this technique can decrease oxygen consumption, change the electrical activity of the brain, slow the metabolism, decrease blood lactate, lower body temperature, and slow the heart rate.

- *Biofeedback–Autogenic Relaxation Training*—Biofeedback training utilizes machines that monitor certain physiological processes of the body and provide visual or auditory evidence of what is happening to normally unconscious bodily functions. When combined with autogenic training, subjects have learned to relax and reduce the electrical activity in their muscles, lower blood pressure, decrease heart rate, change their brain waves, and decrease headaches, asthma attacks, and stomach acid secretion. Biofeedback is helpful in treat-

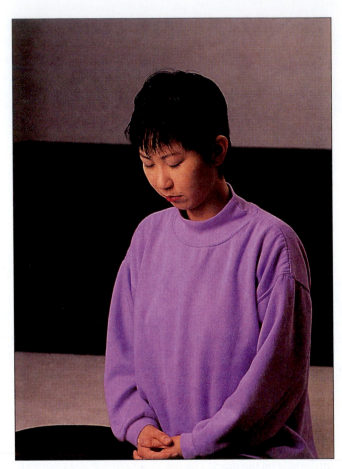

Prayer and meditation can reduce physical symptoms of stress and can help you cope.

ing phobias, stage fright, drug abuse, sexual dysfunction, stuttering, and other psychological problems.

- *Imagery*—Thinking autogenic phrases, you can visualize such feelings as "sinking into a mattress or pillow," or you can think of being a "limp, loose-jointed puppet with no one to hold the strings." You can imagine being a "half-filled sack of flour resting on an uneven surface" or pretend to be "a sack of granulated salt left out in the rain, melting away." Some people seem to respond better to the concept of "floating" than to feeling "heavy." It also includes visualizing pleasant, relaxing scenes as mentioned in the description of "The Quick Fix." You attempt to place yourself in the scene and experience all of the sounds, colors, and scents. Whatever the image you wish to conjure, imagery can help take your mind off anxieties and distractions and, at the same time, release unwanted tension in the muscles using the principle of "mind over matter."

- *Prayer*—Recent studies have shown that prayer can decrease blood pressure for many people and can be a source of internal comfort. It can have other calming effects that are associated with reduced distress. It can also provide confidence to function more effectively, thereby reducing stresses associated with ineffectiveness at work or in other situations.

Some Facts about Muscle Tension and Sleep

> There are a variety of techniques that can reduce muscle tension.

One of the symptoms of stress is muscle tension. Muscle tension can lead to pain, which in turn can negatively influence quality of life, especially for older adults. Various procedures typically used by physical therapists (e.g., ultrasound, heat, cold, and massage) can be helpful in relieving muscle tension. Care should be taken to ensure that these procedures are used properly, typically by experts. Recently, the National Institutes of Health concluded that acupuncture has value in relieving muscle tension and associated pain. Again, it is important that the person administering the treatment have appropriate credentials. Most of the treatments described here are for the relief of already existing muscle tension. They are passive techniques that may give relief to symptoms but may do little to eliminate the cause of the problem.

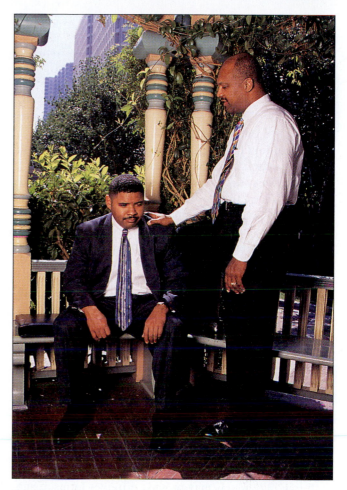

Social support can help a person cope with stress.

> Stress can impair sleep and lack of sleep can be a source of stress.

One of the effects of negative stress is insomnia or inability to sleep. Business pressures, worries about college exams, concerns for loved ones who are ill, and other stressors can cause insomnia. On the other hand, lack of sleep is a stressor itself. Using the coping strategies described in this concept can help people who have insomnia. A common myth is that older people need less sleep than younger people. The amount of sleep you need does not change with age. There are other factors that should also be considered. Some guidelines follow:

- Check with your doctor about medications. Some medicines, such as weight loss pills and decongestants, contain caffeine, ephedrine, or other ingredients that interfere with sleep.
- Avoid tobacco use. Nicotine is a stimulant and can interfere with sleep.
- Avoid excess alcohol use. Alcohol may make it easier to get to sleep but may be a reason why you wake up at night and stay awake.
- Exercise late in the day but do not do vigorous activity right before bedtime.
- Sleep in a room that is cooler than normal.
- Avoid hard-to-digest foods late in the day. Fatty and spicy foods should be avoided.
- Avoid large meals late in the day or right before bedtime. A light snack before bedtime should not be a problem for most people.
- Avoid too much liquid before bedtime.
- Avoid naps during the day.
- Go to bed and get up at the same time each day.

Social Support and Stress Management: The Facts

Social support is important for effective stress management.

Social support has been found to play an important role in coping with stress. Social support has been linked to faster recovery from various medical procedures. One study of athletic injuries has shown that people who were the most stressed were injured more often, and those who had the poorest support system were the most likely to be injured. While the mechanism for this effect is not understood, it is clear that social support plays a major role in stress management. Social support can assist in both active and passive forms of coping. Friends and family can provide very concrete advice that can help solve a problem, and they can also provide moral support and encouragement.

Social support can come from a variety of sources.

Everyone needs someone to turn to for support when feeling overwhelmed. Support can come from friends, family members, clergy, a teacher, a coach, or a professional counselor. Different individuals may provide different forms of support. The goal is to identify and nurture relationships that can provide this type of support. In turn, it is important to look for ways to support and assist others.

There is a variety of types of social support.

Social support can generally be divided into three main components: informational, material, and emotional. Informational (technical support) refers to tips, strategies, or advice that can help a person get through a specific stressful situation. For example, a parent, friend, or coworker may offer insight into how they once resolved similar problems. Material support refers to direct assistance to get a person through a stressful situation. An example would be providing a loan to help pay off a short-term debt. Lastly, emotional support refers to encouragement or sympathy that a person provides to help another cope with a particular challenge. For some stressors all three types of

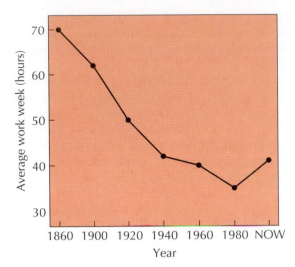

Figure 2

Decreases in working time since 1860.

Compiled from several sources.

social support may be helpful; for others only one or two may be needed.

Obtaining good social support requires close relationships.

While we live in a social environment, it is often difficult to ask people for help. Sometimes the nature and severity of our problems may not be apparent to others. Other times, friends may not want to offer suggestions or insight because they don't want to appear too pushy. To obtain good support, it is important to develop quality personal relationships with several individuals. These individuals will be able to tell when you are stressed and will be willing to help you at times when you need help the most.

The Facts about Work and Leisure

The amount of time the average person spends at work has increased rather than decreased in the last two decades.

Since 1860, the amount of hours typically spent in work decreased dramatically (see Figure 2). The most recent statistics, however, indicate a trend toward increased work time. A major reason for this recent increase is that more people now hold second jobs than in the past. Also, some jobs of modern society have increasing rather than decreasing time demands. For example, medical doctors and other professionals often work more hours than the 35–44 hours that the majority of people work. Also nearly three times as many married women with children work full time now as compared with 1960.

Experts have referred to young adults as the "overworked Americans" because they work several jobs, maintain dual roles (full-time employment coupled with normal family chores), or they work extended hours in demanding professional jobs. A recent Gallup poll shows that the great majority of adults have "enough time" for work, chores, and sleep but not enough time for friends, self, spouse, and children. When time is at a premium, the factors most likely to be negatively affected are personal health, relationships with children, and marriage or romantic relationships.

It is easy to see that work pressures can be stressful. This suggests a need to manage time effectively and to find activities that are enjoyable during free time.

Unenjoyable work detracts from a person's sense of well-being and quality of life.

Many people enjoy the hours they spend at work more than the hours off the job. It is interesting to note, however, that satisfaction at work has dramatically decreased in the last 50 years. The number of people who enjoy work more than nonwork time was twice as high in 1950 as it is in the 1990s. As indicated in the previous concept, disagreements at work and work overload are the second and fourth leading causes of stress. Nevertheless, work is still important to well-being as indicated by the fact that more than 73 percent of all adults would continue to work even if they had enough money to live without working.

Job satisfaction is important to quality living, but an overcommitment to work can result in decreased well-being. In spite of the fact that most young adults feel that they do not have enough free time, the majority say work is more important than recreation. Few (14 percent) would cut their income to have more leisure time.

All nonwork time is *not* free time.

Among some workers, the demands of "other duties" have increased, allowing fewer hours of truly free time each year. **Committed time** has increased for many people, including traveling to and from work, spending extra time at work-related activities that is unpaid, managing the home and care in addition to work outside the home, and transporting the children.

Free time is very important to the average person.

Most people say that **free time** is important, but surveys indicate that more than half of all adults feel that they get too little of it. Many adults report that they get too little time for **recreation** or to simply relax and "do nothing" (leisure).

Recreation and leisure are important contributors to wellness (quality of life).

www.mhhe.com/hper/physed/clw/student/

Leisure is time spent "doing things I just want to do" or "doing nothing." Recreation, on the other hand, is often purposeful. Both leisure and recreation can contribute to stress reduction and wellness, though leisure activities are not done specifically to achieve these benefits.

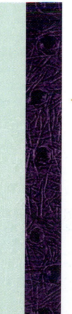

Social Support Any behavior that assists another person in addressing a specific need

Committed Time Time that is committed to specific activity or purpose.

Free Time Time not committed to work or other duties of the day.

Recreation Recreation literally means creating something anew. In this book, it refers to something that you do for your amusement or for fun to help you divert your attention and to refresh yourself (re-create yourself).

Leisure Time that is free from the demands of work is often called leisure time. Leisure is more than free time; it is also an attitude. Leisure activities need not be means to ends (purposeful) but are ends in themselves.

The value of recreation and leisure in the busy lives of people in Western culture is evidenced by the emphasis public health officials place on availability and accessibility of recreational facilities in the future.

To achieve wellness and stress-reduction benefits, recreation should provide a sense of play.

Play is done of one's own free will. It is most often done for fun or intrinsic rather than extrinsic reasons. Activities performed for material things such as trophies and medals can be considered recreational as long as the principal reason for doing the activity is a sense of fun and playfulness. If the activity is done primarily for extrinsic reasons, it may not provide wellness benefits and is probably not true recreation. For example, playing golf to impress the boss is an extrinsic reason that may increase life stress rather than decrease it.

There are many meaningful types of recreation.

www.mhhe.com/hper/physed/clw/student/

Many recreational activities involve moderate to vigorous physical activity. If fitness is the goal, these activities should be chosen. Involvement in nonphysical activities also constitutes recreation. For example, reading is a participation activity that can contribute significantly to other wellness dimensions, such as emotional/mental and spiritual. Passive involvement (spectating) is a third type of participation.

Passive participation has been criticized by some people who feel that active participation is an important ingredient of meaningful recreation. Experts are quick to point out that spectating can be very refreshing and meaningful. For example, watching a good play at the theater qualifies as meaningful recreation and could be true leisure. Likewise, active participation in community theater can be meaningful recreation. To achieve the wellness benefits of recreation, liberal participation and meaningful passive involvement (spectating) are encouraged. Involvement as a spectator does not preclude active participation. However, since free time available for recreation is often limited, excessive spectating can result in decreased active participation. Recent statistics indicate that much of the increase in recreational spending over the past five years is associated with physical activities as evidenced by dramatic increases in money spent for golfing, fitness and sports club memberships, and bowling.

Television viewing has its limitations but is not without its advantages as a recreational activity.

Television is a free-time activity that deserves special mention. Evidence presented elsewhere in this book shows that people who spend a great deal of time watching television tend to be fatter and less physically active than people who spend less time watching television. On the other hand, 58 percent of adults feel that watching television is a "good" use of free time. Nevertheless, as many as four in 10 people feel that they watch too much television. According to a recent Gallup poll, television is still the favorite way to spend an evening for most Americans, and more people feel that television is good rather than bad for society. Like other activities, it can qualify as leisure and recreation, and for many people can be useful in stress reduction.

The Facts about Time Management

Effective time management is essential to adapting to the stresses of modern living.

Many people in our culture lead stress-filled lives and see the need for lifestyle changes but fail to carry out their plans for various reasons. Most often mentioned is the lack of time. "I would like to exercise, but I don't have the time." "My two jobs don't allow me as much time as I would like to spend with my family." "I know I need to relax and enjoy myself, but I just can't find the time." You may never find time to do all of the things you want to do, but you can learn to manage time more effectively to help you cope with the stresses of daily living. In Lab 19E you will get the opportunity to practice the time-management skills outlined in the section that follows.

There are some steps that can be followed to help you manage your time effectively.

Step 1—Establish Priorities

Analyze what you value in life. Most Americans indicate that they want to reduce time spent in work-related activities and spend more time in recreation, at leisure, and with family or friends. Make a list of your priorities. Are these priorities currently being met? Are there activities for which you would like to have more time? Are there people with whom you would like to spend more time?

Step 2—Monitor Your Current Time Use

What we say we value does not always provide the basis for the way we spend our time. Keep a daily log of actual time expenditures to help you see how you could save time to devote to activities you value.

Step 3—Analyze Your Current Time Use

Each day has only 24 hours, and time available for daily activities is fixed. To have more time for priorities, schedules must be modified. Analysis of daily logs can help you determine how you spend your time. Ask yourself these questions:

* *In what activities can I spend less time?* Be honest. It's easy to say you'll spend less time on work, but can you really do it? Sometimes committed time other than work can be the problem. For example, some joggers spend so much time running that they have less time to spend with family.
* *What can I do to reduce time spent in these activities?* Maybe you can "kill two birds with one stone." For example, recreational time could be used to build fitness. Recreational time could also be family time (e.g., jog with the family). The key is finding activities that truly fulfill priorities for everyone involved. Finding work or recreational activities closer to home may save time.

Step 4—Make a Schedule

Writing a daily schedule can help you use time more effectively. This will allow you to enjoy life as a result of meeting priorities and spending time doing the things that enrich life for you and others important to you. A schedule should not be a rigid plan; it should be flexible enough to allow spontaneous activities.

If you cannot adhere to your time schedule, it should be modified. Your plan may not be realistic, and trying to adhere to it could cause you stress. In that case, the schedule is a problem rather than a solution to a problem.

Committed time can also be free time. It is possible to make a commitment to reserve time for activities that are important to you. Taking the time to "re-create" yourself or to enjoy family and friends is important. Sometimes the only way to "find the time" is to plan for it. Charts for helping

you manage time effectively are provided in Lab 19E accompanying this concept.

Strategies for Action: Steps for Stress Management

There are some steps that you can follow to effectively manage stress.

Because everyone responds differently to stressful situations, stress management is a highly individual process. What works for one person may not work for you. The following facts provide steps to manage stress.

The first step in managing stress is to recognize the causes and to be aware of the symptoms.

You need to recognize the situations in your life that are the stressors. Try to identify the things that make you feel "stressed-out." Everything from minor irritations, such as traffic jams, to major life changes, such as births, deaths, or job loss, can be stressors. Or a stress overload of just too many demands on your time can make you feel that you are no longer in control. You may feel so overwhelmed that you become depressed.

Make yourself aware of how your body feels when you are under stress. Are your muscles beginning to tighten? Are you gritting your teeth, gripping the steering wheel tightly, drumming your fingers, tapping your foot, or hunching your shoulders? Can you feel your heart beating faster, your breathing rate becoming faster and more shallow? Are you perspiring, shaking, or getting a headache? By being aware of your most common stressors you will have a better chance of avoiding them or learning how to cope with them. In Lab 19A you will have the opportunity to evaluate muscle tension.

Play Play is something one does of his/her own free will. The play experience is fun, intrinsically rewarding, and a self-absorbing means of self-expression. It is characterized by a sense of freedom or escape from life's normal rules.

The second step is to use some type of relaxation technique or coping strategy for relief of stress.

www.mhhe.com/hper/physed/clw/student/

When you are aware of what stress does to your body, you can do something to relieve those symptoms immediately as well as on a regular and more long-term basis. While there is no magic cure for stress or tension, there are a variety of therapeutic approaches that may be effective in helping you cope with stress. These approaches can slow your heart and respiration, relax tense muscles, clear your mind, and help you relax mentally and emotionally. Perhaps most importantly, these techniques can improve your outlook and help you better cope with the stressful situation. In Lab 19B you will perform a progressive relaxation program. Performing Lab 19B only once will not prepare you to use relaxation techniques effectively. Remember, learning to relax is a skill that must be practiced.

Some treatments are less desirable than others because they act only as "crutches" or "fire extinguishers" and do not get at the root of the problem. Hypnosis may lead to fantasy and dependency. Alcoholic beverages, tranquilizers, and painkillers may give temporary relief and may be prescribed by a physician as part of the treatment, but they do not resolve the problem and may even mask symptoms or cause further problems such as addiction. Drugs do not provide a long-term solution to chronic stress or tension. Contrary to vitamin and mineral advertisements, there are no proven benefits to supplementing the diet with vitamin C or so-called "stress" vitamin formulations. Several different passive relaxation techniques were described earlier, such as massage, heat, deep breathing, and music.

Of course, using coping strategies and finding social support as described earlier in the concept are critical to successful stress management. In Lab 19C you will assess some of your current coping strategies. In Lab 19D you will assess your current support system to help you determine ways in which you can improve it.

The third step is to seek solutions for avoiding or controlling the stress in your life.

While some stressors are unavoidable, much of the stress that we face on a daily basis is self-inflicted and may be somewhat preventable. By taking active control over your lifestyle, you can reduce your risks of experiencing additional stress. Seeking balance and moderation in your lifestyle are good guides toward minimizing stress. Give some priority to proper rest, recreational activities, and diversion in order to prevent burnout. Diversion can be a temporary change from one activity to another (e.g., change from studying to mowing the lawn) or a change of scenery.

Depending on your situation and personality, reducing future exposure to stress may require additional changes in your work habits or interaction style. For example, if you are a person who responds to stress by working harder, then better time management may be an important way to prevent additional stress. If you are a person who can't say no, then assertiveness training may be beneficial. You may even need a change of job or a vacation.

The fourth step is to be as fit and healthy as possible.

The more fit and healthy you are, the better able you are to cope with stress. Selye suggested that physical fitness serves as an inoculation against stress; others have called it a "buffer." A healthy diet and proper rest also are important in managing stress. Leading a healthy lifestyle can help you cope with current stressors and can also help you avoid additional stress in the future

Web Review

Web review materials for Concept 19 are available are at *www.mhhe.com/hper/physed/clw/student/*.

American Institute of Stress
   www.stress.org
American Psychological Association
   www.apa.org
National Institute of Mental Health
   www.gopher.nimh.nih.gov/
Stress Management Education
   www.unl.edu/stress/mgmt

Suggested Readings

Blonna, R. *Coping with Stress in a Changing World.* St. Louis, MO: WCB/McGraw-Hill, 1996.

Coleman, D., and Gurin, J., eds. *Mind/Body Medicine.* Fairfield, OH: Consumer Reports Books, 1993.

Corbin, D. E. (ed.). *Perspectives: Stress Management.* Boulder, CO: Coursewise Publishing Co., 1999.

Girdano, D. and Everly, G. *Controlling Stress and Tension: A Holistic Approach* (5th ed.). Englewood Cliffs, NJ: Prentice-Hall, 1996.

Greenberg, J. S. *Comprehensive Stress Management,* 6th ed. Dubuque, IA: McGraw-Hill, 1999.

Jacobson, E. *You Must Relax.* New York: McGraw-Hill, 1978.

O'Grady, D. *Taking the Fear Out of Change.* Rainier, WA: Adams Publishing, 1995.

Ortal, M. and Sherman, C. "Exercise Against Depression," *Physician and Sportsmedicine* 26(10)(1998):55.

Petruzzello, et al. "A Meta-Analysis on the Anxiety-Reducing Effects of Acute and Chronic Exercise," *Sports Medicine* 11(1991):143–182.

Selye, H. *The Stress of Life,* 2d ed. New York: McGraw-Hill, 1978.

U.S. Department of Health and Human Services. *Healthy People 2010 Objectives: Draft for Comment.* Washington, DC: U.S. Department of Health and Human Services, 1998, Objectives Chapter 23: Mental Health and Mental Disorders.

Williams, R. and Williams, V. *Anger Kills: 17 Strategies for Controlling Hostility that Can Harm You.* New York: Times Books/Random House, 1994.

Lab 19A: Evaluating Neuromuscular Tension

Name	**Section**	**Date**

Purpose: To learn to recognize signs of excess muscle tension.

Procedure:
1. Choose a partner. Designate one partner as the subject and the other as the tester.
2. The subject should lie supine in a comfortable position and consciously try to relax.
3. The tester should kneel beside the subject's right hand and remain very still and quiet while the subject is concentrating.
4. After 5 minutes have elapsed, the tester should observe the subject for signs of tension in Part A of Chart 1 and check "yes" or "no" for symptoms of visual tension.
5. Quietly and gently, the tester should grasp the subject's right wrist with his or her fingers, and slowly raise it about 3 inches from the floor, letting it hinge at the elbow, then let the hand drop. Observe the signs of tension outlined in Part B of Chart 1. *Caution:* Make no movement or sound to disturb your partner's concentration and relaxation. Check Chart 1, Section B, manual systems of tension.
6. You may wish to repeat this after another minute or two.
7. Arouse the subject at the end of the testing and total the number of "yes" checks.
8. Find the rating in Chart 2 and record it on the back of this sheet.
9. Change roles and repeat the evaluation with a new subject and tester.
10. Answer the questions in the Results and Conclusions and Implications section.
11. If time permits, perform the exercises from Table 1 in the concept.

Results:

Check one circle for each of the following questions.

Yes	No	
◯	◯	Were you aware of your own tension?
◯	◯	Was it more difficult to relax than you expected?
◯	◯	Did your awareness of your partner make it more difficult to concentrate?
◯	◯	Could you concentrate on your breathing without altering its rhythm?
◯	◯	Could you learn to release muscular tension and help manage your stress with additional practice?
◯	◯	Could you learn to release tension while sitting or standing with your eyes open?
◯	◯	Do you think your score today is typical of your normal tension level?

Chart 1 Signs of Tension Observed by Tester

Visual Symptoms	No	Yes
Frowning	◯	◯
Twitching	◯	◯
Eyelids fluttering	◯	◯
Breathing	◯	◯
shallow	◯	◯
rapid	◯	◯
irregular	◯	◯
Mouth tight	◯	◯
Swallowing	◯	◯

Manual Symptoms	No	Yes
Assistance (subject helps lift arm)	◯	◯
Resistance (subject resists movement)	◯	◯
Posturing (subject holds arm in raised position)	◯	◯
Perseveration (subject continues upward movement)	◯	◯

Total score equals sum of "yes" checks [ ]

Chart 2 Tension-Relaxation Rating Scale

Classification	Total Score
Excellent (relaxed)	0
Very good (mild tension)	1–3
Good (moderate tension)	4–6
Fair (tense)	7–9
Poor (marked tension)	10–12

Record Your Tension-Relaxation Rating [ ]

Conclusions and Implications:

In several sentences, describe the implications this lab has for you in terms of your daily life (e.g., sleeping, studying, taking exams, performing on stage, etc.)?

Lab 19B: Relaxing Tense Muscles

Name	Section	Date

Purpose: To learn how to relax tense muscles.

Procedure:

Part I

1. Lie on your back in a quiet, nondistracting atmosphere while you are learning this relaxation technique. (Later, you will want to be able to use the technique in public, everyday situations, while you are at work, or any time you are under stress.) Get as comfortable as possible. Close your eyes.

2. Do the Contract-Relax Exercise Routine for Relaxation. Contract the muscles to a moderate level of tension (do not use maximum contractions) as you inhale for 5 to 7 seconds. Study where you are feeling the tension. Try to keep the tension isolated to the designated muscle group without allowing it to spill over to other muscles. Use the dominant side of the body first; repeat on the nondominant side.

3. Next, release the tension completely, instantly relaxing the muscles, and exhale. Extend the feeling of relaxation throughout your muscles for 20 to 30 seconds before contracting again. Think of relaxation words like "warm," "calm," "peaceful," and "serene."

4. If time permits, you should practice each muscle group two to five times (until tension is gone) before proceeding to the next group. In a class, you may only have time for one trial. For home practice, do the routine twice a day for 15 minutes.

Contract-Relax Exercise Routine for Relaxation

1. Hand and forearm—Contract your right hand, making a fist; hold 3 counts; relax and keep letting go 6–10 counts. Repeat, then do left fist, then both fists.

2. Biceps—Flex both elbows and contract your biceps; hold 3 counts; relax and continue relaxing 6–10 counts. Repeat.

3. Triceps—Extend both elbows, contract the triceps on the back of the arm. Hold 3 counts; relax 6–10 counts. Repeat.

4. Relax both hands, forearms, and upper arms.

5. Forehead—Raise your eyebrows and wrinkle your forehead; hold 3 counts; relax and continue relaxing 6–10 counts.

6. Cheeks and nose—Make a face; wrinkle your nose and squint; hold 3 counts; relax and continue relaxing 6–10 counts.

7. Jaws—Clench your teeth 3 counts; relax 6–10 counts.

8. Lips and tongue—With teeth apart, press lips together and press tongue to roof of mouth; hold 3 counts; relax 6–10 counts.

9. Neck and throat—Push head backward while tucking chin, pushing against floor or pillow if lying down; if sitting, push against high chairback; hold 3 counts; relax for 6–10 counts.

10. Relax forehead, cheeks, nose, jaws, lips, tongue, neck, and throat. Relax hands, forearms, and upper arms.

11. Shoulder and upper back—Hunch shoulders to ears; hold 3 counts; relax 6–10 counts.

12. Relax lips, tongue, neck, throat, shoulders, and upper back.

13. Abdomen—Suck in abdomen; hold 3 counts; relax 6–10 counts.

14. Lower back—Contract and arch the back; hold 3 counts; relax 6–10 counts.

15. Thighs and buttocks—Squeeze your buttocks together and push your heels into the floor (if lying down) or against a chair rung (if sitting); hold 3 counts; relax 6–10 counts.

16. Relax shoulders and upper back, abdomen, lower back, thighs, and buttocks.

17. Calves—Pull instep and toes toward shins; hold 3 counts; relax 6–10 counts.

18. Toes—Curl toes; hold 3 counts; relax 6–10 counts.

19. Relax every muscle in your body.

Note: Eventually, you should progress to a combination of muscle groups and gradually eliminate the "contract" phase of the program. Refer to Jacobson (1978) or Greenberg (1996).

Part II Perform each of the relaxation exercises that follow (see page 365 for pictures).

1. **Neck Stretch**—Roll the head slowly in a half-circle from 9:00 to 8:00 to 7, 6, 5, 4, and 3, then reverse from 3 to 9. Close your eyes and feel the stretch. Do *not* make a full circle by tipping the head back. Repeat several times.

2. **Shoulder Lift**—Hunch the shoulders as high as possible (contract) and then let them drop (relax). Repeat several times. Inhale on the lift; exhale on the drop.

3. **Trunk Stretch and Drop**—Stand and reach as high as possible; tiptoe and stretch every muscle, then collapse completely, letting knees flex and trunk, head, and arms dangle. Repeat two or three times. Inhale on the stretch and exhale on the collapse.

4. **Trunk Swings**—Following the trunk stretch and drop, remain in the "drop" position and with a minimum of muscular effort, set the trunk swinging from side to side by shifting the weight from one foot to the other, letting the heels come off the floor alternately. Keep the entire body (especially the neck) limp.

5. **Tension Contrast**—With arms extended overhead, lie on your side. Tense the body as stiff as a board, then let go and relax, letting the body fall either forward or backward in whatever direction it loses balance. Continue letting go for a few seconds after falling and allow yourself to feel like you are still sinking. Repeat on the other side.

Results:

  Did you find the relaxation exercises effective?

  Do you think you would find them useful as part of your normal daily routine or as a "quick fix" for stress?

  Did you find the contract-relax exercise routine relaxing?

  Do you think you would find it useful as part of your normal daily routine or as a "quick fix" for stress?

Conclusions and Implications:
In several sentences, discuss whether or not you feel that relaxation exercises will be a part of your wellness program.

Lab 19C: Evaluating Coping Strategies

Name	**Section**	**Date**

Purpose: To learn how to use appropriate coping strategies that work best for you.

Procedures:

1. Think of five recent stressful experiences that caused you some concern, anxiety, or distress. Describe these situations in chart 1. Then use chart 2 to make a rating for changeability, severity, and duration. Assign one number for each category for each situation.
2. In chart 3 place a check for each coping strategy that you used in coping with each of the five situations you described.
3. Answer the questions in the Conclusions and Implications section.

Results:

Chart 1 Stressful Situations

Think of five different recent stressful situations. Appraise each situation and assign a score (changeable, severity, duration) using the scale in chart 2.

	Briefly describe the situation.	Changeable	Severity	Duration
1.				
2.				
3.				
4.				
5.				

Chart 2 Appraisal of the Stressful Situations

Use this chart to rate the five situations you described above. Assign a number for changeability, severity, and duration for each situation in Chart 1.

	1.	2.	3.	4.	5.
Was the situation changeable?	Completely within my control	Mostly within my control	Both in and out of my control	Mostly out of my control	Completely outside of my control
What was the severity of the stress?	Very minor	Fairly minor	Moderate	Fairly major	Very major
What was the duration of the stress?	Short-term (weeks)	Moderately short	Moderate (months)	Moderately long	Long (months to year)

Chart 3 Coping Strategies

Directions: Place a check for each coping strategy you used for each of the five situations you described.

Think about your response to the five stressful situations you recently experienced and check the strategies that you used each situation.	Situation	Situation	Situation	Situation	Situation
Coping Strategy	1	2	3	4	5
1. I apologized or corrected the problem as best I could.					
2. I ignored the problem and hoped that it would go away.					
3. I told myself to forget about it and grew as a person from the experience.					
4. I tried to make myself feel better by eating, drinking, or smoking.					
5. I prayed or sought spiritual meaning from the situation.					
6. I expressed anger to try to change the situation.					
7. I took active steps to make things work out better.					
8. I used music, images, or deep breathing to help me relax.					
9. I tried to keep my feelings to myself and kept moving forward.					
10. I pursued leisure or recreational activity to help me feel better.					
11. I talked to someone who could provide advice or help me with the problem.					
12. I talked to someone about what I was feeling or experiencing.					

Conclusions and Implications:

1. In several sentences, discuss the coping strategies you used. Were they the ones you used the most? The ones you typically use? Were they effective? Would you consider other strategies in the future?

Lab 19D: Evaluating Levels of Social Support

Name	Section	Date

Purpose:
To evaluate your level of social support and to identify ways that you can find additional support.

Procedures:
1. Use chart 1 to get personal social support scores. Answer each question. Place number of answers in score box. Sum these questions for each score.
2. In the Results section, record your scores and rate your social support (use chart 2 for ratings).
3. Use chart 2 to evaluate the quality and nature of your social support network.
4. Answer the questions in the Conclusions and Implications section.

Chart 1 Social Support Questionnaire

The following questions assess various aspects of social support. Base your answer on your actual degree of support, not on the type of support that you would like to have. Place a check in the space that best represents what is true for you.

	Not True	Somewhat True	Very True	
	1	2	3	Score
1. I have close personal ties with my relatives.				
2. I have close relationships with a number of friends.				
3. I have a deep and meaningful relationship with a spouse or close friend.				
Access to social support score:				
4. I have parents and relatives who take the time to listen and understand me.				
5. I have friends or co-workers whom I can confide in and trust when problems come up.				
6. I have a nonjudgmental spouse or close friend who supports me when I need help.				
Degree of social support score:				
7. I feel comfortable asking others for advice or assistance.				
8. I have confidence in my social skills and enjoy opportunities for new social contacts.				
9. I am willing to open up and discuss my personal life with others.				
Getting social support score:				

Scores and Ratings (Use chart 2 to obtain ratings).

Access to social support score [   ]   Rating [   ]

Degree of social support score [   ]   Rating [   ]

Getting social support score [   ]   Rating [   ]

Total social support score [   ]   Rating [   ]
(sum of three scores)

Results:

Chart 2 Rating Scale for Social Support		
Rating	**Item Scores**	**Total Score**
High	8–9	24–27
Moderate	6–7	18–23
Low	Below 6	Below 18

Conclusions and Implications:

1. In several sentences, discuss your overall social support. Do you think your scores and ratings are a true representation of your social support?

2. In several sentences, describe any changes you think you should make to improve your social support system. If you do not think change is necessary, explain why.

Lab 19E: Time Management

Name	**Section**	**Date**

Purpose: To help you learn to manage time to meet personal priorities.

Procedure:
1. Follow the four steps outlined in chart 1 in the Results section.
2. Answer the questions in the Conclusions and Implications section.

Results:

Chart 1 Time Management

Step 1: Establishing Priorities

1. Check circles that reflect your priorities from the list below. Add priorities as necessary.

2. Rate each of the priorities you checked. Use a 1 for highest priority, a 2 for moderate priority, and 3 for low priority.

Check Priorities	*Rating*	*Check Priorities*	*Rating*	*Check Priorities*	*Rating*
◯ more time with family		◯ more time with boy/girlfriend		◯ more time with spouse	
◯ more time for leisure		◯ more time to relax		◯ more time to study	
◯ more time for work success		◯ more time for physical activity		◯ more time to improve myself	
◯ more time for other recreation		◯ other _____		◯ other _____	

Step 2: Monitor Current Time Use

1. On the daily calendar, keep track of daily time expenditure.

2. Write in exactly what you did for each time block.

7–9 A.M.	9–11 A.M.	11 A.M.–1 P.M.	1–3 P.M.
3–5 P.M.	5–7 P.M.	7–9 P.M.	9–11 P.M.

Chart 1 Time Management *(continued)*

Step 3: Analyze Your Current Time Use

Where can I spend less time? (write below)

Where do I need to spend more time? (write below)

Step 4: Make a Schedule. Write in Your Planned Activities for the Day.

7–9 A.M.	9–11 A.M.	11 A.M.–1 P.M.	1–3 P.M.
3–5 P.M.	5–7 P.M.	7–9 P.M.	9–11 P.M.

Conclusions and Implications:

In several sentences, discuss how you might modify your schedule to find more time for important priorities.

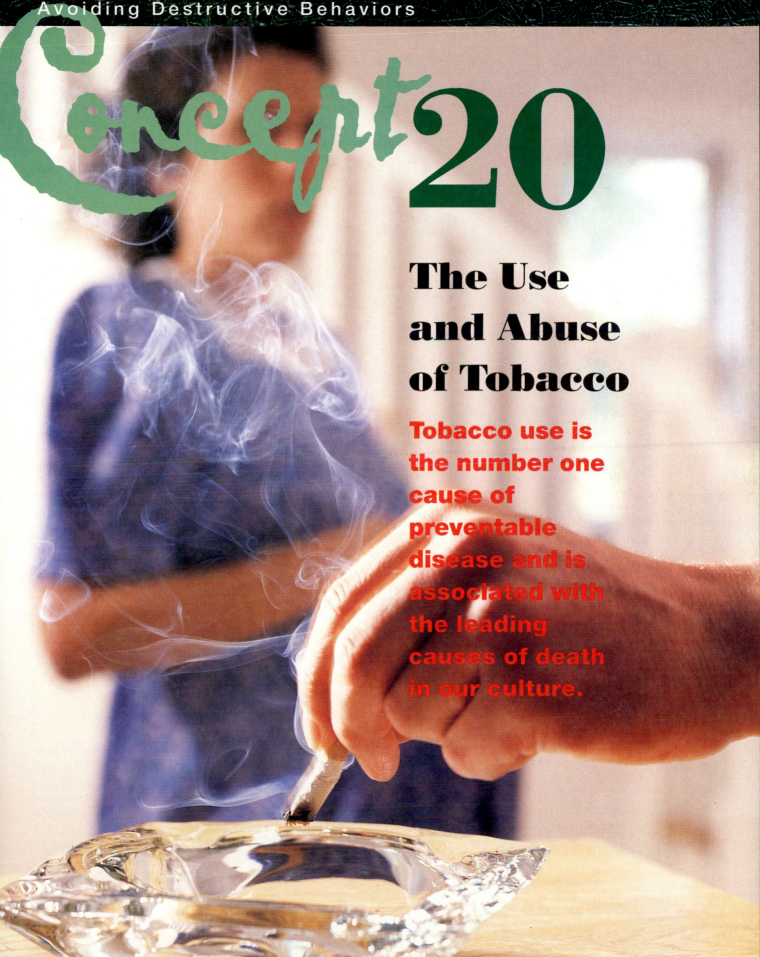

Concept 20

The Use and Abuse of Tobacco

Tobacco use is the number one cause of preventable disease and is associated with the leading causes of death in our culture.

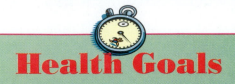

Health Goals

for year 2010

Reduce disease, disability, and death related to tobacco use and exposure to secondhand smoke.

Prevent initiation of tobacco use.

Reduce proportion of people who use tobacco products (especially pregnant women, new mothers, young people, and military personnel).

Reduce exposure to secondhand smoke.

Change social norms and environments that support tobacco use.

Increase proportion of smokers who have stopped for a day.

Increase proportion of smokers who have stopped for a month.

Increase education to decrease tobacco use.

Introduction

Tobacco is the number one cause of preventable mortality in the United States. It is linked to most of the leading causes of death and also leads to a variety of other chronic conditions. Rates of smoking in the United States have decreased in recent decades due to better awareness and a changed social norm concerning smoking and tobacco use. Despite the progress, smoking is still a major public health problem. Estimates suggest that there are approximately 62 million smokers in the United States. The majority of smokers would prefer to quit but find it too difficult to free themselves from the grip of nicotine addiction. This concept will review the health risks of tobacco use and provide practical guidelines for quitting.

The Facts about Tobacco and Nicotine

Tobacco and its smoke contain over 400 noxious chemicals, including 200 known poisons and 50 carcinogens.

Tobacco smoke contains both gases and particulates. During one phase of burning tobacco (the gaseous phase), a variety of gases dangerous to humans are released. The most dangerous is carbon monoxide. This gas binds onto hemoglobin in the bloodstream and thereby limits how much oxygen can be carried in the bloodstream. The regular exposure to carbon monoxide by smokers contributes to the "winded" feeling that smokers experience during physical activity. While not likely from smoking, overexposure to carbon monoxide can be fatal.

The other phase that occurs when tobacco is burned is the particulate phase. This phase releases a variety of particulates that contain a variety of carbon-based compounds referred to as tar. Many of these compounds are known to be **carcinogenic.** Cigarettes have nearly 2,000 times more benzene contamination than the Perrier water that was recalled years ago because it had benzene levels that were above health standards. Nicotine is also inhaled during the particulate phase of smoking. Nicotine is a highly addictive and poisonous chemical (often used in insecticides). It has a particularly broad range of influence and is a potent and powerful psychoactive **drug** that affects the brain and alters mood and behavior (see next fact).

Nicotine is the addictive component of tobacco.

When smoke is inhaled, the nicotine reaches the brain in seven seconds, where it acts on highly sensitive receptors and provides a sensation that brings about a wide variety of responses throughout the body. At first there is an increase in heart and breathing rates. Blood vessels constrict, peripheral circulation (especially to the hands and feet) slows down, and blood pressure increases. (New users may experience dizziness, nausea, and headache.) Then, feelings of tension and tiredness are relieved.

After a few minutes, the feeling wears off and a rebound or **withdrawal** effect occurs. The smoker may feel depressed and irritable and have the urge to smoke again. **Addiction** occurs with continued use. Nicotine is one of the most addictive drugs known—even more addictive than heroin or alcohol.

Nicotine has varying effects on mood and arousal.

Nicotine can act as a stimulant or a sedative, depending upon the smoker's circumstances. As a stimulant, nicotine may cause the smoker to experience an energetic feeling. On the other hand, it may increase the alpha waves in the brain and trigger the release of endorphins, producing feelings of relaxation. Whether it acts as a stimulant or sedative depends on the dose, the smoker's metabolism, the amount of stress the smoker is experiencing, and the time of day. It tends to stimulate in the morning and sedate in the afternoon.

Smokeless chewing tobacco is as addictive (and maybe more so) as smoking and produces the same kind of withdrawal symptoms upon quitting.

Chewing tobacco comes in a variety of forms including loose leaf, twist, or plug form. Rather than being smoked, the "chaw," "wad," or "quid" stays in the mouth for several hours, where it mixes with saliva and is absorbed into the bloodstream. Smokeless tobacco contains about seven times more nicotine than cigarettes, and more of it is absorbed because of the length of time the tobacco is in the mouth. It also contains a higher level of carcinogens than cigarettes.

Snuff, a form of smokeless tobacco, comes in either dry or moist forms. Dry snuff is powdered tobacco mixed with flavorings, designed to be "sniffed," "pinched," or "dipped." Moist snuff is used the same way, but it is moist, finely cut tobacco in a loose form or in a teabag–like packet. It comes in a variety of flavors. Experts believe that the flavoring of smokeless tobacco is designed to attract young users.

The Health Risks of Tobacco: The Facts

Smoking is the most preventable cause of death in our society.

www.mhhe.com/hper/physed/clw/student/
Smoking is the leading known cause of lung cancer (causing 90 percent of all lung cancer deaths) and is related to seven other cancers. The American Cancer Society estimates that tobacco usage contributes to over 30 percent of all cancer deaths. The American Heart Association also classifies smoking as a major risk factor for cardiovascular disease. Chemicals in tobacco smoke increase blood pressure, promote atherosclerosis, and increase the clotting of blood, which can lead to a heart attack. Smokers are five times more likely to suffer heart attacks in their 30s and 40s than nonsmokers. Among other adult age groups, the risk of a heart attack is doubled in smokers who smoke more than a pack a day. In addition to these major risks, smokers are at an increased risk for a variety of other medical problems (see Table 1).

Overall, smoking causes over 400,000 deaths per year; that is, about 1,000 people die per day of the health problems related to smoking. This is more Americans than were killed in World War II. It is not just an American problem. Worldwide, 2.5 to 3 million people die annually from smoking. According to the World Health Organization, smoking causes 20 percent of all deaths in the United States.

Table 1 Unhealthy Effects of Smoking

- It is the number one avoidable cause of mortality in the United States
- It is the number one cause of lung cancer deaths in the United States
- It is the number one cause of cancer in women.
- It is the number one cause of cancer of the esophagus (especially when combined with alcohol).
- It is the number one cause of cancer of the kidney.
- It is the number one cause of pancreatic cancer.
- It increases risk of cancer of the oral cavity.
- It increases risk of cancer of the larynx.
- It increases risk of fatal breast cancer.
- It increases risk of leukemia.
- It increases risk of cancer of the urinary bladder.
- It increases risk of heart attack and heart disease.
- It increases risk of atherosclerosis.
- It increases risk of Type II diabetes.
- It increases risk of stomach ulcers.
- It increases risk of chronic bronchitis and emphysema.
- It increases risk of miscarriage, infant death, and other complications in pregnant women.
- It causes 88 million more days of sickness per year than for nonsmokers.
- Every cigarette shortens a smoker's life by 1 minute.
- It decreases the HDL in the blood.

The health risks from tobacco are directly related to overall exposure.

In past years, tobacco companies denied that there was conclusive proof of the harmful effects of tobacco products. Now, in the face of overwhelming medical evidence, tobacco officials have finally conceded that tobacco is

Carcinogen A substance thought to promote or facilitate the growth of cancerous cells.

Drug Any biologically active substance that is foreign to the body and is deliberately introduced to affect its functioning.

Withdrawal A temporary illness precipitated by the lack of a drug in the body of an addicted person.

Addiction A drug-induced condition in which a person requires frequent administration of a drug in order to avoid withdrawal.

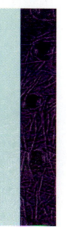

harmful to health. It is now clear that the more you use the product (the more doses), the greater the health risk. Several factors determine the dosage: (1) the number of cigarettes smoked; (2) the length of time one has been smoking; (3) the strength (amount of tar, nicotine, etc.) of the cigarette; (4) the depth of the inhalation; and (5) the amount of exposure to other lung-damaging substances (e.g., asbestos). The greater the exposure of smoke, the greater the risk.

Cigar and pipe smokers have lower death rates than cigarette smokers but still are at great risk.

Cigar and pipe smokers usually inhale less and therefore have less risk of heart and lung disease, but cigarette smokers who switch to cigars and pipes tend to continue inhaling the same way and may not decrease their risk appreciably. Cigar and pipe smoke contains most of the same harmful ingredients of cigarette smoke, sometimes in higher amounts, so smokers who do inhale have an even greater risk of dying from lung or heart disease. The little cigars that resemble cigarettes tend to be inhaled like cigarettes, so they are especially dangerous because of a very high nicotine and tar content.

Cigar and pipe smokers have higher risks of cancer of the mouth, throat, and larynx than the cigarette smoker. Pipe smokers are especially at risk for lip cancer. Pipe smoking is less acceptable socially because of the strong odor and more irritating smoke, but cigar smoking has become quite trendy in recent years. Some people seem to associate the smoking of cigars with power and influence. Cigars pollute the air much more than cigarettes. One study has shown that in 30 minutes, one cigar can pollute the air more than 42 cigarettes.

All smokers pollute the air that everyone must breathe.

When a smoker lights up, individuals around him or her are exposed to **secondhand** smoke. Secondhand smoke is a combination of both **mainstream** and **sidestream** smoke. Sidestream smoke is considered more dangerous than mainstream smoke because it contains higher concentrations of 13 carcinogens, plus other harmful substances, including nicotine, tar, and carbon monoxide. Its carbon monoxide levels are reported to be from two to fifteen times greater than in the mainstream smoke. Carbon monoxide robs the blood of oxygen. Offices where smoking is allowed may have triple the amount of nicotine level considered hazardous. Emphysema, hypertension, and chronic bronchitis have been related to large doses of cadmium (a carcinogen).

The odor of tobacco smoke presents an additional environmental irritant. It clings to hair, skin, and clothes. Smokers tend to be unaware of the odor because of their

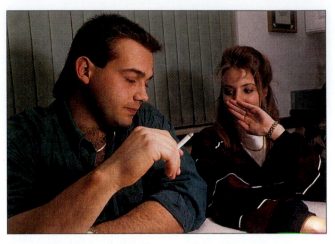

Secondhand smoke makes us all involuntary smokers.

impaired sense of smell, but to the nonsmoker it is irritating and offensive. While smokeless tobacco does not pollute the air like smoking, most nonusers dislike the spitting and the bad breath of users.

Secondhand smoke poses a significant health risk

www.mhhe.com/hper/physed/clw/student/

Nonsmokers who must breathe secondhand smoke are in fact "involuntary" or "passive" smokers and can suffer serious health problems, especially if they are repeatedly exposed to tobacco smoke over long periods of time. The Environmental Protection Agency (EPA) estimated as many as 3,800 lung cancer deaths per year could be attributed to secondhand smoke. Passive smoking has also been found to increase the risk of heart attacks, causing 35,000–40,000 deaths per year in the United States. The EPA suggested a direct link between secondhand smoke and asthma. It is believed that smoke accounts for serious respiratory ailments in as many as 200,000 children. The National Center for Health Statistics found that children in nonsmoking households are likely to be healthier and miss fewer days of school than children who live with smokers. Evidence also indicates that the divorce rate is significantly higher among smokers than nonsmokers. Because of these effects, the EPA has classified secondhand smoke as a serious environmental problem.

While not technically considered as secondhand exposure, smoking during pregnancy can also harm a developing fetus or newborn baby. Studies suggest that smoking contributes to increased rates of premature births. Mothers who smoke are also found to be less likely to nurse their baby, and if they do nurse, the duration of nursing tends to be less than for nonsmoking women.

Table 2 Health Risks of Smokeless
Tobacco

Smokeless tobacco increases the risk of:

- Oral cavity cancer (cheek, gum, lip, palate). It increases the risk by 4–50 times, depending on length of time used.
- Cancer of the throat, larynx, and esophagus.
- Precancerous skin changes.
- High blood pressure.
- Rotting teeth, exposed roots, premature tooth loss, worn-down teeth.
- Ulcerated, inflamed, infected gums.
- Slow healing of mouth wounds.
- Decreased resistance to infections.
- Arteriosclerosis, myocardial infarction, and coronary occlusion.
- Widespread hormonal effects, including increased lipids, higher blood sugar, and more blood clots.
- Increased heart rate.

Smokeless tobacco has similar health risks to other forms of tobacco.

Some smokers switch to smokeless tobacco because of the misconception that it is a safe substitute for cigarette, cigar, and pipe smoking. While smokeless tobacco does not lead to the same respiratory problems as smoking, the other health risks may be even greater because smokeless tobacco has more nicotine and higher levels of carcinogens. Because it comes in direct contact with body tissues, the health consequences are far more immediate than those from smoking cigarettes. One-third of teenage users have receding gums, and about half have precancerous lesions, 20 percent of which can become oral cancer within five years. Some of the health risks of smokeless tobacco are listed in Table 2.

The Facts about Tobacco Usage

Smoking was an accepted part of our culture, but the social norm has changed greatly in recent years.

www.mhhe.com/hper/physed/clw/student/

Tobacco was one of the primary cash crops among the 13 original colonies of the United States. While smoking has always been a part of our culture, the industrialization and marketing in the mid-

dle of the twentieth century led to tremendous social acceptance of smoking. As paradoxical as it may sound, cigarettes were once provided to airline passengers for free when they boarded planes. The release of the *Surgeon General's Report* on smoking in 1964 and an aggressive and well-funded anti-smoking campaign from various public health agencies have contributed to greatly reduced smoking rates in our country. Rates in the United States have declined from a high of over 50 percent in the 1950s to current levels of about 27 percent. Worldwide, the rates of smoking are much higher than they are in the United States. For example, in China, 75 percent of adult males are smokers.

The use of smokeless tobacco is not as prevalent as smoking, but the National Institute of Drug Abuse estimates 22 million Americans (mostly males) have used it. Clearly more men use smokeless tobacco than women. Also young people are among the frequent users. The percentage of smokeless tobacco users ranges widely from state to state. For example, over 23 percent of West Virginians used smokeless tobacco, whereas the percentage of users in the District of Columbia is close to zero.

Most tobacco users begin "using" during adolescence and find it hard to quit.

www.mhhe.com/hper/physed/clw/student/

The initiation of smoking is viewed as a pediatric problem by most public health experts. According to a recent report from the Centers for Disease Control, 6,000 people every day under the age of 19 try their first cigarette. At least 3,000 adolescents a day reach adulthood (over the age of 19) as confirmed cigarette smokers. Overall, 90 percent of smokers began before the age of nineteen. This is the group that finds it most difficult to break the habit later in life.

While tremendous progress has been made in recent years to reduce the prevalence of smoking, some evidence suggests that the rates of smoking are on the rise among adolescents. The percentage of adolescents (ages 12–17) who reported trying a cigarette increased by 30 percent from 1988 to 1996. The percentage of adolescents who reported daily use increased by 50 percent during that same time

Secondhand smoke A combination of mainstream and sidestream smoke.

Mainstream smoke Smoke that is exhaled after being filtered by the smoker's lungs.

Sidestream smoke Smoke that comes directly off the burning end of the cigarette/cigar/pipe.

span. Much of the blame for tobacco use among adolescents has been attributed to the tobacco industry. According to former Surgeon General C. Everett Koop, the tobacco industry has a marketing budget of more than $5 billion per year. Reports from internal tobacco documents released during lawsuits indicate that much of this marketing is focused on youth. In general, the tobacco industry portrays tobacco use as fun, macho, stylish, sexy, and the "cool" thing to do. Studies show that 60 percent of high school juniors and 40 percent of high school seniors do not believe there is a risk in smoking or using smokeless tobacco.

Smokeless tobacco use also begins early in life. Fifty percent of the users report that they started before the age of 13. There is some indication of a recent increase in use. The nationwide use of smokeless tobacco among 8–12 graders has ranged from a low of 3.3 percent to a high of 4.4 percent in 1997.

Health-problems associated with tobacco use have resulted in legal settlements for damages.

Over 40 states have sued the tobacco industry to recoup funds spent by Medicaid for people with smoking-related diseases. Several states have reached settlements of hundreds of millions of dollars. A federal settlement has not been reached, so individual states are continuing with their lawsuits. In the Minnesota case, millions of pages of tobacco industry documents were made public, and they revealed that in many instances the tobacco industry was targeting youth in their marketing, despite years of denial.

A variety of factors have been found to influence a person's decision to begin or quit smoking.

www.mhhe.com/hper/physed/clw/student/
The reasons for starting smoking are varied, but strikingly similar to reasons given for using alcohol and other drugs (see Table 3). Once a person starts, he or she will typically find it difficult to quit. While a variety of smoking cessation programs are available, several studies have found that increasing the price of cigarettes is the most successful method of reducing smoking among youth. A recent survey of 35,000 high school students revealed that 38 percent felt that higher prices for cigarettes would help to reduce teen smoking.

Weight loss is not a good reason for smoking.

It is believed that more than a few people, especially young girls, begin smoking because they feel that it will help them

Table 3 Why Young People Start Using Tobacco
• Peer influence.
• Social acceptance.
• Desire to be "mature."
• Desire to be "independent."
• Desire to be like their role models.
• It looks appealing in advertisements.

control their weight and body fatness. It is known, for example, that models and dancers have a high incidence of smoking, and the desire to keep weight down is given as a common reason. Some smokers feel that they are unable to quit because they fear gaining weight. The evidence shows that people who smoke do not have a lower weight over the long term than nonsmokers. People who fear weight gain should especially not begin smoking, and those who currently smoke may need psychological help when quitting smoking to help overcome fears about weight gain.

There is a tendency for people who smoke cigarettes to also use alcohol, marijuana, and hard drugs.

More smokers use other drugs than do nonsmokers. This is particularly true of the college age (18–25). The reasons are not clear, but it may be that people who do not smoke have a better understanding of the health risks, have better self-esteem, and have better support systems of family and friends. Also they may have learned how to say no without giving in to the pressures and lures that make the smokers use tobacco in the first place (Table 3).

Strategies for Action: The Facts about Quitting

The addictive nature of nicotine makes it difficult to quit using tobacco.

When a person first stops using tobacco, some of the withdrawal symptoms listed in Table 4 occur. Because people react differently, a person may experience only a few or all of the symptoms. The length of time it takes to recover from the symptoms varies from days to weeks or months. Most

Table 4 Tobacco Withdrawal Symptoms

- Craving for tobacco
- Anxiety
- Headaches
- Gastrointestinal discomfort
- Mood changes
- Irritability
- Difficulty sleeping
- Difficulty concentrating
- Tremors
- Changes in appetite
- Craving for sweets

people do not succeed the first time they try to quit. The important thing is to keep trying, because most people who try will eventually succeed. More than 46 million Americans have quit smoking.

There are some techniques and strategies that increase the probability of breaking the nicotine addiction.

The following tips should be useful to those who wish to quit using tobacco:

- You must want to quit. This is the most important thing. The reasons could be for health, family, money, etc.
- Remind yourself of the reasons. Each day, repeat to yourself the reasons for not using tobacco.
- Decide how to stop. Some ways to stop include counseling, attending formal programs, quitting with another smoker friend, going "cold turkey" (abruptly), quitting gradually. More people succeed "cold turkey" than with the gradual approach.
- Remove reminders and temptations. Get rid of ashtrays, tobacco, etc.
- Use substitutes and distractions. Substitute low-calorie snacks or chewing gum, change your routine, try new activities, and sit in nonsmoking areas.
- Don't worry about gaining weight. If you gain a few pounds, it is not as detrimental to your health as continuing to smoke.
- Get support. Try a formal "quit smoking program." Examples include "Freedom from Smoking" (American Lung Association) and "Fresh Start" (American Cancer Society). Many state, county, and local health

departments, as well as colleges and universities, have programs. Seek support from friends and relatives.

- Consider a "crutch." If you choose to taper off, you may want to consider a product that requires a prescription, such as a nicotine transdermal patch or nicotine chewing gum.
- Alternative tobacco products *may* help. Low-tar or ultra-low-tar cigarettes have helped some people stop smoking. They can, however, be just as harmful as regular cigarettes if use continues. Some people have used clove cigarettes, but some experts feel these may be more harmful than regular cigarettes because of immediate harmful effects to the lungs. Realistically, it is likely that repeated and prolonged exposure to any type of smoke would be harmful to human health.

The good news is that when you quit, you may feel better right away and your body will eventually heal most of the damage.

You will begin to feel more energetic, the coughing will stop, you will suddenly begin to taste food again, and your sense of smell will return. Your lungs will eventually heal and look like the lungs of a nonsmoker. Your risk of lung cancer will return to that of the nonsmoker in about 15 to 20 years. There is life after smoking!

 ## Web Review

Web review materials for Concept 20 are available are at *www.mhhe.com/hper/physed/clw/student/*.

American Cancer Society
   www.cancer.org

American Lung Association
   www.lungusa.org

Agency for Health Care Policy and Research
   www.ahcpr.gov

American Dental Association
   www.ada.gov

American Heart Association
   www.amhrt.org

CDC Tobacco Information
   www.cdc.gov/nccdphp/osh/tobacco.htm

Suggested Readings

American Cancer Society. "CPSII Adds to Breast Cancer Knowledge." *CPSII Newsletter* 11(1)(1994):1.

American Cancer Society. "CPSII and Tobacco Control." *CPSII Newsletter* 12(1995):1.

American Heart Association. "Active and Passive Tobacco Exposure: A Serious Pediatric Health Problem." *Circulation* (November 1995).

Bowles, W., et al. "Abrasive Particles in Tobacco Products: A Possible Factor in Dental Attrition." *Journal of the American Dental Association* 126(1995):327.

Centers for Disease Control. "Cigarette Smoking Among Adults." *Journal of the American Medical Association* 273(1995):369.

Centers for Disease Control and Prevention. "Incidence of Initiation of Cigarette Smoking— United States, 1965–1996." *Morbidity and Mortality Weekly Report* (October 1998).

Flegal, K., et al. "The Influence of Smoking Cessation on the Prevalence of Overweight." *The New England Journal of Medicine* 333(1995): 1166.

Glantz, S. A., and Parmley, W. W. "Passive Smoking and Heart Disease: Mechanism and Risk." *Journal of the American Medical Association* 273(1995):1047.

Gunby, P. "World No-Tobacco Day Targets Sports and the Arts." *Journal of the American Medical Association* 275(16)(1996):1220.

Hammond, K., et al. "Occupational Exposure to Environmental Tobacco Smoke." *Journal of the American Medical Association* 274(1995): 956.

"Hooked on Tobacco: The Teen Epidemic." *Consumer Reports* 60(3)(1995): 142.

Jinot, J., and Bayard, S. "Respiratory Health Effects of Passive Smoking: EPA's Weight of Evidence Analysis." *Journal of Clinical Epidemiology* 47(1994):339.

Kluger, R. *Ashes to Ashes: America's Hundred-Year Cigarette War, the Public Health, and the Unabashed Triumph of Philip Morris.* New York: Vintage Books, 1997.

National Center for Health Statistics. *Health, United States, 1998: With Socioeconomic Statistics and Health Chartbook.* Hyattsville, MD: National Center for Health Statistics, 1998.

Parish, S., et al. "Cigarette Smoking, Tar Yield and Non-Fatal Myocardial Infarction." *British Medical Journal* 333(1995):471.

Payne, W. A. and Hahn, D. B. *Understanding Your Health* (5th ed.). St. Louis: WCB/McGraw-Hill, 1998, Chapter 9: Rejecting Tobacco Use.

"Secondhand Smoke: Is It a Hazard?" *Consumer Reports* 60(1)(1995):142.

Straus, R. H. "Spittin' Image: Breaking the Sports-Tobacco Connection." *Physician and Sportsmedicine* 19(1991):46–48.

U.S. Department of Health and Human Services. *Healthy People 2010 Objectives: Draft for Comment.* Washington, DC: U.S. Department of Health and Human Services, 1998, Objectives Chapter 3: Tobacco.

Wichmann, S. A., and Martin, D. R. "Sports and Tobacco: The Smoke Has Yet to Clear." *Physician and Sportsmedicine* 19(1991):125–31.

Lab 20A: Use and Abuse of Tobacco

Name	**Section**	**Date**

Purpose:

To help you understand the risks of diseases (such as heart disease and cancer) associated with the use of tobacco or exposure to tobacco byproducts.

Procedure:

1. Read the Tobacco Use Risk Questionnaire (chart 1).
2. Answer the questionnaire based on your tobacco use or exposure.
3. Record your scores in the Results section.

Results:

What is your Tobacco Risk score? ☐ (total from chart 1)

What is your Tobacco Risk rating? ☐ (see chart 2)

Chart 1 Tobacco Use Risk Questionnaire

Circle one response in each row of the questionnaire. Determine a point value for each response using the point values in the first row of the chart. Sum the numbers of points for the various responses to determine a Tobacco Use Risk score.

Categories	Points				
	0	**1**	**2**	**3**	**4**
Cigarette Use	Never smoked		1–10 cigarettes a day	11–40 cigarettes a day	40+ cigarettes a day
Pipe and Cigar Use	Never smoked	Pipe occasional use	Cigar infrequent daily use	Cigar or pipe frequent daily use	Cigar heavy use
Smoking Style	Don't smoke		No inhalation	Slight to moderate inhalation	Deep inhalation
Smokeless Tobacco Use	Do not use	Occasional use– not daily	Daily use– one use per day	Daily use– multiple use per day	Heavy use– repetitious multiple use daily
Secondhand or Sidestream Smoke	No smokers at home or in workplace	Smokers at workplace but not at home	Smokers at home but not workplace	Smokers at home and at workplace	
Years of Tobacco Use	Never used	1 or less	2–5	5–10	10+

NOTE: Different forms of tobacco use pose different risks for different diseases. This questionnaire is designed to give you a general idea or risk associated with use and exposure to tobacco by products.

Chart 2 Tobacco Use Risk Questionnaire Rating Chart

Rating	Score
Very high risk	16+
High risk	7–15
Moderate risk	1–6
Low risk	0

Conclusions and Implications:

1. In several sentences, discuss your personal risk. If your risk is low, discuss some implications of the behavior of other people that affect your risk, including what can be done to change these risks. If your risk is above average, what changes can be made to reduce your risk?

2. In several sentences, discuss how you feel about public laws designed to curtail tobacco use. Discuss your point of view, either pro or con.

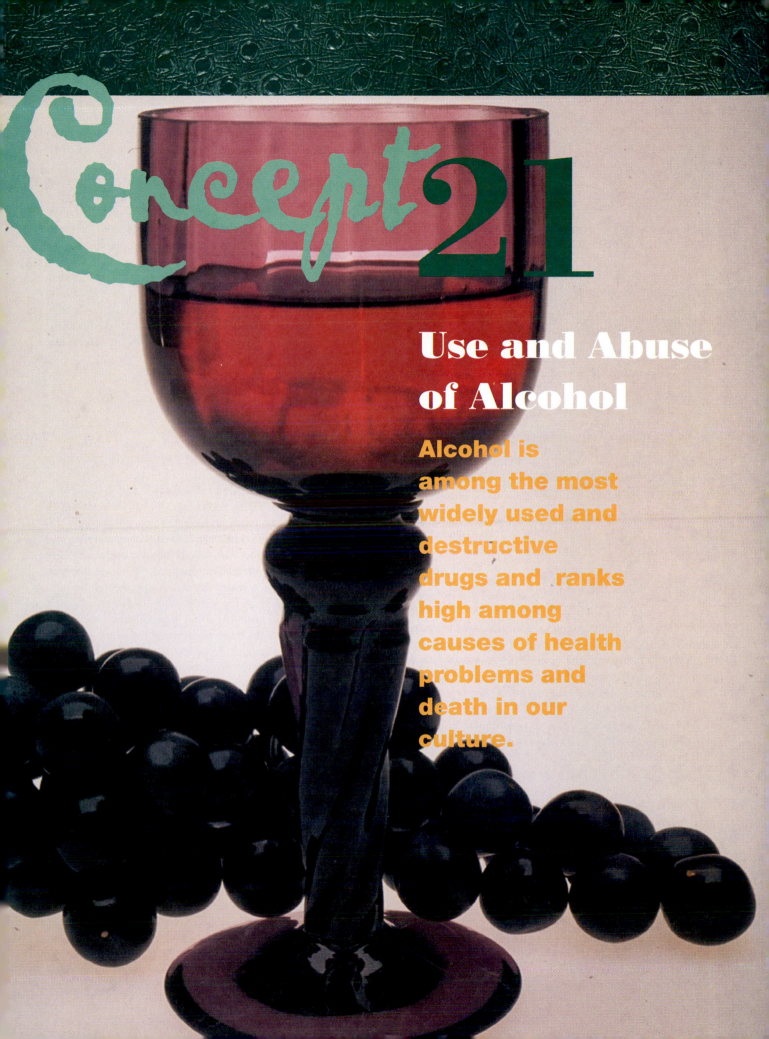

Concept 21

Use and Abuse of Alcohol

Alcohol is among the most widely used and destructive drugs and ranks high among causes of health problems and death in our culture.

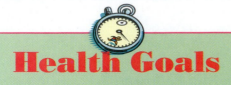

Health Goals

for year 2010

Reduce alcohol- and drug-related deaths and injuries from auto crashes.

Reduce rate of cirrhosis deaths.

Reduce rate of reported alcohol use especially among youth.

Reduce binge drinking especially among college students.

Reduce annual alcohol consumption.

Increase screening and treatment among those with alcohol problems.

Increase alcohol abuse education.

Increase number of states using .08 as the legal blood alcohol concentration (BAC).

Introduction

Alcohol is the most widely used and destructive drug in the United States. If all of the deaths caused by this drug are counted, it is the third major health problem in the United States. It is second only to tobacco as a cause of premature death in this country. It is considered to be more destructive than tobacco because of the devastating results of drinking and driving (or operating other vehicles) and because of the consequences of increased crime, physical and sexual abuse, and destroyed family relationships that are often associated with overindulgence in alcohol. It is estimated that at least two-thirds of all adults drink alcoholic beverages and 13.7 million are alcoholics.

The Facts about Alcohol and Alcoholic Beverages

Alcoholic beverages contain ethanol (ethyl alcohol), an intoxicating and addictive drug that is most often misused in the United States.

The active **drug** in alcoholic beverages (ethanol) is a toxic chemical, but unlike methanol (wood alcohol) and isopropyl (rubbing alcohol), it can be consumed in small doses. As a drug, it is classified as a depressant. By depressing the central nervous system, alcohol often makes people more relaxed and uninhibited. For this reason, alcohol is often referred to as a "social lubricant."

Alcoholic beverages have been consumed by humans for thousands of years—written records in Egyptian hieroglyphics warned against the overconsumption of alcohol. Unfortunately, many people in our culture (particularly college students) view drunkenness as a rite of passage and an expectation. Indeed, there are more synonyms for the word drunk or **intoxication** than for any other word in the English language. This illustrates the importance that we give to overconsumption. Fortunately, as people mature, they tend to realize that consumption of alcohol does not live up to the expectations that are voiced by their peers and in advertising.

Alcoholic beverages have varying concentrations of alcohol but often have similar amounts per serving.

The amount of alcohol in distilled spirits (liquor) and wine is listed on the label as its "proof." (Labels on beer and wine coolers are not presently required to list this.) The proof represents approximately double the percentage of alcohol in the beverage; for example, 90 proof gin is about 45 percent alcohol. Different beverages have different alcohol content, and they also may vary by brand. Beer is usually the lowest percentage at 3–6 percent, depending on state regulations. Wine has approximately 12–22 percent, whereas vodka, gin, scotch, brandy, cognac, and whiskey are the highest, with 40–52 percent.

Beverages are usually served in proportions such that a drink of any one of the three categories (beer, wine, or liquor) contains the same amount of alcohol. Beer is usually served in a 12-ounce can, bottle, or mug. A typical glass of wine holds 4 ounces, and a shot of liquor is 1 and one quarter ounce. Even though the percentage of alcohol in the beverages differs, the drinks would be equivalent in alcohol because each would contain about 15 ml of alcohol (see Figure 1).

The effect of alcohol on the body depends on many factors.

Alcohol is absorbed directly into the bloodstream through the walls of the stomach and the small intestines. It then concentrates in various organs in proportion to the amount of water each contains. The brain has a high water content, so much of the alcohol goes there, where it depresses the central nervous system. The rate and magnitude of the effects on an individual depend upon (1) the drinker's level of fatigue; (2) his/her mood; (3) what and how much food is in the stomach; (4) other drugs/medications consumed; (5) body size/weight; (6) rate of consumption; (7) type of beverage; and (8) individual body chemistry/genetic predisposition. In general, the

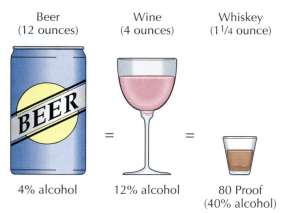

Beer (12 ounces) — 4% alcohol = Wine (4 ounces) — 12% alcohol = Whiskey (1 1/4 ounce) — 80 Proof (40% alcohol)

Figure 1

Alcohol content of drinks.

SOURCE: Data from the U.S. Surgeon General and the Government Printing Office.

Figure 2 Maximum Blood Alcohol Level.

Your Weight in Pounds	Drinks Consumed in One Hour				
	1	2	3	4	5
100	0.038%	0.076	0.114	0.152	0.190
120	0.032	0.064	0.096	0.128	0.160
140	0.027	0.054	0.081	0.108	0.135
160	0.024	0.048	0.072	0.096	0.120
180	0.021	0.042	0.063	0.084	0.105
200	0.019	0.038	0.057	0.076	0.095
220	0.017	0.034	0.051	0.068	0.085
240	0.016	0.032	0.048	0.064	0.080

Note: Percentages obtained by dividing the number 3.8 by the body weight in pounds. This factor takes into account various English-to-metric and other conversion factors, the body's typical weight-percentage of blood (per pound of body weight) in which the alcohol will be mixed, and the proportion of alcohol that will wind up in the blood.

more and faster one drinks, the greater the effect. Differences in effects are apparent between genders even when differences in body size are considered. One reason for this is that women have lower amounts of body water so a given amount of alcohol will represent a greater percentage of the volume of the blood in their bloodstream. Another factor is that women have lower amounts of the enzymes needed to process alcohol. Thus, alcohol stays in the bloodstream longer before being broken down.

There is evidence that some people develop tolerance to some of the effects of alcohol. While tolerance is often something that individuals boast about, studies suggest that **tolerance** may increase a person's risk for alcoholism.

> The body cannot usually process alcohol as fast as it is consumed.

Alcohol in the bloodstream is eventually oxidized in the liver. Under normal conditions, the liver can process up to 0.25 ounces of alcohol an hour. Because the average alcoholic beverage contains 0.5 ounces of alcohol, it takes approximately 2 hours to completely process a drink. If the rate of alcohol consumption is greater than the rate at which it is processed, the alcohol content in the bloodstream begins to increase. The amount of alcohol in the blood is measured as a percentage and is referred to as "blood alcohol content" (BAC). This figure is used by law enforcement officials to determine if a driver is legally intoxicated.

Studies show there is an increased risk in driving when the BAC is between 0.01 and 0.04 percent. A BAC of .04 percent is approximately half a drink if you weigh 120 pounds and one drink if you weigh 160 (see Figure 2). A BAC of 0.10 percent is the level at which driving becomes illegal in most states, although many states have adopted laws making 0.08 percent the legal limit (a national health goal). In many states, if the driver is under age 21, the legal limit is 0.01 percent

since people under 21 are not supposed to be drinking anyway. While rates of alcohol removal vary by size, the decrease in BAC is approximately 0.015 percent per hour. Thus, a long time is required to process even small amounts of alcohol.

The Facts about the Health and Behavioral Consequences of Alcohol

> The health effects of alcohol consumption depend on the amount that is consumed.

Alcohol consumed in moderation (i.e., two or fewer drinks per day for men and one or fewer drinks per day for women) has been found to reduce risks of cardiovascular disease. The reason for this is that alcohol consumed in these moderate amounts can raise the levels of high-density lipoproteins

Drug Any biologically active substance that is foreign to the body and is deliberately introduced to affect its functioning.

Intoxication Drunkenness, or blood alcohol level above 0.10 percent (legal intoxication in most states), though national health goals recommend a .08 percent standard.

Tolerance The phenomenon of requiring more and more alcohol over time to achieve the desired effect.

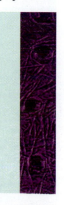

(HDLs), which are referred to as "good cholesterol." Alcohol consumed in greater amounts is associated with a variety of health problems. For example, as few as three drinks per day for men or two drinks per day for women increases the risk of cirrhosis of the liver. Excessive alcohol consumption has also been linked to various heart problems. Women are twice as vulnerable as men to the heart-destroying effects of too much alcohol because they metabolize alcohol differently than men. There are an estimated 100,000 deaths from alcohol use each year. Some of these are sudden deaths in healthy people! These and other health problems related to alcohol consumption are summarized in Table 1.

> The greatest danger of alcohol occurs when the drinker gets behind the wheel of a motor vehicle.

www.mhhe.com/hper/physed/clw/student/
Alcohol-related traffic crashes are the leading cause of death and spinal cord injury for young Americans. The driver's likelihood of causing a highway acci-

dent increases significantly at a BAC of 0.04 percent (approximately the level reached by a 150-pound man who has 1–2 drinks in an hour) (see figure 2). When the BAC reaches 0.10 percent, the chances have increased by 600 percent. In a government survey, 70 percent of college students reported driving while under the influence at least once in the past year, and 22 percent said they had done it five times or more. Two out of five Americans will be involved in an alcohol-related auto crash at some time in their lives. In the United States, someone is killed in an alcohol-related crash every 30 minutes. The effects of alcohol on driving performance are listed in Table 2.

> Extreme alcohol consumption can result in alcohol poisoning and death.

Every year, several college students, usually as a hazing stunt, drink themselves to death by consuming too much alcohol too fast. The body has a natural protective mechanism that normally prevents acute alcohol poisoning (vomiting or passing out). However, if the alcohol is consumed too quickly, this mechanism does not have a chance to be utilized. A BAC of 0.4–0.5 percent (approximately 20–25 drinks) would typically be fatal in most individuals.

The Facts About Alcohol Consumption and Alcohol Abuse

> The Surgeon General has expressed serious concern about the amount of alcohol drunk in the United States and the consequences of alcohol consumption.

It is estimated that each year Americans drink 378 million gallons of distilled spirits (liquor), 540 million gallons of

Table 1 Unhealthy Effects of Alcohol Consumption

Increased risk of
- High blood pressure
- Stroke
- Cardiac arrhythmias
- Blood clotting diseases
- Cirrhosis of the liver
- Cancer:

stomach	tongue	liver
pharynx	pancreas	larynx
colon	esophagus	breast

- Death
- Impaired immune system
- Problems in the reproductive system:
  infertility
  hormonal imbalance
  menstrual disturbance
- Fetal alcohol syndrome (in pregnant women):
  low birth weight
  physical defects
  brain damage/mental retardation
  heart defects
  stunted growth
- Malnutrition
- Decreased health-related physical fitness

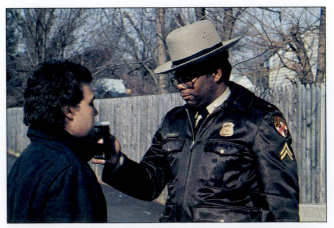

Alcohol-related crashes are the leading cause of death for young people.

Table 2   The Effects of Blood Alcohol Content (BAC) on Driving

BAC 0.02%

- Vision impaired: less ability to see objects in motion; less ability to monitor multiple objects
- Lowered attention span
- Reaction time slows
- Less critical of own actions

BAC 0.05–0.06%

- Reaction time noticeably reduced
- Reduced inhibitions (taking unnecessary chances)
- Visual abilities decrease; side vision impaired approximately 30%
- Superficial feelings of relaxation
- Judgment is the first function to be impaired
- Braking distance is extended
- Diminished ability to maneuver through narrow spaces
- Lowered attention span
- Coordination impaired
- Information processing impaired
- Impaired driving performance at moderate speed

BAC 0.08%

- Slower reflexes and reaction time
- Poor coordination
- Seriously impaired vision, especially at night
- Overconfidence in driving ability
- Emotions are exaggerated
- Thinking and reasoning powers impaired
- Less ability to concentrate
- Judgments dulled: careless
- Hinders muscle control and coordination
- Distances are misjudged
- Braking distance exceeded farther
- Reduced inhibitions (taking unnecessary chances)
- Impaired driving performances at low speeds
- Possible steering inaccuracy
- Increased use of accelerator and brake
- Less able to see dimly lit objects

Developed by Alaska Chapter of MADD and reprinted in the *Orange County (CA) Chapter Newsletter,* Winter 1989–1990, page 5. Reprinted by permission of MADD/Orange County, CA and MADD/Anchorage, AK.

wine and wine coolers, and 6 billion gallons of beer. Two-thirds of the adult population drink alcoholic beverages, and one in 10 has a chance of becoming an alcoholic. According to one report, 90 percent of all drinkers consume 50 percent of the alcohol served–which means the other 10 percent are very heavy drinkers, consuming the remaining 50 percent.

College students drink more than the rest of society and are more at risk for alcohol problems than other segments of the population.

www.mhhe.com/hper/physed/clw/student/

 Approximately 85 percent of college students drank alcohol at least once during the past year, with 41 percent of the students engaged in heavy drinking (five or more consecutive drinks). At one-third of the colleges surveyed, half the students went on drinking binges. In the last half of the last decade, there was a 33% increase in the number of students who drank with the specific intent of getting drunk. Alcoholic beverage consumption on campuses exceeds that of soft drinks, coffee, tea, milk, and juices put together.

The average annual consumption of alcoholic beverages for college students is more than 34 gallons per person, and they spend more than $4.2 billion on alcohol (more than is spent on operating campus libraries and college scholarships and fellowships by all colleges in the United States combined). The excess consumption of alcohol on college campuses contributes to increased sexual and physical assaults, increased absenteeism, and increased vandalism. Because fraternities and sororities have traditionally had higher rates of alcohol consumption, many are revising their rules and policies to help prevent alcohol-related problems. Those organizations that have not cooperated with campus regulations have been punished or banned from some campuses.

Alcohol-related problems cost American society an estimated $116–136 billion annually.

www.mhhe.com/hper/physed/clw/student/

 Alcohol is believed to account for 100,000 deaths per year. Approximately 360,000 students who are now in college will eventually lose their lives due to drinking. National studies conclusively link heavy drinking among youths to physical fights, destroyed property, job troubles, and troubles with the law. Drinking is usually a factor in date rapes and gang rapes. College administrators unanimously

Table 3 Social Problems Associated with Alcohol Abuse

Problems	Percentage of Cases That Are Alcohol Related
• Suicides	33
• All deaths from auto accidents	40
• All deaths from accidents, suicides, murders	50
• All deaths from boating accidents	60
• Deaths from drownings	69
• Deaths from falls	17–53
• Sexual assaults	72
• Child abuse	60
• Family violence	80
• College academic problems	34
• Deaths from college sorority/fraternity hazings	90
• College undergraduates reporting unplanned sexual activity (at least one instance)	29

Table 4 Why People Start Drinking

- Peer pressure
- Need to belong and to be accepted
- Media depiction of drinking
- Advertising depiction of drinking
- Lack of knowledge about its effects
- Easy access (especially at home)
- Absence of strong religious attachment
- Male bonding (especially in college)
- Cultural traditions at college
- Social "lubrication"
- It makes them "feel good"

agree that it is the cause of most campus crime. A list of some of the alcohol-related problems that contribute to the costs to society are listed in Table 3 with their percentage of incidence.

> The reasons given for starting to drink alcohol are the same or similar to those given for starting to use other drugs; however, the reasons for starting are not necessarily the reasons for continuing to use alcohol.

Peer pressure and the desire to be accepted are probably the two main reasons people take their first few drinks (usually as a young teenager). Other important influences include the portrayal of drinking as being macho, fun, cool, sexy, mature, elegant, and "the thing to do" by role models in the media (magazines, movies, television) and in advertising in newspapers and magazines, on billboards, at sports events, and so on. The alcohol industry focuses much of its advertising at young audiences and admits it contributes to underage drinking. It markets heavily on college campuses.

In one study, college newspaper space devoted to alcohol advertisements was approximately twenty times greater than the space devoted to books and forty times greater than that devoted to soft drinks. It is estimated that 10 percent of the revenue of the alcohol industry comes from college students. Some college newspapers have prohibited the advertising of alcoholic beverages.

Another factor contributing to the decision of youth to drink is failure to understand the health effects of alcohol and lack of knowledge about the alcoholic content of beverages. A national survey found that junior high and high school students could not identify the beverage that contained the most alcohol when shown beer (4 percent alcohol), malt beverage coolers (4–8 percent), wine coolers (1.5–6.5 percent), mixed drink coolers (4 percent), fruit-flavored wine, such as Cisco (20 percent), and nonalcoholic, fruit-flavored mineral water (0 percent). More than one-third did not know that Cisco contained alcohol.

Table 4 lists the most common reasons people give for starting to drink. Reasons people continue to drink (in addition to addiction) include boredom, rebellion, to get drunk, to reduce inhibitions, etc. The main reasons can be summarized as personal (e.g., to escape, to forget, to produce mood changes) and social (e.g., to go along with others and to facilitate social interaction).

> There is no sure way to predict who will become addicted to alcohol because each person is born with a different level of risk.

Alcoholism is a disease, and it may take a little or a lot of alcohol to trigger it. Some people seem to have a genetic predisposition for it. There is a one in 10 chance that a person who drinks will become an alcoholic, but for children of alcoholics the chances may be as high as 40–50 percent.

Women are more at risk than men because of their lighter weight, and the fact that they metabolize alcohol differently than men. They suffer greater physiological damage from the disease. The death rate among women alcoholics is 50–100 percent higher than for men alcoholics.

It all begins with the first drink. Then there is the social drinking, and later it is used as an escape from stress. The more one drinks, the greater the tolerance for alcohol and the more required to feel the effect—and the cycle continues. Many

Table 5 Warning Signs of Alcohol Abuse

- Needing a drink to start the day
- Making excuses for drinking
- Sneaking drinks
- Frequent absences from work or school
- Drinking alone
- Gulping drinks
- Financial difficulties
- Guilt feelings after drinking episodes
- Loss of ambition
- Lack of concern for family's welfare
- Memory loss
- Shabby appearance
- Mood changes
- Chronic hangovers

Table 6 People Who Should not Drink

- People under age 21 (legal age)
- Athletes striving for peak performance
- Women trying to get pregnant or who are pregnant or nursing
- Alcoholics or recovering alcoholics
- People with a family history of alcoholism
- People with a medical or surgical problem and/or on medications
- Psychiatric patients or persons experiencing severe psychosis
- People driving vehicles or operating dangerous machinery or involved in public safety
- People conducting serious business transactions or study

people mistakenly believe that the ability to "hold one's liquor" is an advantage, but actually those who can "hold their liquor" tend to drink more alcohol, placing them at greater physiological risk.

There are certain warning signs of alcohol abuse that the drinker should be aware of (but may deny).

Friends and family can help the person recognize these symptoms because the more that are present, the greater the likelihood of alcoholism. Table 5 lists the warning signs of alcohol abuse.

The best advice for preventing alcohol problems is not to start drinking, but if you do, there are some positive steps you can take.

Alcoholics need professional help and strong support from friends and family, but they have to want to stop drinking for themselves and must take the proper steps themselves. Some friends and family do not help them by denying the problem, nagging them about it, or covering it up for them.

To stop drinking, you may need to find some nondrinking friends and, if necessary, get a job or go to another college where you can get away from the people who influence you to drink. And you may have to practice ways to say no so others get the message that you mean it. You may need to get some professional help with assertiveness skills and how to improve your self-esteem. It is important that you develop leisure skills to avoid boredom. Exercise and sports can make you feel good, help you to become more fit and

healthy, fill your leisure time, and expose you to new friends. Some professional sources of help include the National Council on Alcoholism (1-800-NCA-Call), Alcoholics Anonymous (AA), and the National Clearinghouse for Alcohol and Drug Abuse Information (Box 2345, Rockville, MD, 20852). Your local health department can also refer you to local support and/or rehabilitation groups. The yellow pages of your telephone book list a number of professional help groups (look under Alcohol, Drugs, and Addiction).

Strategies for Action: The Facts about Responsible Drinking and Hosting

Some people should not drink at all, and most people who do drink should drink less.

While moderate alcohol consumption may be safe for some individuals, Dr. Ernest Noble (former director of the National Institute of Alcohol Abuse and Alcoholism) believes that some people should abstain completely (see Table 6).

For people who choose to drink, a large study of both men and women concludes that drinking should be limited to no more than 1–3 drinks per week. In the study on women, it

Alcoholism The loss of control over drinking behavior and/or the lack of ability to refrain from becoming intoxicated.

was found that the only women who benefited from light drinking were those over 50 with at least one risk factor for heart trouble.

If you drink, be a responsible drinker and avoid intoxication.

If you drink (at a party, for example), follow these guidelines:

- Limit alcoholic beverages to no more than one every hour and a half, or two or three drinks over a course of a four- or five-hour party (to stay within the legal BAC). *Note:* Between alcoholic beverages, you may wish to carry a nonalcoholic beverage to sip and to prevent friends from pressing a new drink on you.
- Sip the drink slowly.
- Eat foods rich in protein and starch to slow the absorption of alcohol in the blood.
- Choose non-carbonated drinks (rather than carbonated) for slower absorption.
- Measure your alcohol in a jigger (people who guess use too much).
- Never drink and drive. Choose a designated driver (who will not drink) before you go to the party.
- Don't participate in drinking games or hazing involving drinking.

Contrary to popular opinion, you cannot prevent intoxication by eating a meal or having a glass of milk before drinking alcohol. Neither can you sober up faster by drinking coffee, taking a cold shower, or walking.

If you are giving a party at which alcohol will be served, be a responsible host/hostess.

- Encourage guests to bring a designated driver.
- Secure safe transportation for those who are intoxicated. Do not let them drive.
- Have plenty of nonalcoholic beverages and high-protein and starchy foods available for the guests.
- Tactfully remove alcoholic beverages from the hands of guests who overindulge. (You might give them a job to do and/or substitute a non-alcoholic drink.)
- Close the bar an hour or two before the party ends.

Web Review

Web review materials for Concept 21 are available are at *www.mhhe.com/hper/physed/clw/student/*.

Alcoholics Anonymous
   http://www.alcoholics-anonymous.org
Betty Ford Center
   www.bettyfordcenter.org
Mothers Against Drunk Driving (MADD)
   www.gran-net.com/madd/madd.htm
National Clearinghouse for Alcohol and Drug Information
   www.health.org
National Institute on Alcohol Abuse and Alcoholism
   http://www.niaaa.nih.gov
Students Against Drugs and Alcohol
   www.sada.org

Suggested Readings

"Alcohol and Tolerance." *Alcohol Alert* No. 28 PH356 April 1995. National Institute on Alcohol Abuse and Alcoholism.

"Alcohol Related Impairment." *Alcohol Alert* No. 25 PH351 July, 1994. National Institute on Alcohol Abuse and Alcoholism.

Bonham, B. J., et al. "Binge Drinking in College." *Journal of the American Medical Association* 273(1995):1903.

Centers for Disease Control and Prevention. "Frequent Alcohol Consumption Among Women of Childbearing Age." *Journal of the American Medical Association* 271(1994):1820.

"Drinking and Driving," *Alcohol Alert* No. 31 PH362 January 1996. National Institute on Alcohol Abuse and Alcoholism.

Eigen, L. D. "Alcohol Practices, Policies and Potentials of American Colleges and Universities: An OSAP White Paper." Washington, D.C.: Office for Substance Abuse and Prevention; Alcohol, Drug Abuse and Mental Health Administration; U.S. Department of Health and Human Services, 1991.

Fuchs, C. S., et al. "Alcohol Consumption and Mortality Among Women." *New England Journal of Medicine* 332(1995):1245.

National Center for Health Statistics. *Health, United States, 1998: With Socioeconomic Statistics and Health Chartbook.* Hyattsville, MD: National Center for Health Statistics, 1998.

Payne, W. A. and Hahn, D. B. *Understanding Your Health* (5th ed.). St. Louis: WCB/McGraw-Hill, 1998, Chapter 8: Using Alcohol Responsibly.

U.S. Department of Health and Human Services (1998). Healthy People 2010 Objectives: Draft for Comment. Washington, D.C.: U.S. Department of Health and Human Services, Objectives Chapter 26: Substance Abuse.

Lab 21A: Blood Alcohol Level

Name	**Section**	**Date**

Purpose: To learn to calculate your (or a friend's) blood alcohol level (BAC).

Procedures:

1. Assume a drink is a 12-ounce can or bottle of 4 percent beer or a 4-ounce glass (a small glass) of 12 percent alcohol (wine), or a mixed drink with a 1-ounce shot glass (jigger) of 100 proof liquor (or one and one-fourth of a jigger of 80 proof).

   Case A: Assume you consumed two drinks within 40 minutes.

   Case B: Assume you consumed two drinks over a period of one hour and twenty minutes.

   Case C: Assume you had two six-packs of beer (12 cans) over five hours.

   Case D: Same as C, but if you weigh fewer than 150 pounds, assume you weigh 50 pounds more than you now weigh, and if you weigh more than 150 pounds, assume you weigh 50 pounds less.

2. Divide 3.8 by your weight in pounds to obtain your "BAC maximum per drink," or refer to chart 1. You should obtain a number between 0.015 and 0.04 (based on one drink in 40 minutes). Use the formula below to determine BAC over time.

$$\text{Approximate BAC over time} = \frac{(3.8 \times \# \text{ of drinks})}{(\text{body weight})} - \frac{[0.01 \times (\# \text{ min.} - 40)]}{40}$$

3. After 40 minutes have passed, your body will begin eliminating alcohol from the bloodstream at the rate of about 0.01 percent for each additional 40 minutes. Multiply the number of drinks you've had by your "BAC maximum per drink" and subtract 0.01 percent from the number for each 40 minutes that have passed since you began drinking—but don't count the first 40 minutes. Compute your BAC for cases A, B, C, and D.

   Example: Case A. Mary weighs 100 pounds. $\dfrac{3.8 \times 2}{100} = \dfrac{7.6}{100} = 0.076\% \text{ BAC}$

   Case B. Mary takes 80 minutes. $0.076\% - \dfrac{[0.01 \times (80 - 40)]}{40} = 0.066\% \text{ BAC}$

4. Record your results below by writing the formula and computing the BAC for each case.

Results:

Case A $\dfrac{(3.8 \times \underline{\quad} \ \# \text{ drinks})}{\underline{\quad} \text{ lbs.}} = \underline{\quad} \% \text{BAC}$

Case B $\dfrac{(3.8 \times \underline{\quad} \ \# \text{ drinks})}{\underline{\quad} \text{ lbs.}} - \dfrac{[0.01 \times (\underline{\quad} \# \text{ min.} - 40)]}{40} = \text{BAC}\left(\quad\right) - \left(\quad\right) = \underline{\quad} \% \text{BAC}$

Case C $\dfrac{(3.8 \times \underline{\quad} \ \# \text{ drinks})}{\underline{\quad} \text{ lbs.}} - \dfrac{[0.01 \times (\underline{\quad} \# \text{ min.} - 40)]}{40} = \text{BAC}\left(\quad\right) - \left(\quad\right) = \underline{\quad} \% \text{BAC}$

Case D $\dfrac{(3.8 \times \underline{\quad} \ \# \text{ drinks})}{\underline{\quad} \text{ lbs.}} - \dfrac{[0.01 \times (\underline{\quad} \# \text{ min.} - 40)]}{40} = \text{BAC}\left(\quad\right) - \left(\quad\right) = \underline{\quad} \% \text{BAC}$

1. Would you be able to drive legally according to your state laws? Place an X over your answer.

   Case A. (Yes) (No)

   Case B. (Yes) (No)

   Case C. (Yes) (No)

   Case D. (Yes) (No)

2. Would you be able to drive legally if the Health Goals for the Year 2010 (.08) were put into effect? Place an X over your answer.

   Case A. (Yes) (No)

   Case B. (Yes) (No)

   Case C. (Yes) (No)

   Case D. (Yes) (No)

Conclusions and Implications: In several sentences, discuss what you have learned from doing this activity.

Chart 1 Maximum Blood Alcohol Level (%)*

Your Weight in Pounds	Drinks Consumed in One Hour				
	1	2	3	4	5
100	0.038%	0.076	0.114	0.152	0.190
120	0.032	0.064	0.096	0.128	0.160
140	0.027	0.054	0.081	0.108	0.135
160	0.024	0.048	0.072	0.096	0.120
180	0.021	0.042	0.063	0.084	0.105
200	0.019	0.038	0.057	0.076	0.095
220	0.017	0.034	0.051	0.068	0.085
240	0.016	0.032	0.048	0.064	0.080

*Note: Percentages obtained by dividing the number 3.8 by the body weight in pounds. This factor takes into account various English-to-metric and other conversion factors, the body's typical weight-percentage of blood (per pound of body weight) in which the alcohol will be mixed, and the proportion of alcohol that will wind up in the blood.

Lab 21B: Perceptions about Alcohol Use

Name	Section	Date

Purpose: To help you better understand perceptions about drinking behaviors.

Procedures:
1. Think of a person you care about. Do not identify this person on this lab report.
2. Answer each of the questions in the questionnaire below as honestly as possible, evaluating the behavior of the person you have identified.
3. At another time, when you do not have to submit your results, you should answer the questions about yourself.
4. Answer the questions in the Conclusions and Implications section.

Results

	Never	Sometimes	Frequently	Too Often
1. How often does the person drink?	○	○	○	○
2. How often do the friends of the person drink?	○	○	○	○
3. How often does the person miss class or work associated with drinking?	○	○	○	○
4. How often does the person have personal or social problems associated with drinking?	○	○	○	○
5. How often does the person deny drinking too much? (only for those who you consider to drink too often)	○	○	○	○

Conclusions and Implications:
1. In several sentences, discuss the drinking behavior of the person you identified. Do you think your ratings give an accurate picture of the person? Do you think the person you rated has a problem with alcohol?

2. In several sentences, discuss the drinking behavior of the person's friends. Do the friends promote drinking or not?

3. In several sentences, discuss things that you could do to help a friend or loved one solve a drinking problem.

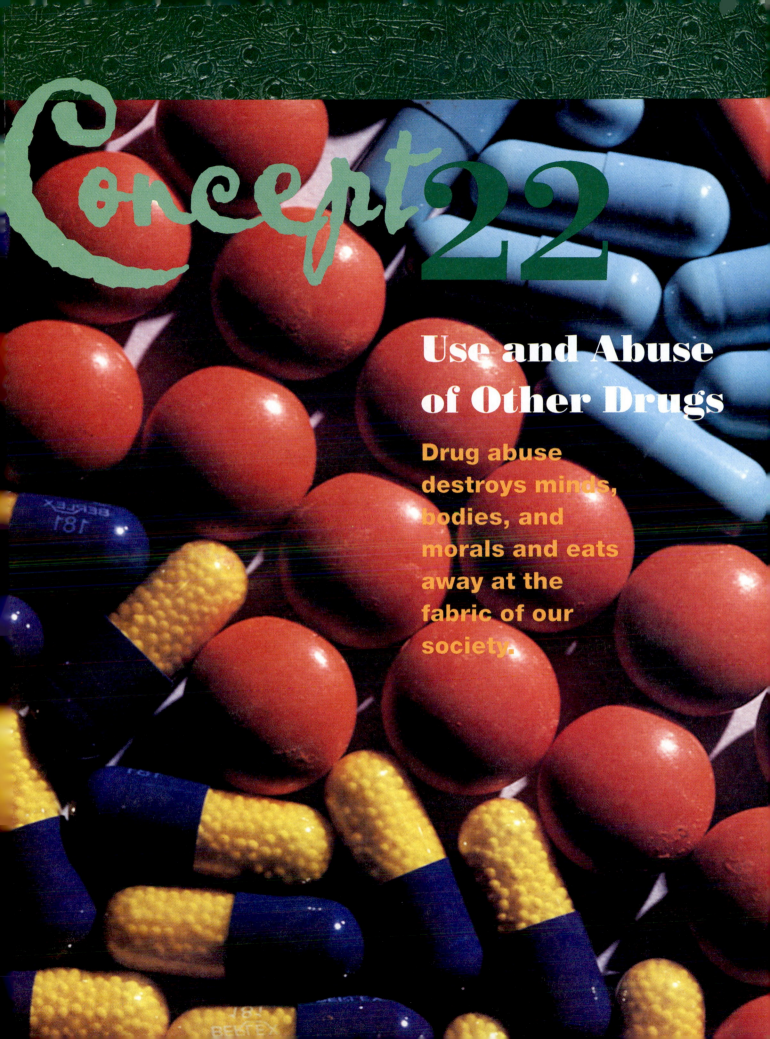

Concept 22

Use and Abuse of Other Drugs

Drug abuse destroys minds, bodies, and morals and eats away at the fabric of our society.

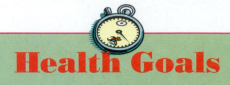

Health Goals

for year 2010

Reduce drug related deaths.

Reduce drug related hospital emergencies.

Reduce rate of reported drug use especially among youth.

Reduce steroid use especially among youth.

Increase screening and treatment among those with drug problems.

Increase substance abuse education.

Reduce suicide and suicide attempts especially among youth.

Reduce incidence of depression and resulting loss of quality of life.

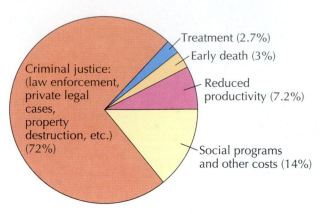

Figure 1

The estimated cost of drug abuse (percent of total costs).

SOURCE: Data from the National Institutes on Drug Abuse, Department of Health and Human Services.

Introduction

About a third of college students currently use illegal drugs, up from a low of 29 percent in 1991, but far below the 56.2 percent who had used an illicit drug in 1980. A study at the University of Southern California estimated that if current trends continue, the cost of drug abuse to the United States will exceed $150 billion by the first few years of the new millennium. In the late 1990s, an estimated million-and-a-half people were arrested each year for drug offenses—including sale, distribution, and possession. This is a tremendous cost to society. Tobacco and alcohol—the two most commonly used drugs in the United States—are discussed in other concepts. This concept discusses the misuse and abuse of other drugs, with emphasis on the illegal, so-called "street drugs".

The Facts about Drugs

The abuse of **drugs** is a particularly serious problem with youth but also invades the workplace.

Many adolescents are at a high risk of **drug abuse.** For example, annually there are over 14,000 deaths from drug-induced causes. Over 142,000 people are admitted to med-

ical emergency rooms as a result of cocaine complications. Because of problems with low productivity at the worksite, a large percentage of American businesses now conduct employee drug tests. Among the problems of drug-abusing employees are more frequent absences, erratic performance, increased violence and stealing, bad judgment, and increased accidents that often endanger others.

Drug abuse in the United States costs in excess of $150 billion annually.

Estimates by the Department of Health and Human Services suggest that the costs of drug abuse in our society are huge. Figure 1 illustrates the proportion of costs resulting from factors such as law enforcement expenditures, social programs, and reduced productivity.

Most of the medical establishment considers addiction to be a disease.

Addiction has been studied and continues to be studied by neuroscientists and geneticists. There is strong evidence that susceptibility to addiction has some genetic components. Nevertheless, the addicted person must accept some personal responsibility for control of his or her own personal circumstances, just as a diabetic must learn self-care activities to help control the disease.

Ten to 15 percent of Americans who use psychoactive drugs are susceptible to physical dependence or addiction. They will lose control over when they use drugs and how much they use, and many will die without outside help. Addiction is called a primary psychosocial and biogenetic disease by most of the medical establishment. **Habituation** to drugs also poses problems to the individual and to society. Guidelines for treatment apply to both addiction and habituation.

Table 1 Depressants ("Downers," Sedatives)

Examples	Physiological Effects	Psychological Effects
• Alcohol • Sedatives (e.g., Valium, Xanax, meprobamate, sleeping pills, methaqualone) • Rohypnol ("Roofies")	• In small doses slow the heart and respiration. • In large doses act as a poison and damages every organ system. • Quick sedation: vomiting; loss of motor and neurological control, combined with alcohol can lead to coma and death.	• Initially: stimulation, lowered inhibitions, excited talking, sense of well-being. • After prolonged use: depression, loss of coordination, drop in energy level, mood swings, confusion, euphoria. • Amnesia.

It is generally believed that drug use begins with smoking cigarettes.

The graduation from one drug (such as tobacco or alcohol) to another drug (such as cocaine or heroin) is commonly called the "gateway concept," and tobacco, alcohol, and marijuana are referred to as the "gateway drugs." Of course, most people who smoke or drink alcohol will not go on to take illicit drugs, but it is rare for nonsmokers and drinkers to use illegal drugs. The average age for starting cigarettes is estimated to be about 12 and for alcohol and marijuana about 13. In general, the younger a person is when he or she starts using drugs, including nicotine and alcohol, the more likely that person is to use illegal drugs and the more likely he or she is to become physically dependent on drugs. One in three college students uses marijuana, about four out of 100 has tried cocaine, and about one in 125 has used cocaine in the past 30 days. The connection between the three gateway drugs and illegal drugs is fairly strong, and it emphasizes the importance of discouraging young people from using them.

Drugs may be classified in several ways, but the mood-altering or psychoactive drugs are the ones we hear about most.

Mood-altering and **psychoactive drugs** may be placed in five major groups: (1) depressants, (2) narcotics, (3) stimulants, (4) hallucinogens, and (5) designer drugs. (A sixth category of misused and abused drugs is prescription drugs.) Drugs in the same group have similar effects. Narcotics are actually depressants, but because the word *narcotics* is so widely used in law enforcement and in society in general, they are generally given their own category. Each of the five categories of drugs is discussed in this concept, and the effects are described in Tables 1 through 5. The effects are classified as either physiological or psychological (meaning primarily affecting the body versus primarily affecting behavior).

Because the effects of drugs can vary with each individual and with different doses, it is only possible to generalize about the effects in the tables that follow.

Some examples of depressants (also known as sedatives or "downers") are alcoholic drinks and prescription drugs such as Valium, Xanax, meprobamate (brand names include Miltown or Equanil), sleeping pills, and methaqualone.

Depressants come in the form of pills, liquids, or injectables (see Table 1). In small doses, they slow the heart rate and respiration. In larger doses (for example, alcohol), they act as a poison and damage every organ system in the body. In large enough doses they can depress heart beat and respiration

Addiction A drug-induced condition in which a person requires frequent administration of a drug in order to avoid withdrawal; also referred to as physical dependence.

Drug Any biologically active substance that is foreign to the body and is deliberately introduced to affect its functioning.

Drug Abuse The use of a drug to an extent that it produces impairment of social, psychological, or physiological functioning.

Habituation The state of psychological dependence on a drug.

Psychoactive Drug Any drug that produces a temporary change in the physiological functions of the nervous system, affecting mood, thoughts, feelings, or behavior.

Table 2 Narcotics

Examples	Physiological Effects	Psychological Effects
• Codeine • Morphine • Methadone • Heroin (also called smack, junk, tar, and H)	• Narcotics: blockage of pain, chronic constipation, depressed respiration, redness and irritation of nostrils, nausea, lowered sexual drive, impaired immune system. • Heroin causes blood clots, bacterial endocarditis, serum hepatitis, brain abscess, HIV infection (from shared needles). In pregnant users, high risk of miscarriage, stillbirths, birth defects, toxemia, addicted babies.	• Narcotics: euphoria and feeling of pleasure. Nontherapeutic doses may result in mental distress, such as fear and nervousness. In heavy users, drowsiness and apathy may occur.

resulting in death, if quick intervention is not available. In terms of their effect on behavior, the user might at first feel stimulated, despite the actual depressant effect, because the drugs lower inhibitions. The user may talk more excitedly and experience a temporary sense of well-being. Depression, loss of coordination, drop in energy level, mood swings, and confusion occur after prolonged use. Rohypnol (10 times more powerful than Valium) is a legal medication in some countries, but not the United States. It is becoming a popular street drug known as the "date rape drug" because the rapist usually slips it in his date's drink. Women should not leave their drinks unattended nor accept drinks from strangers. Other "downers" include barbiturates (also called reds, yellow jackets, pink ladies, rainbows) and Quaaludes. Quaaludes (also known as ludes, methqualone and juicers) were the "drug of the '80s" and were manufactured for medicinal uses. Despite their removal from the market as a legal drug, they are still available on the illegal market.

Narcotics abuse, including heroin, codeine, morphine, opium, and methadone, like other illegal drugs can be fatal if taken in large quantities.

Narcotics are either smoked, injected, sniffed, or swallowed (see Table 2). Heroin has no legal medical use in the United States and has a very high rate of addiction. It is three times stronger than morphine and the other medicinal narcotics. Narcotics are all opium poppy derivatives or synthetics that emulate them. The *narco-* part of the word derives from the Greek word for sleep, because of its sleep-inducing properties.

Every narcotic, legal or illegal, is a potential poison. Although rare, a single dose can be fatal. A large percent of all deaths related to narcotic abuse is caused by overdose, impurities of the drug, or mixing the drug with other depressants such as alcohol. The mixing of drugs in the same or similar categories can produce a "heightened" physiological effect known as synergism or the **synergistic effect.** The combined use makes drug taking far more dangerous. The

same is true among some prescription and over-the-counter drugs—when used in combination, they can be dangerous.

Injection drug use and sexual contact with injection drug users account for 71 percent of AIDS cases among adult and adolescent women. One-quarter of the deaths are caused by violence associated with drug trafficking.

Stimulants, also called "uppers," include nicotine, cocaine, amphetamines (diet and pep pills), "ice," "meth," and even caffeine.

Some effects of stimulants are described in Table 3. One of these stimulants—cocaine—comes in powder form ("coke") and a rocklike form ("crack"). It is inhaled, injected, or smoked. If crack is snorted, it might be used several months or even years before becoming addicted. In contrast, when it is smoked it produces a very intense and instant "high" that lasts only eight to 20 minutes. The user can become addicted much more rapidly. The low cost of "crack" has contributed to its abuse.

"Ice" (also known as XTC) is a purified methamphetamine. It comes in rock form or powder. As a powder, it is usually smoked in a glass pipe or cigarette. It is a very powerful stimulant with a "high" that lasts from eight to 30 hours. No other drug damages the body as much as "ice"! It may be sold as pure methamphetamine or as a mixture of heroin, crack, and methadrine.

Designer drugs are made in laboratories and have many of the same properties as the drugs they simulate, such as pain relievers, anesthetics, or amphetamines.

Designer drugs (see Table 4) are modifications of illegal or restricted drugs, made by underground chemists who create street drugs that are not specifically listed as controlled.

Table 3 Stimulants

Examples	Physiological Effects	Psychological Effects
• Nicotine • Cocaine (also called coke or crack) • Amphetamines and methamphetamines (also called speed, crank, bennies, whites, dexies); diet and pep pills • Ice (also called glass, L.A. glass, hot ice, or super ice)	• Stimulants: excite central nervous system; increase blood pressure, respiration, and heart rate (sometimes resulting in convulsions and stroke); reduce appetite; highly addictive; overdose is fatal; with increased use: dizziness, headaches, sleeplessness; with long-term use: progressive brain damage, malnutrition, HIV infection (from shared needles). • Cocaine: sore throat, hoarseness, shortness of breath (leads to bronchitis and emphysema), eyes dilate, seeing "lights" around objects. May become addicted the first time. • Ice: extreme energy, thrashing about and running aimlessly, sleeplessness, seizures, flushed skin, constricted pupils.	• Stimulants: initially, feeling of being invincible, alertness, outgoing, excited; with increased use: feeling of anxiety; with long-term use: hallucinations, psychosis. • Crack: intense euphoria, then crushing depression, intense feeling of self-hate; as it wears off: depression and sadness, intense anxiety about where to get more drugs, vicious, aggressive, paranoid. • Ice: major effect is toxic psychosis; euphoria, delusions of grandeur, think they are invincible, violent when provoked. • Cocaine: initial rush of energy, feeling confident; as it wears off: depression, moodiness, irritability, severe mental disorders.

Table 4 Designer Drugs

Examples	Physiological Effects	Psychological Effects
• China white	• Designer drugs: depress blood pressure, depress respiration, relax muscles, relieve pain. • Nausea, slurred speech, loss of appetite, depressed blood pressure, relaxed muscles, relieves pain.	
• MDMA (also called ecstasy, XTC, or Adam)	• MDMA: irregular heartbeat, intensifies heart problems, causes exhaustion, liver damage, sometimes brain damage, dilates pupils, dry mouth/throat, nervousness, muscle tension, may deplete neurotransmitters, causes brain damage in animals.	• MDMA: feelings of calm and relaxation, feeling of great insight, may lead to psychosis and psychological burnout even at moderate doses.
• DOM (also called STP, Serenity, or Peace)		• DOM: low-dose, high-velocity trips that last a full day or more, high potential for panic reactions.
• DOB	• DOB: can trigger spasms in blood vessels, shutting down blood flow to arms and legs.	
• TMA		• At low dose: produces mescalinelike effects; at high dose: increased aggression, anger, paranoia.
• PMA		• PMA: triggers panic attacks, fatal dose is equivalent to mild dose of mescaline, is believed to have long-term harmful effects on appetite, sleep, mood, impulsiveness and other mental functions.

They are created by changing the molecular structure of an existing drug to create a new substance. Since these drugs are being created all of the time, the effect that they might have is unknown. In the past, some have killed the people who take them, some have paralyzed people, and some have

Synergistic Effect The joint action of two or more drugs that greatly increase the effects of each.

Table 5 Hallucinogens (Psychedelics)

Examples	Physiological Effects	Psychological Effects
	• Hallucinogens usually: elevate blood pressure, dilate pupils, cause dizziness.	• Hallucinogens: all signs and symptoms very similar to state of temporary insanity and can lead to recurrent and even permanent insanity. Hallucinations, distorted sense of space/time, "bad trips" (panic attacks, delusions, paranoia) that can return as flashbacks months later.
• LSD (also called acid, pearly gates, wedding bells, micro-dot, heavenly blue, royal blue, or window pane, scrambler, blotter acid)	• LSD: changes chromosomes and may result in birth defects of babies of users; bad trips, confusion, flashback.	• LSD: vivid hallucinations, feelings of overlapping/merging of the senses, expanded consciousness and mystical experiences, stimulated awareness and desire, confusion, flashback.
• PCP (also called crystal tea, angel dust, or hog, sugargrass, superkools, stardust, sherms)	• PCP: accumulates in fat cells and may remain in body longer than most drugs; impairs immune system, poor coordination, weight loss, speech problems, heart and lung failure, irreversible brain damage, convulsions, coma, and death.	• PCP: Insensitivity to pain can lead to death; euphoria, depersonalization, hallucinations, delirium, amnesia, tunnel vision, loss of control, and violent behavior.
• Marijuana (also called pot, grass, weed, ganja, bhang, Mary Jane, hash, joint, reefer)	• Marijuana long-term use: bronchitis, emphysema and lung cancer, bloodshot eyes, heart disease, infertility, and sexual dysfunction, permanent memory loss (brain damage).	• Marijuana: may not hallucinate; pleasant relaxed feeling; giddiness; self-preoccupation; less precise thinking; task performance impaired; inertia develops; with prolonged use: may be withdrawn and apathetic, have anxiety reactions, paranoia. Eventually, decreased motivation and enthusiasm, reduced ability to absorb and integrate effectively, scholastic performance profoundly impaired.
• Inhalants (solvents, aerosols, and nitrites, also known as poppers, rush, and laughing gas)	• Inhalants: slow reaction time; maybe headache, nausea, and vomiting; can cause seizure, brain damage, suffocation, heart attack, and death; double vision; sensitivity to light; dizziness; loss of coordination; weakness; numbness; irregular heartbeat; maybe liver and kidney failure; maybe bone marrow damage.	• Inhalants: giddiness, overexcitement, less inhibition, feelings of being all-powerful; powerfulness soon fades and leaves irritability.

been innocuous. The people who take these drugs are human guinea pigs. Designer drugs are a class of drugs often associated with "raves," all-night underground dance parties frequented by teens and college students.

There are thousands of variations of amphetamines alone, and new drugs are continuously being concocted in illegal labs. These drugs are often extremely potent and can be contaminated or "botched" in the laboratory so that one dose can seriously damage or kill the user. The risk of overdose or adverse side effects is high.

Ecstasy is often used in all-night clubs called "raves."

MDMA (methylenedioxymethamphetamine) or Ecstasy is known as a hallucinogenic stimulant and is inhaled, injected, or swallowed. Methamphetamine (meth) is a type of amphetamine easily manufactured by amateur chemists. Because of this, it is a popular drug. Meth use in California, in the Southwest, and in many parts of the Midwest has increased considerably in recent years. Meth used to be associated with long-distance truckers or college students cramming for exams, but some housewives use meth for energy, and young people at clubs and raves use it to fight fatigue so they can dance all night. Even in the drug-using 1970s, the word on the street was that "meth is death." Ecstasy, the amphetamine, is different from the Herbal Ecstasy.

> Drugs that cause the user to have hallucinations are called hallucinogens or "psychedelics."

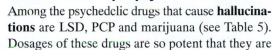

www.mhhe.com/hper/physed/clw/student/

Among the psychedelic drugs that cause **hallucinations** are LSD, PCP and marijuana (see Table 5). Dosages of these drugs are so potent that they are measured in micrograms (a microgram is one-millionth of a gram, and a gram is approximately equivalent to the weight of a standard paper clip). These drugs are not addictive, but users may develop a tolerance to them thus requiring increasingly larger doses. A less-known drug in this category is peyote cactus buttons, which are chewed. They are used legally by some American Indians in religious rites.

Marijuana use became widespread in the 1960s, and there is still political pressure among special interest groups to make it legal; however, the current street marijuana can be three to 10 times more potent than the marijuana of the 1960s. And extensive research has shown that it can have far-reaching effects.

Inhalants are sometimes listed separately because their effects are so serious. They reach the brain in seconds, and the effect lasts only a few minutes. They come in three types: (1) solvents—such as glue, gasoline, paints, paint thinner, typewriter correction fluid, lighter fluid, shoe polish, and liquid wax; (2) aerosols, such as hair spray, air fresheners, insect spray, and spray paint; and (3) nitrites, including amyl nitrite, nitrous oxide ("laughing gas"), and butyl nitrite (a room odorizer or liquid incense). They are most often abused by preteens and early teens. Long term use has been shown to cause brain damage.

The Facts about Misuse or Abuse of Prescriptions and Over-the-Counter Medications

> Many people unknowingly become drug abusers or misusers by failing to carefully follow the prescription on their medications.

Two of the most prevalent occurrences of abuse are taking prescription drugs (medications) with alcohol or with other medications and taking one medication in quantities out of proportion to the needs for which it was originally prescribed. An example is the use of Prozac. Prozac is often described as the "prescription drug of the decade." It was introduced by Eli Lilly in 1987 and since then it has been used by more than 20 million people. While the medication is useful taken in appropriate doses for appropriate conditions, critics note that many people use the product in combination with other medications creating dangerous drug interactions and take it in doses in excess of those prescribed. Depressants are another example of drugs that have a synergistic effect with other drugs that can cause death.

> Accidental misuse of prescriptions and medications is common and dangerous.

An unwitting abuse of drugs, particularly among the elderly, is overdosing because of forgetfulness. A particular problem is taking a medication two times. People who have vision problems may not be able to read labels so they guess at the proper dosage. Other people take several prescriptions at the same time for different ailments, and sometimes these come from different doctors who are unaware that the patient is being treated by another physician. These drugs may interact dangerously or have a synergistic effect.

Accidental misuse can also occur if drugs are taken from the medicine cabinet at night in the dark or if medications are stored in unlabeled bottles so that the wrong drug is taken. Using outdated drugs can also lead to problems. After a medication is no longer needed, any remaining part of it should be destroyed. Because people react differently to drugs, it is possible to become addicted to a prescription drug even when you follow the directions.

The Public Citizen's Health Research Group (PCHRG) notes how prescription drugs can contribute to drug-induced conditions (see Table 6).

> Anabolic steroids are prescription drugs that are being sold now on the black market and are being widely misused and abused.

www.mhhe.com/hper/physed/clw/student/

Government studies estimate that there are one million steroid users in the United States (also see concepts on muscle fitness and quackery). Approximately 2 percent of teenagers have used steroids by the time they graduate from high school. Anabolic steroids are also known as "roids," "juice," and "sauce." Users are likely to misuse or abuse other drugs and frequently share needles, increasing risk of disease transmission. Recent studies show habituation often occurs with use of this drug.

Hallucinations Seeing, feeling, and/or hearing imaginary things or seeing things in a distorted way.

Table 6 Incidence of Problems with Prescription Drugs

Number of Drugs and Potential Problems	Number of People and Potential Problems
• 119 drugs can cause sexual dysfunction.	• 61,000 develop drug-induced Parkinson's disease.
• 105 drugs can cause hallucinations or psychoses.	• 32,000 older adults fall and break their hips due to side effects of drugs.
• 88 drugs can cause constipation.	• 1,500 older adults die as a result of drug-induced falls.
• 86 drugs can cause depression.	• 16,000 automobile crashes are caused by adverse drug reactions.
• 65 drugs can cause dementia.	• 163,000 older adults develop memory problems because of inappropriate use of prescription drugs.
• 46 drugs can contribute to falls and hip fractures.	• 659,000 people are hospitalized because of adverse reactions to drugs.
• 29 drugs can cause Parkinson's disease.	• 9.6 million older adults suffer adverse drug reactions each year.
• 22 drugs can contribute to auto accidents.	
• 18 drugs can cause insomnia.	

Reprinted with the permission of PocketBooks, a Division of Simon & Schuster from *Best Pills, Worst Pills,* By Wolfe, et. al, 1999.

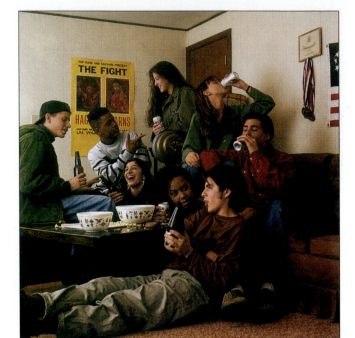

Peer pressure contributes to drug use and abuse.

- Decreased oxygen to the baby and possibly a fetal stroke.
- Low birth weight and shorter babies.
- Babies are often born addicted and undergo withdrawal symptoms.
- Increased risk of sudden infant death syndrome.
- Increased risk of learning disabilities, as well as delayed motor, speech, and language development.

Women who are pregnant or trying to get pregnant or who are nursing infants can cause serious harm to the fetus or baby by using drugs, even prescription drugs.

The National Institute on Drug Abuse (NIDA) conducted the National Pregnancy and Health Survey—a national assessment of the extent of drug use by women during pregnancy—and estimated that 5.5 percent of the 4 million women who gave birth each year in the United States used illegal drugs while they were pregnant. Taking drugs during pregnancy can result in a variety of conditions.

- Premature separation of the placenta from the womb and hemorrhage, threatening the lives of both the baby and the mother. (Cocaine use makes mothers twice as likely to have this problem as women on other drugs, and four times as likely as women not on drugs.)
- Miscarriage resulting from increased blood pressure and increasing uterine contractions. Birth defects also occur.

Drugs can reduce inhibitions and interfere with clear thinking about sexual activity.

Drugs put the user at greater risk for unwanted and/or unprotected sex and its consequences—unwanted pregnancies and sexually transmitted disease. There is a misconception that being on drugs makes you sexier. On the contrary, drugs are more likely to have the opposite effect. If you are under the influence of a substance, you may think you are cute and sexy, when in fact you may just be loud and obnoxious to others. The drug also may make you feel bolder or more aggressive or may make you give in to pressure and do things you normally would not do.

The effects of specific drugs are described elsewhere in this concept, but remember they can affect sexual development for the rest of your life. Men can have lowered sperm count or develop feminine characteristics from taking drugs like steroids, and women may have menstrual problems. It is also worth reiterating that HIV can be contracted from contaminated needles as well as from sexual activity.

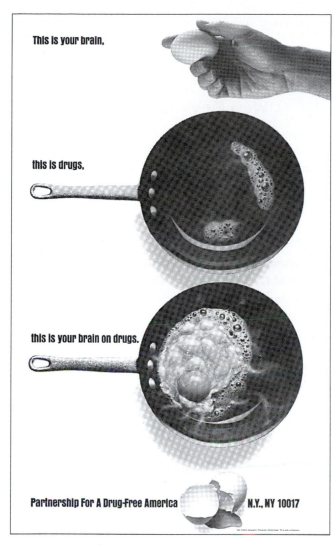

This is your brain,

this is drugs,

this is your brain on drugs.

Partnership For A Drug-Free America   N.Y., NY 10017

Any questions?

There are some risk factors that make one more likely to misuse or abuse drugs.

www.mhhe.com/hper/physed/clw/student/
The potential for addiction depends on attitude, ease of access, method of use, purpose of use, mental state, and physiological or genetic sensitivity. For example, the risk is greater if one has used drugs (including alcohol) recreationally and thinks there is no problem with that. If drugs are readily available—perhaps in the home, dormitory, or sorority/frat house, on campus, or at work—one is more apt to become a user. If when you use a drug you choose the fastest method of getting high, you are in great danger of becoming addicted. Having a history of child abuse or other childhood traumas increases your risk, as do feelings of stress, loneliness, anxiety, and other mental pain. Finally, there seems to be a genetic tendency such that if other members of your family have been alcoholics or abused other drugs, your chances of becoming addicted are significantly greater.

Note: It is possible to get an accidental "trip" by tasting a substance to see what it is, or by putting your hands in your mouth after handling drugs or drug paraphernalia. Remember, for some people, the first trip is the one that starts the addiction. With some drugs, for some people, the first trip is the last! If you don't use drugs, you can't get addicted.

The reasons given for using drugs are very similar to the reasons given for using alcohol and tobacco.

Typically, the reasons people give when asked why they use drugs or how they got started include the following:

- Peer pressure (i.e., "Everyone is doing it"; even though in most cases the majority of people aren't using drugs).
- It makes young people feel grown up.
- "I just want to see what it is like (to experiment)."
- To have fun.
- "It makes me feel good."
- As a rebellion against parents or authority.
- To cope with pressure/stress.
- To take a risk (thrill-seeking).

National controversies abound regarding the best methods to deal with drug problems.

www.mhhe.com/hper/physed/clw/student/
Although most Americans believe that drug abuse is a huge problem, there is widespread controversy about which are the best methods of dealing with the problem. Some examples of issues currently being debated are the effectiveness of antidrug media campaigns, the legalization of drugs for medicine, needle exchange programs, and drug testing. Only time and quality research will allow us to answer questions about these issues.

Strategies for Action: The Facts about Getting Help

The best way to avoid problems associated with drug use is not to try illegal drugs and to be careful in the use of legal drugs.

The information presented in this concept clearly indicates that starting to take a drug for reasons other than managing your own good health increases the risk of taking more drugs in the future. Most readers of this book have already made the decision not to take illegal drugs and will follow the guidelines presented earlier concerning how to avoid misusing legal drugs. Nevertheless, at some time in the lives of most people, medication will be taken. It is important to continually be aware of what you are taking and why. You need to monitor the use of medications to be sure that you are using them as directed and not in combination with other medications that may result in dangerous synergistic effects.

One of the characteristics needed to resist peer pressures to use drugs is healthy self-esteem. You need to believe that you are important. It is also essential to learn skills to cope with problems and stress (see the concept on stress management). Using a responsible process to make decisions is another skill that needs to be acquired. Knowing the effects and risks of drugs should help you to make more responsible decisions. To combat peer pressure, the ability to clearly and effectively say "no" is necessary. Be assertive. And finally, you need to choose friends whose values support, rather than undermine, your own.

> People who have a problem with a drug typically will need help to develop some skills and personal characteristics to avoid resuming old behavior patterns.

Denial is a difficult obstacle to overcome and a frequent problem of the abuser. Until it is confronted and controlled, recovery cannot begin. But once the first step is taken, help is available. The first step is recognizing that help is needed. In Lab 22A you will have the opportunity to evaluate the behavior of a friend or loved one to determine if the person needs help. If a person needs help, he or she needs to talk to someone who can be trusted, perhaps a friend or relative or maybe you can help. You may be able to help the person seek help from a referral source such as an employee assistance program, family or university physician or hospital, or your city or county health department. These sources help get the person into a rehab program or support group. Some of the better-known, nationwide programs include Alcoholics (or Narcotics or Cocaine) Anonymous and Al-Anon Family Groups. Another option is to look in the yellow pages of the telephone book for rehab programs operated by public and private agencies. Still another possibility is to call a hotline, and someone will direct you to help in your area. Three of these include:

- National Institute on Drug   (1-800-662-HELP)
  Abuse (NIDA) Hotline
- Cocaine Helpline   (1-800-COCAINE)
- Just Say No International   (1-800-258-2766)

At a later time it would be wise to answer the questions in Lab 22A for yourself rather than for a friend or loved one. This will allow you to determine if you might need help.

 ## Web Review

Web review materials for Concept 22 are available are at *www.mhhe.com/hper/physed/clw/student/*.

Web of Addiction
   www.well.com/user/woa
Cocaine Anonymous World Services
   www.ca.org
Drug Free Resource Net
   www.drugfreeamerica.com
National Clearinghouse for Alcohol and Drug Information
   www.health.org
National Institute on Drug Abuse
   www.nida.nih.gov
Students Against Drugs and Alcohol (SADA)
   www.sada.org

Suggested Readings

Fields, R. *Drugs in Perspective.* (3rd ed.). St. Louis: WCB/McGraw-Hill, 1998.

Payne, W. A. and Hahn, D. B. *Understanding Your Health* (5th ed.). St. Louis: WCB/McGraw-Hill, 1998, Chapter 7: Living Drug Free.

Pinger, R., Payne, W. A., Hahn, D. B., and Hahn, E. J. *Drugs: Issues for Today* (3rd ed.). St. Louis: WCB/McGraw-Hill, 1998.

Schwenk, T. L. "Psychoactive Drugs and Athletic Performance," *Physician and Sportsmedicine.* 25(1)(1997):32.

U.S. Department of Health and Human Services. (1998). *Healthy People 2010 Objectives: Draft for Comment.* Washington, DC: U.S. Department of Health and Human Services, Objectives Chapter 26: Substance Abuse.

Wolfe, S. M., Sasich, L. D., Hope, R., and Public Citizen Health Research Group. *Best Pills, Worst Pills.* New York: PocketBooks, 1999.

Lab 22A: Use and Abuse of Other Drugs

Name	**Section**	**Date**

Purpose: To help you to evaluate a friend or family member's behavior and potential for becoming an abuser of drugs. If this report is submitted to an instructor, be sure *not* to identify by name the person you are evaluating.

Procedure: Answer these questions to determine if the person you are evaluating could be an abuser of medications. Place an X over the answer that applies.

A. Prescription Drug Abuse

(Yes) (No)   1. Does he/she take more medicine than prescribed per dosage?

(Yes) (No)   2. Does he/she feel more nervous than ever when the medicine wears off?

(Yes) (No)   3. Does he/she hoard medicine?

(Yes) (No)   4. Does he/she gulp pills?

(Yes) (No)   5. Does he/she hide the amount of medicine taken from friends, family or his/her doctors?

(Yes) (No)   6. Does his/her doctor know he/she has other doctors, and do they have a list of all the medications he/she is taking from all sources (dentist, family physician, specialists)?

The more questions to which you answered "yes," the more likely he/she is to be a drug abuser.

B. Risk Factors for Becoming Addicted

(Yes) (No)   1. Have any members of his/her family ever abused drugs?

(Yes) (No)   2. Was he/she abused as a child, or did he/she go through other trauma during childhood?

(Yes) (No)   3. Is he/she now undergoing unusual stress or mental pain?

(Yes) (No)   4. Does he/she have easy access to drugs?

(Yes) (No)   5. Has or does he/she used drugs recreationally?

(Yes) (No)   6. If he/she has or now uses drugs recreationally, did or does he/she choose the fastest method of getting a "hit"?

The more "yes" answers you have, the greater his/her risk of addiction. (Remember that alcohol is a drug, too.)

C. Signs and Symptoms That a Problem with Drugs Exists

(Yes) (No)   1. Does he/she use drugs as an escape or to help cope with a stressful situation?

(Yes) (No)   2. Does he/she become depressed easily?

(Yes) (No)   3. Does he/she use drugs the first thing in the morning?

(Yes) (No)   4. Has he/she ever tried to quit and resumed using again?

(Yes) (No)   5. Does he/she do things under the influence of a drug that he/she would not normally do?

(Yes) (No) 6. Has he/she had any drug-related "close calls" with the police, or any arrests?

(Yes) (No) 7. Does he/she think a party or social gathering isn't fun unless drugs are served?

(Yes) (No) 8. Does he/she feel proud of an increased tolerance to drugs?

(Yes) (No) 9. Does he/she use drugs when alone?

(Yes) (No) 10. Has or does he/she use a wide variety of drugs?

(Yes) (No) 11. Is he/she constantly thinking about being high?

(Yes) (No) 12. Does he/she avoid people or places that oppose usage?

(Yes) (No) 13. Has his/her friends, family, teachers, or employer expressed concern about his/her use?

(Yes) (No) 14. Is his/her usage causing him/her to neglect responsibilities?

(Yes) (No) 15. Has he/she ever had blackouts or lack of memory of drug use or other events?

(Yes) (No) 16. Has he/she stolen to get money for drugs?

(Yes) (No) 17. Has he/she seriously considered that he/she might have a drug problem?

The more questions to which you answer "yes," the more likely he/she is to have a serious problem with drugs.

Results:

A. Does he/she abuse prescription drugs (medications)?　　(Yes) (No)
    (Questions A 1–6)

B. Is he/she at considerable risk for addiction?　　(Yes) (No)
    (Questions B 1–6)

C. Does he/she have a serious problem with drugs?　　(Yes) (No)
    (Questions C 1–17)

Conclusions and Implications:

In several sentences, discuss a plan of action that could be taken by a person who has a problem with misuse of over-the-counter drugs, prescription drugs, or illegal drugs. Discuss specific things you could do to help a person with a problem.

* At some point you may want to answer the questions yourself.

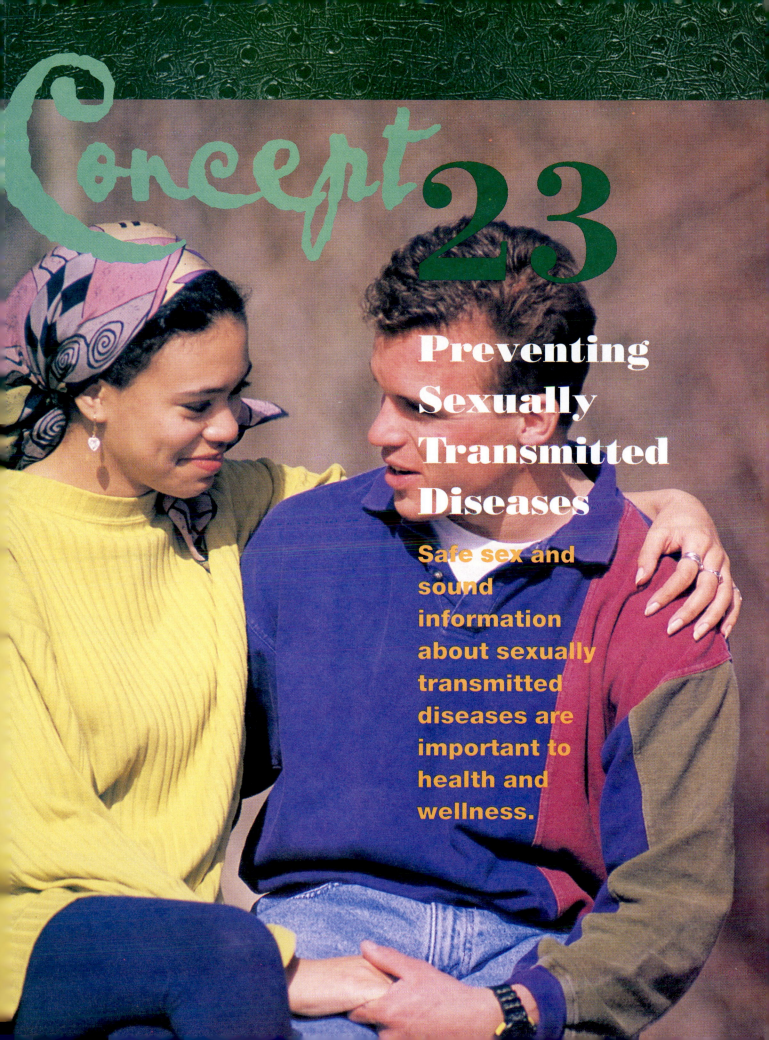

Concept 23

Preventing Sexually Transmitted Diseases

Safe sex and sound information about sexually transmitted diseases are important to health and wellness.

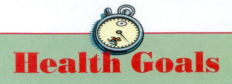

Health Goals

f o r   y e a r   2 0 1 0

Reduce incidence of Chlamydia, gonorrhea, syphilis, herpes simplex, HPV, and PID.

Increase screening and treatment for STDs including HIV.

Reduce new cases of STD and HIV (including prenatal infections).

Reduce number of diagnosed cases of AIDS.

Increase use of methods to prevent HIV and STD infection.

Increase STD education and public information.

Increase treatment rate among HIV positive and reduce death rate for HIV infected.

Increase years of quality living among those with HIV/AIDS.

Introduction

The sexual experience is an interpersonal one that influences the actions and behaviors of many people. It is basic to family life and fundamental to the reproduction of the human species. Approached responsibly, the human sexual experience contributes to wellness and quality of life in many ways. When approached irresponsibly, it can result in disease and personal and interpersonal suffering. Responsible decision making requires sound information regarding the symptoms, causes, and treatments of sexually transmitted diseases (STDs).

General Facts

The healthy sexual experience can contribute to wellness in many ways.

Because it is interpersonal, the human sexual experience is a social one. It affects many more people than a sexual partner. Personal beliefs have much to do with the feelings that participants have toward the sexual experience; thus, spiritual wellness is influenced. Because the sexual experience is often emotionally charged, emotional wellness is also affected. Clearly, intellectual decisions are made concerning the experience, so intellectual well-being is a factor to consider as well. The sexual act is a physical experience that can be pleasurable but that has many long-lasting physical consequences. All five wellness dimensions are involved in decisions concerning participation in, the meaningfulness of, and the long-term consequences of the sexual experience. The healthy sexual experience requires sensitive and thoughtful consideration of the consequences.

Decisions concerning sexual behavior have lifelong consequences.

Positive consequences of a sexual experience include pleasure, childbearing, and an enriched, happy family life. Negative lifelong consequences can include unwanted pregnancy, emotional and physical stress, and strained social relationships, among others. Unsafe sex also takes a toll in disease and death for large numbers of people worldwide.

Unsafe sexual activity can result in disease, poor health, and much pain and suffering.

Until the 1940s, **sexually transmitted diseases (STDs)** were a leading cause of death. The discovery of penicillin and other antibiotics, and improved public health practices, lowered the death rate from STDs, but they remained a significant health problem. In 1991, STDs became one of the 10 leading causes of death in the United States, principally because of the high death rate from **acquired immune deficiency syndrome (AIDS)** caused by the **human immuno-deficiency virus (HIV).** In 1998, STDs dropped from the top ten list, primarily because of the effectiveness of recently developed drugs in reducing the death rate from HIV/AIDS. STDs, including HIV/AIDS, will continue to be a leading health problem in the future if better prevention programs are not implemented.

Each year, millions of Americans, mostly teenagers and young adults, are affected by STDs. One-quarter of teenagers who are sexually active need treatment for STDs annually. Of the more than 50 different STDs, Chlamydia is the most prevalent, but most cases can be treated with early diagnosis and early treatment. Other common STDs are syphilis, gonorrhea, genital herpes, genital warts, pubic lice, and hepatitis B and C. HIV/AIDS is the most serious STD because it is deadly and there is no known cure, only a treatment that suppresses the condition.

In addition to the general national health goals designed to prevent, control, and reduce STDs, specific goals include increasing STD education in schools and colleges, extending regulations to protect workers, and improving services through community agencies designed to help the general public.

The Facts about HIV/AIDS

> Of all STDs, HIV/AIDS poses the most significant health threat to the nation and the world.

www.mhhe.com/hper/physed/clw/student/

Health experts indicate that we are in the midst of a worldwide HIV/AIDS epidemic. Many experts say that the AIDS epidemic has become larger than the plague. The United Nations says 30 million people are infected with HIV worldwide—two-thirds of them in Africa. In 1997, there were 6 million new HIV infections worldwide. The good news is that HIV infections have slowed in 44 countries, though the rate of increased infection in the United States has remained fairly steady in recent years.

The first known cases of AIDS were identified in 1981, and in 1984, HIV was identified as the cause. Though it dropped from the top 10 causes of death, it is still a leading cause of potential years of lost life in the United States. HIV/AIDS is still the fifth leading killer of people in the 25–44 age group. As noted above, the rate of HIV infection has not decreased significantly; only the death rate has. The decreased death rate from HIV/AIDS noticed in the United States has not been apparent in underdeveloped countries. This is primarily because they do not have access to the types of medicines available in this country. HIV/AIDS is now one of the leading infectious diseases of death in the world. Each year more than two million people die of AIDS, about the same number who die of malaria, another major global killer.

> Minorities and women are populations in which the incidence of HIV/AIDS is increasing disproportionately.

What was once thought to be a disease of males, especially gay men, is now increasingly a female condition in the United States. Because of a recent change in the clinical case definitions from when HIV was first discovered, many more women are classified as having AIDS than in previous years. In the past, AIDS was defined by many specific ailments among HIV-positive individuals. Because women have different ailments associated with HIV (cervical cancer, recurrent pneumonia, and pulmonary tuberculosis), some women were being denied new and experimental treatments available to men. The revised definition of AIDS includes these ailments so 26 conditions and a low **CD4+ cell** count are now used to define it. For this reason, more women qualify for treatment, but more women are also included as having AIDS. Currently, about one-fifth of all AIDS cases are among women (up from 7 percent in 1985). Experts also believe that HIV is underreported among women because the symptoms are less apparent for women than for men, so the disease is often undiagnosed.

HIV/AIDS is also a major problem among minority groups. Rates of infection among African Americans (eight times the risk) and Hispanics (four times the risk) show disproportionately higher HIV/AIDS rates than non-Hispanic whites. The disproportionate risk among minorities has resulted in the development of multimillion-dollar governmental programs to fight HIV/AIDS among African American and Hispanic populations.

Though incidences of HIV infection are greatest among the young, recent evidence suggests that older adults are not free of risk. One study in a county in Florida showed a high incidence of new infection among adults 50 and over. This suggests that some older adults may not be aware of their risk and are not taking appropriate precautions to prevent infection.

> HIV is the virus that causes AIDS.

A test of **serostatus** can indicate if a person is seropositive. When a person "tests seropositive" for HIV, it means that a blood test has indicated the presence in the body of the HIV. HIV invades the body's immune system cells, even killing them. This results in damage to the immune system and the body's ability to fight infections. One of the principal problems is that HIV causes immune suppression by directly invading

Sexually Transmitted Diseases (STD) Disease for which a primary method of transmission is sexual activity.

Acquired Immune Deficiency Syndrome (AIDS) An HIV-infected individual is said to have AIDS when he/she has developed certain opportunistic infections (for example, pneumonia, tuberculosis, yeast infections, or other infections) or when their CD4+ cell count drops below 200.

Human Immunodeficiency Virus (HIV) A virus that causes a breakdown of the immune system among humans, resulting in the inability of the body to fight infections. It is a precursor to AIDS.

CD4+ Cell A type of cell that protects against infections and that instigates the body's immune response. HIV kills these cells so a high count usually means better health; also known as T helper cell.

Serostatus A blood test indicating the presence of antibodies the immune system creates to fight disease. A seropositive status indicates that a person has antibodies to fight HIV and is HIV positive.

and killing CD4+ helper cells. When too many of these cells (also called **T helper cells**) are destroyed, the body cannot fight opportunistic infections effectively.

What all of this means is that the immune system can no longer function properly, thereby making the seropositive person more susceptible to various types of diseases and disorders. **Antibodies** in the blood that normally fight infections are ineffective in stopping the HIV from invading the body. Though it is not clear exactly why HIV affects the immune system as it does, the stages of HIV are better understood than in the past. First, HIV infects the body. Over time, white blood cells are damaged, and antibodies become ineffective. Depending on time elapsed and individual variance in the progression of the disease, AIDS may develop or no symptoms may appear (see Figure 1). After HIV enters the body, it takes several months before enough antibodies are developed to be able to detect its presence. Newer tests are available, which detect a portion of the HIV virus known as P24. These tests may prove to be an improvement over those of the past, but they are more expensive. One reason that HIV is so widely transmitted is that in the early stages, before it can be confirmed by testing, HIV can be transmitted. If untreated, five of 10 of people infected with HIV will develop AIDS within 10 years. Four of 10 who go untreated will develop **AIDS-related complex (ARC),** another illness associated with HIV, and one in 10 will have no apparent ill effects.

An individual has AIDS when he or she is infected with HIV and develops various opportunistic diseases because of impairment of the immune system. Among the conditions that indicate the presence of AIDS are pneumonia, tuberculosis, **Kaposi's sarcoma,** yeast infections, and the previously described conditions for women. Other symptoms include fatigue, swollen glands, rashes, weight loss, and loss of appetite. Those HIV victims who have access to the "cocktail" of drugs used to treat HIV/AIDS can live much longer than previously thought possible. When treated with the "cocktail," many have become free of detectable amounts of HIV as long as they continue the treatments. It should be noted that non-detectable levels of HIV among those infected does not prevent transmission. Apparently virus "reservoirs" exist that allow transmission even when drugs have reduced HIV to undetectable levels. The recent discovery of new strains of HIV have caused concern among public health officials because of the fear that they may be mutations that are resistant to current treatments. More research is necessary to find out to what extent this may become a problem.

Some people possess a "non-progressor or non-pathogenic" strain of HIV. This strain of HIV has a different genetic structure than other strains. Some believe that the study of the genetic structure of this unique HIV strain could be important to finding a cure. Other research involves the study of a group of people from European ancestry. This research has discovered a genetic mutation that causes these people to resist HIV. This mutation apparently occurred as a result of adaptations to the plague in previous centuries. About 2 million Caucasian people of European ancestry

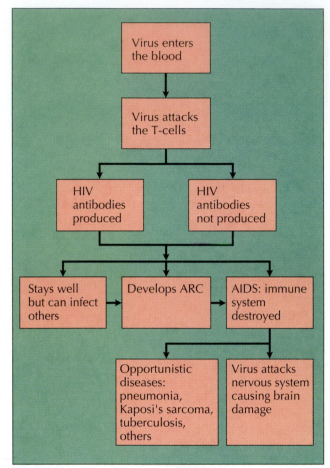

Figure 1
Stages of the HIV infection.

possess this mutation. Experts believe that the study of this mutation may result in a cure for HIV/AIDS.

There is no known cure for AIDS.

www.mhhe.com/hper/physed/clw/student/

For those infected with HIV/AIDS, there is no known cure. However, treatments have been developed to suppress or slow the progress of the disease process. As mentioned earlier, current treatment for HIV/AIDS includes administration of a cocktail of drugs including **AZT,** and other similar drugs as well as **protease inhibitors.** These combination treatments can cost up to $15,000 per year, and the drugs must be taken in a complex sequence. They have many adverse side effects. Of concern is the fact that 95 percent of the HIV-infected people worldwide do not currently have access to the types of drugs that have been effective in lowering death rates.

Many others drugs and treatments are now being studied. For example, the FDA recently approved a drug called Sustiva (chemical name is efavirenz) that is an effective alternative to the cocktail. It provides hope to those who cannot tolerate other drugs and has the advantage of being administered only once each day. Experts emphasize that it is unwise to change treatments to new drugs in midtreatment. This prevents the body from becoming resistant to medication.

A high-priority health goal for the nation is the development of an HIV vaccine. Among the current priorities described by government officials is a vaccine using live virus that can be killed when it starts the body's own immune responses. At the recent World AIDS Conference, vaccine researchers gave the disheartening news that a promising candidate vaccine, tested in monkeys, caused the disease rather than prevented it. On the other hand, a long-term study of another possible vaccine is currently underway. Gene therapy is also being studied as a possible cure for AIDS. An anti-HIV gel for use by women is also under study.

There is some controversy as to when it is best to treat HIV aggressively.

Recent government statements agree that the cocktail of drugs is the most effective treatment for HIV, but there are two camps of experts when it comes to scheduling the treatment. Some recommend "hitting early and hitting hard." This means administering drugs as soon as a seropositive status is confirmed. Others suggest that the treatment should wait until the **viral load** is high. Standards for viral load were recently established by public health officials indicating that treatment should begin when the viral load reaches a level of 10,000 copies of HIV per milliliter of blood. More recent evidence suggests that the values may need to be adjusted downward for women because they have greater risk of opportunistic infections than men for the same viral load.

Those who recommend waiting to treat HIV do so because they feel that early treatment may lead to resistance to the drug prematurely. To date, it is not known how long the HIV/AIDS cocktail can be administered effectively. About 16 percent of people treated since AZT and other similar drugs were first administered have now become resistant to at least one drug in the anti-HIV cocktail. The new public health statement indicates a consensus that all people who have a high viral load, have symptoms of opportunistic infections, or have other evidence of a damaged immune system should begin aggressive treatment.

Many people with HIV do not know they are infected.

Recent public health statistics indicate that many people are HIV positive and do not know it. This complicates efforts to achieve national health goals associated with the condition because HIV can be transmitted by unknowing individuals. Lack of awareness also prevents early treatment.

A blood test, generally eight to 10 weeks or more after exposure, can detect the presence of HIV. More than one test may be necessary to accurately detect HIV in the blood because of the lengthy incubation period. It is especially important that people who are currently at risk or who may have been at risk in recent years be tested to determine if they are seropositive.

The FDA recently approved a home HIV test. This test can be administered anonymously at home and the results received by phone. It has been found to be as accurate as professionally administered tests. Some experts were concerned about home tests because of the consequences of a positive result in the absence of professional consultation. The evidence now shows that taking the home test has led to earlier treatment and has not decreased the number of people who get a non-confidential test from a health care provider. A saliva test for HIV has also been developed, but confirmation should always include a clinical blood test.

Two mechanisms account for most HIV transmission.

The two primary mechanisms responsible for the transmission of HIV are sexual activity and contact with infected blood (sharing needles or transfusion). Among men, the greatest number of new cases result from men having sex with men, though a significant number of cases results from

T helper cells A disease-fighting blood cell that is damaged by the HIV virus; also called a CD4+ cell.

Antibodies Bodies in the bloodstream that react to overcome bacterial and other agents that attack the body.

AIDS-Related Complex (ARC) The development of HIV-related immunodeficiency conditions but not those considered to be AIDS.

Kaposi's Sarcoma A type of cancer evidenced by purple sores (tumors) on the skin.

AZT (Antiviral Drug Zidovudine) The first well-used treatment for people infected with HIV; one of several drugs including ddI, ddC, d4T and 3TC that blocks a protein necessary for the reproduction of HIV. This type of drug is typically part of the "cocktail" of several drugs used to combat HIV.

Protease Inhibitor (PI) A drug that blocks an enzyme called protease that is important in the final states of HIV reproduction. Saquinavir was the first protease inhibitor approved by the FDA, but now several are available. At least one is included in the "cocktail" of drugs used to treat HIV.

Viral Load The level of virus (HIV) in the blood.

heterosexual sex. Among women, risk of transmission is most frequent in heterosexual sex. Worldwide, 75 percent of all AIDS cases are now transmitted by heterosexual sex.

Twenty-one percent of cases are a result of injecting drugs with contaminated needles and most of the rest of the cases are among people who may combine these risk factors. Because of efforts to protect the blood supply, few cases result from contaminated blood. Some cases are transmitted from HIV-infected mothers to children during childbirth. At least one study has shown that Cesarean delivery can reduce the risk of mother-to-baby transmission if the mother is seropositive. Recent evidence has led to the recommendation that infected mothers consider alternatives to breast feeding.

Only a small percentage of health-care workers have become infected from contact with infected blood at medical or dental facilities. It should be noted that those with other STDs such as herpes and syphilis have a greater risk of transmission of HIV than those who do not have these conditions. Though HIV/AIDS is more prevalent among certain populations, it is clear that it can affect any individual who participates in risky behavior.

> **The risk of acquiring HIV/AIDS is reduced if exposure to HIV and to the methods of transmission are avoided.**

A recent National Institutes of Health consensus statement indicated that HIV transmission could be reduced if legislative barriers to needle exchange programs were lifted, if greater emphasis were given to youth education programs about HIV/AIDS, if greater funding were available for treatment of people who abuse drugs, and if educational efforts among high-risk populations were increased. Speakers at a recent World AIDS Conference spoke out in favor of similar recommendations. In this country, not all people agree with these recommendations. Nevertheless, it is important to examine the evidence and make decisions that will help meet national health goals for HIV/AIDS. Worldwide, the money expended on treatment far exceeds the amounts spent on prevention. Experts suggest that if we are to meet national health goals, more effort and money will need to be spent on prevention.

There is evidence that relatively short-term educational sessions with trained counselors can reduce risk of HIV transmission. A seven-week program using small groups and a counselor motivated people to refrain from risky behaviors that increase risk. Other steps that can be taken to lower your risk of HIV infection are presented in Table 1.

> **The HIV/AIDS epidemic is a problem that affects all members of society.**

HIV is not spread through the air or in saliva, sweat, or urine. It does not spread by hugging, sharing foods or bever-

Table 1 Factors Associated with Reducing Risk of HIV/AIDS

- Abstain from sexual activity.
- Limit sexual activity to a noninfected partner. A lifetime partner who never has sex with other people or never uses injected drugs (other than medically administered) is the only "safe" partner.
- Avoid sexual activity or other activity that puts you in contact with another person's semen, vaginal fluids, or blood.
- Use a new condom (latex) every time you have sex, especially with a partner who is not known to be "safe." Know how to use it properly.
- Use a water-based lubricant with condoms, because petroleum-based lubricants increase risk of condom failure.
- Abstain from risky sexual activity, such as anal sex and sex with high-risk people (prostitutes, people with HIV or other STDs).
- Do not inject drugs.
- Never share a needle or drug paraphernalia.
- Get tested for STDs, and seek proper treatment.
- Anal and oral sex places people at higher risk of contracting STDs.
- People who have had an STD have increased risk of HIV/AIDS.

ages, or casual kissing. Contact with phones, silverware, or toilet seats does not cause the spread of HIV.

HIV must invade the blood in order for a person to become infected. People who had blood transfusions prior to 1985 had an increased risk of HIV transmission, but since that time the safety of the blood supply has increased dramatically. There is no danger in donating blood, only in receiving HIV-infected blood. Babies born to women with HIV have increased risk of being HIV infected.

The Facts about Other Sexually Transmitted Diseases

> **The most frequently reported STD in the United States is Chlamydia.**

Chlamydia is the most commonly reported STD. The number of cases increased dramatically in the late 1990s. Infection with *Chlamydia trachomatis* may result in inflammation of the urethra, fallopian tube, and the cervix for females and inflammation of the epididymis for males (located over the testes). It is detected by isolation of a culture (smear).

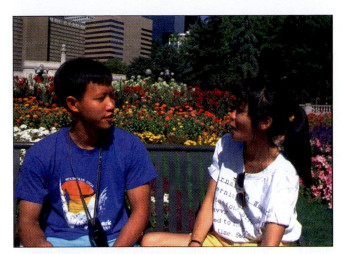

Open communication concerning sexual histories is important in preventing STDs.

Pelvic inflammatory disease (PID) as a result of Chlamydia can result in sterility among female sufferers. Mothers with chlamydia infections can contribute to inflammation of the eyes or pneumonia in their newborns.

Many cases of chlamydia go undetected and experts indicate that annual testing is not adequate for sexually active people. For at-risk sexually active women of childbearing age, two tests per year are recommended.

Another widespread STD is gonorrhea.

www.mhhe.com/hper/physed/clw/student/

Gonorrhea and hepatitis B are the next most frequently reported of all STDs. In the late 1990s, there was a rather dramatic decrease in the number of gonorrhea cases. Although this is a step in the right direction, there is still a need to educate people about prevention. Gonorrhea is a bacterial infection that can be treated with modern antibiotics if detected early. However, recent strains of the gonorrhea organism have become resistant to antibiotics, due to widespread overuse, causing concern among public health officials since some cases are quite difficult to treat.

Sexual activity is the principal method of disease transmission. Penile and vaginal gonorrhea are the most common types. Symptoms usually occur within three to seven days after bacteria enter the system. Among men the most common symptoms are painful urination and penile drip or discharge. Symptoms are less apparent among women, though painful urination and vaginal discharge are not uncommon. Other types of gonorrhea often have fewer symptoms in both sexes. Chills, fever, painful bowel movements, and sore throat are among the most common.

Early detection by a culture or smear test at the site or sites of sexual contact is how the disease is diagnosed. Early

cure is especially important for females because gonorrhea can lead to pelvic inflammatory disease, which can result in infertility.

Hepatitis B is widespread but can be prevented by a vaccine.

Hepatitis B is 100 times more infectious than HIV, so chances of getting hepatitis B from each unsafe sexual encounter is greater. About 200,000 to 300,000 Americans each year get hepatitis B, most of whom are adolescents and young adults. Hepatitis B is common on college campuses.

Hepatitis B may strike silently and damage the liver. In the mildest cases, it may never be detected and it may be gone in six months. Some people develop jaundice or yellowing of the skin and eyes. Still others become carriers for the rest of their lives, infecting others. Some go on to have chronic liver disease such as cirrhosis, a disease that scars the liver. Hepatitis B carriers are 200 times more likely to develop liver cancer than those who do not have the condition. There is no cure for hepatitis B, but there is a vaccine to prevent it. The Centers for Disease Control and Prevention (CDC) and other public health officials recommend widespread use of hepatitis B vaccine for young people to protect them from hepatitis B.

Syphilis is another serious but less commonly contracted STD.

Syphilis was a serious national health problem in the 1940s, when it was 10 times more prevalent than it is now.

Chlamydia A bacterial infection similar to gonorrhea that attacks the urinary tract and reproductive organs.

Pelvic Inflammatory Disease (PID) An infection of the urethra (urine passage) that can lead to infertility among women.

Gonorrhea A bacterial infection of the mucous membranes including the eyes, throat, genitals, and other organs.

Hepatitis B A virus found in body secretions that causes many symptoms including fever, nausea, jaundice (yellow skin and eyes), and liver enlargement.

Syphilis An infection caused by a corkscrew-shaped bacteria that travels in the bloodstream and embeds itself in the mucous membranes of the body, including those of the sexual organs.

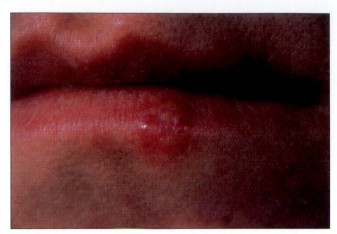

Lip (oral) herpes

During the 1970s and 1980s, there was a dramatic increase in this STD. Fortunately, progress toward the national health goal of reducing the number of syphilis cases has been made. Syphilis was the first STD for which national control measures were initiated. Reported cases of syphilis declined 84 percent nationwide during the 1990s. CDC reports that syphilis continues to have a disproportionate effect on African Americans and people living in the South.

Like gonorrhea, syphilis is a bacterial infection that can be effectively treated with antibiotics. The corkscrew-shaped bacteria cannot live long outside the human organism. However, it can be easily transmitted from person to person through sexual contact. The bacteria then become embedded in the walls of the mucous membranes, where they can be transmitted throughout the body. Syphilis can also be transmitted by an infected mother to her unborn child (congenital syphilis).

Once the bacteria invade the body, it typically takes one to three weeks before syphilis is detected. The symptoms of syphilis include **chancre** sores that generally appear at the primary site of sexual contact, then change from a red swelling to a hardened ulcer on the skin. Even if not treated, the sores disappear after a period of one to five weeks. It is important to get treatment even after this primary phase of the disease because the disease is still present and contagious. After several weeks or longer, secondary symptoms occur, such as a rash, loss of hair, joint pain, sore throat, and swollen glands. Even after these symptoms go away, untreated syphilis lingers in a latent phase. Serious health problems may result, including blindness, deafness, tumors, and stillbirth.

Early detection is important and can be diagnosed from chancre discharge or a blood test several weeks after the appearance of chancres. There is an association between syphilis and the spread of HIV. Apparently the presence of chancres greatly increases the risk of transmitting HIV during sexual activity.

Of all STDs, genital herpes is among the most commonly spread because of a lack of awareness of infection.

Genital herpes, one of the most commonly reported STDs, is caused by the herpes simplex virus (HSV). HSV is a family of many viruses that can produce various disorders in humans, such as shingles and chicken pox. HSV Type 1 is often called lip or oral herpes because it causes cold sores and fever blisters on the lips and the mouth. HSV Type 2 is often referred to as the STD type because it is known to cause genital lesions. These lesions or blisters on the penis, vagina, or cervix usually occur two to 12 days after infection and typically last a week to a month. Swollen glands and headache may also occur.

Though Type 2 HSV is generally referred to as the STD type, it is now known that both Types 1 and 2 HSV can cause genital sores, just as either type can cause lip and oral sores. At present there is no cure for genital sores caused by HSV, though some prescription drugs can help treat the disease symptoms. HSV can remain dormant in the body for long periods of time, and as a result, symptoms can recur at any time, especially after undergoing stress or illness.

Genital herpes is especially contagious when the blisters are present. Condom use or abstinence from sexual activity when symptoms are present can reduce the risk of transmission of the disease. Herpes is more dangerous for women than men because of the association between genital herpes and cervical cancer and the risk of transmitting the disease to the unborn.

Some lesser known STDs are significant health problems.

Genital warts, pubic lice, and **chancroid** are examples of lesser known, but very prevalent, STDs. Some general information about these diseases is presented in Table 2.

Strategies for Action: The Facts

A first step in prevention is to recognize risk. Young people are especially at risk for STDs.

Teens and young adults are especially at risk of getting STDs. College students have high incidences of STDs. In Lab 23A, you will have the opportunity to evaluate the risk of a friend

Table 2 Facts about Lesser Known STDs

Genital Warts (Condylomas)

- Comprise approximately 5% of all reported STDs.
- Are most prevalent in ages 15–24.
- Are caused by the human papilloma virus (HPV).
- Are linked to cervical and genital cancers.
- Are hard and yellow or gray on dry skin.
- Are soft and pink, red or dark on moist skin.
- There is no known culture test.
- Early diagnosis is important (because of association with some forms of cancer).
- The prescription drug Podophyllin is one treatment.

Pubic Lice (Crabs)

- Are pinhead-sized insects (parasites) that feed on the blood of the host.
- Are transmitted by sexual contact and/or contact with contaminated clothes, bedding, and other washable items.
- Symptoms include itching; some people have no symptoms.
- Can be controlled by using medicated lotion and shampoos, and by washing contaminated bedding, etc.
- Do *not* transmit other STDs.

Chancroid

- Is caused by bacteria.
- Is more commonly seen in men than in women, particularly uncircumcised males.
- Symptoms include one or more sores or raised bumps on the genitals.
- Can result in progressive ulcers occurring on the genitals. Sometimes the ulcers persist for weeks or months.
- Can be successfully treated with certain antibiotics.

gest that 70 percent are sexually active by age 20, yet few have used condoms.

- Experimenting with lifestyles. Young people are likely to experiment with drugs (especially alcohol, which contributes to lower inhibitions and poor judgment) and unplanned sex, thus increasing risk of STDs in this population.
- Instant gratification. Many young people believe that sex should be entirely spontaneous. They fear what their partner might say if he/she is prepared to have sex and has protection available. They also feel that they cannot pass up an opportunity to have sex. It must be now.
- Inability to talk about sexual issues. It is easier for some young people to be sexually active than it is for them to truly communicate with each other about commitments and protection.

STDs can be considered as lifestyle-related conditions.

Most of the risk of STD infection can be eliminated by adopting healthy lifestyles as noted in Table 1. We can control behaviors associated with high risk. Only children born to mothers with STDs and young children who are not in control of their own behavior lack the ability to alter lifestyles to reduce risk of STDs. A cure for STDs such as HIV/AIDS is a top-priority national health goal. But until cures are found, prevention through healthy lifestyles is a key. Sound health practices among those who are infected are also critical to meeting national goals. It is important to remember that people do not develop an immunity to STDs

or loved one. You may also want to evaluate your own risk using the STD Risk Questionnaire. Probable reasons for the high risk among teens and young adults are presented here.

- Perceived immortality. Many teens feel that disease is something that happens to other people, not to them. For example, one study indicated that a large proportion of teens do not feel that they are the "kind of person who would get AIDS."
- Risky sexual activity. Evidence suggests that teens and young adults often do not follow the STD guidelines presented earlier in this concept. For example, data sug-

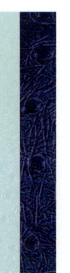

Chancre A sore or lesion commonly associated with syphilis.

Genital Herpes A viral infection that can attack any area of the body but often causes blisters on the genitals.

Genital Warts Warts, caused by a virus, that grow in the genital/anal area (also called condyloma).

Pubic Lice Lice that attach themselves to the base of pubic hairs; also called crabs.

Chancroid A bacterial infection resulting in sores or ulcers on the genitals; different from chancres associated with syphilis.

from previous exposures, and people can have more than one STD at a time. Indeed, having one STD often places a person at risk of getting another STD.

> Removing factors that contribute to fear of discrimination may increase our effectiveness in dealing with the HIV/AIDS epidemic and the high incidence of other STDs.

Public health sources indicate that some people are reluctant to seek medical assistance, even when symptoms of STDs are present, for fear that detection will result in discrimination. Among the common fears are loss of employment or housing, descrimination in hiring or housing, rejection for medical treatment, and loss of educational opportunities. Overcoming fear of STDs and reducing discrimination among those who may be infected are important steps to reducing the incidence of STDs. The development of self-tests for HIV/AIDS makes it possible to be tested without fear of discrimination. It is important that sources of confidential testing for other STDs become available and that people with STDs inform their sexual partner(s) so they can seek testing and treatment, if needed.

> Hotlines are available to help people who want information concerning STDs such as HIV/AIDS.

The following national AIDS hotlines are toll-free and allow the caller to retain anonymity:

(English) 1-800-342-AIDS (342-2437)

(Spanish) 1-800-344-SIDA (344-7432)

The CDC's national STD hotline (1-800-227-8922) is a toll-free number that provides information for a variety of STDs.

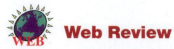 **Web Review**

Web review materials for Concept 23 are available are at *www.mhhe.com/hper/physed/clw/student/*.

American Social Health Association
   http://www.ashastd.org

CDC Center for STD Prevention
   www.cdc.gov/nchstp/od/nchstp.html

CDC National Prevention Information Network
   http://www.cdcpin.org

Harvard AIDS Institute
   www.hsph.harvard.edu/organizations/hai /home.html

Suggested Readings

Altamn, L. K. "AIDS Meeting Ends with Little Hope of Breakthrough. *The New York Times* (July 4, 1998):5.

Clark, J. R. "Sexually Transmitted Disease: Detection, Differentiation, and Treatment." *Physician and Sportsmedicine* 25(1)(1997):76.

Clements, M. "Sex in America Today," *Parade Magazine* (Aug. 7, 1994):4.

HIV/AIDS Surveillance Report. Atlanta: U.S. Department of Health and Human Services, Public Health Service, 8(2)(1998).

Hochhauser, M., and Rothenberger, J. *AIDS Education.* St. Louis: WCB/McGraw-Hill, 1996.

Lappé, M. *The Tao of Immunology.* New York: Plenum, 1997.

McGinnis, J. M., and Lee, P. R. "Healthy People 2000 at Mid Decade." *Journal of the American Medical Association* 273(1995):1123.

National Institutes of Health. Interventions to Prevent HIV Risk Behaviors, *NIH Consensus Statement* 15(2)(1997):1.

Payne, W. A., and Hahn, D. B. *Understanding Your Health* (5th ed.). St. Louis: WCB/McGraw-Hill, 1998, Chapter 13.

U. S. Department of Health and Human Services. *Healthy People 2010 Objectives: Draft for Comment.* Washington, DC: U. S. Department of Health and Human Services, 1998, Objectives Chapter 25: Sexually Transmitted Diseases and Objectives Chapter 21: HIV.

Lab 23A: Sexually Transmitted Disease Risk Questionnaire

Name	Section	Date

Purpose: To help you understand the risks of contracting a sexually transmitted disease.

Procedure:
1. Read the Sexually Transmitted Disease Risk Questionnaire.
2. Answer the questionnaire based on information about someone you know who might be at high risk of contracting an STD.
3. Record the scores in the Results section for the person for whom the questionnaire was answered but do *not* include the person's name on the lab sheet. Use the scores to make a rating (chart 2) and draw conclusions.
4. You may also wish to answer the questionnaire based on your own information but do *not* record your personal results on the lab sheet. Use these scores strictly for your own personal information.

Chart 1 Sexually Transmitted Disease Risk Questionnaire

Directions: Mark an X over one response in each row of the questionnaire. Determine a point value for each response using the values in the circles. Sum the numbers of points for the various responses to determine a STD risk score.

			Points		
Categories	**0**	**1**	**3**	**5**	**8**
Feelings about prevention	Able to talk with future partner about STDs. (0)	Find it hard to discuss STDs with a possible partner. (1)			
Behaviors	Never engages in sexual activity. (0)		Sexual activity with one partner, well-known to him/her. (3)	Sexual activity with one partner, not well-known to him/her. (5)	Sexual activity with multiple partners and/or high-risk individuals. (8)
Behavior of friends	Most friends do not engage in unsafe sexual activity. (0)	Many friends engage in unsafe sexual activity. (1)			
Contraception	Not sexually active. (0)	Would use condom to prevent STD. (1)		Would sometimes use condom to prevent STD. (5)	Would never use condom to prevent STD. (8)
Other	Does not use drugs. (0)				Uses injected drugs in unsafe manner. (8)

Chart 2 Risk Questionnaire Rating Chart

Rating	Score
High risk	9+
Above average risk	7–8
Moderate risk	4–6
Low risk	0–3

Results:

What is the person's STD risk score [   ] (total from STD Risk Questionnaire)

What is the person's STD rating? [   ] (See STD Risk Questionnaire Rating Chart)

Conclusions and Implications: Of course, risk varies with different types of STDs. However, this questionnaire will give you an idea of an individual's "general" risk for most STDs. Answer the following questions about the risk of the person you scored and rated.

1. In several sentences, explain which STD do you think this person should be especially concerned about? Why?

2. What specific recommendations would you have for the person for whom you filled out this questionnaire?

Concept 24

Preventing Other Health Threats through Lifestyle Changes

Many diseases and conditions that cause pain, suffering, and premature death in modern society are associated with unhealthy lifestyles.

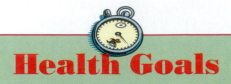

Health Goals

for year 2010

Reduce cancer deaths.

Reduce sun overexposure.

Increase the number of cancer survivors who live five years or more after diagnosis.

Reduce incidence and diagnosis of Type II diabetes.

Reduce death rates from diabetes and disabilities associated with diabetes.

Decrease incidence of depression.

Increase healthy and active days.

Decrease incidence of and deaths from heart disease and stroke, especially among women.

Decrease incidence of high blood pressure and high blood fat levels.

Increase screening and availability of medical treatment for a variety of health threats.

Eliminate health disparities.

Improve air quality, ensure safe water, and reduce environmental waste and hazards.

Reduce unintentional injuries (focus on head and spinal cord) from all sources including firearms, drowning, pedestrian, bicycle and auto accidents, and fires.

Reduce violence and abuse.

Introduction

Each year, many deaths and much pain and suffering could be prevented by altering lifestyles associated with various diseases and health threats. Heart disease, the leading cause of death and stroke (third leading cause of death), and osteoporosis were discussed in the concept on health benefits of physical activity so they will not be discussed here. Among the conditions that are discussed in this concept are cancer, bronchitis/emphysema, injuries, diabetes, and emotional disorders (including suicide), and Syndrome X, a recently identified metabolic condition. Cancer is second only to heart disease among the leading causes of death. Deaths from heart disease have decreased in recent years, but deaths from cancer have increased. If this trend continues, cancer will soon become the leading cause of death in North America. Injuries, diabetes, and suicide all rank among the top ten leading causes of death in our society.

The Facts about Cancer

Cancer is a group of more than 100 different diseases.

According to the American Cancer Society, cancer is a group of many different conditions characterized by abnormal, uncontrolled cell growth that will ultimately invade the blood and lymph tissues and spread throughout the body if not treated. Throughout the human body, new cells are constantly being created to replace older ones. For reasons unknown, abnormal cells sometimes develop that are capable of uncontrolled growth. **Benign tumors** are generally not considered to be cancerous because their growth is restricted to a specific area of the body by a protective membrane. Treatment is important because any tumor can interfere with normal bodily functioning. Once removed, a benign tumor typically will not return.

Malignant tumors are called **carcinomas** because they are capable of uncontrolled growth that can cause death to tissue. Malignant cells invade healthy tissues and deplete them of nutrition and interfere with a multitude of tissue functions. In the early stages of cancer, malignant tumors are located in a small area and can be more easily treated or removed. In advanced cancer, the cells invade the blood or lymph systems and travel throughout the body (**metastases**). When this occurs, cancer becomes much more difficult to treat. Early detection is very important in the treatment and cure of cancer. One method of detecting a tumor is to take a **biopsy** of suspicious lumps in the breasts, testicles, or other parts of the body.

Cancer is a leading killer in our society.

www.mhhe.com/hper/physed/clw/student/

Cancer is the second leading cause of death in our society. After a rise in incidence in the early 1990s, there has been a small decrease in cancer deaths in recent years. Still, one of every five deaths in the United States is caused by some form of cancer. One of three people now living will have cancer at some time in his/her life. It is the cause of much suffering and accounts for a large portion of the money spent on health care. Other diseases, such as heart disease and stroke, have decreased in recent years, but for cancer such dramatic declines have not occurred. Lung cancer is one type of cancer that has increased in the past few decades. This increase is at least

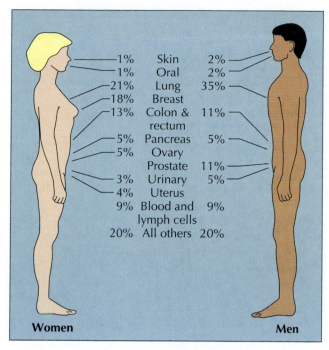

Figure 1
Cancer incidence by site and sex.
SOURCE: Data from the American Cancer Society.

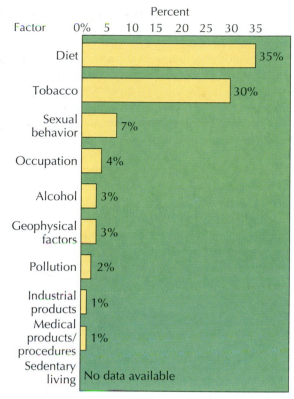

Figure 2
Lifestyle and environmental cancer risk factors.
SOURCE: Data from the American Cancer Society.

part of the reason why cancer rates are so high in North America.

> ## Of the more than 100 forms of cancer, four account for more than half of all illness and death.

The four types of cancer that account for the majority of deaths are lung cancer, colorectal cancer, breast cancer, and prostate cancer (see Figure 1). For women aged 50–60, breast cancer is the most prevalent form of cancer. Prostate cancer risk for men is especially high after age 55. Cancer risk among African Americans is higher than among Caucasians. Nonmalignant skin cancer (**melanoma**) is the most common form of cancer in the United States, but because it can be relatively easily detected and treated if discovered early, it is not among the leading cancer killers.

> ## Many factors are associated with increased risk of cancer; among them is unhealthy lifestyles.

Genetics, environment, and lifestyle are general categories of risk factors associated with cancer. People who have a family history of cancer have a greater risk than those who have no family history. Whereas genetic factors are not within your personal control, many environmental and lifestyle factors are. Figure 2 illustrates the contribution of various lifestyle and environmental factors to cancer mortality. Controlling these risk factors can considerably reduce cancer risk.

Benign Tumor A slow-growing tumor that does not spread to other parts of the body.

Malignant Tumor Malignant means "growing worse." A malignant tumor is one that is considered to be cancerous and will spread throughout the body if not treated.

Carcinoma A malignant or invasive form of tumor.

Metastases The spread of cancer cells to other parts of the body.

Biopsy Removal of a tissue sample that can be checked for cancer cells.

Melanoma Cancer of the cells that produce skin pigment.

Among the lifestyle behaviors that can be changed to reduce cancer risk are performing regular physical activity and eating well. Because the relationship between physical activity and cancer was discussed at length in the concept on the health benefits of physical activity, this relationship will be discussed only briefly here. It is now known that sedentary living is a risk factor for several types of cancer. People who are active have less risk of colorectal, breast, and reproductive system cancer. Being active is important, in part, because it improves fitness. Recent studies have shown that individuals with low levels of fitness have a greater risk of death from cancer than those with good levels of fitness. The importance of good nutrition has been discussed previously. However, it bears repeating that eating well, including decreasing fat and increasing complex carbohydrate consumption (more fiber in diet), are factors that can reduce cancer risk. The importance of a positive attitude cannot be discounted. People with a "fighting spirit" and who hold out hope have less reoccurrence of cancer than people with less positive attitudes.

Tobacco use has been shown to cause cancer of a variety of types. About 30 percent of all cancers are related to tobacco use, especially lung cancer and oral cancer. The decreases in smoking from 1965 to the present have been dramatic, but the rate of decrease has not been as great among women as men. According to the Department of Health and Human Services, a sharper decline in smoking among women is necessary or women will be faced with more cancer than men in the twenty-first century. Lung cancer deaths continue to exceed death rates from breast cancer among women. The recent decline in smoking among men has resulted in a decline in lung cancer deaths in this population.

Examples of some of the less well-known risk categories include geophysical (radiation), pollution (PCB, a byproduct of the plastic industry), industrial products (asbestos, DDT, and 2-4-5-T [also known as Agent Orange]), and medical products (X-rays). Substances contained in many of these products are considered to be **carcinogens** because exposure to them causes cancer. Avoiding exposure to or consumption of carcinogens reduces the risk of cancer.

Recognizing early warning signals can help reduce the risk of cancer.

The acronym CAUTION will help you remember these early warning signs. Look for the following:

C = Changes in bowel or bladder habits

A = A sore that does not heal

U = Unusual bleeding or discharge

T = Thickening or lump in the breast or elsewhere

I = Indigestion or difficulty swallowing

O = Obvious change in a wart or mole

N = Nagging cough or hoarseness

Table 1 Strategies for Preventing Cancer

- Eat a healthy diet: reduce fat to less than 30%, increase complex carbohydrates, decrease simple carbohydrates, avoid junk food, and eat green and yellow vegetables.
- Eliminate tobacco use: cigarettes, other smoking, and smokeless tobacco.
- Perform regular activity: be physically fit, do daily exercise, and avoid obesity.
- Reduce sun and ultraviolet light exposure: use sunscreen, wear protective clothing, and avoid exposure to sun and tanning lights.
- Do regular self-screening and medical testing.
- Avoid carcinogens in food (such as sodium nitrate in bacon) and in other sources (such as insecticides).
- Use moderation if you drink alcohol.
- Avoid breathing polluted air.
- Avoid excessive X-rays.
- Have a positive attitude and a "fighting spirit."

There are several strategies that can be followed to help prevent cancer.

The national health goals focus on altering lifestyles to improve health and well-being. Some of the strategies that can help prevent cancer are shown in Table 1.

Regular self-examinations and periodic medical tests can help reduce risk of cancer.

Self-examination is one screening method that can detect cancer early. In addition, regular medical tests should be sought. Table 2 lists some of the tests that should be performed and provides guidelines as to frequency and the type of individual who could most benefit from the test. The national health goal report indicates that we have made progress in several areas of cancer screening in recent years including increased rate of **mammograms** and **Pap tests** among women, and **fecal occult blood tests** for both men and women. A recently developed "Thin Prep" Pap test has been developed. It finds more abnormal cells than traditional tests, but is more expensive. In Lab 24B information is presented to help you perform breast and testicular self-exams.

Many forms of cancer can be cured.

A total of 51 percent of people who have had cancer survive five years after detection, at which time they are considered to be cured if they are symptom-free. This survival rate is well

Table 2 Cancer Screening Guidelines

Test or Procedure	Sex	Age	Frequency
Cancer checkup (exam for cancers of the thyroid, testicles, prostate, ovaries, lymph nodes, mouth, and skin)	Men/women	20 to 40 Over 40	Every 3 years Every year
Testicle self-evaluation	Men	Over 20	Every month
Digital rectal exam for prostate cancer	Men	Over 40	Every year
Fecal occult blood test (sample of stool examined for the presence of blood)	Men/women	Over 50	Every year
Sigmoidoscopy (examination of a portion of the large intestine)	Men/women	50 and over	Every 3 to 5 years
Pap test	Women	Sexually active women over 18 should have an annual Pap test and pelvic exam	
Pelvic exam	Women		
Breast self-exam	Women	20 and over	Every month
Breast exam by physician	Women	Over 20	Every year
Mammogram	Women	35 to 39 40 to 49 50 and over	Baseline Every 1 to 2 years Every year
Endometrial tissue sample (sample of tissue from the lining of the uterus)	Women	At menopause for women at high risk (history of infertility, obesity, failure to ovulate, abnormal uterine bleeding, or estrogen therapy)	At menopause for women at high risk
Skin cancer check	Men/women	At any age if at high risk because of lengthy exposure to the sun	As recommended by your physician. See your doctor if changes occur in warts or moles.

Sᴏᴜʀᴄᴇ: Data from the American Cancer Society.

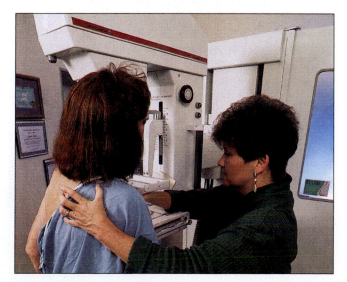

Cancer risk can be reduced by periodic medical tests and self-screening.

above the 38 percent rate several decades ago. The increased survival rate is no doubt due to new and effective methods of treatment not available years ago, but experts believe that preventive measures have also improved and are also responsible. Early detection is critical to chances of a cure. This points out the importance of self-exams and regular medical check-ups.

Carcinogen A substance that tends to produce a tumor or cancer. Examples include asbestos fibers and various substances in tobacco.

Mammogram An X-ray of the breast.

Fecal Occult Blood Test (FOBT) A test to check if there is blood in stool (fecal matter).

Pap Test A test of cells of the cervix to detect cancer or other conditions.

The Facts about Diabetes

There are several classifications of diabetes that cause health risk to many individuals.

Glucose is a sugar in the blood that is a source of energy. Normally, glucose levels range from 50 to 100 mg per each 100 ml of blood. Diabetes is a disease that occurs when the blood glucose is chronically high. There are as many as 30 different reasons for high blood sugar. Therefore, diabetes is really many different diseases, not just one. There is no cure for diabetes, but in most cases it can be controlled with proper medication and a healthy lifestyle.

Insulin, a hormone produced by the pancreas, regulates the glucose in the blood. When a person's body fails to produce adequate insulin and the individual needs to take insulin (oral or injection) to regulate blood-glucose levels, he or she is said to have **Type I diabetes.** About 5 percent of all diabetics have Type I diabetes, and this condition is typically diagnosed before the age of 30.

Type II diabetes is typically non-insulin dependent and can often be controlled with significant lifestyle changes and drugs other than insulin. Nearly 95 percent of all diabetics have Type II diabetes. About 10.5 million diabetics have been diagnosed and another 5.5 million are unaware of their condition. A third and relatively rare form of diabetes is referred to as gestational diabetes mellitus. This occurs when high blood-sugar levels occur in pregnant women previously not known to have diabetes. This condition is present in about 3 percent of all pregnancies and can have implications for the fetus and may or may not result in a diabetes state after pregnancy. There are other forms of diabetes but they are rare.

There is a familial predisposition to both Type I and Type II, though the predisposition is greater for Type I diabetes. Some people with Type II diabetes do not produce enough insulin to regulate their blood-sugar levels, but more commonly they are insensitive to insulin, so the body cannot effectively use available blood sugar.

Diabetes and related conditions are a leading cause of death in our society.

www.mhhe.com/hper/physed/clw/student/
People with diabetes have a shortened life span as well as many short-term and long-term complications associated with the disease. It is especially important for them to recognize their illness because proper medication and changes in lifestyle can greatly reduce the complications of the disease and the death rate associated with it.

African Americans and Native Americans are especially at risk of diabetes. Not only is the death rate higher among these groups, but so are the health problems associated with the disease. Unlike heart diseases and cancers for which we have made progress toward national health goals of reducing disease rates, there has actually been an increase in the incidence of diabetes in the last decade.

Diabetes is associated with other health problems.

People with diabetes have an increased risk of additional health problems. For example, diabetes is considered to be a risk factor for heart disease and high blood pressure. Diabetics have a higher rate of kidney failure (including the need for kidney transplants and kidney dialysis), a high incidence of blindness, and a high incidence of lower limb amputation. Women with diabetes also have a high rate of pregnancy complications.

Lifestyle changes can help reduce the symptoms and complications typically associated with diabetes.

Three of the national health goals for the year 2010 reflect lifestyle changes that can help reduce health problems associated with diabetes. These goals are:

- Reduce overweight (fatness) in the general population. Reducing body fat is probably the most significant way to reduce the incidence of diabetes in our society.
- Increase daily physical activity. Regular exercise results in calories expended and is one way to help reduce overfatness. It also helps regulate blood-sugar levels and helps body cells become more sensitive to insulin.
- Reduce dietary fat intake, increase intake of complex carbohydrates, and decrease total calorie intake. Particularly important is the value of a sound diet in reducing body fatness.

There has been some recent progress in increasing daily activity levels, but not for totally sedentary people. Furthermore, there has actually been an increase in the incidence of overweight people over the last decade. Health experts suggest that diabetes is a "big problem that will get bigger in the future." It is considered a "wasteful" disease because lifestyle changes that are possible for most people could greatly reduce the incidence of Type II diabetes.

Once diabetes is recognized, adherence to a treatment program is essential to prevent related conditions.

www.mhhe.com/hper/physed/clw/student/
Controlling weight, eating properly, and performing regular exercise can help prevent the symptoms of Type II diabetes, in particular. In addition to these strategies, adherence to a regular medication schedule and stress management are important. However, if symptoms

such as nausea, fatigue, weakness, excessive thirst, and loss of weight occur, as they often do in Type I diabetics, or if blurred vision, numbness of the limbs, and skin or gum infections occur, medical help should be sought. A **glucose tolerance test** can be performed to help detect the existence of diabetes. Early diagnosis resulting from attention to the symptoms described above can expedite successful treatment. A national health goal is to increase the rate of diagnosis and to increase the number of diabetics who get regular blood lipid assessments, blood pressure checks, and foot and eye examinations. The incidence of amputations and blindness is high among diabetics who go untreated.

The Facts about Other Health Threats

Injuries are a major cause of death and suffering.

Not only are injuries the fifth leading cause of death among people of all ages; they claim more lives than chronic and infectious diseases among people aged 40 and younger. The major causes of injuries are shown in Table 3.

Injuries also account for much pain and suffering. Of all hospital stays, one in six results from a nonfatal injury. Injury rates are higher among males than females, and they are quite high among ethnic and racial minority groups. Since 1990, the number of deaths caused by unintentional injuries and by work-related injuries has decreased.

Changes in lifestyles can reduce injury rates.

A major conclusion of the Public Health Service is that the prevention of injuries requires the combined efforts of many fields, including health, education, transportation, law, engineering, architecture, and safety science.

The second major conclusion of the Public Health Service is that alcohol is "intimately associated" with the causes and severity of injuries. Other lifestyle behaviors are also associated with reducing injury incidence, and some of the steps that can be taken to reduce these injuries are listed in Table 4.

Table 3 Major Causes of Injuries

- Motor vehicle crashes
- Falls
- Poisoning
- Drowning
- Residential fires

SOURCE: Data from the Public Health Service.

Table 4 Steps to Reduce Injuries

Reduce Motor Vehicle Accidents

- Do not drive while under the influence of alcohol.
- Increase use of shoulder seat belts and air bags.
- Reduce driving speed.
- Use motorcycle helmets.
- Improve safety of off-road vehicles.
- Increase safety programs for pedestrians and cyclists.
- Establish more effective licensing for very young and older drivers.

Improve Home and Neighborhood Environments

- Enact laws requiring new handguns be designed to minimize discharge by children.
- Extend laws requiring sprinkler systems in homes with high risk of fire.
- Increase presence of functional smoke detectors in homes.
- Increase injury education in schools.
- Wear effective face, head, eye, and mouth protection in sports, including helmets for cycling.
- Improve pool and boat safety education.
- Learn cardiopulmonary resuscitation.
- Properly mark poisons and prescription drugs.
- Properly package and store poisons and prescription drugs (childproof).
- Shift to nontoxic fuels for cooking.
- Provide poison education for children and older populations.

Insulin A hormone that regulates blood-sugar levels.

Type I Diabetes A chronic metabolic disease characterized by high blood-sugar (glucose) levels associated with the inability of the pancreas to produce insulin; also called insulin-dependent diabetes mellitus (IDDM) or juvenile-onset diabetes.

Type II Diabetes A chronic metabolic disease characterized by high blood sugar, usually not requiring insulin therapy: also called non-insulin dependent diabetes mellitus (NIDDM) or adult-onset diabetes.

Glucose Tolerance Test A test used to diagnose diabetes. It consists of a blood-sugar measurement following the ingestion of a standard amount of sugar (glucose) after a period of fasting.

Improved occupational safety could help reduce injury rates.

Many of the nation's health goals focus on improving occupational safety, especially among construction, health care (nurses, etc.), farm, transportation, and mine workers. (For more details, see "Healthy People 2010" in Suggested Readings.)

Many mental disorders pose threats to health and wellness.

The health goals for the nation identify suicide, schizophrenia, and depression as the most serious mental disorders needing attention. (Though the Public Health Service uses the term "mental disorders," they are sometimes called emotional disorders.) Other common mental disorders are sleep disturbances, panic disorders, antisocial personality disorders, fears, and phobias.

Mental disorders result in loss of life, injury, and inability to function, and they cost the public millions of dollars annually.

Nearly one in 10 among the adult population suffers from a mental disorder that limits ability to function effectively and requires special assistance. Depression and other mood disorders affect one in 20 people. These disorders cost $73 billion annually, primarily from loss of productivity. The most serious outcome of mental disorders is suicide (30,000 annually). In the last 10 years, progress has been made in reducing suicide (a national health goal).

Reducing the incidence of suicide and serious injury from suicide attempts is an important national health goal.

Suicide attempts are common among all age groups. Men are more likely to attempt and commit suicide than women. Among male teenagers, it is the second leading cause of death, and male teenagers with antisocial personality disorders are especially susceptible.

Depression is closely associated with suicide, as are alcohol and drug abuse. Inability to cope with stressful life events may contribute to suicide. Examples of precipitating

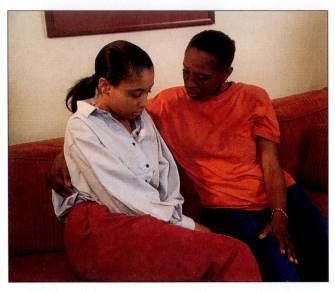

The help of a professional is often necessary to treat depression.

events are divorce, separation, loss of a loved one, unemployment, and financial setbacks.

The best chance for reducing suicides appears to be early detection and treatment of mental disorders such as depression. Professional help should be sought, and as many concerned people as possible should be recruited to help the suicidal individual seek professional assistance. Experts suggest that threats of suicide must not be taken lightly.

Depression is a common mental disorder that can usually be treated effectively.

www.mhhe.com/hper/physed/clw/student/

At some time in life, most people occasionally feel depressed or "blue." This type of depression is usually not a mental disorder. People with clinical depression (classified as a mental disorder) have chronic feelings of guilt, hopelessness, low self-esteem, and dejection. They frequently have trouble sleeping, loss of appetite, lack of interest in social activities, lack of interest in sex, and inability to concentrate.

Among the lifestyle changes that can help relieve symptoms are regular exercise, increased social contact, realistic goal setting, and removing oneself from situations that contribute to depression. These changes, however, may need to be accompanied by professional therapy and/or medication. Helping an individual to change lifestyles and to seek professional help are important because depression is often associated with suicide.

Sleep disorders can often be helped by lifestyle changes.

Sleep disorders, especially insomnia (long-term problems with sleep) can result in depression and other dysfunctions. Physiological problems in the brain can cause sleep disorders, but often they are a result of depression, stress, chronic pain, or abuse of alcohol/drugs. Some sleep disorders require professional help. However, there are some things you can do to prevent insomnia. Examples include creating a healthy sleeping environment, avoiding excessive caffeine or alcohol, exercising regularly, and using stress-management techniques. Establishing a regular routine for sleeping can also be helpful and should include regular sleeping hours and a stress-reduction time before retiring.

Syndrome X is a newly identified health problem that can be modified with lifestyle changes.

www.mhhe.com/hper/physed/clw/student/

Syndrome X is a name given to a metabolic problem that exists when a person possesses several or all of the following: high blood pressure; high LDL levels; low HDL levels; high levels of other blood fats; resistance to insulin; high levels of insulin in the blood; high body fat levels; and high amounts of fat in the abdominal region. This complex of risk factors predisposes a person to many different medical conditions including heart disease, diabetes, and cancer. More and more researchers are finding that the risk factors for one disease are also risk factors for others. Syndrome X illustrates this fact.

Men typically have risk profiles associated with Syndrome X, especially as age increases. Hispanic, Native American, and some other ethnic minorities are also more likely to have Syndrome X profiles. Recent evidence suggests that postmenopausal women develop many of the characteristics of Syndrome X yet may not receive the same medical advice as males. Of course, medical help is a must for people with Syndrome X characteristics. However, healthy lifestyles help alter many of Syndrome X risk factors, which can have multiple benefits in terms of reduced incidence of a variety of diseases and in improving quality of life and sense of well-being.

Strategies for Action: The Facts

Self-assessments and regular medical exams can help you determine if you need help with various health problems.

Just as the fitness assessments you completed earlier in this book helped you build a profile that will help you improve your fitness, regular self-assessments can help you identify and prevent common health problems. Regular medical exams that include the tests outlined in Table 2 as well as those described in other sections of this concept will help you identify problems that can be treated and cured with early diagnosis. In Lab 24A, you will have the opportunity to assess your cancer risk. In Lab 24B, you will learn to do self-exams to help you resist breast and testicular cancer.

Staying current with new health information can help you identify and get treatment for health problems.

Information about various health problems changes rapidly as new methods of treatment and prevention become available. It is important to learn ways to stay current on health topics. Web Review contains addresses for websites of reputable health organizations that will help you stay abreast of current information.

Adhering to sound medical advice is important to disease prevention and treatment.

Many people in our culture have a fear of disease. Too many avoid medical advice because of this fear. Many of the conditions described in this concept, especially cancer and diabetes, can be managed or cured with early diagnosis and proper treatment. Once a plan of treatment is outlined, it is important to stick with it.

Web Review

Web review materials for Concept 24 are available are at *www.mhhe.com/hper/physed/clw/student/*.

American Cancer Society

http://www.cancer.org

American Diabetes Association

www.diabetes.org

American Heart Association

www.amhrt.org

CDC Diabetes Home Page

www.cdc.gov/nccdphp/ddt/ddthome.htm

Environmental Protection Agency

www.epa.gov

National Cancer Institute

http://www.nci.nih.gov/

National Center for Environmental Health

www.cdc.gov/nceh/oncehhom.html/

National Institute of Environmental Health Sciences

www.niehs.nih.gov

National Institute of Mental Health (NIMH)

http://gopher.nih.gov/

Suggested Readings

Corbin, C. B. and Pangrazi, R. P. (ed.) *Towards a Better Understanding of Physical Fitness and Activity.* Scottsdale, AZ: Holcomb-Hathaway, 1999, Chapters 9, 10, 11.

Payne, W. A. and Hahn, D. B. *Understanding Your Health* (5th ed.). St. Louis: WCB/McGraw-Hill, 1998, Chapters 10, 11, 12, 19, and 20.

Ransdell, L. B., et al. "Syndrome X: A Postmenopausal Woman's Hidden Nemesis." *Journal of Women and Aging* 9 (1/2) 1997, 53.

U. S. Department of Health and Human Services. *Healthy People 2010 Objectives: Draft for Comment.* Washington, DC: U. S. Department of Health and Human Services, 1998, Objectives Chapters 5, 7, 8, 17, 18, 19, 20, 23, and 24.

Lab 24A: Determining Your Cancer Risk

Name	**Section**	**Date**

Purpose: To make you aware of your cancer risk for various types of cancer.

Procedures:
1. Answer the questions in the six-part questionnaire for the various forms of cancer.
2. Record the number of "yes" answers for each form of cancer in the Results section.
3. Use chart 1 to determine ratings and record the ratings in the Results section.
4. Answer the questions in the Conclusions and Implications section.

Results: Directions: Mark an X over your answer to each question.

Skin Cancer Risk Factor

Do you frequently work or play in the sun for long periods of time? Yes No

Do you or have you worked near industrial exposure (coal mine, radioactivity)? Yes No

Do you have a family history of skin cancer? Yes No

Do you have fair skin? Yes No

Lung Cancer Risk Factor

Do you smoke? Yes No

Do you or have you worked near industrial exposure (coal mine, radioactivity)? Yes No

Do you have a family history of cancer? Yes No

Do you work in a place that allows smoking, such as a bar, or live in a home with smokers? Yes No

Colorectal Cancer Risk Factor

Do you eat a lot of fat? Yes No

Do you avoid foods that are high in fiber? Yes No

Do you have a family history of colon or rectal cancer? Yes No

Have you noticed blood in your stool? Yes No

Breast Cancer Risk Factor

Do you have a family history of breast cancer? Yes No

Are you sedentary? Yes No

Are you a female over 35 who has not had children? Yes No

Have you ever detected lumps or cysts in your breasts? Yes No

Uterine/Cervical Cancer Risk Factor* (Females)

Do you regularly have bleeding between periods? Yes No

Is your body fat level high? Yes No

Did you have early intercourse and multiple sexual partners? Yes No

Have you had viral infections of the vagina such as herpes? Yes No

*Because of the personal nature of several questions, do not record results if turned in to an instructor.

Prostate Cancer Risk Factor (Males)

Do you eat a high-fat or low-fiber diet? Yes No

Are you a male over 50 years of age? Yes No

Have you had a positive PSA test? Yes No

Has a digital rectal exam shown an enlargement of the prostate? Yes No

Cancer Type	Score	Rating
Breast		
Uterine/cervical (women)*		
Colorectal		
Skin		
Lung		
Prostate (men)		

*Do not record results if handed in to an instructor.

Chart 1: Cancer Risk Ratings

Score	Rating
4	High risk
3	Relatively high risk
2	Lower risk
0–1	Low risk

Conclusions and Implications: In several sentences, discuss the type or types of cancer for which you are at greatest risk and why. Also, discuss the lifestyles you could modify to reduce your risk.

Lab 24B: Breast and Testicular Self-Exams

Name	**Section**	**Date**

Purpose: To help you learn to do breast and testicular self-exams.

Procedures:
1. Females should read the procedures for breast self-exams. Note: Males should also be aware of abnormal lumps in their breasts.
2. Males should read the procedures for testicular self-exams.
3. After reading the directions, perform the self-exam.
4. If you find lumps or nodules contact a physician.
5. This procedure should be done monthly. The breast exam is best done a day or two after the end of menstrual flow. For this lab, it can be done at any time.
6. It is not necessary to record your results here. Do answer the questions in the Conclusions and Implications section.

Testicular Self-Exam (Men)

1. Using both hands, grasp one testicle between the thumb and first finger.
2. Roll the testicle gently with the thumb and first finger feeling for lumps or nodules.
3. Examine the other testicle using the same procedure.
4. If you find a lump or nodule consult a physician. Note: A lump or nodule may not be a result of disease but this can only be determined by a physician.

Breast Self-Exam (Women and Men)

1. Lie down on your back. Place a pillow or towel under one shoulder and place the arm overhead.
2. With the opposite hand, gently move the fingers over the breast. Use a circular motion (see picture) to probe for lumps starting in a large circle and continuing to probe in smaller and smaller circles. Examine every part of your breast including your nipple. A band of firm tissue along the lower part of the breast is normal. If you have questions, consult your physician.
3. Finally squeeze each nipple gently between the thumb and first finger. If you notice blood or clear discharge, contact a physician.

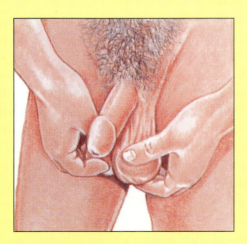

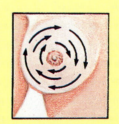 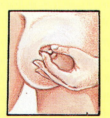

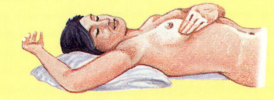

4.   Repeat on the other breast. If you notice any lumps, report it to a physician.
5.   Periodic exams before a mirror can be helpful. With the arms above the head, look for any changes in breast (from your normal). Repeat with the hands on the hips—flex the chest muscles. Again look for any changes from normal.

Conclusions and Implications: In several sentences, discuss the effectiveness of the procedure you performed. Do you think that the directions provided were adequate for you to perform the self-exam effectively? Do you think you will perform this self-exam on a regular basis? What could be done to motivate you and others to do regular self-exams?

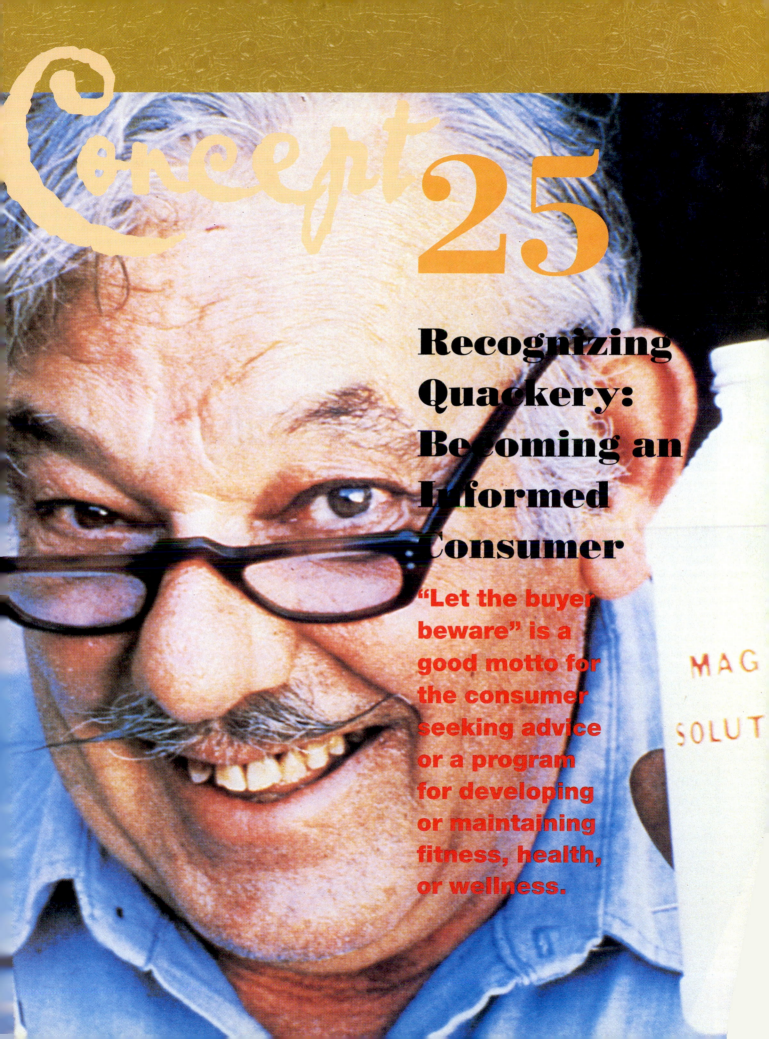

Concept 25

Recognizing Quackery: Becoming an Informed Consumer

"Let the buyer beware" is a good motto for the consumer seeking advice or a program for developing or maintaining fitness, health, or wellness.

MAG

SOLUT

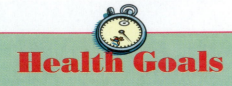

Introduction

People have always searched for the fountain of youth and the easy, quick, and miraculous route to health and happiness. This search has included the area of physical fitness, especially physical activity, nutrition, and weight loss. Because of the popularity of these subjects, the mass media have made it possible to convey as much misinformation as information. All people should seek the truth to protect their health as well as their pocketbooks. This concept discusses some myths and separates fact from fancy.

The Facts about Physical Activity

Physical activity has many benefits, but it is not a cure all.

There are numerous benefits of physical activity, many of which have been described throughout this book, but physical activity is not a **panacea.** Some media accounts would have you believe the impossible. People who contemplate beginning a fitness or weight-reducing program are reminded of the following:

- The most satisfactory way to lose weight is to combine caloric reduction and physical activity. There is no fast and easy way.

- Exercise will not change the size of bony structures (e.g., ankles).
- Exercise will not change the size of glands (e.g., breasts); however, chest/bust girth may be increased by strengthening chest muscles.
- Exercise does not break up fatty deposits, though it does burn calories, thus fat will eventually be burned.
- Exercise does not ensure good posture or good health, but it does help attain or maintain these attributes.
- There is no such thing as "effortless exercise."

Physical activity is not effective in promoting physical fitness unless it meets the appropriate threshold of training.

Some popular literature suggests that only a few minutes of physical activity each day is necessary to develop total physical fitness. Research, however, indicates that total fitness (cardiovascular fitness, strength, muscular endurance, flexibility, and desirable body composition) can be attained only through considerable effort. As mentioned previously, exercise must be of sufficient frequency, intensity, and for a sufficient length of time for each part of health-related physical fitness to be effective. Programs that promise complete fitness but do not meet the necessary levels for frequency, intensity, and time should be strongly questioned.

Contrary to some claims, hatha yoga is not a good program for developing comprehensive physical fitness.

Some advocates of hatha yoga claim that regular practice of the asanas (positions) will bring about many benefits. There is no scientific evidence to support most of these claims. Hatha yoga will not help you lose weight, trim inches, remove flab, improve endurance, maintain proper circulation, strengthen glands and organs, or improve complexion as is claimed. Neither will it cure diseases nor conditions such as arthritis, the common cold, diabetes, gallstones, nor menstrual disorders as claimed by some advocates.

Hatha yoga is considered useful for improving flexibility, although some positions are contraindicated (see concept on safe exercises). Hatha yoga is also useful in reducing stress reactions and in promoting neuromuscular relaxation. In some cases, it may be effective in lowering blood pressure in hypertensives. If a person has very weak muscles to begin with, mild (static) strengthening and muscular endurance may develop from assuming and holding the positions.

Getting rid of cellulite does not require a special exercise, diet, cream or device, as some books and advertisements insist.

Cellulite is ordinary fat with a fancy name. You do not need a special treatment or device to get rid of it. In fact, there is no special "remedy." Fat is fat. To decrease fat, reduce calories and do more physical activity.

Spot reducing, or losing fat from a specific location on the body, is not possible. It is a fallacy.

When you do physical activity, calories are burned and fat is recruited from all over the body in a genetically determined pattern. You cannot selectively exercise, bump, vibrate, or squeeze the fat from a particular spot. If you were flabby to begin with, local exercise could strengthen the local muscles, causing a change in the contour and the girth of that body part. But exercise affects the muscles, not the fat on that body part. General aerobic exercises are the most effective for burning fat, but you cannot control where the fat comes off.

Surgically sculpting the body with implants and liposuction to acquire physical beauty will not give you physical fitness and may be harmful.

Rather than doing it the hard way, an increasing number of people are having their "love handles" removed surgically and fake calf and pectoral muscles implanted to improve their physique. Liposuction is not a weight loss technique, but rather a contouring procedure. Like any surgery, it is not without risks. There have been fatalities and there is a risk of infection, hematoma, skin slough, and other conditions.

Muscle implants give a muscular appearance, but they do not make you stronger or more fit. The implants are not really muscle tissue, but rather silicon gel or saline such as that used in breast implants, or a hard substitute. Some complications can occur, such as infection and bleeding, but also, some physicians believe the calf implant may put pressure on the calf muscles and cause them to atrophy. A better way to improve physique and fitness is proper exercise.

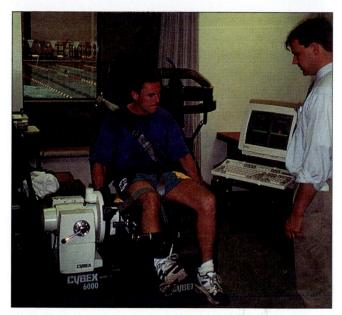

Doing machine exercises can help you recover from injury, but you must provide the movement—not the machine.

The use of hand weights and wrist weights while walking, running, dancing, or bench-stepping can increase the energy cost but requires caution.

The practice of carrying small weights (1–3 pounds) while performing aerobic dance, walking, or other aerobic exercise has been found to increase the metabolic cost of the exercise. When the weight is simply carried, the effect is negligible, but when the arms are pumped (bending the elbow and raising the weight to shoulder height and then extending the elbow as the arm swings down), the energy output can increase enough to make a walk comparable to a slow jog. For the person who does not want to walk or jog faster or farther, it could be an effective way of burning more calories or increasing fitness. It may be better to use wrist weights than to carry a weight, since the act of gripping causes an increase in the diastolic blood pressure. Hand weights or wrist weights are more effective than ankle weights if they do not alter your gait pattern.

It has been suggested that for step-aerobics (bench-stepping), weights should be limited to intermediate and advanced

Panacea   A cure-all; a remedy for all ills.

steppers only and that they not exceed 1–2 pounds. Up to a point, the aerobic intensity can be increased by adding height to the bench. There are hazards to consider in using weights. Coronary patients and people with high blood pressure should be aware that using weights increases both the systolic and diastolic blood pressures. Aerobic dance participants may find it wise to keep the weights below shoulder level if they aggravate the shoulder joint. Anyone with shoulder or elbow joint problems such as arthritis should use weights with caution.

The Facts about Passive Exercise and Passive Devices

Passive exercise is not effective in weight reduction, spot reduction, increasing strength, or increasing endurance.

www.mhhe.com/hper/physed/clw/student/
Passive exercise or devices come in a variety of forms.

WEB

- *Rolling machines*—These ineffective wooden or metal rollers, operated by an electric motor, roll up and down the body part to which they are applied. They do not remove, break up, or redistribute fat.
- *Vibrating belts*—These wide canvas or leather belts may be designed for the chin, hips, thighs, or abdomen. Driven by an electric motor, they jerk back and forth, causing loose tissue of the body part to shake. They do not have any beneficial effect on fitness, fat, or figure, and they are potentially harmful if used on the abdomen (especially if used by women during pregnancy, menstruation, or while an IUD is in place). They might also aggravate a back problem.
- *Vibrating tables and pillows*—Some of these quack devices are actually called toning tables. Contrary to advertisements, these passive devices will not improve posture, trim the body, reduce weight, nor will they develop muscle **tonus.** For some people, vibration can help induce relaxation.
- *Continuous Passive Motion (CPM) Tables*—The CPM table is motor driven, but unlike the vibrating table it moves body parts repeatedly through a range of motion. Tables are designed to do such things as passively extend the leg at the hip joint, raise the upper trunk in a sit-up–like motion, or rotate the legs while the client lies relaxed. Many of the same false claims are made for it as for the vibrating table. It also claims to remove cellulite, increase circulation and oxygen flow, and eliminate excess water retention. None of these claims is true, but the table might be justified in claiming to maintain the range of motion in certain body parts for people who cannot move themselves. A similar concept is incorporated in small, portable

machines used in hospitals and rehabilitation centers to maintain range of motion in the legs of knee surgery patients, maintain integrity of the cartilage, and decrease the incidence of thrombosis. Certainly the normal, healthy person has nothing to gain from using such a device.

- *Motor-driven cycles and rowing machines*—Like all mechanical devices that do the work for the individual, these motor-driven machines are not effective in a fitness program. They may help increase circulation, and some may even help maintain flexibility, but they are not as effective as active exercise. *Nonmotorized cycles and rowing machines* are very good equipment for use in a fitness program.
- *Massage*—Whether done by a masseur/masseuse or by a mechanical device, massage is passive, requiring no effort on the part of the individual. It can help increase circulation, induce relaxation, prevent or loosen adhesions, retard muscle atrophy, and serve other therapeutic uses when administered in the clinical setting for medical reasons. However, massage has no useful role in a physical fitness program and will not alter your shape. There is no scientific evidence that it can hasten nerve growth, remove subcutaneous fat, or increase athletic performance. Some athletes (e.g., cyclists) find that it aids in recovery from exercise.
- *Electrical muscle stimulators*—Neuromuscular electrical stimulators cause the muscle to contract involuntarily. In the hands of qualified medical personnel, muscle stimulators are valuable therapeutic devices. They can increase muscle strength and endurance selectively and aid in the treatment of edema. They can also help prevent atrophy in a patient who is unable to move, and they may decrease spasticity and contracture, but in a healthy person they do not have the same value as exercise. The multiple muscle group stimulation as done in the so-called "toning" clinics or spas has been proven ineffective for muscle strengthening. These devices can be harmful when used improperly and may induce heart attacks; complicate gastrointestinal, orthopedic, kidney, and other disorders; and aggravate epilepsy, hernias, and varicose veins. They should never be used by the layperson and have no place in a reducing or fitness program.
- *Weighted belts*—Claims have been made that these belts reduce waists, thighs, and hips when worn for several hours under the clothing. In reality, they do none of these things and have been reported to cause actual physical harm. When used in a progressive resistance program, wristlet, anklet, or laced-on weights can help produce an overload and, therefore, develop strength or endurance.
- *Inflated, constricting, or nonporous garments*—These garments include rubberized inflated devices ("sauna belts" and "sauna shorts") and paraphernalia that are airtight plastic or rubberized. Evidence indicates that their girth-reducing claims are *unwarranted*. If exercise is performed while wearing such garments, the exercise,

not the garment, may be beneficial. You cannot squeeze fat out of the pores nor can you melt it!

- *Body wrapping*—Some reducing salons, gyms, or clubs advertise that wrapping the body in bandages soaked in a "magic solution" will cause a permanent reduction in body girth. This so-called treatment is pure quackery. Tight, constricting bands can temporarily indent the skin and squeeze body fluids into other parts of the body, but the skin or body will regain its original size within minutes or hours. The solution is usually similar to epsom salts, which can cause fluid to be drawn from tissue. The fluid is water, not fat, and is quickly replaced. Body wrapping may be dangerous to your health; at least one fatality has been documented.

- *Elastic tights*—These are often worn by athletes such as cyclists for the purpose of decreasing chaffing of the skin. There have been some claims that the tights helped improve venous return and thus recovery from exercise. However, studies have shown that the recovery-response of those who wear tights is no different from those who do not wear them.

> Having a good tan is often associated with being fit and looking good, but getting tanned can be risky business.

www.mhhe.com/hper/physed/clw/student/
Tanning salons may claim their lamps are safe because they emit only UV-A rays, but these rays can age the skin prematurely and make it look wrinkled and leathery. It may also increase the cancer-producing potential of UV-B rays and cause eye damage. Since there is no warning sign of redness, there is danger of overdosing. Thirty minutes of exposure to UV-A can suppress the immune system. Tanning devices can also aggravate certain skin diseases. The **FDA** advises against the use of any suntan lamp. It is dangerous to use tanning accelerator lotions with the lamps because they can promote burning of the skin. Tanning pills are an even worse choice. They can cause itching, welts, hives, stomach cramps, and diarrhea, and can decrease night vision. Tanning in the sun is also hazardous because it damages the skin, making it age prematurely. It may cause skin cancer. It is best to use products with sun blockers if you must spend long periods in the sun.

The Facts about Baths

> Saunas, steam baths, whirlpools, and hot tubs are not effective in weight reduction or in the prevention and cure of colds, arthritis, bursitis, backaches, sprains, or bruises.

Baths do not melt off fat; fat must be metabolized. The heat and humidity from baths may make you perspire, but it is water, not fat, oozing from the pores.

The effect of such baths is largely psychological, although some temporary relief from aches and pains may

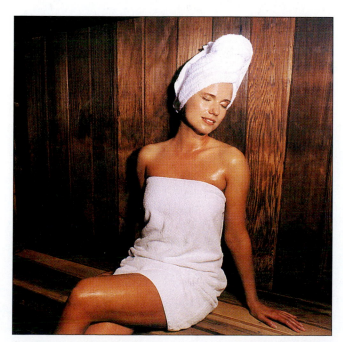

Saunas or other baths may help you relax, but they do not result in fat loss or fitness improvement.

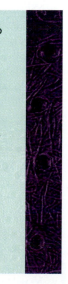

Passive Exercise A type of exercise in which no voluntary muscle contraction occurs; some outside force moves the body part with no effort by the person.

Tonus The most frequently misused and abused term in fitness vocabularies. Tonus is the tension developed in a muscle as a result of passive muscle stretch. Tonus cannot be determined by feeling or inspecting a muscle. It has little or nothing to do with the strength of a muscle.

FDA Abbreviation for the Food and Drug Administration: a federal agency that recommends and enforces government regulations regarding certain foods and drugs.

result from the heat. The same relief can be had by sitting in a tub of hot water in your bathroom.

Various baths are potentially dangerous and should be used and maintained properly.

The following guidelines/precautions should be considered before using a sauna, steam bath, whirlpool, or hot tub:

- Take a soap shower before and after entering the bath.
- Don't wear makeup or skin lotion/oil.
- Wait at least an hour after eating before bathing.
- Cool down after exercise before entering the bath to avoid overheating.
- Drink plenty of water before or during the bath to avoid dehydration.
- Don't wear jewelry.
- Don't sit on a metal stool; do sit on a towel in the steam or sauna bath.
- Don't bathe alone.
- Don't drink alcohol before bathing.
- Get out immediately if you become dizzy; feel hot, chilled, or nauseous; or get a headache.
- Get approval from your physician if you have heart disease, low or high blood pressure, a fever, kidney disease, or diabetes, are obese or pregnant, or are on medications (especially anticoagulants, stimulants, hypnotics, narcotics, or tranquilizers).
- Prolonged use can be hazardous for the elderly or for children.
- Don't exercise in a sauna or steam bath.
- Skin infections can be spread in a bath; make certain it is cleaned regularly and that the hot tub or whirlpool has proper pH and chlorination.
- Follow these recommendations on temperature and duration of stay:

Sauna: should not exceed 190°F (88°C) and duration should not exceed 10 to 15 minutes.

Steam bath: should not exceed 120°F (49°C) and duration should not exceed 6 to 12 minutes.

Whirlpool/hot tub: should not exceed 100°F (37°C) and duration should not exceed 5 to 10 minutes.

The Facts about Quacks

You can usually tell the difference between an expert and a quack because a quack does not use scientific methods.

A good example of this fact is seen in a study that attempted to obtain documentation for products claiming to enhance athletic performance. It was found that there was no published scientific evidence to support the promotional claims of 42 percent of the products. Thirty-two percent had some scientific documentation but were marketed in a misleading manner, and 21 percent were without any human clinical trials.

Some of the ways to identify quacks, frauds, and rip-offs are to look for these clues:

- They do not use the scientific method of controlled experimentation that can be verified by other scientists.
- To a large extent, they use testimonials and anecdotes to support their claims rather than scientific methods. There is no such thing as a valid testimonial. Anecdotal evidence is no evidence at all.
- They advise you to buy something you would not otherwise have bought.
- They have something to sell.
- They claim everyone can benefit from the product or service they are selling. There is no such thing as a simple, quick, easy, painless remedy/tonic or other concoction that is good for many ailments or useful for conditions for which medical science has not yet found a remedy.
- They promise "quick," "miraculous" results. There is no such thing as a perfect no-risk treatment.
- The claims for benefits are broad, covering a wide variety of conditions.
- They may offer a money-back guarantee. A guarantee is only as good as the company.
- They may claim the treatment or product is approved by the FDA. *Note:* Federal law does not permit the mention of the FDA in any way that suggests marketing approval.
- They may claim the support of experts, but the experts are not identified.
- The ingredients or materials in the product may not be identified.
- They may claim there is a conspiracy against them by "bureaucrats," "organized medicine," the FDA, the **AMA,** and other experts and governmental bodies. Never believe a doctor who claims the medical community is persecuting him/her or that the government is suppressing a wonderful discovery.
- Their credentials may be irrelevant to the area in which they claim expertise.
- They use scare tactics, such as "if you don't do this, you will die of a heart attack."
- They may appear to be a sympathetic friend who wants to share with you a "new discovery."
- They may quote from a scientific journal or other legitimate source, but they misquote or quote out of context to mislead you; or they may mix a little bit of truth with a lot of fiction.
- They may cite research or quote from individuals or institutions that have questionable reputations for scientific truth.
- They may claim it is a "new discovery" (usually it is said to have originated in Europe). There is never a great medical breakthrough that debuts in an obscure

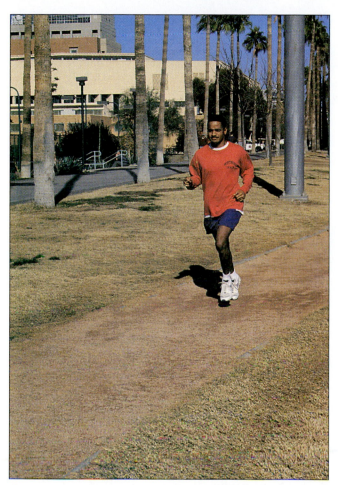

Changing your lifestyle, rather than "quick solutions" is the key to health, fitness and wellness.

magazine or tabloid. There are no secret cures or magic formulae that have not been recognized by the scientific community, a picture on the cover of *Time* magazine, nomination for a Nobel prize, etc.

- The product or organization named is often similar to that of a famous person or creditable institution (e.g., the Mayo diet had no connection with the Mayo Clinic).
- They often sell products through the mail, which does not allow you to examine the product personally. There are no miracle products available only by mail order or from a single source.

There are some common-sense precautions one can take to avoid being a victim of a rip-off.

The following suggestions can help protect you:

- Read the ad carefully, especially the small print.
- Do not send cash; use a check, money order, or credit card so you'll have a receipt.

- Do not order from a company with only a P.O. box, unless you know the company.
- Do not let high-pressure sales tactics make you rush into a decision.
- Do not order from a company requiring use of an 800 telephone number and a credit card (they may be trying to avoid federal statutes).
- When in doubt, check out the company through your Better Business Bureau (BBB).
- If you have a complaint, write to the company first, but keep a copy of all receipts, checks, and correspondence.
- If that fails, write to the Direct Marketing Association. You may also report to the BBB, postmaster (if it was a mail order), state attorney general, and/or the Federal Trade Commission (FTC).

The Facts about Equipment

The consumer who plans to purchase exercise equipment should keep in mind certain guidelines to get the most for the money.

The following suggestions will help you select equipment:

- Unless you are wealthy or just like to collect gadgets, there is no need to buy a lot of exercise equipment. A complete fitness program can be carried out with *no* equipment. If you learn to depend upon equipment, you may eventually feel that you cannot exercise unless you are at home or at a gym.
- If you do not like jogging or swimming, and you hate calisthenics, then the minimal equipment you may want to consider is a bicycle (regular or stationary), tread-mill, or rowing machine for cardiovascular fitness; and a set of weights, pulleys, or isokinetic device for strength and endurance.
- Consult an expert if you want to know the effectiveness of a product. Individuals with college or university degrees in physical education, physical therapy, kinesiotherapy, and kinesiology should be able to give you good advice.
- Buy from a well-established, reputable company that will not disappear overnight and will back up warranties. Avoid mail-order products. If the product is not available in a retail store where it can be examined, you probably should not buy it.
- You get what you pay for. Buying an inexpensive, poorly produced product will result in dissatisfaction in the long run.

AMA Abbreviation for the American Medical Association.

The Facts about Health Clubs

It is not necessary to join a club, spa, or salon to develop fitness, but if you are considering joining such an establishment, make your choice with care.

The consumer should observe these precautions before becoming a member of a club, spa, or salon:

- Do not expect "miraculous" results as advertised.
- Be prepared to haggle over price and to resist a very hard sell for a long-term contract.
- Choose a no-contract, pay-as-you-go establishment if possible. Otherwise, choose the shortest term contract available.
- If there is a contract, read the fine print carefully and look for:
  - the interest rate;
  - "confession of judgment" clauses waiving your right to defend yourself in court;
  - noncancelable clauses;
  - "holder-in-due-course" doctrines allowing the establishment to sell your contract to a collection agency;
  - a waiver of the establishment's liability for injury to you on the premises.
- Consult with an independent expert if you have questions about the programs offered by the establishment.
- Do not accept diets, drugs, or food supplements from the club. Your physician will prescribe these if they are needed.
- You do not have to conform to the program the club suggests for you. Do not perform dangerous exercises, or passive exercises, or participate in fraudulent "treatments." Choose only those activities that meet the criteria explained in this book.
- Refuse to be pestered by solicitations for new members.
- Make a trial visit to the establishment during the hours when you would normally expect to use the facility to determine if it is open, if it is overcrowded, if the equipment is available, if the attendants are selling rather than assisting, and if you would enjoy the company of the other patrons.
- Determine the qualifications of the personnel, especially of the individual responsible for your program. Is he or she an expert as defined previously?
- Make certain the club is a well-established facility that will not disappear overnight.
- Check its reputation with the Better Business Bureau in your area.

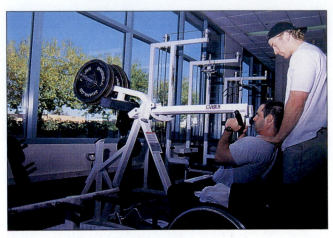

Visit a health club before you join.

- Investigate the programs offered by the YMCA/YWCA, local colleges and universities, and municipal park and recreation departments. These agencies often have excellent fitness classes at lower prices than commercial establishments and usually employ qualified personnel. For weight loss, investigate franchised clubs, such as Weight Watchers or TOPS, or affiliate with a university or a hospital-based program.

The Facts about Dietary Supplements

The burden of proof about the effectiveness of food supplements rests with the consumer.

The passage of the Dietary Supplements Health and Education Act in 1994 shifted the burden of providing assurances of product effectiveness from the FDA to the food supplement industry, which really means it shifted to you—the consumer. Food supplements are typically not considered to be drugs, so they are not regulated. Unlike drugs and medicines, food supplements need not be proven effective or even safe to be sold in stores. To be removed from stores, they must be proven ineffective or unsafe. This leaves consumers vulnerable to false claims. Many experts suggest that quackery has increased significantly since 1994 when the Act was passed.

The Act had at least one positive effect. Food supplement labeling must now be truthful and nonmisleading. Claims concerning disease prevention, treatment, or diagnosis must be substantiated in order to appear on the product. Unfortunately, the act did not limit false claims if they are not on the product label. The result has been the removal of claims from labels in favor of claims on separate literature often called "third-party" literature because the label makes no claims, and the seller makes no written claims (second party). Rather the seller provides claims in literature by other people (third party). The literature is distributed separately from the product, thus allowing sellers to make unsubstantiated claims for products. Also the law does not prohibit unproven verbal claims by sales people. It is now up to the consumer to make decisions about the safety and effectiveness of food supplements so it is especially important to be well-informed.

> **Recent legislation designed to regulate food supplements has not been effective in protecting the consumer.**

www.mhhe.com/hper/physed/clw/student/

Since the Dietary Supplements Health and Education Act was passed in 1994, the sales of various supplements has increased dramatically. Some supplements that are thought to enhance performance are called ergogenic aids and were discussed previously in the concept on muscle fitness and the concept on nutrition. Vitamins and mineral supplements were also discussed in the concept on nutrition. Herbal or botanical supplements have also become popular in recent years. Some of the products receiving considerable media attention in recent years are St. John's Wort, Ginseng, Ginkgo, and Saw Palmetto. Information illustrating the claims and potential problems associated with taking herbal supplements is available in Webshow.

www.mhhe.com/hper/physed/clw/student/

A recent report in the *New England Journal of Medicine* (suggested reading Angell, 1998) indicates that the recent increase in food supplement sales ($8 billion a year in 1994 and $12 billion a year by 1997) has resulted in more than a few cases of serious illnesses including lead poisoning, nausea, vomiting, diarrhea, abnormal heart rhythms, impotence, and lethargy. Six reports in the journal address the topic of food supplements that are unregulated suggesting that "alternative treatments should be subjected to scientific testing no less rigorous than that required for advocating unproven and potentially harmful treatments." One of the reports indicates that nearly one-third of the samples of one herbal product tested in California contained dangerous chemicals and drugs not listed on the label. These reports show the importance of asking questions before buying or taking any supplement.

Some questions that should be asked about food supplements are presented in Table 1. It would be wise to ask yourself these questions and to get answers before you consider using a food supplement.

The Facts about Fitness Books, Magazines, and Articles

> **All fitness books do not provide scientifically sound, accurate, and reliable information.**

Because publishers are motivated by profit and publishing is a highly competitive field, the choice of material to be printed is often selected on the basis of how popular, famous, or attractive the author is, or how sensational or unusual his or her ideas are. Movie stars, models, TV personalities, and even Olympic athletes are rarely experts in biomechanics, anatomy and physiology, exercise, and other foundations of physical fitness. Having a good figure/physique, being fit, or having gone through a training program does not, in itself, qualify a person to advise others.

If you have read the facts presented in the other concepts, you should be able to distinguish between fact and fiction. To assist you further, however, there are 10 guidelines listed in Lab 25A. These might help you evaluate whether or not a book, magazine, or article on exercise and fitness is valid, reliable, and scientifically sound. If the answer to each of the questions is not "yes," then you should be suspicious of the material. If in doubt, ask one or more experts, or contact the American Alliance of Health, Physical Education, Recreation and Dance (AAHPERD) or the American College of Sports Medicine (ACSM) (see WebReview). These organizations will refer your question to an appropriate expert.

Strategies for Action: The Facts

> **Being a good consumer requires time, information, and effort.**

www.mhhe.com/hper/physed/clw/student/

With time and effort, you can gain the information you need to make good decisions about products and services that you purchase. In Lab 25A, you will get the opportunity to evaluate an exercise device, a food supplement, a book, or a magazine article. In Lab 25B, you will evaluate a health/wellness or fitness club. Taking the time to investigate a product will help you save money and help you avoid making poor decisions that affect your health, fitness, and wellness. The labs are designed to give you practice in being a good consumer. When you are making real decisions about products or services, it is a good idea to begin your investigation well in advance of the day when a decision is to be made. Sales people often suggest

Table 1 Questions and Comments about Food Supplements

Questions	Comments
Does the government regulate this product to be sure that it is safe and effective?	Since 1994, food supplements can be sold without proof that they are effective. The government does not test food supplements to ensure effectiveness or safety. The FDA must prove the product to be harmful or ineffective to remove it from the market. It is much harder to prove a product ineffective than to provide evidence that it is effective.
Is there evidence to support claims for supplement?	The evidence should be based on research with normal people, not evidence based on a population of subjects who have medical problems or nutritional deficiencies. Third-party information often cites research out-of-context and based on inappropriate studies of atypical, not normal, people.
What are the active ingredients?	If the active ingredient really works, there will be research to show its effectiveness. Of course, if it works, then it is much like a medicine and has similar side effects. Sellers of supplements often suggest the product works, but that it has no side effects that are associated with medicines. Both cannot be true. For example, Cholestin is a variety of red yeast—a natural product. It contains lovastatin, the same active ingredients in medicines for lowering cholesterol. While the product works, it has now been banned by the FDA as an over-the-counter supplement because it has the same active ingredient as medicine and has the same side effects. The regulation of this product by the FDA has been challenged in the courts by the supplement industry. The decision of the courts will have consequences for future regulation of supplements.
What are the possible side-effects and risks of taking the supplement?	As noted above, if a product works as well as a medicine, it probably has the same side effects. If you know the active ingredient, you will know more about the side effects.
Are there possible interactions associated with taking the supplement?	When you take a medicine, you consult a physician or pharmacist about drug interactions. Supplements may interact with other supplements or medicines.
What are the long-term effects of taking the supplement?	Because supplements are not regulated, there has been little research about long-term effects of products. For example, melatonin is a hormone that is used for insomnia. Hormones have strong effects on the body and little is known about melatonin's long-term effects. Consider alternative solutions to long-term use of an unstudied supplement.
Are you sure the product is what it claims to be and that the size of the dose is appropriate?	U. S. Pharmacopeia (USP) is a private nonprofit organization that developed uniform standards for medicines and other health-care products. This organization set standards for vitamins and minerals to assure quality and purity as well as appropriate size and strength of a standard unit of the product (dose size and strength). When standards are developed, the USP label will ensure that the product is what it says it is. As many as two or three dozen herbal products are currently being evaluated to determine appropriate dose size. Products with the USP label that fail to meet standards will be removed from stores. Without the USP label, you are at the mercy of the company that produces the product. The deaths associated with L-tryptophan, an amino acid supplement, occurred because of contaminants (Peak-X) in the unregulated product.
Who makes the product?	In the absence of regulations, the reputation of the company that makes the product is very important. Have complaints been made against the company? Have there been health problems with their products? How long has the company been in business? Large pharmaceutical companies are now beginning to sell supplements because of the high profit margin. Using a product from a large drug company is more likely to ensure that a product is what it is supposed to be but it does not ensure that the product is effective.
Is the cost worth the potential benefits?	The costs of dietary supplements are typically quite high. For example, protein supplements may cost as much as $1.00 a gram. The cost per gram in good food such as protein in a chicken breast is typically a few cents per gram. Most experts suggest that even the most effective supplements have relatively small effects at a very high cost.
Is the source of your information about the supplement reliable and accurate?	Avoid verbal information about products, especially information from the seller. Be wary of third-party literature or research in obscure journals. Be wary of those who discredit sound medical advice or information from regulatory agencies such as the FDA.

that "this offer is only good today." They know that people often make poor decisions when under time pressure, and they want you to make a decision today so that they won't lose a sale.

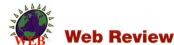 ## Web Review

Web review materials for Concept 25 are available are at *www.mhhe.com/hper/physed/clw/student/*.

Agency for Health Care Policy and Research
www.ahcpr.gov/clinic

American Medical Association Health Insight
www.ama-assn.org/consumer.htm

Center for Science in the Public Interest
www.cspinet.org

Medscape
www.medscape.com

National Council for Reliable Health Information (NCRHI)
www.ncahf.org

Office of Dietary Supplements
http://odp.od.nih.gov/ods/default.html

Quackwatch
www.quackwatch.com

Suggested Readings

Angell, M., and Kassirer, J. P. "Alternative Medicine: The Risks of Untested and Unregulated Remedies." *New England Journal of Medicine* 339(12)(1998):839.

Armsey, T. D., and Green, G. A. "Nutrition Supplements: Science vs. Hype. *Physician and Sportsmedicine* 25(6)(1997):76.

Barrett, S., and Jarvis, W., eds. *The Health Robbers: A Close Look at Quackery in America.* Buffalo, NY: Prometheus Books, 1993.

Cardinal, B. J. "Rating the Clubs: A Health and Fitness Center Consumer Checklist." *American Fitness* (Sept./Oct. 1994).

Clarkson, P. M. "The Skinney on Weight Loss Supplements and Drugs: Winning the War Against Fat." *ACSM's Health and Fitness* 2(4)(1998):18.

deLateur, B. J., and Lehmann, J. F. "Therapeutic Exercise to Develop Strength and Endurance." In Kotke, S., and Lehman, O., eds. *Krusen's Handbook of Physical Medicine and Rehabilitation,* 4th ed. Philadelphia: W.B. Saunders, 1990, 480–495.

"Health Clubs: The Right Choice." *Consumer Reports* 61(1996):27.

"Health Spas, Exercise Clubs, etc." *Information for Prudent Consumers.* Loma Linda, CA: National Council Against Health Fraud, 1994.

Kuntzleman, C. T., and Wilkerson, R. "A Primer to Recommending Home Aerobic Equipment." *ACSM's Health and Fitness Journal* 1(6)(1997):24.

Lake, D. A. "Neuromuscular Stimulation: An Overview and Its Implications in the Treatment of Sports Injuries." *Sports Medicine* 13(1992):320–336.

National Council for Reliable Health Information Newsletter. Published every other month, it contains articles that give objective information about health products and food supplements. NCRHI, P. O. Box 1276, Loma Linda, CA 92354.

"Shearing the Suckers." *Consumer Reports,* (February 1986):87.

Lab 25A: Practicing Consumer Skills: Evaluating Products

Name	**Section**	**Date**

Purpose: To evaluate an exercise device, a book, or an article.

Procedure:
1. Mark an X in the circle by the product you are evaluating in chart 1. Choose an exercise device, book/magazine or food supplement.
2. Use the appropriate section of chart 1 to answer questions about the product you have chosen to evaluate.
3. Total the marks for the product. The higher the score, the more likely the product is effective.
4. Answer the questions in the Conclusions and Implications section.

Results:

Chart 1 Questions to Ask about Exercise Devices, Books/Magazines, and Food Supplements

Directions: Place an x over the product you evaluated. Place an X over each true statement.

Exercise Device	Book/Magazine	Food Supplement
1. The exercise device requires effort consistent with the FIT formula.	1. The credentials of the author are sound. He/she has a degree in an area related to the content of the book or magazine.	1. The seller is not the prime source of product information.
2. The exercise device is safe and the exercise done using the device is safe.	2. The facts in the article are consistent with the facts described in this book.	2. The seller has been in business for a long time and has a good reputation.
3. There are no claims that the device uses exercise that is effortless.	3. The authors do not claim "quick" or "miraculous" results.	3. There is scientific evidence of product effectiveness.
4. Exercise using the device is fun or is a type that you might do regularly.	4. There are no claims about the spot reduction of fat.	4. There is clear evidence about the side effects of the active ingredients.
5. There are no claims using gimmick words such as tone, cellulite, quick, or spot fat reduction.	5. The author is not selling a product described in the article.	5. The long-term effectiveness and safety of the product are cited.
6. The seller's credentials are sound.	6. Reputable experts are cited.	6. You are sure of the content of the product.
7. The product does something for you that cannot be done without it.	7. The article does not promote unsafe exercises or products.	7. You have information that the manufacturer is reputable.
8. You can return the device if you do not like it (the seller has been in business for a long time).	8. New discoveries from exotic places are not cited.	8. The known benefits are worth the cost.
9. The cost of the product is justified for the potential benefits.	9. The article does not rely on testimonials by nonexpert, famous people.	9. There is evidence that you can get benefits from this product that cannot be obtained in good food.
10. The device is easy to store or you have a place to permanently use the equipment without storing it.	10. The author does not make claims that the AMA, FDA, or other legitimate organization is trying to suppress information.	10. There are no claims that use quack words, or claims about conspiracies against the product by reputable organizations.

Conclusions and Implications:

1.   Describe the product or the article in the appropriate space below.

Exercise Device:

Name of device:

Description and manufacturer:

Book or article

Author(s)

Journal article or book title:

Journal name or name of publisher:

Date of publication:

Food supplement

Name of supplement:

Puported benefit:

Manufacturer/seller:

Suggested dose and active ingredient:

Total number of X's for device, book/magazine or food supplement.

2.   In several sentences, give your assessment of the product or article. Did it score well on the questions in Chart 1? Would you use/buy the product or article/book? Explain.

Lab 25B: Evaluating a Health/Wellness or Fitness Club

Name	Section	Date

Purpose: To practice evaluating a health club. (Various combinations of the words *health, wellness,* and *fitness* are often used for these clubs.)

Procedure:

1. Visit a club and pretend to be interested in becoming a member. (*Note:* Only one or two class members should go to each club to avoid suspicion.)
2. Listen carefully to all that is said and ask lots of questions (without exposing your real motives).
3. Look carefully all around you as you are given the tour of the facilities; ask what the exercises or the equipment does for you or ask leading questions such as, "Will this take inches off my hips?", etc.
4. As soon as you leave the club, rate it using chart 1. Space is provided for notes in chart 1.

Chart 1 Health Club Evaluation Questionnaire

Directions: Place an x over a yes or no answer. Make notes as necessary.

	Yes	No	Notes
1. Were claims for improvement in weight, figure/physique, or fitness realistic?	◯	◯	
2. Was a long-term contract (1–3 years) encouraged?	◯	◯	
3. Was the sales pitch high-pressure to make an immediate decision?	◯	◯	
4. Were you given a copy of the contract to read at home?	◯	◯	
5. Did the fine print include objectionable clauses?	◯	◯	
6. Did they ask you about medical readiness?	◯	◯	
7. Did they sell diet supplements as a sideline?	◯	◯	
8. Did they have passive equipment?	◯	◯	
9. Did they have cardiovascular training equipment or facilities (cycles, track, pool, aerobic dance)?	◯	◯	
10. Did they make unscientific claims for the equipment, exercise, baths, or diet supplements?	◯	◯	
11. Were the facilities clean?	◯	◯	
12. Were the facilities crowded?	◯	◯	
13. Were there days and hours when facilities were open but would not be available to you?	◯	◯	
14. Were there limits on the number of minutes you could use a piece of equipment?	◯	◯	
15. Did the floor personnel closely supervise and assist clients?	◯	◯	
16. Were the floor personnel qualified "experts"?	◯	◯	
17. Were the managers/owners qualified "experts"?	◯	◯	
18. Has the club been in business at this location for a year or more?	◯	◯	

Results:

1. Score the chart as follows:
   A. Give one point for each "no" answer for items 2, 3, 5, 7, 8, 10, 12, and 13, and place the score in the box.

   Total A [ ]

   B. Give one point for each "yes" answer for items 1, 4, 6, 9, 11, and 18 and place the score in the box.

   Total B [ ]

   Total A and B above and place the score in the box.

   Total A and B [ ]

   C. Give one point for each "yes" answer on 15, 16, and 17 and place the score in the blank.

   Total C [ ]

2. A total score of 12–15 points on items A and B suggests the club rates at least "fair" compared to other clubs.
3. A score of 3 on item C indicates that the personnel are qualified and suggests that you could expect to get accurate technical advice from the staff.
4. Regardless of the total scores, you would have to decide the importance of each item in the questionnaire to you personally, as well as evaluate other considerations such as cost, location, personalities of the clients and the personnel, and so on, to decide if this would be a good place for you or your friends to join.

Conclusions and Implications: In the space below, use several sentences to discuss your conclusion about the quality of this club and whether you think it would fit your needs if you wanted to belong.

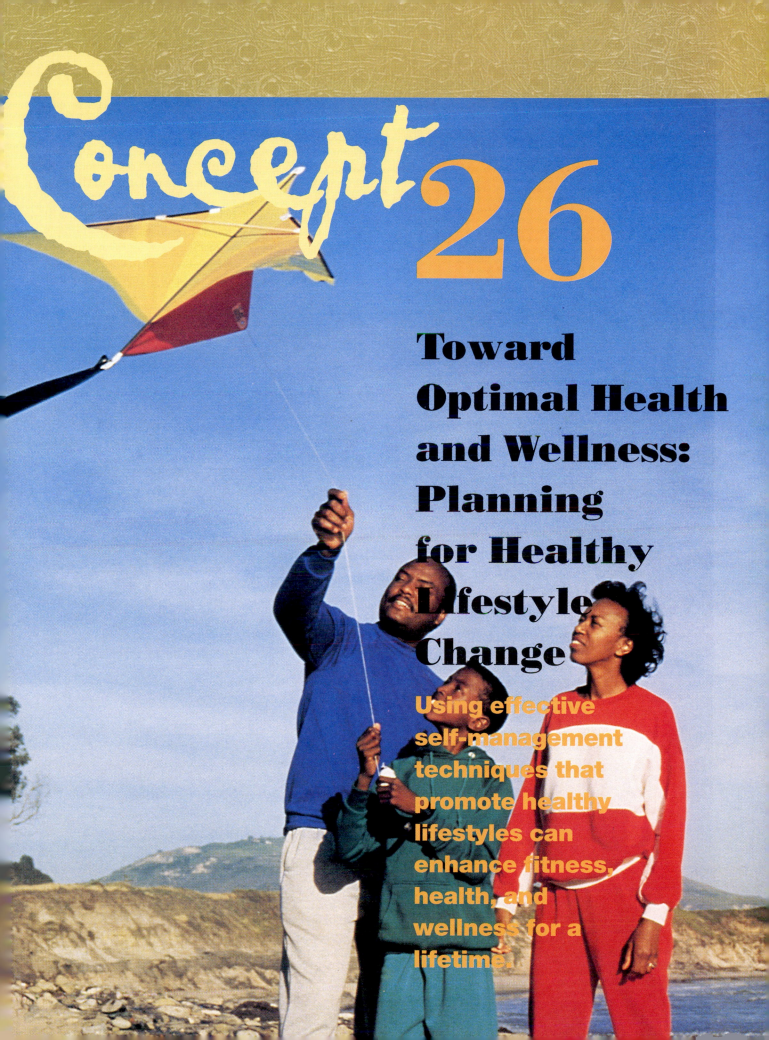

Concept 26

Toward Optimal Health and Wellness: Planning for Healthy Lifestyle Change

Using effective self-management techniques that promote healthy lifestyles can enhance fitness, health, and wellness for a lifetime.

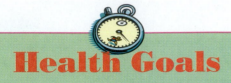

Health Goals
for year 2010

Increase quality and years of healthy life.

Increase healthy and active days.

Eliminate health disparities.

Increase adoption and maintenance of appropriate daily physical activity.

Promote health by improving dietary factors and nutritional status.

Promote healthy and safe communities.

Promote availability of high quality health information.

Increase availability of health care and counseling for mental health problems.

Avoiding destructive behaviors.

Introduction

The two primary health goals for the nation for the year 2010 are increasing the quality and years of life and eliminating health disparities so that all people can attain fitness, health, and wellness. The focus of this book has been on making changes in three priority lifestyles: performing adequate physical activity, eating well, and managing stress. In this concept, you will get information about other lifestyle changes that can affect health, fitness, and wellness and help all people achieve national health goals. You will have the opportunity to tie together all of the information presented in previous concepts to help you plan for a lifetime of healthy active living.

Increasing Years and Quality of Life: The Facts

Living a longer life is an important health goal.

Throughout this book, evidence has been presented to show how practicing healthy lifestyles can reduce risk of illness and contribute to longer life. You have learned that some of the factors that contribute to longer life and reduced risk of illness are out of your control (see Figure 1). Examples are heredity, poor medical care, and environmental factors. On the other hand, you know that healthy lifestyles are factors you can control and they have an enormous effect on health and length of life (see Figure 1).

It is important to note that virtually all people will be ill at some time in life. The key is to reduce the days of illness to a minimum. One of the specific goals for the nation is to increase the number of **healthy days** each of us experiences. Healthy days are typically measured using **self-rated health.**

Attaining wellness as evidenced by "quality of life" is a universal goal.

www.mhhe.com/hper/physed/clw/student/

The focus of the national health goals for the year 2010 is to increase not only the years of life, but to increase the years of **quality of life.** Quality of life is an indicator of the positive component of health. Though the 2010 goals continue to emphasize treatment of illness and rehabilitation for people with disabilities, a new emphasis is placed on prevention of disease and disability and the promotion of wellness as indicated by quality of life. The Department of Health and Human Services uses various indicators to determine the extent to which the goal of increasing quality and years of healthy life has been achieved for all people. As noted in the previous section, one indicator is self-rated health. The intent is to increase the proportion of the population who subjectively rate their health as good or better on most days of the year. If self-rated health is regularly good, a person will have a high frequency of healthy days. Also of importance is having a high frequency of **activity days** or days in which you can do your normal activities without restriction.

In summary, the goals for the nation and the goals of this book are to help readers achieve optimal health and wellness as evidenced by freedom from disease, the ability to function effectively on a daily basis, and a high quality of life including happiness and life satisfaction.

Community quality of life is important to personal quality of life.

Though national health goals focus on the individual, it is important to understand that community quality of life is also important. National goals have been directed at providing "livable" communities that provide an environment in which personal quality of life can thrive. Participation by citizens in community activities is essential if efforts to attain quality of life for all people are to be successful.

Healthy lifestyles

1. Regular physical activity
2. Eating well
3. Managing stress
4. Avoiding destructive habits
5. Practicing safe sex
6. Adopting good safety habits
7. Learning first aid
8. Adopting good personal health habits
9. Seeking and complying with medical advice
10. Being an informed consumer
11. Protecting the environment

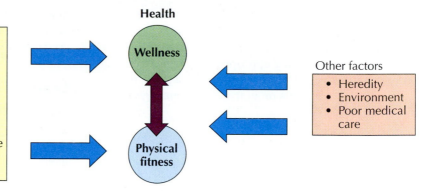

Figure 1

Factors influencing health, wellness, and physical fitness.

Good fitness is important to both health and wellness.

Physical fitness is a state of being that results from healthy lifestyles, particularly regular physical activity. Fitness is neither health nor wellness, but possessing fitness enhances health and wellness. As noted throughout this book, having health-related physical fitness can help you reduce disease risk. Fitness is also crucial to wellness and quality of life. Evidence shows that fitness can help people to excel in performances that enhance quality of life. It allows you to do the daily work activities without fatigue and allows you to enjoy leisure time activities that enrich life. As people grow older, there are added benefits of fitness. Good fitness allows older adults to function independently in daily life activities such as driving a car and performing daily tasks without restriction.

Healthy Lifestyles: The Facts

Adhering to healthy lifestyles is essential to increasing quality and years of healthy life.

Lifestyles and behaviors are in your control. If you make changes and adhere to them, good things will happen. Some of the important healthy lifestyles are listed in Figure 1 and are summarized in the following section.

Participating in Physical Activity Regularly

As noted throughout this book, regular physical activity is associated with the reduced risk of many diseases. Regular physical activity is a positive addiction. It is habit-forming,

but the result of the habit is positive, not negative. Regular exercise can be fun and can improve the quality of life. It is interesting to note that people who exercise regularly are more likely to adopt other healthy lifestyles. For example, regular exercisers are more likely than sedentary individuals to visit a physician for preventive examinations, practice preventive dentistry, and wear seat belts.

Eating Properly (Good Nutrition)

Good eating habits can help you feel and look your best. Failure to eat properly can result in many health problems. It has been shown that six of the 10 leading causes of death in North America are linked to improper nutrition. Millions of teenagers and adults regularly modify

Activity Days A self-rating of the number of days (per week or month) a person feels that he/she can perform usual daily activities successfully and in good health.

Healthy Days A self-rating of the number of days (per week or month) a person considers himself or herself to be in good or better than good health.

Quality of Life A term used to describe wellness. An individual with quality of life can enjoy the activities of life with little or no limitation and can function independently. Individual quality of life requires a pleasant and supportive community quality of life.

Self-Rated Health A subjective measure of daily health and wellness.

their diet in an attempt to assume control of the way they look and their health. Unfortunately, many of these dietary modifications have a negative rather than positive impact on health. Making appropriate changes in eating patterns is the key. Eating properly is a goal that is achievable (see concepts on nutrition and managing diet and activity).

Managing Stress

Nearly 30 million professionals and executives who rank among the highest in annual earnings indicate that they would like to find a way to get away from their steady diet of stress and tension. Reducing stress in your life and learning to cope with stress are associated with feelings of well-being and an improved quality of life. Stress reduction is possible for most people with alterations in lifestyle (see concepts on stress and health and on stress management).

Avoiding Destructive Habits

Among the most destructive habits are the use of tobacco and alcohol and the abuse of drugs. Once they are adopted, these habits are exceptionally difficult to eliminate, but there are ways to help. These are lifestyle or health behaviors over which you have personal control, but breaking habits takes the assistance of others (see concepts on use and abuse of tobacco, alcohol, and drugs).

Practicing Safe Sex

Though sexually transmitted diseases (STDs) are not currently among the top 10 killers, they are the source of much pain and suffering. Healthy lifestyles are the key to prevention of the most common STDs (see concept on STDs).

Adopting Good Safety Habits

Accidents are a major cause of death in North America, accounting for more than six percent of all deaths in the United States. In addition, they result in many disabilities and problems that can detract from good health and wellness. All accidents cannot be prevented, but it is possible to adopt habits that greatly reduce the risk of accidents. Deaths from automobile accidents can be greatly reduced by regular use of seat belts. The proper maintenance of play and work equipment can greatly reduce injury and death rates. Many children die each year from water-related accidents that can be prevented by proper supervision, the use of proper safety devices such as life jackets, and knowledge of cardiopul-

monary resuscitation. Proper storage of guns, use of smoke alarms, proper use of ladders, and proper maintenance of cars, motorcycles, and bicycles can also reduce accident risk.

Learning First Aid

Many deaths could be prevented if those at the site of emergencies were able to administer first aid. Because they can prevent death, all people should be familiar with cardiopulmonary resuscitation (CPR) and the Heimlich maneuver for assisting a person who is choking. Many agencies give extensive classes in first aid taught by qualified experts. It is best to learn these procedures in such a class. First aid for minor injuries and poisoning and for control of bleeding are other important procedures.

Adopting Good Personal Health Behaviors

Many of the healthy lifestyles already discussed are good personal health habits. There are other simple personal health behaviors that are important to optimal health. These behaviors may be considered elementary because they are often taught in school and at home at a very young age. Still, there are many adults who fail to adopt these behaviors on a regular basis. Examples include regular brushing and flossing of the teeth; care of ears, eyes, and skin; proper sleep habits; proper innoculations for disease prevention; and good posture. Health behaviors that prevent sexually transmitted diseases are also important.

Seeking and Complying with Medical Advice

Some people purposely avoid seeking the advice of a physician because they fear that something may be wrong. This occurs in spite of the evidence that delay in treatment greatly increases the risk of death for many diseases that can be cured or controlled. In addition to medical exams for unhealthy people beginning exercise, regular preventive medical exams are important. After age 40, a yearly preventive exam is recommended for all people. Young adults probably need a regular medical examination less often, but a regular examination is important for all people to help in the early diagnosis of problems. For women (especially after age 40), regular self-examination for breast cancer is recommended, as are periodic mammograms and Pap tests. For men, regular testicular exams and a prostate test are recommended. Other important behaviors that should be considered are listed below:

- Be familiar with the symptoms of the most common medical problems in our culture.

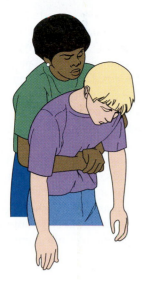

Learn first aid, such as the Heimlich maneuver.

- If symptoms are present, seek medical help. Many deaths could be prevented if the early warning signs of medical problems were heeded.
- If medical advice is given, comply. It is not uncommon for people to stop taking medicine when symptoms stop rather than taking the full amount of medicine prescribed.
- If you doubt the advice given, seek a second opinion.

Being an Informed Consumer

Each year too many people purchase health services and products that are ineffective and often dangerous. Extensive advertising of quack health products, often by celebrities, bombards all of us. It is important to investigate so-called health products and services of all kinds (see concept on quackery).

Protecting the Environment

A recent national poll indicated that 70 percent of the adult population felt that the public was not concerned enough about the environment. In fact, more than half felt that there was an immediate need to take drastic action to protect the environment. Concern for the environment has increased in recent years as indicated by the fact that more than eight of 10 households now indicate that they voluntarily recycle newspapers, glass, or aluminum. We have not been as actively involved in other lifestyle changes that would help protect the environment (e.g, carpool, reduce water use).

Unlike lifestyle behaviors such as regular physical activity or managing stress, behaviors that help protect the environment may not have immediate wellness benefits. Experts are quick to point out, however, that protecting the environment may be one of the most important things that we can do over time to guarantee quality of living for our children and the generations to come.

Managing Time and Priorities Effectively

Central to the concept of wellness are working efficiently and making a significant contribution to society. Working effectively requires a commitment of time. A social contribution requires time for special causes, and social wellness requires a commitment of time to family and friends. Similarly, each of the other dimensions of wellness requires a time commitment. A healthy lifestyle is one that allocates time efficiently to insure that appropriate time is allocated to appropriate priorities. Time and priority management can lead to behaviors that contribute to each wellness dimension, and ultimately to total wellness (see concept on stress management).

One positive lifestyle change often leads to another.

If you make one significant lifestyle change to enhance wellness you are likely to make other changes. For example, people who begin a regular physical activity program and adhere to it over a period of time are also likely to make modifications in diet and adopt effective stress-reduction procedures. People who smoke are more likely to stop if they have been successful in becoming a regular exerciser or a healthy eater.

The wellness lifestyle seems to be contagious. The key is to start slowly to increase the chance of success. Remember, a critical goal for the year 2010 is increasing quality of life for all people. This is best accomplished by altering lifestyles in a consistent and regular manner. The nation's health leaders believe that a commitment by each individual combined with scientific knowledge, professional skills, community support, and political effort will enable each of us to achieve our potential to live full, active lives.

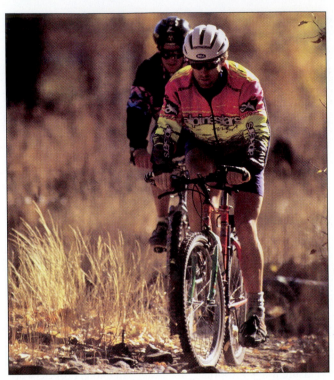

Making one lifestyle change, such as becoming more physically active, can lead to other healthy lifestyle changes.

Adhering to behaviors supported by scientific principles will do a lot to promote optimal wellness. But health promotion is also an art. Accordingly, pursuit of optimal wellness requires social and personal purpose. For example, interactions with friends, family, and community contribute to wellness, as do expressing and receiving love, having hope of better things to come, having a sense of charity to promote the community good, and having a personal sense of purpose.

Being compassionate, understanding, and supportive of family, friends, and coworkers will strengthen the bonds in your relationships and contribute to higher levels of social wellness. Meaningful relationships cannot be formed overnight; Instead, they require persistent effort over an extended period of time. Similarly, to gain high levels of spiritual wellness, dedication and commitment to the principles of your particular religion or spiritual doctrine are necessary. Spiritual enlightenment and understanding cannot be attained without committed effort and focus on these behaviors.

The basic truth in all of these examples is that you can't get something for nothing. The benefits of wellness require continued commitments and efforts, but the benefits are well worth the effort. The "products" are health, wellness and physical fitness. These outcomes occur when you do the "processes" or healthy lifestyle behaviors associated with each of the dimensions of wellness summarized in Table 1.

The Art of Achieving Health and Wellness: The Facts

> Having insight to the different dimensions of wellness can help you adopt healthy lifestyles.

www.mhhe.com/hper/physed/clw/student/
Health, including wellness, is something that most people desire, but achieving it is more challenging. Having a clear understanding of what you want to achieve in the areas of health and wellness can also help you change behavior to achieve your personal goals. The American Journal of Health Promotion defines health promotion as the "science and art of helping people change their lifestyle to move toward a state of optimal health." Adopting the healthy lifestyles discussed in the previous section of this concept would constitute adherence to the science of health promotion.

Strategies for Action: The Facts

> Sometimes bad things happen to good people, but good things are likely to happen to those who make an effort to alter lifestyles.

Healthy lifestyle adherence is under your control. But all factors that influence your fitness, health, and wellness are not under your control. As noted on several occasions in previous concepts, factors such as heredity and quality of health services are not always in your personal control. Even people who do all of the right things will have health problems. Still, the best way to make a difference in your own health and wellness is to take control of the things over which you have control. Making an effort to control these factors is the closest thing to the proverbial fountain of youth.

Table 1   Dimensions of Wellness: Processes and Products

Dimension of Wellness	Process or Behavior	Product or Outcome
Physical wellness	Pursuing behaviors that are conducive to good physical health (being physically active and maintaining a healthy diet).	Development of good physical fitness and good physical health that provides some freedom from disease.
Social wellness	Being supportive of family, friends, and co-workers and practicing good communication skills.	Development of a strong social support system and satisfying relationships.
Emotional wellness	Balancing work and leisure and responding proactively to challenging or stressful situations.	Development of a positive outlook on life and freedom from emotional illness and stress.
Intellectual wellness	Challenging yourself to continually learn and improve in your work and personal life.	Development of satisfying career, hobbies, or pursuits that provides a sense of meaning or purpose.
Spiritual wellness	Praying, meditating, or reflecting on life.	Development of a philosophy or spiritual relationship that guides your life's pursuits.
Total wellness	Taking responsibility for your own health and happiness.	Quality of life.

Adopting a new way of thinking can help you achieve health, fitness, and wellness.

The determination as to whether a person is healthy, fit, or well is often subjective. The tendency of many is to make comparisons to other people. Such comparisons often result in setting personal standards that are impossible to achieve. Trying to achieve the body fatness of a model seen on TV is not realistic nor healthy for most people. Expecting to be able to perform like a professional athlete is not something that most of us can achieve. It is for this reason that the standards for fitness, health, and wellness in this book are based on health criteria rather than comparative criteria. As you began your study on this book, you were introduced to the HELP philosophy. Adhering to this philosophy can help you adopt a new way of thinking. This philosophy suggests that each person should use health (H) as the basis for making decisions rather than comparisons to others. This is something that everyone (E) can do for a lifetime (L). This allows each of us to set personal (P) goals that are realistic and possible for each person to attain.

The new way of thinking simply allows each of us to be successful on our own terms rather than comparing ourselves to others in ways that make success impossible. As you set personal health, fitness, and wellness goals, consider using a new way of thinking.

Assessing your current stage of change for a variety of lifestyles will help you determine goals for the future.

www.mhhe.com/hper/physed/clw/student/
The stages of change model described in the first concept provides the basis for assessing your current behaviors related to a variety of lifestyles. Research suggests that people can be at a level of maintenance for one behavior and at a precontemplation level for another. In Labs 26A and 26B, you will have the opportunity to rate your current stage of change for a variety of lifestyle behaviors.

Table 2 Self-Management Skills

• Self-assessment	• The ability to administer and interpret assessments of health, fitness, and wellness.
• Self-monitoring skills	• The ability to keep records of your adherence to activity, good eating, or other lifestyles.
• Goal setting	• The ability to set realistic and attainable goals for modifying lifestyles.
• Planning skills	• The ability to plan for healthy lifestyles based on personal self-assessments and goals.
• Balancing attitudes	• The ability to develop more good than bad attitudes about healthy lifestyles.
• Overcoming barriers	• The ability to practice healthy lifestyles even when barriers make it difficult.
• Consumer skills	• The ability to make good consumer decisions based on the facts rather than misinformation.
• Finding social support	• The ability to find support from other people.
• Preventing relapse	• The ability to prevent relapsing into unhealthy lifestyles after making positive changes.
• Coping skills	• The ability to cope with stressful situations and to adopt a positive outlook on life.
• Managing time	• The ability to use time wisely to achieve personal goals.
• Performance skills	• The ability to perform skills that enhance fitness and health, such as sports and recreation skills and stress-management skills.

Self-management skills can help you adopt and adhere to healthy lifestyles.

In earlier concepts you learned about a variety of self-management skills. These skills are summarized again in Table 2. If you are to alter your behaviors to improve fitness, health, and wellness, it is important that you practice these self-management skills. You have had the opportunity to practice them in a variety of labs in this book.

Self-management skills have been shown to very effective. They are based on sound theory and research. You may want to review these skills and the theories on which they are based (see concept on self-management). You will use many of the self-management skills to develop comprehensive lifetime physical activity plans and to make plans to change to other healthy lifestyles.

Self-planning is one of the most important self-management skills.

In a number of labs, you have had the opportunity to plan for a variety of different physical activities in the physical activity pyramid. In Lab 26A, you will plan a comprehensive physical activity program using self-management skills you have practiced previously. In this case, you will plan for all types of activities in the pyramid. In Lab 26B you will use self-management skills to plan for changing other lifestyles. The steps in program planning for physical activity were described in a previous concept. These steps are reviewed in Table 3. They can be used in planning for other healthy lifestyles as well (see Lab 26B).

In the end, it is what you do that counts!

Throughout this book, lifestyle modification has been endorsed as a means of achieving optimal health, fitness, and wellness. An underlying and consistent thread in all of the concepts has been an emphasis on the behavior rather than the outcome. This philosophy is best expressed as "focusing on the process instead of the product." *If you do the process, the product follows,* to the extent that is possible for a person with your heredity. Develop a plan and stick to it.

Sometimes lifestyle changes cannot be made without the assistance of others.

As already noted, support of friends and family can be very important in helping you to accomplish lifestyle changes. However, there are some lifestyle changes that may require the assistance of a professional. If your attempts to change your lifestyle meet with failure, don't set yourself up for repeated failure. Get help!

Table 3 Steps in Program Planning

1. Clarify your reason for making a lifestyle change.
2. Identify your needs using self-assessment.
3. Set realistic and achievable goals.
4. Select the lifestyles you plan to change.
5. Prepare a written plan.
6. Keep records of progress.

Most colleges have programs through their health center that provide free, confidential assistance or referral. Many businesses now have Employee Assistance Programs (EAP). The programs have counselors who will help you or your family members find help with a particular problem. The EAP staff are dedicated to help you without revealing personal information to your employer. These programs have a strong record for helping people with problems ranging from small to very serious, such as drug addiction or smoking cessation. Many other programs and support groups are now available to help you change your lifestyle. For example, most hospitals and many health organizations now have hotlines that provide you with referral services for establishing healthy lifestyles.

 Web Review

Web review materials for Concept 26 are available arc at *www.mhhe.com/hper/physed/clw/student/.*

American Alliance for Health Physical Education Recreation and Dance
www.aahperd.org

American College of Sports Medicine
www.acsm.org

Canada's Healthy Living Guide
http://healthylivingguide.com

Canada's Physical Activity Guide
http://paguide.com

Morbidity and Mortality Weekly Reports
www.cdc.gov/epo/mmwr/mmwr.html

National Institute of Alcohol Abuse and Alcoholism
www.niaaa.nih.gov

National Institute of Drug Abuse
www.nida.hih.gov

National Institute of Environmental Health Sciences
www.niehs.nih.gov

Suggested Readings

American College of Sports Medicine. *ACSM's Guidelines for Exercise Testing and Exercise Prescription,* 5th ed. Baltimore, MD: Williams and Wilkins, 1995.

American College of Sports Medicine. "The Recommended Quantity and Quality of Exercise for Developing and Maintaining Cardiorespiratory and Muscular Fitness in Healthy Adults." *Medicine and Science in Sports and Exercise* 22(1990):2.

Bryan, C. X., Peterson, J. A., and Franklin, B. A. "Fountain of Youth." *Fitness Management* 14(10)(1998):44.

Corbin, C. B., and Pangrazi, R. P. (Editors). *Towards a Better Understanding of Physical Fitness and Activity.* Scottsdale, AZ: Holcomb-Hathaway, 1009/

Maddux, J. E. "Habit, Health, and Happiness." *Journal of Sport & Exercise Psychology* 19(1997):331.

National Center for Health Statistics. *Health, United States, 1998: With Socioeconomic Statistics and Health Chartbook.* Hyattsville, MD: National Center for Health Statistics, 1998.

Pate, R., et al. "Physical Activity and Public Health." *Journal of the American Medical Association* 273(1995):402.

Payne, W. A., and Hahn, D. B. *Understanding Your Health* (5th ed.). St. Louis: WCB/McGraw-Hill, 1998.

U. S. Department of Health and Human Services. *Physical Activity and Health: A Report of the Surgeon General.* Atlanta, GA: U. S. Department of Health and Human Services, 1996.

U. S. Department of Health and Human Services. *Healthy People 2010 Objectives: Draft for Comment.* Washington, DC: U. S. Department of Health and Human Services, 1998.

Lab 26A: Planning Your Personal Physical Activity Program

Name	**Section**	**Date**

Purpose: To establish a comprehensive plan of lifestyle physical activity and to self-monitor progress in your plan. Note: You may want to re-read the concept on planning for physical activity before completing this lab.

Procedures:

Step 1. Establishing your reasons.

In the spaces provided below, list several of your principal reasons for doing a comprehensive activity plan.

1.

2.

3.

4.

5.

6.

Step 2. Identify your needs using fitness self-assessments and ratings of stage of change for various activities.

In Chart 1, rate your fitness by darkening a box by the appropriate rating for each part of fitness. Use your results obtained from previous labs or perform the self-assessments again to determine your ratings. If you took more than one self-assessment for one component of physical fitness, select the rating that you think best describes your true fitness for that fitness component. If you were unable to do a self-assessment for some reason, check the "no results" box.

Chart 1 Rating for Self-Assessments

Health-Related Fitness Tests	High Performance Zone	Good Fitness Zone	Marginal Zone	Low Zone	No Results
1. Cardiovascular: Twelve-Minute Run (chart 3, page 120)	○	○	○	○	○
2. Cardiovascular: Step Test (chart 2, page 119)	○	○	○	○	○
3. Cardiovascular: Bicycle Test (chart 5, page 121)	○	○	○	○	○
4. Cardiovascular: Walking Test (chart 5 & 6, page 119)	○	○	○	○	○
5. Flexibility: Sit and Reach (chart 1, page 162)	○	○	○	○	○
6. Flexibility: Shoulder Flexibility (chart 1, page 162)	○	○	○	○	○
7. Flexibility: Hamstring/Hip Flexibility (chart 1, page 162)	○	○	○	○	○
8. Flexibility: Trunk Rotation (chart 1, page 162)	○	○	○	○	○
9. Strength: Isometric Grip (chart 3, page 199)	○	○	○	○	○
10. Strength: 1 RM Upper Body (chart 2, page 199)	○	○	○	○	○

Chart 1 *(Continued)*

Health-Related Fitness Tests	Rating				
	High Performance Zone	Good Fitness Zone	Marginal Zone	Low Zone	No Results
11. Strength: 1 RM Lower Body (chart 2, page 199)	◯	◯	◯	◯	◯
12. Muscular Endurance: Curl-Up (chart 4, page 200)	◯	◯	◯	◯	◯
13. Muscular Endurance: 90-degree push-up (chart 4, page 200)	◯	◯	◯	◯	◯
14. Muscular Endurance: Flexed Arm Support (chart 5, page 200)	◯	◯	◯	◯	◯
15. Fitness Rating: Skinfold (chart 4, page 293)	◯	◯	◯	◯	◯
16. Body Mass Index (chart 8, page 295)	◯	◯	◯	◯	◯

Skill-Related Fitness and Other Self-Assessments	Rating				
	High Performance Zone	Good Fitness Zone	Marginal Zone	Low Zone	No Results
1. Agility (chart 1, page 267)	◯	◯	◯	◯	◯
2. Balance (chart 2, page 268)	◯	◯	◯	◯	◯
3. Coordination (chart 3, page 268)	◯	◯	◯	◯	◯
4. Power (chart 4, page 268)	◯	◯	◯	◯	◯
5. Reaction Time (chart 5, page 269)	◯	◯	◯	◯	◯
6. Speed (chart 6, page 269)	◯	◯	◯	◯	◯
7. Fitness of the Back (chart 2, page 242)	◯	◯	◯	◯	◯
8. Posture (chart 2, page 245)	◯	◯	◯	◯	◯

Summarize Your Fitness Ratings Using the Results Above	Rating				
	High Performance Zone	Good Fitness Zone	Marginal Zone	Low Zone	No Results
Cardiovascular	◯	◯	◯	◯	◯
Endurance	◯	◯	◯	◯	◯
Strength	◯	◯	◯	◯	◯
Flexibility	◯	◯	◯	◯	◯
Body fatness	◯	◯	◯	◯	◯
Skill-related fitness	◯	◯	◯	◯	◯
Posture and fitness of the back	◯	◯	◯	◯	◯

Rate your stage of change for each of the different types of activities from the physical activity pyramid. Make an X over the circle beside the stage that best represents your behavior for each of the five types of activity in the lower three levels of the pyramid. A description of the various stages is provided below to help you make your ratings.

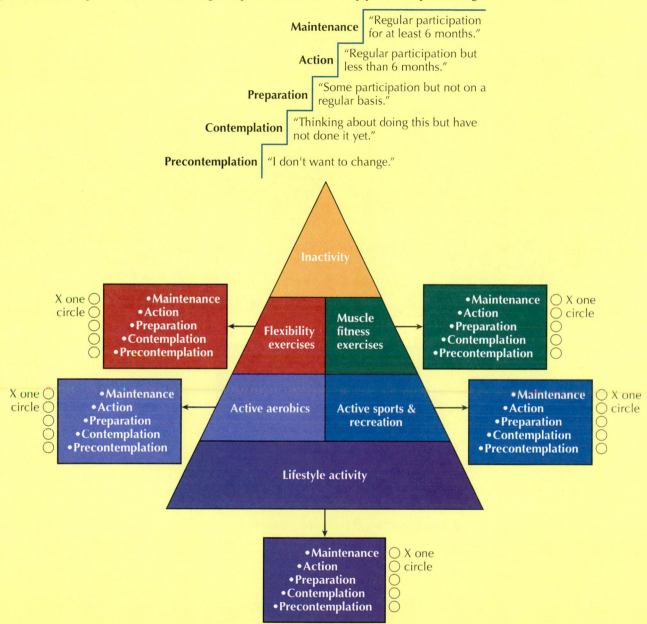

Maintenance | "Regular participation for at least 6 months."

Action | "Regular participation but less than 6 months."

Preparation | "Some participation but not on a regular basis."

Contemplation | "Thinking about doing this but have not done it yet."

Precontemplation | "I don't want to change."

Inactivity

X one circle
- Maintenance
- Action
- Preparation
- Contemplation
- Precontemplation

Flexibility exercises

Muscle fitness exercises

- Maintenance
- Action
- Preparation
- Contemplation
- Precontemplation
X one circle

X one circle
- Maintenance
- Action
- Preparation
- Contemplation
- Precontemplation

Active aerobics

Active sports & recreation

- Maintenance
- Action
- Preparation
- Contemplation
- Precontemplation
X one circle

Lifestyle activity

- Maintenance
- Action
- Preparation
- Contemplation
- Precontemplation
X one circle

Step 3. Set realistic and achievable goals.

In step 1, you wrote down some general reasons for developing your physical activity plan. Setting goals requires more specific statements of goals that are realistic and achievable. For people who are at the contemplation or preparation stages for a specific type of activity, it is recommended that you write only short-term physical activity goals (no more than 4 weeks). Those at the action or maintenance levels may choose short-term goals to start with or, if you have a good history of adherence, choose long-term goals (longer than 4 weeks). Precontemplators are not considered because they would not be doing this activity.

Chart 2

Physical Activity Goals. Place an X over the appropriate circle for the number of days of the week and the number of weeks for each type of activity. Write the number of exercises or activities you plan in each of the five areas.

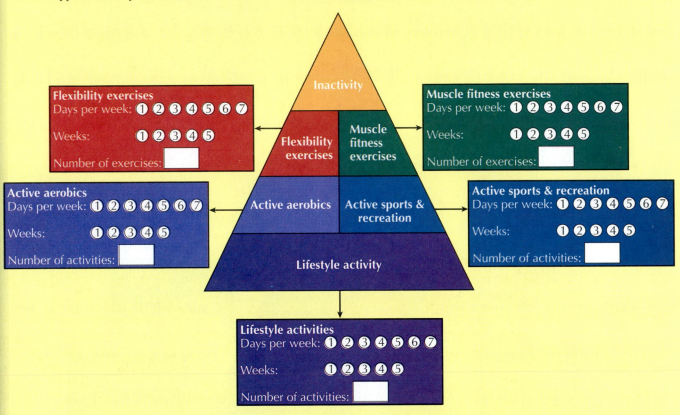

Flexibility exercises
Days per week: ① ② ③ ④ ⑤ ⑥ ⑦
Weeks: ① ② ③ ④ ⑤
Number of exercises: ___

Muscle fitness exercises
Days per week: ① ② ③ ④ ⑤ ⑥ ⑦
Weeks: ① ② ③ ④ ⑤
Number of exercises: ___

Active aerobics
Days per week: ① ② ③ ④ ⑤ ⑥ ⑦
Weeks: ① ② ③ ④ ⑤
Number of activities: ___

Active sports & recreation
Days per week: ① ② ③ ④ ⑤ ⑥ ⑦
Weeks: ① ② ③ ④ ⑤
Number of activities: ___

Lifestyle activities
Days per week: ① ② ③ ④ ⑤ ⑥ ⑦
Weeks: ① ② ③ ④ ⑤
Number of activities: ___

Physical Fitness Goals (for people at action or maintenance only). Write specific physical fitness goals in the space provided below. Indicate when you expect to accomplish the goal (in weeks). Examples include: improving the 12-minute run to a specific score, being able to perform a specific number of push-ups, attaining a specific BMI, or being able to achieve a specific score on a flexibility test.

Part of Fitness	Description of Specific Performance	Weeks to Goal

Steps 4. Selecting activities.

In chart 3, indicate the specific activities you plan to perform from each area of the physical activity pyramid. If the activity you expect to perform is listed, note the number of minutes or reps/sets you plan to perform. If the activity you want to perform is not listed, write the name of the activity or exercise in the space designated as "other." For lifestyle activities, active aerobics, and active sports and recreation, indicate the length of time the activity will be performed each day. For flexibility and muscle fitness exercises, indicate the number of repetitions for each exercise.

Chart 3 Lifetime Physical Activity Selections

√	Lifestyle Activities	Min/day	√	Active Aerobics	Min/day	√	Active Sports and Recreation	Min/day
	Walking			Aerobic exercise machines			Basketball	
	Yard work			Bicycling			Bowling	
	Active house work			Circuit training or calisthenics			Golf	
	Gardening			Dance or step aerobics			Karate/Judo	
	Social dancing			Hiking or backpacking			Mountain climbing	
	Occupational activity			Jogging or running (or walking)			Raquetball	
	Wheeling in wheelchair			Skating/cross-country skiing			Skating	
	Bicyling to work or store			Swimming			Softball	
	Other:			Water activity			Skiing	
	Other:			Other:			Soccer	
	Other:			Other:			Softball	
	Other:			Other:			Volleyball	
	Other:			Other:			Other:	
	Other:			Other:			Other:	
	Other:			Other:			Other:	

√	Flexibility Exercises	Reps/Sets	√	Muscle Fitness Exercises	Reps/Sets	√	Exercises for Back and Neck	Reps/set
	Calf stretcher			Bench or seated press			Back saver stretch	
	Hip and thigh stretcher			Biceps curl			Single knee to chest	
	Sitting stretcher			Triceps curl			Low back stretch	
	Hamstring stretcher			Lat pull down			Hip/Thigh stretch	
	Back stretcher (leg hug)			Seated rowing			Pelvic tilt	
	Trunk twister			Wrist curl			Bridging	
	Pectoral stretch			Knee extension			Wall slide	
	Arm stretch			Heel raise			Pelvic stabilizer	
	Other:			Half-squat Skiing			Neck rotation	
	Other:			Lunge			Isometric neck ex.	
	Other:			Toe press			Chin tuck	
	Other:			Crunch or reverse curl			Trapezius stretch	
	Other:			Other:			Other:	
	Other:			Other:			Other:	
	Other:			Other:			Other:	

Step 5. Prepare a written plan.

Place a check in the shaded boxes for each activity you will perform for each day you will do it. Indicate the time of day you expect to perform the activity or exercise (Example: 7:30 to 8 AM or 6 to 6:30 PM).

In the spaces labeled "Warm-Up Exercises" and "Cool-Down Exercises," check the warm-up and cool-down exercises you expect to perform. Indicate the number of reps you will use for each exercise.

Chart 4 My Physical Activity Plan

√	Monday	Time	√	Tuesday	Time	√	Wednesday	Time
	Lifestyle activity			Lifestyle activity			Lifestyle activity	
	Active aerobics			Active aerobics			Active aerobics	
	Active sports/rec.			Active sports/rec.			Active sports/rec.	
	Flexibility exercises*			Flexibility exercises*			Flexibility exercises*	
	Muscle fitness exercises*			Muscle fitness exercises*			Muscle fitness exercises*	
	Back/neck exercises*			Back/neck exercises*			Back/neck exercises*	
	Warm-up exercises			Warm-up exercises			Warm-up exercises	
	Other:			Other:			Other:	
√	**Thursday**	**Time**	**√**	**Friday**	**Time**	**√**	**Saturday**	**Time**
	Lifestyle activity			Lifestyle activity			Lifestyle activity	
	Active aerobics			Active aerobics			Active aerobics	
	Active sports/rec.			Active sports/rec.			Active sports/rec.	
	Flexibility exercises*			Flexibility exercises*			Flexibility exercises*	
	Muscle fitness exercises*			Muscle fitness exercises*			Muscle fitness exercises*	
	Back/neck exercises*			Back/neck exercises*			Back/neck exercises*	
	Warm-up exercises			Warm-up exercises			Warm-up exercises	
	Other:			Other:			Other:	
√	**Sunday**	**Time**	**√**	**Warm-Up Exercises**	**Reps**	**√**	**Cool-Down Exercises**	**Reps**
	Lifestyle activity			Walk or jog 1–2 min.			Walk or jog 1–2 min.	
	Active aerobics			Calf stretcher			Calf stretcher	
	Active sports/rec.			Hamstring stretcher			Hamstring stretcher	
	Flexibility exercises*			Leg hug			Leg hug	
	Muscle fitness exercises*			Sitting side stretch			Sitting side stretch	
	Back/neck exercises*			Zipper			Zipper	
	Warm-up exercises			Other:			Other:	
	Other:			Other:			Other:	

*Perform the specific exercises you checked in chart 3.

Step 6. Keep records of progress.

Make copies of chart 4 (one for each week that you plan to keep records). Each day, make a check by the activities you actually performed. Include the times when you actually did the activities in your plan. Periodically check your goals to see if they have been accomplished. At some point, it will be necessary to re-establish your goals and to create a revised activity plan.

Results:

After performing your plan for a specific period of time, answer the questions in the space provided.

How long have you been performing the plan?

Conclusions and Implications:

1. In several sentences, discuss your adherence to the plan. Have you been able to stick with the plan? If so, do you think it is a plan you could do for a lifetime? If not, why do you think you are unable to do your plan?

2. In several sentences, discuss how you might modify your plan in the future.

3. In several sentences, discuss your goals for your program. Do you think you will meet your goals? Why or why not?

Lab 26B: Planning for Healthy Lifestyle Change

Name	**Section**	**Date**

Purpose: To establish goals for healthy lifestyle change and to self-monitor progress in your plan.

Procedures and Results

Step 1. Establishing your reasons for your proposed lifestyle change.

In the spaces provided below, list several of your principal reasons for doing a comprehensive lifestyle plan.

1.   4.

2.   5.

3.   7.

Step 2. Identify your needs using self-assessments and ratings of stage of change for various lifestyles.

In chart 1, rate your stage of change for each of the lifestyles by placing an X over the stage that best represents your behavior. A description of the various stages is provided below to help you make your ratings. Note: You are not asked to rate your stage of change for your sexual behaviors and destructive behaviors because this is very personal information. You may wish to rate your stage of change for these lifestyles for your own personal information.

In various labs you have performed, you have made self-assessments regarding your stage of change for a variety of lifestyles. For example, you may have assessed the content of your diet or assessed the stress in your life. Use the information from these labs as you assess your current stage of change for the various healthy behaviors in chart 1.

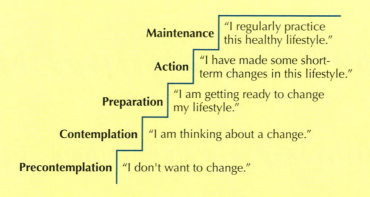

Maintenance — "I regularly practice this healthy lifestyle."

Action — "I have made some short-term changes in this lifestyle."

Preparation — "I am getting ready to change my lifestyle."

Contemplation — "I am thinking about a change."

Precontemplation — "I don't want to change."

Chart 1 States of Change Questionnaire

Lifestyle	Pre-contemplation	Contemplation	Preparation	Action	Maintenance
Eating properly	○	○	○	○	○
Managing stress	○	○	○	○	○
Adopting safety habits	○	○	○	○	○
Learning first aid	○	○	○	○	○
Adopting personal health behaviors	○	○	○	○	○
Protecting the environment	○	○	○	○	○
Managing time	○	○	○	○	○
Seeking and complying with medical advice	○	○	○	○	○
Becoming an informed consumer	○	○	○	○	○
Other:	○	○	○	○	○

Step 3. Set realistic and achievable goals

In step 1, you wrote down some general reasons for making lifestyle changes. Setting goals requires more specific statements of goals that are realistic and achievable. In chart 2, select two or three different lifestyles in which you would like to make change. Beside the lifestyle, list specific goals that you would like to achieve.

Focus on lifestyle or behavior changes. Contemplators and people at the preparation stage should set short-term goals (four weeks or less). Those already at the action or maintenance stage you may want to establish long-term goals.

Chart 2 Setting Goals for Various Lifestyles

Lifestyle	Goal 1	Weeks to Goal	Goal 2	Weeks to Goal
Eating properly				
Managing stress				
Adopting safety habits				
Learning first aid				
Adopting personal health behaviors				
Protecting the environment				
Managing time				
Seeking and complying with medical advice				
Becoming an informed consumer				
Other:				

Steps 4 and 5. Selecting Activities and Making a Written Plan

In chart 3, check the specific activities you will do to meet your goals. Write a plan for meeting your goal. If appropriate, indicate where you will meet the goal. For example, if you are planning to learn first aid, indicate the place of the first aid class. Indicate the days of the week that you will do the activity. For example, if you are going to modify diet, indicate on what days the behavior will be modified (use the "MTWTFSS" columns).

Chart 3 A Written Plan for Changing Lifestyle Behaviors

√	Lifestyle	Plan for Meeting Goal	Where	M	T	W	T	F	S	S
	Eating properly									
	Managing stress									
	Adopting safety habits									
	Learning first aid									
	Adopting personal health behaviors									
	Protecting the environment									
	Managing time									
	Seeking and complying with medical advice									
	Becoming an informed consumer									
	Other:									

Step 6. Keep Records of Progress

Make extra copies of chart 3 (one for each week that you plan to keep records). Each day, make a check in the box for the day on which you carried out your plan. Periodically check your goals to see if they have been accomplished. At some point it will be necessary to re-establish your goals and to create a revised plan.

Results:

After performing your plan for a specific period of time, answer the questions in the space provided.

How long have you been performing the plan? [   ]

Conclusions and Implications:

1. In several sentences, discuss your adherence to the plan. Have you been able to stick with the plan? If not, why do you think you are unable to do your plan? Is it necessary for this plan to be done all of your life to be effective? If so, do you think it is a plan you could do for a lifetime?

2. In several sentences, discuss how you might modify your plan in the future.

3. In several sentences, discuss your goals for your program. Do you think you will meet your goals? Why or why not?

Appendix A

Metric Conversion Chart

Approximate Conversions from Metric to Traditional Measures

Length
  centimeters to inches: cm $\times$ .39 = in
  meters to feet: m $\times$ 3.3 = ft
  meters to yards: m $\times$ 1.09 = yd
  kilometers to miles: km $\times$ 0.6 = mi

Mass (Weight)
  grams to ounces: g $\times$ 0.0352 = oz
  kilograms to pounds: kg $\times$ 2.2 = lbs

Area
  square centimeters to square inches: $cm^2 \times 0.16 = in^2$
  square meters to square feet: $m^2 \times 11.11 = ft^2$
  square meters to square yards: $m^2 \times 1.02 = yd^2$

Volume
  milliliters to fluid ounces: ml $\times$ 0.03 = fl oz
  liters to quarts: 1 $\times$ 1.06 = qt
  liters to gallons: 1 $\times$ 0.264 = gal

Approximate Conversions from Traditional to Metric Measures

Length
  inches to centimeters: in $\times$ 2.54 = cm
  feet to meters: ft $\times$ .3048 = m
  yards to meters: yd $\times$ 0.92 = m
  miles to kilometers: mi $\times$ 1.6 = km

Mass (Weight)
  ounces to grams: oz $\times$ 28.41 = gm
  pounds to kilograms: lbs $\times$ 0.45 = kg

Area
  square inches to square centimeters: $in^2 \times 6.5 = cm^2$
  square feet to square meters: $ft^2 \times 0.09 = m^2$
  square yards to square meters: $yd^2 \times 0.76 = m^2$

Volume
  fluid ounces to mililiters: fl oz $\times$ 29.573 = ml
  quarts to liters: qt $\times$ 0.95 = 1
  gallons to liters: gal $\times$ 3.8 = 1

Appendix B

Metric Conversions of Selected Charts and Tables

Chart 1 — Twelve-Minute Run Test (Scores in Meters)

Men (Age)				
Classification	**17–26**	**27–39**	**40–49**	**50+**
High-performance zone	2880+	2560+	2400+	2240+
Good fitness zone	2480–2779	2320–2559	2240–2399	2000–2239
Marginal zone	2160–2479	2080–2319	2000–2239	1760–1999
Low zone	< 2160	< 2080	< 2000	< 1760

Women (Age)				
Classification	**17–26**	**27–39**	**40–49**	**50+**
High-performance zone	2320+	2160+	2000+	1840+
Good fitness zone	2000–2319	1920–2159	1840–1999	1680–1839
Marginal zone	1840–1999	1680–1919	1600–1839	1520–1679
Low zone	< 1840	< 1680	< 1600	< 1520

Chart 2 Isometric Strength Rating Scale (kg)

Classification	Left Grip	Right Grip	Total Score
Men			
High-performance zone	57+	61+	118+
Good fitness zone	45–56	50–60	95–117
Marginal zone	41–44	43–49	84–94
Low zone	<41	<43	<84
Women			
High-performance zone	34+	39+	73+
Good fitness zone	27–33	32–38	59–72
Marginal zone	20–26	23–31	43–58
Low zone	<20	<23	<43

Suitable for use by young adults between 18 and 30 years of age. After 30, an adjustment of 0.5 of 1 percent per year is appropriate because some loss of muscle tissue typically occurs as you grow older.

Chart 3 Power Rating Scale

Classification	Men	Women
Excellent	68 cm+	60 cm+
Very good	53–67 cm	48–59 cm
Good	42–52 cm	37–47 cm
Fair	31–41 cm	27–36 cm
Poor	<32 cm	<27 cm

Chart 4 Reaction Time Rating Scale

Classification	Score in inches	Score in cenimeters
Excellent	More than 21"	53+
Very good	19"–21"	48–52
Good	16"–18 3/4"	41–47
Fair	13"–15 3/4"	33–40
Poor	Below 13"	<33

Chart 5 Speed Rating Scale

Classification	Men		Women	
	Yards	Meters	Yards	Meters
Excellent	24+	22+	22+	20+
Very good	22–23	20–21.9	20–21	18–19.9
Good	18–21	16.5–19.9	16–19	14.5–17.9
Fair	16–17	14.5–16.4	14–15	13–14.4
Poor	<16	<14.5	<14	<13

Appendix C

Calorie Guide to Common Foods

Beverages

Coffee (black)	0
Coke (12 oz.)	137
Hot chocolate, milk (1 cup)	247
Lemonade (1 cup)	100
Limeade, diluted to serve (1 cup)	110
Soda, fruit flavored (12 oz.)	161
Tea (clear)	0

Breads and Cereals

Bagel (1 half)	76
Biscuit (2″ × 2″)	135
Bread, pita (1 oz.)	80
Bread, raisin (1/2″ thick)	65
Bread, rye	55
Bread, white enriched (1/2″ thick)	64
Bread, whole wheat (1/2″ thick)	55
Bun (hamburger)	120
Cereals, cooked (1/2 cup)	80
Corn flakes (1 cup)	96
Corn grits (1 cup)	125
Corn muffin (2 1/2″ diam.)	103
Crackers, graham (1 med.)	28
Crackers, soda (1 plain)	24
English muffin (1 half)	74
Macaroni, with cheese (1 cup)	464
Muffin, plain	135
Noodles (1 cup)	200
Oatmeal (1 cup)	150
Pancakes (1–4″ diam.)	59
Pizza (1 section)	180
Popped corn (1 cup)	54
Potato chips (10 med.)	108
Pretzels (5 small sticks)	18
Rice (1 cup)	225
Roll, plain (1 med.)	118
Roll, sweet (1 med.)	178
Shredded wheat (1 med. biscuit)	79
Spaghetti, plain cooked (1 cup)	218
Tortilla (1 corn)	70
Waffle (4 1/2″ × 5″)	216

Dairy Products

Butter, 1 pat (1 1/2 tsp.)	50
Cheese, cheddar (1 oz.)	113
Cheese, cottage (1 cup)	270
Cheese, cream (1 oz.)	106
Cheese, Parmesan (1 tbsp.)	29
Cheese, Swiss natural (1 oz.)	105
Cream, sour (1 tbsp.)	31
Frozen custard (1 cup)	375
Frozen yogurt, vanilla (1 cup)	180
Ice cream, plain (prem.) (1 cup)	350
Ice cream soda, choc. (large glass)	455
Ice milk (1 cup)	184
Ices (1 cup)	177
Milk, chocolate (1 cup)	185
Milk, half-and-half (1 tbsp.)	20
Milk, malted (1 cup)	281
Milk, skim (1 cup)	88
Milk, skim dry (1 tbsp.)	28
Milk, whole (1 cup)	166
Sherbet (1 cup)	270
Softserve cone (med.)	335
Whipped topping (1 tbsp.)	14
Yogurt (1 cup)	150

Desserts and Sweets

Cake, angel (2″ wedge)	108
Cake, chocolate (2″ × 3″ × 1″)	150
Cake, plain (3″ × 2 1/2″)	180
Chocolate, bar	200–300
Chocolate, bitter (1 oz.)	142
Chocolate, sweet (1 oz.)	133
Chocolate, syrup (1 tbsp.)	42
Cocoa (1 tbsp.)	21
Cookies, plain (1 med.)	75
Custard, baked (1 cup)	283
Doughnut (1 large)	250
Gelatin, dessert (1 cup)	155
Gelatin, with fruit (1 cup)	170
Gingerbread (2″ × 2″ × 2″)	180
Jams, jellies (1 tbsp.)	55
Pie, apple (1/7 of 9″ pie)	345
Pie, cherry (1/7 of 9″ pie)	355
Pie, chocolate (1/7 of 9″ pie)	360
Pie, coconut (1/7 of 9″ pie)	266
Pie, lemon meringue (1/7 of 9″ pie)	302
Sugar, granulated (1 tsp.)	27
Syrup, table (1 tbsp.)	57

Fruit

Apple, fresh (med.)	76
Applesauce, unsweetened (1 cup)	184
Avocado, raw (1/2 peeled)	279
Banana, fresh (med.)	88
Cantaloupe, raw (1/2, 5″ diam.)	60
Cherries (10 sweet)	50
Cranberry sauce, unsweetened (1 tbsp.)	25
Fruit cocktail, canned (1 cup)	170
Grapefruit, fresh (1/2)	60
Grapefruit juice, raw (1 cup)	95
Grape juice, bottled (1/2 cup)	80
Grapes (20–25)	75
Nectarine (1 med.)	88
Olives, green	72
Olives, ripe (10)	105
Orange, fresh (med.)	60
Orange juice, frozen diluted (1 cup)	110
Peach, fresh (med.)	46
Peach, canned in syrup (2 halves)	79
Pear, fresh (med.)	95
Pears, canned in syrup (2 halves)	79
Pineapple, crushed in syrup (1 cup)	204
Pineapple (1/2 cup fresh)	50
Prune juice (1 cup)	170
Raisins, dry (1 cup)	26
Strawberries, fresh (1 cup)	54
Strawberries, frozen (3 oz.)	90
Tangerine (2 1/2″ diam.)	40
Watermelon, wedge (4″ × 8″)	120

Meat, Fish, Eggs

Bacon, drained (2 slices)	97
Bacon, Canadian (1 oz.)	62
Beef, hamburger chuck (3 oz.)	316
Beef, pot pie	560
Beef steak, sirloin or T-bone (3 oz.)	257
Beef and vegetable stew (1 cup)	185
Chicken, fried breast (8 oz.)	210
Chicken, fried (1 leg and thigh)	305
Chicken, roasted breast (2 slices)	100
Chili, without beans (1 cup)	510
Chili, with beans (1 cup)	335
Egg, boiled	77
Egg, fried	125
Egg, scrambled	100
Fish and chips (2 pcs. fish; 4 oz. chips)	275
Fish, broiled (3″ × 3″ × 1/2″)	112
Fish stick	40
Frankfurter, boiled	124
Ham (4″ × 4″)	338
Lamb (3 oz. roast, lean)	158
Liver (3″ × 3″)	150
Luncheon meat (2 oz.)	135
Pork chop, loin (3″ × 5″)	284
Salmon, canned (1 cup)	145
Sausage, pork (4 oz.)	510
Shrimp, canned (3 oz.)	108
Tuna, canned (1/2 cup)	185
Veal, cutlet (3″ × 4″)	175

Nuts and Seeds

Cashews (1 cup)	770
Coconut (1 cup)	450
Peanut butter (1 tbsp.)	92
Peanuts, roasted, no skin (1 cup)	805
Pecans (1 cup)	752
Sunflower seeds (1 tbsp.)	50

Sandwiches
(2 slices of bread—plain)

Bologna	214
Cheeseburger (small McDonald's)	300
Chicken salad	185
Egg salad	240
Fish filet (McDonald's)	400
Ham	360
Ham and cheese	360
Hamburger (small McDonald's)	260
Hamburger, Burger King Whopper	600
Hamburger, Big Mac	550
Hamburger (McDonald's Quarter Pounder)	420
Peanut butter	250
Roast beef (Arby's Regular)	425

Sauces, Fats, Oils

Catsup, tomato (1 tbsp.)	17
Chili sauce (1 tbsp.)	17
French dressing (1 tbsp.)	59
Margarine (1 pat)	50
Mayonnaise (1 tbsp.)	92

Mayonnaise-type (1 tbsp.)	65	Beans, navy (1 cup)	642	Peas, field ($^1/_2$ cup)	90
Vegetable, sunflower, safflower oils		Beans, pork and molasses (1 cup)	325	Peas, green (1 cup)	145
(1 tbsp.)	120	Broccoli, fresh cooked (1 cup)	60	Pickles, dill (med.)	15
		Cabbage, cooked (1 cup)	40	Pickles, sweet (med.)	22
Soup, Ready to Serve (1 cup)		Cauliflower (1 cup)	25	Potato, baked (med.)	97
Bean	190	Carrot, raw (med.)	21	Potato, french fried (8 stick)	155
Beef noodle	100	Carrots, canned (1 cup)	44	Potato, mashed (1 cup)	185
Cream	200	Celery, diced raw (1 cup)	20	Radish, raw (small)	1
Tomato	90	Coleslaw (1 cup)	102	Sauerkraut, drained (1 cup)	32
Vegetable	80	Corn, sweet, canned (1 cup)	140	Spinach, fresh, cooked (1 cup)	46
		Corn, sweet (med. ear)	84	Squash, summer (1 cup)	30
Vegetables		Cucumber, raw (6 slices)	6	Sweet pepper (med.)	15
Alfalfa sprouts ($^1/_2$ cup)	19	Lettuce (2 large leaves)	7	Sweet potato, candied (small)	314
Asparagus (6 spears)	22	Mushrooms, canned (1 cup)	28	Tomato, cooked (1 cup)	50
Bean sprouts (1 cup)	37	Onions, french fried (10 rings)	75	Tomato, raw (med.)	30
Beans, green (1 cup)	27	Onions, raw (med.)	25		
Beans, lima (1 cup)	152				

Appendix D

Calories of Protein, Carbohydrates, and Fats in Foods*

Food No./Food Choice	Total Calories	Protein Calories	Carbohydrate Calories	Fat Calories
Breakfast				
1. Scrambled Egg (1 lg)	111	29	7	75
2. Fried Egg (1 lg)	99	26	1	72
3. Pancake (1–6^W)	146	19	67	58
4. Syrup (1 T)	60	0	60	0
5. French Toast (1 slice)	180	23	49	108
6. Waffle (7-inch)	245	28	100	117
7. Biscuit (medium)	104	8	52	44
8. Bran Muffin (medium)	104	11	63	31
9. White Toast (slice)	68	9	52	7
10. Wheat Toast (slice)	67	14	52	6
11. Peanut Butter (1 T)	94	15	11	68
12. Yogurt (8 oz. plain)	227	39	161	27
13. Orange Juice (8 oz.)	114	8	100	6
14. Apple Juice (8 oz.)	117	1	116	0
15. Soft Drink (12 oz.)	144	0	144	0
16. Bacon (2 slices)	86	15	2	70
17. Sausage (1-link)	141	11	0	130
18. Sausage (1 patty)	284	23	0	261
19. Grits (8 oz.)	125	11	110	4
20. Hash Browns (8 oz.)	355	18	178	159
21. French Fries (reg.)	239	12	115	112
22. Donut Cake	125	4	61	60
23. Donut Glazed	164	8	87	69
24. Sweet Roll	317	22	136	159
25. Cake (medium slice)	274	14	175	85
26. Ice Cream (8 oz.)	257	15	108	134
27. Cream Cheese (T)	52	4	1	47
28. Jelly (T)	49	0	49	0
29. Jam (T)	54	0	54	0
30. Coffee (cup)	0	0	0	0
31. Tea (cup)	0	0	0	0
32. Cream (T)	32	2	2	28
33. Sugar (t)	15	0	15	0
34. Corn Flakes (8 oz.)	97	8	87	2
35. Wheat Flakes (8 oz.)	106	12	90	4
36. Oatmeal (8 oz.)	132	19	92	21
37. Strawberries (8 oz.)	55	4	46	5
38. Orange (medium)	64	6	57	1
39. Apple (medium)	96	1	86	9
40. Banana (medium)	101	4	95	2
41. Cantaloupe (half)	82	7	73	2
42. Grapefruit (half)	40	2	37	1
43. Custard Pie (slice)	285	20	188	77
44. Fruit Pie (slice)	350	14	259	77
45. Fritter (medium)	132	11	54	67
46. Skim Milk (8 oz.)	88	36	52	0
47. Whole Milk (8 oz.)	159	33	48	78
48. Butter (pat)	36	0	0	36
49. Margarine (pat)	36	0	0	36

Food No./Food Choice	Total Calories	Protein Calories	Carbohydrate Calories	Fat Calories
Lunch				
1. Hamburger (reg. FF)	255	48	120	89
2. Cheeseburger (reg. FF)	307	61	120	126
3. Doubleburger (FF)	563	101	163	299
4. 1/4 lb. Burger (FF)	427	73	137	217
5. Doublecheese Burger (FF)	670	174	134	362
6. Doublecheese Baconburger (FF)	724	138	174	340
7. Hot Dog (FF)	214	36	54	124
8. Chili Dog (FF)	320	51	90	179
9. Pizza, Cheese (slice FF)	290	116	116	58
10. Pizza, Meat (slice FF)	360	126	126	108
11. Pizza, Everything (slice FF)	510	179	173	158
12. Sandwich, Roast Beef (FF)	350	88	126	137
13. Sandwich, Bologna	313	44	106	163
14. Sandwich, Bologna-Cheese	428	69	158	201
15. Sandwich, Ham-Cheese (FF)	380	91	133	156
16. Sandwich, Peanut Butter	281	39	118	124
17. Sandwich, PB and Jelly	330	40	168	122
18. Sandwich, Egg Salad	330	40	109	181
19. Sandwich, Tuna Salad	390	101	109	180
20. Sandwich, Fish (FF)	432	56	147	229
21. French Fries (reg. FF)	239	12	115	112
22. French Fries (lg. FF)	406	20	195	191
23. Onion Rings (reg. FF)	274	14	112	148
24. Chili (8 oz.)	260	49	62	148
25. Bean Soup (8 oz.)	355	67	181	107
26. Beef Noodle Soup (8 oz.)	140	32	59	49
27. Tomato Soup (8 oz.)	180	14	121	45
28. Vegetable Soup (8 oz.)	160	21	107	32
29. Small Salad, Plain	37	6	27	4
30. Small Salad, French Dressing	152	8	50	94
31. Small Salad, Italian Dressing	162	8	28	126
32. Small Salad, Bleu Cheese	184	13	28	143
33. Potato Salad (8 oz.)	248	27	159	62
34. Cole Slaw (8 oz.)	180	0	25	155
35. Macaroni and Cheese (8 oz.)	230	37	103	90
36. Taco Beef (FF)	186	59	56	71
37. Bean Burrito (FF)	343	45	192	106
38. Meat Burrito (FF)	466	158	196	112
39. Mexican Rice (FF)	213	17	160	36
40. Mexican Beans (FF)	168	42	82	44
41. Fried Chicken Breast (FF)	436	262	13	161
42. Broiled Chicken Breast	284	224	0	60
43. Broiled Fish	228	82	32	114
44. Fish Stick (1 stick FF)	50	18	8	24
45. Fried Egg	99	26	1	72
46. Donut	125	4	61	60
47. Potato Chips (small bag)	115	3	39	73
48. Soft Drink (12 oz.)	144	0	144	0

*Notes:
1. FF by a food indicates that it is typical of a food served in a fast food restaurant.
2. Your portions of foods may be larger or smaller than those listed here. For this reason you may wish to select a food more than once (i.e., two hamburgers) or select only a portion of a serving (i.e., divide the calories in half for a half portion).
3. An oz. equals an ounce or 28.4 grams.
4. T = Tablespoon and t = teaspoon.
The principal reference for the calculation of values used in this appendix were the *Nutritive Value of Foods,* published by the United States Department of Agriculture, Washington, D.C., Home and Gardens Bulletin, No. 72, although other published sources were consulted, including Jacobson, M., and S. Fritschner, *The Fast-Food Guide* (an excellent source of information about fast foods), New York, Workman Publishing Company.

Food No./Food Choice	Total Calories	Protein Calories	Carbohydrate Calories	Fat Calories
49. Apple Juice (8 oz.)	117	1	116	0
50. Skim Milk (8 oz.)	88	36	52	0
51. Whole Milk (8 oz.)	159	33	48	78
52. Diet Drink (12 oz.)	0	0	0	0
53. Mustard (t)	4	0	4	0
54. Catsup (t)	6	0	6	0
55. Mayonnaise (T)	100	0	0	100
56. Fruit Pie	350	14	259	77
57. Cheese Cake	400	56	132	212
58. Ice Cream (8 oz.)	257	15	108	134
59. Coffee (8 oz.)	0	0	0	0
60. Tea (8 oz.)	0	0	0	0

Dinner

Food No./Food Choice	Total Calories	Protein Calories	Carbohydrate Calories	Fat Calories
1. Hamburger (reg. FF)	255	48	120	89
2. Cheeseburger (reg. FF)	307	61	120	126
3. Doubleburger (FF)	563	101	163	299
4. 1/4 lb. Burger (FF)	427	73	137	217
5. Doublecheese Burger (FF)	670	174	134	362
6. Doublecheese Baconburger (FF)	724	138	174	412
7. Hot Dog (FF)	214	36	54	124
8. Chili Dog (FF)	320	51	90	179
9. Pizza, Cheese (slice FF)	290	116	116	58
10. Pizza, Meat (slice FF)	360	126	126	108
11. Pizza, Everything (slice FF)	510	179	173	158
12. Steak (8 oz.)	880	290	0	590
13. French Fried Shrimp (6 oz.)	360	133	68	158
14. Roast Beef (8 oz.)	440	268	0	172
15. Liver (8 oz.)	520	250	52	218
16. Corned Beef (8 oz.)	493	242	0	251
17. Meat Loaf (8 oz.)	711	228	35	448
18. Ham (8 oz.)	540	178	0	362
19. Spaghetti, No Meat (13 oz.)	400	56	220	124
20. Spaghetti, Meat (13 oz.)	500	115	230	155
21. Baked Potato (medium)	90	12	78	0
22. Cooked Carrots (8 oz.)	71	12	59	0
23. Cooked Spinach (8 oz.)	50	18	18	14
24. Corn (one ear)	70	10	52	8
25. Cooked Green Beans (8 oz.)	54	11	43	0
26. Cooked Broccoli (8 oz.)	60	19	26	15
27. Cooked Cabbage	47	12	35	0
28. French Fries (reg. FF)	239	12	115	112
29. French Fries (lg. FF)	406	20	195	191
30. Onion Rings (reg. FF)	274	14	112	148
31. Chili (8 oz.)	260	49	62	148
32. Small Salad, Plain	37	6	27	4
33. Small Salad, French Dressing	152	8	50	94
34. Small Salad, Italian Dressing	162	8	28	126
35. Small Salad, Bleu Cheese	184	13	28	143
36. Potato Salad (8 oz.)	248	27	159	62
37. Cole Slaw (8 oz.)	180	0	25	155
38. Macaroni and Cheese (8 oz.)	230	37	103	90
39. Taco Beef (FF)	186	59	56	71
40. Bean Burrito (FF)	343	45	192	106
41. Meat Burrito (FF)	466	158	196	112
42. Mexican Rice (FF)	213	17	160	36
43. Mexican Beans (FF)	168	42	82	44
44. Fried Chicken Breast (FF)	436	262	13	161

Food No./Food Choice	Total Calories	Protein Calories	Carbohydrate Calories	Fat Calories
45. Broiled Chicken Breast	284	224	0	60
46. Broiled Fish	228	82	32	114
47. Fish Stick (1 stick FF)	50	18	8	24
48. Soft Drink (12 oz.)	144	0	144	0
49. Apple Juice (8 oz.)	117	1	116	0
50. Skim Milk (8 oz.)	88	36	52	0
51. Whole Milk (8 oz.)	159	33	48	78
52. Diet Drink (12 oz.)	0	0	0	0
53. Mustard (t)	4	0	4	0
54. Catsup (t)	6	0	6	0
55. Mayonnaise (T)	100	0	0	100
56. Fruit Pie (slice)	350	14	259	77
57. Cheese Cake (slice)	400	56	132	212
58. Ice Cream (8 oz.)	257	15	108	134
59. Custard Pie (slice)	285	20	188	77
60. Cake (slice)	274	14	175	85

Snacks

Food No./Food Choice	Total Calories	Protein Calories	Carbohydrate Calories	Fat Calories
1. Peanut Butter (1 T)	94	15	11	68
2. Yogurt (8 oz. plain)	227	39	161	27
3. Orange Juice (8 oz.)	114	8	100	6
4. Apple Juice (8 oz.)	117	1	116	0
5. Soft Drink (12 oz.)	144	0	144	0
6. Donut, Cake	125	4	61	60
7. Donut, Glazed	164	8	87	69
8. Sweet Roll	317	22	136	159
9. Cake (medium slice)	274	14	175	85
10. Ice Cream (8 oz.)	257	15	108	134
11. Soft Serve Cone (reg.)	240	10	89	134
12. Ice Cream Sandwich Bar	210	40	82	88
13. Strawberries (8 oz.)	55	4	46	5
14. Orange (medium)	64	6	57	1
15. Apple (medium)	96	1	86	9
16. Banana (medium)	101	4	95	2
17. Cantaloupe (half)	82	7	73	2
18. Grapefruit (half)	40	2	37	1
19. Celery Stick	5	2	3	0
20. Carrot (medium)	20	3	17	0
21. Raisins (4 oz.)	210	6	204	0
22. Watermelon (4″ × 6″ slice)	115	8	99	8
23. Chocolate Chip Cookie	60	3	9	48
24. Brownie	145	6	26	113
25. Oatmeal Cookie	65	3	13	49
26. Sandwich Cookie	200	8	112	80
27. Custard Pie (slice)	285	20	188	77
28. Fruit Pie (slice)	350	14	259	77
29. Gelatin (4 oz.)	70	4	32	34
30. Fritter (medium)	132	11	54	67
31. Skim Milk (8 oz.)	88	36	52	0
32. Diet Drink	0	0	0	0
33. Potato Chips (small bag)	115	3	39	73
34. Roasted Peanuts (1.3 oz.)	210	34	25	151
35. Chocolate Candy Bar (1 oz.)	145	7	61	77
36. Choc. Almond Candy Bar (1 oz.)	265	38	74	164
37. Saltine Cracker	18	1	1	16
38. Popped Corn	40	7	33	0
39. Cheese Nachos	471	63	194	214

Appendix E

Canada's Food Guide to Healthy Eating

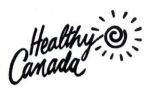

Health and Welfare Canada   Santé et Bien-être social Canada

CANADA'S
Food Guide
TO HEALTHY EATING

Enjoy a variety
of foods from each
group every day.

Choose lower-
fat foods
more often.

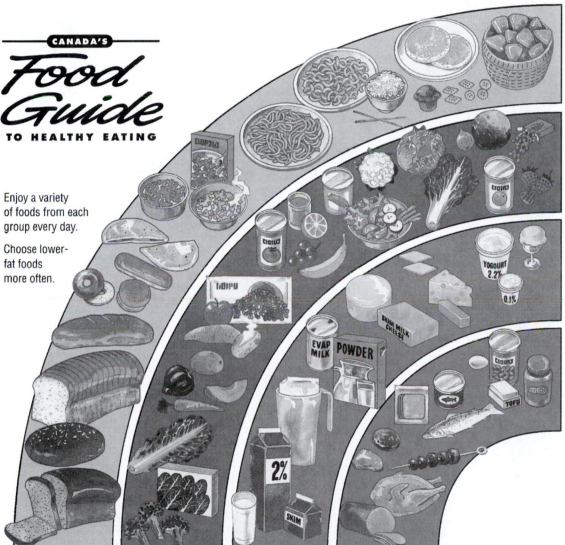

Grain Products
Choose whole grain
and enriched
products more
often.

Vegetables & Fruit
Choose dark green and
orange vegetables and
orange fruit more often.

Milk Products
Choose lower-fat
milk products more
often.

Meat & Alternatives
Choose leaner meats,
poultry and fish, as well
as dried peas, beans and
lentils more often.

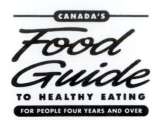

Different People Need Different Amounts of Food

The amount of food you need every day from the 4 food groups and other foods depends on your age, body size, activity level, whether you are male or female and if you are pregnant or breast-feeding. That's why the Food Guide gives a lower and higher number of servings for each food group. For example, young children can choose the lower number of servings, while male teenagers can go to the higher number. Most other people can choose servings somewhere in between.

Grain Products
5-12
SERVINGS PER DAY

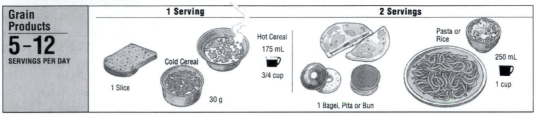

1 Serving — Cold Cereal, Hot Cereal 175 mL 3/4 cup, 1 Slice, 30 g
2 Servings — Pasta or Rice 250 mL 1 cup, 1 Bagel, Pita or Bun

Vegetables & Fruit
5-10
SERVINGS PER DAY

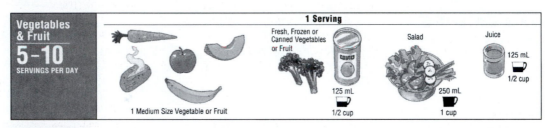

1 Serving — 1 Medium Size Vegetable or Fruit; Fresh, Frozen or Canned Vegetables or Fruit 125 mL 1/2 cup; Salad 250 mL 1 cup; Juice 125 mL 1/2 cup

Milk Products
SERVINGS PER DAY
Children 4–9 years: 2–3
Youth 10–16 years: 3–4
Adults: 2–4
Pregnant & Breast-feeding Women: 3–4

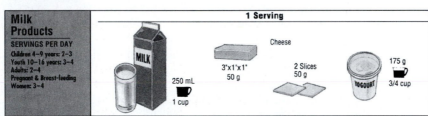

1 Serving — MILK 250 mL 1 cup; Cheese 3"x1"x1" 50 g, 2 Slices 50 g; YOGOURT 175 g 3/4 cup

Meat & Alternatives
2-3
SERVINGS PER DAY

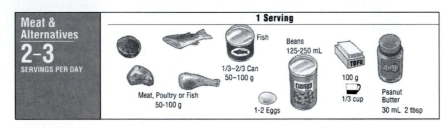

1 Serving — Meat, Poultry or Fish 50-100 g; Fish 1/3–2/3 Can 50–100 g; 1-2 Eggs; Beans 125-250 mL 1/3 cup; TOFU 100 g; Peanut Butter 30 mL 2 tbsp

Other Foods

Taste and enjoyment can also come from other foods and beverages that are not part of the 4 food groups. Some of these foods are higher in fat or Calories, so use these foods in moderation.

Enjoy eating well, being active and feeling good about yourself. That's VITALITé

© Minister of Supply and Services Canada 1992   Cat. No. H39-252/1992E   No changes permitted. Reprint permission not required.
ISBN 0-662-19648-1

Selected References

WEB **www.mhhe.com/hper /physed/clw/student/** Additional references available at this address.

ACSM. (1997). Position Stand on the Female athlete triad. *Medicine and Science in Sports and Exercise* 29(5):1997):i.

ACSM's Health and Fitness Journal 2(2)(1998): entire issue. This issue contains 11 articles dealing with the health benefits of physical activity.

Agosti, R. "Reduce Risk of Activity Induced Injury." *ACSM's Health and Fitness* 2(2)(1998):28.

Aisenbrey, J., and J. L. DePaepe. "A Review of Osteoporosis Research: Implications for Exercise Education and Future Inquiry." *Clinical Kinesiology* 46(1992):2–12.

Alaimo, K. et al. "Dietary Intake of Vitamins, Minerals, and Fiber of Persons Ages 2 Months and Over in the United States." *Vital and Health Statistics: Advance Data* 258(1994):1.

Albert, C. M. et al. "Fish Consumption and Risk of Sudden Cardiac Death." *Journal of the American Medical Association* 279(1)(1998):23.

"Alcohol and Cognition." *Alcohol Alert.* Washington, DC: National Institute on Alcohol Abuse and Alcoholism, 1989. Produced for the U.S. Department of Health and Human Services; Public Health Service; Alcohol, Drug Abuse, and Mental Health Administration.

Alcohol and Health. Seventh Special Report to the U.S. Congress from the Secretary of Health and Human Services, NIAAA. Rockville, MD; U.S. Department of Health amd Human Services, 1990.

"Alcohol and Tolerance." *Alcohol Alert.* Nov. 28 PH356 April, 1995, National Institute on Alcohol Abuse and Alcoholism.

"Alcohol Related Impairment." *Alcohol Alert.* No. 25 PH351 July, 1994, National Institute on Alcohol Abuse and Alcoholism.

Alderman, M. H. et al. "Dietary Sodium Intake and Mortality." *Lancet* 351(9105)(1998):781.

Aleshire, P. "Fourteen in State Tell of Side Effects from Diet Aid L-Tryptophan." *The Arizona Republic,* November 15, 1989.

Alon, G., et al. "Comparison of the Effects of Electrical Stimulation and Exercise on Abdominal Musculature." *Journal of Orthopaedic and Sports Physical Therapy* 8(1987):567.

Alsop, K. "Potential Hazards of Abdominal Exercises." *Journal of Physical Education, Recreation and Dance* 42(1971):89.

Alter, M. J. *Sports Stretch.* Champaign, IL: Human Kinetics Publishers, 1990.

Alter, M. J. *Science of Flexibility.* Champaign, IL: Human Kinetics, 1996.

Alvarado, D. "Survey of Exercises Determines Skating a High-Risk Activity." *The Arizona Republic* (June 11, 1992):D7.

American Alliance of Health, Physical Education, Recreation and Dance. 1900 Association Drive, Reston, VA 22091.

American Cancer Society, "CPSII and Tobacco Control," *CPSII, Newsletter* 12(1995):1.

American Cancer Society. *Cancer Statistics 1999.* www.cancer.org/cancerinfo/ specific.a8p.

American College of Sports Medicine and American Dietetics Association. "Joint Statement on Diabetes Mellitus and Exercise." *Medicine and Science in Sports and Exercise* 29(12)(1997):992.

American College of Sports Medicine. *ACSM's Guidelines for Exercise Testing and Prescription,* 5th ed. Baltimore, MD: Williams and Wilkins, 1995.

American College of Sports Medicine. Position Stand on Heat and Cold Illness During Distance Running. *Medicine and Science in Sports and Exercise* 28(12)(1996):i.

American College of Sports Medicine. "Exercise and Physical Activity for Older Adults." *Medicine and Science in Sports and Exercise* 30(6),(1998):992.

American College of Sports Medicine. "Position Stand on Exercise and Fluid Replacement." *Medicine and Science in Sports and Exercise* 28(1),(1996):i.

American College of Sports Medicine. "Proper and Improper Weight Loss Programs." *Medicine and Science in Sports and Exercise* 15(1983):ix.

American College of Sports Medicine. "The Recommended Quantity and Quality of Exercise for Developing and Maintaining Cardiorespiratory and Muscular Fitness in Healthy Adults." *Medicine and Science in Sports and Exercise* 22(1990):2.

American College of Sports Medicine. "The Recommended Quantity and Quality of Exercise for Developing and Maintaining Cardiorespiratory and Muscular Fitness, and Flexibility in Healthy Adults." *Medicine and Science in Sports and Exercise* 30(6)(1998):975.

American Heart Association (Greater Long Beach Chapter). "Stress—Bona Fide A.H.A. Risk Factor." *Heart Lines* 41(1984):1.

American Heart Association. *1999 Heart & Stroke Statistical Update.* www.amhrt.org/ catalog/scientifc-catpage70.html

American Heart Association. "A Statement on Exercise: Benefits and Recommendations for Physical Activity Programs for All Americans." *Circulation* 91(1995), 580.

American Heart Association. "Active and Passive Tobacco Exposure. A Serious Pediatric Health Problem." (Scientific Statement) *Circulation* Nov. (1995).

Andersen, R. E. et al. "Effects of Lifestyle Activity Vs. Structured Aerobic Exercise in Obese Women." *Journal of the American Medical Association* 281(4)(1999):335.

Androstenedione et al: "Nonprescription Steroids." *Physician and Sports Medicine* 26(11)(1998):15.

Angell, M. and Kassirer, J. P. "Alternative Medicine: The Risks of Untested and Unregulated Remedies." *New England Journal of Medicine* 339(12)(1998):839.

"Are Sports Drinks Better Than Water?" *Physician and Sportsmedicine* 20(1992):33.

Armsey, T. D. & Green, G. A. "Nutrition Supplements: Science vs. Hype." *Physician and Sports Medicine* 25(6)(1997):76.

"Athletes Find Health Food Supplements Big Trouble." *Toronto Star,* Nov. 15, 1995.

Ascherio, A., et al. "Dietary Intake of Marine n–3 Fatty Acids, Fish Intake, and the Risk of Coronary Disease Among Men. " *The New England Journal of Medicine* 332(1995):977.

Ashton-Miller, J. A., and A. B. Schultz. "Biomechanics of the Human Spine and Trunk." *Exercise and Sports Sciences Reviews* 16(1988):169–204.

Auble, T. E., et al. "Aerobic Requirement for Moving Handweights through Various Ranges of Motion While Walking." *Physician and Sportsmedicine* 15(1987):133.

Babbitt, D. "Training Theory: Periodization." *American Track and Field* (1998), Summer.

Baily, D. A., et al. "Growth, Physical Activity and Bone Mineral Acquisition." *Exercise and Sport Sciences Reviews* 24(1996):233.

Ballor, D. et al. "Exercise Training Enhances Fat-Free Mass Preservation During Diet Induced Weight Loss: A Meta Analysis." *International Journal of Obesity* 18(1994):35.

Barnard, R. J. "The Heart Needs a Warm-Up Time." *Physician and Sportsmedicine* 4(1976):40.

Basmajian, J. V. *Therapeutic Exercise.* 5th ed. Baltimore: Williams & Wilkins, 1990.

Bazzoli, A. S. "Chronic Back Pain: A Common Sense Approach." *American Journal of Physical Medicine and Rehabilitation* 71(1992):53–54.

Berlin, J., et al. "A Meta-analysis of Physical Activity in the Prevention of Heart Disease." *American Journal of Epidemiology* 132(1990):612.

"Beta Carotine Pills: Should You Take Them?" *University of California at Berkeley Wellness Letter* 12(April 1996):1.

Biddle, S. J. H. and Fox, K. R. "Motivation for Physical Activity and Weight Management." *International Journal of Obesity* 22 (Supplement 2)(1998)S:39.

Bindman, R., et.al. "Multistate Evaluation of Anonymous HIV Testing and Access to Medical Care." *Journal of the American Medical Association* 280(16)(1998):1416.

Black, D. R., and M. E. Burckes-Miller. "Male and Female College Athletes: Use of Anorexia Nervosa and Bulimia Nervosa Weight Loss Methods." *Research Quarterly for Exercise and Sports* 59(1988):252.

Blair, S. N., and A. Oberman. "Epidemiological Analysis of Coronary Heart Disease." *Cardiology Clinics* 5(1987):271.

Blair, S. N., and R. S. Paffenbarger. "Physical Activity and Risk of Cancer." (ab.) *Medicine and Science in Sports and Exercise* 19(1987):418.

Blair, S. N. & Connelly, J. C. "How Much Physical Activity Should We Do? The Case for Moderate Amounts and Intensities of Physical Activity." *Research Quarterly for Exercise and Sport* 67(2)(1996):193.

Blair, S., et al. "Physical Activity and Health: A Lifestyle Approach." *Medicine, Exercise, Nutrition and Health* 1(1992):54.

Blair, S., et al. "Physical Fitness and All-Cause Mortality." *Journal of the American Medical Association* 262(1989):2395.

Blonna, R. *Coping with Stress in a Changing World.* St. Louis, MO: WCB/McGraw-Hill, 1996.

Bonham, B. J., et al. "Binge Drinking in College." *Journal of the American Medical Association* 273(1995):1903.

Bouchard, C. et al. *Genetics of Fitness and Physical Performance.* Champaign, IL: Human Kinetics, 1997.

Bouchard, C. "Heredity and the Path to Overweight and Obesity." *Medicine and Science in Sports and Exercise* 23(1991):285.

Bouchard, C., et al. "Genetics of Aerobic and Anaerobic Performances." *Exercise and Sport Sciences Reviews* 20(1992):27.

Bourey, R. E., et al. "Interactions of Exercise, Coagulation, Platelets, and Fibrinolysis: A Brief Review." *Medicine and Science in Sports and Exercise* 20(1988):439.

Bova, A. A. & Sherman, C. "Active Control of Hypertension." *Physician and Sports Medicine* 26(4)(1998):45.

Brittenham, G. "Plyometric Exercise: A Word of Caution." *Journal of Physical Education, Recreation and Dance* (Jan. 1992):20–23.

Bronson, F. H. & Matherne, C. M. "Exposure to Anabolic-Androgenic Steroids Shortens Life Span for Male Mice:" *Medicine and Science in Sports and Exercise* 29(5)(1997):615.

Brower, K. J., et al. "Evidence for Physical and Psychological Dependence on Anabolic Androgenic Steroids in Eight Weight Lifters." *American Journal of Psychiatry* 147(1990):510–12.

Brunick, T. "Choosing the Right Shoe." *Physician and Sportsmedicine* 18(1990):104.

Buckwalter, J. A. "Decreased Mobility in the Elderly: The Exercise Antidote." *Physician and Sports Medicine* 25(9)(1997):138.

Burney, M. W. & Brehm, B. A. "The Female Athlete Triad." *Journal of Physical Education Recreation and Dance* 69(9)(1998):29.

Buroker, K. C., and J. A. Schwane. "Does Post-Exercise Static Stretching Alleviate Delayed Muscle Soreness?" *Physician and Sportsmedicine* 17(1989):65.

Burstein, G. R., et al. "Incident Chlamydia Trachomatis Infections Among Inner City Adolescent Females." *Journal of the American Medical Association* 280(6)(1999):521.

Byers, T. "Body Weight and Mortality." *New England Journal of Medicine* 334(1996):723.

Byers, T. "Dietary Trends in the United States." *Cancer* 72(1993):1015.

CDC. "The Cost Effectiveness of Screening for Type II Diabetes." *Journal of the American Medical Association* 280(20)(1999):1957.

Cailliet, R. *Knee Pain and Disability.* 3d ed. Philadelphia: F. A. Davis, Co., 1992.

Cailliet, R. *Low Back Pain Syndrome.* 5th ed. Philadelphia: F. A. Davis, Co., 1994.

Cailliet, R. *Neck and Arm Pain.* 3d ed. Philadelphia: F. A. Davis, Co., 1991.

Cailliet, R. *Shoulder Pain.* 3d ed. Philadelphia: F. A. Davis, Co., 1995.

Cailliet, R. *Soft Tissue Pain and Disability.* 2d ed. Philadelphia: F. A. Davis, Co., 1988.

"Calcium: Vital for Women and Men." *Consumer Reports on Health* 6(1994):13.

Califano, J. A. Jr. "The Wrong Way to Stay Slim." *New England Journal of Medicine* 333(1995):1214.

Campaigne, B. N. "Exercise and Type I Diabetes." *ACSM's Health and Fitness Journal* 2(4)(1998):35.

Campaigne, B. N. "Provide Physical Activity Precautions for Clients with Diabetes." *ACSM's Health and Fitness* 2(2)(1998):18.

Campbell, W. et al. "Increased Energy Requirements and Changes in Body Composition With Resistance Training in Older Adults." *American Journal of Clinical Nutrition* 60(1994):167.

"Can One Train Cardiorespiratory and Muscular Fitness Simultaneously?" (Editorial). *Canadian Journal of Sport Science* 16(1991):167–68.

"Can Your Mind Heal Your Body?" *Consumer Reports* (Feb. 1993):107.

Cardinal, B. J. "Rating the Clubs: A Health and Fitness Center Consumer Checklist."*American Fitness* Sept./Oct. 1994.

Carpenter, C. C. J. et al. "Antiretroviral for HIV Infection in 1998: Updated Recommendations." *Journal of the American Medical Association* 280(1)(1998):78.

Carpenter, D. M. and Nelson, B. W. "Low Back Strengthening for the Prevention and Treatment of Low Back Pain." *Medicine and Science in Sports and Exercise* 31(1)(1999):18.

Casperson, C. J., et al. "Physical Activity, Exercise, and Physical Fitness: Definitions and Distinctions for Health-Related Research." *Public Health Reports* 100(1985):126.

Centers for Disease Control. "Cigarette Smoking Among Adults." Epidemiology Branch, Office on Smoking Health. National Center for Chronic Disease Prevention and Health Promotion. *Journal of the American Medical Association* 273(1995):369.

Centers for Disease Control. *HIV/AIDS Surveillance Report.* Atlanta, GA: U.S. Department of Health and Human Services, 1991.

Centers for Disease Control. *Morbidity and Mortality Weekly Report* 39(1990):110.

Chambers, M. "Exercise: A Prescription for a Good Night's Sleep?" *Physician and Sportsmedicine* 19(1991):107.

Chase, L. A., Corbin, C. B. and Rutherford, W. "Self measured vs Expert Measaured Skinfolds of College Aged Females." *J. British Journal of Physical Education:* Research Supplement. 12(1992):9.

Cherkin, D. C. et al. "A Comparison of Physical Therapy, Chiropractic Manipulation and Providing of an Educational Book for Treatment of Patients with Low Back Pain." *New England Journal of Medicine* 339(15)(1998):1021.

Chodak, G. W., et al. "Routine Screening for Prostate Cancer Using the Digital Rectal Examination." *Progress and Clinical and Biological Research* 269(1988):87.

Chu, D. A. *Jumping Into Plyometrics, 2e.* Champaign, IL: Human Kinetics, 1998.

Clark, J. R. "Sexually Transmitted Disease: Detection, Differentiation, and Treatment." *Physician and Sports Medicine* 25(1)(1997):76.

Clark, K. "Water, Sports Drinks, Juice, or Soda?" *ACSM's Health and Fitness Journal* 2(5)(1998):41.

Clark, N. "How to Gain Weight Healthfully." *Physician and Sportsmedicine* 19(1991):53.

Clark, N. "Protein Myths: The Meat of the Matter." *Sportcare and Fitness* 2(1989):53.

Clark, N. "Water: The Ultimate Nutrient." *Physician and Sportsmedicine* 23(1995):21.

Clarkson, P. M. "The Skinny on Weight Loss Supplements and Drugs: Winning the War Against Fat." *ACSM's Health and Fitness Journal* 2(4)(1998):18.

Clarkson, P. M. "Minerals, Exercise Performance and Supplementation." *Journal of Sport Sciences* 9(1991):91.

Clements, M. "Sex in America Today." *Parade Magazine* (August 7, 1994):4.

Clouet, D., K. Asghar, and R. Brown. "Mechanisms of Cocaine Abuse and Toxicity." Rockville, MD: National Institute on Drug Abuse (1988):ix. Research Monograph 88, U.S. Department of Health and Human Services, Public Health Service.

Cohen, J. S., et al. "Hypercholesterolemia in Male Power Lifters Using Anabolic-Androgenic Steroids." *Physician and Sportsmedicine* 16(1988):49.

Cohen, S. "Psychosocial Models of the Role of Social Support in the Etiology of Physical Disease." *Health Psychology* 7(1988), 269–297.

Cohne, O. J. & Fauci, A. S. "HIV/AIDS in 1998: Gaining the Upper Hand." *Journal of the American Medical Association* 280(1)(1998):87.

Coleman, D., and J. Gurin. Eds. *Mind/Body Medicine.* Consumer Reports Books, Fairfield, OH: 1993.

Coleman, E. "Carbohydrate Unloading." *Physician and Sports Medicine* 25(2)(1997):97.

Colucci, D., et al. "Comparison of Static versus PNF Stretching on Shoulder ROM in Intercollegiate Baseball Players." *Athletic Training* 24(1989):116.

Commandre, F. A., et al. "Lumbar Spine, Sport and Actual Treatment." *Journal of Sports Medicine and Physical Fitness* 31(1992):129–35.

Cooper, E. "Statement on Physical Activity and Heart Disease." American Heart Association News Release. July 1, 1992, pp.1–2.

Corbin, C. B., and R. Lindsey. *Fitness for Life.* 4th ed. Glenview, IL: Scott, Foresman and Co., 1997.

Corbin, C. B., and R. Pangrazi. "Are American Children and Youth Fit?" *Research Quarterly for Exercise and Sport* 63(1993):96.

Corbin, C. B., and R. Pangrazi. "The Health Benefits of Exercise." *Research Digest for Physical Activity and Fitness* 1(1993):1.

Corbin, C. B., and R. P. Pangrazi. Answers to Questions: How Much Physical Activity is Enough? *Journal of Physical Education Recreation and Dance* 67(1996):33.

Corbin, C. B. & Pangrazi, R. P. (Editors), *Towards a Better Understanding of Physical Fitness and Activity.* Scottsdale, AZ: Holcomb-Hathaway, 1999.

Corbin, C. B. & Pangrazi, R. P. "Physical Activity for Children and Youth" *Journal of Physical Education Recreation and Dance* 67(4)(1996):38.

Corbin, C. B. & Pangrazi, R. P. "Physical Activity Pyramid Rebuffs Peak Exercise." *ACSM's Health and Fitness Journal* 2(1)(1998):12.

Corbin, C. B. & Pangrazi, R. P. "What You Need to Know About the Surgeon General's Report on Physical Activity and Health." *President's Council on Physical Fitness and Sports Research Digest* 2(6)(1996):1.

Corbin, D. E., and J. Metal-Corbin. *Reach for It: A Handbook of Health, Exercise and Dance Activities, for Older Adults.* 2d ed. Dubuque, IA: E. Bowers, 1990.

Corbin, D. E. (ed.). *Perspectives: Stress Management.* Boulder, CO: Coursewise Publishing Co., 1999.

Cordain, L., et al. "The Effects of an Aerobic Running Program on Bowel Transit Time." *Journal of Sports Medicine* 26(1986):101.

Cornacchea, J., and S. Barrett. *Consumer Health* 5th ed. C. V. Mosby, 1993.

Couldry, W., et al. "Carotid vs. Radial Pulse Counts." *Physician and Sportsmedicine* 10(1982):67.

Cowart, V. S. "Dietary Supplements." *Physician and Sportsmedicine* 20(1992):189.

Cowart, V. S. "Can Exercise Help Women with PMS?" *Physician and Sportsmedicine* 17(1989):169.

Cox, M. H. "Exercise for Coronary Artery Disease." *Physician and Sports Medicine* 25(12)(1997):27.

Curran, J. W., et al. "Epidemiology of HIV Infection and AIDS in the United States." *Science* 239(1988):610.

Curry, S. J. et al. "Use and Cost Effectiveness of Smoking Cessation Services Under Four Insurance Plans in an HMO." *New England Journal of Medicine* 339(10)(1998):673.

Davidson, M. H. et al. "Weight Control and Risk Factor Reduction in Obese Subjects Treated for 2 Years with Orlistat." *Journal of the American Medical Association* 280(3)(1999):281.

DeMarco, H. M. et al. "Pre-Exercise Carbohydrate Meals: Application of the Glycemic Index." *Medicine and Science in Sports and Exercise* 31(1),(1999):164.

DePiccoli, B., et al. "Anabolic Steroid Use in Body Builders: An Echocardiographic Study of Left Ventricle Morphology and Function." *International Journal of Sports Medicine* 4(1991):408–12.

Derosiers, "New Clues Found to How Some People Live with HIV." *Science* 270(1995):917.

Detels, R. et al. "Effects of Potent Antiretroviral Therapy on the Time to AIDS in Men Known to Have HIV Infection Duration." *Journal of the American Medical Association* 280(17)(1998):1497.

DiClemente, R. J., et al. "Adolescents and AIDS: A Survey of Knowledge, Attitudes, and Beliefs about AIDS in San Francisco." *American Journal of Public Health* 76(1986):1443.

DiClemente, R. J. "Prevention of Sexually Transmitted Infections Among Adolescents: A Clash of Ideology and Science." *Journal of the American Medical Association* 279(19)(1998):1574.

DiPietro, L. "Physical Activity, Body Weight, and Adiposity: An Epidemiological Perspective." *Exercise and Sport Sciences Reviews* 23(1995):275.

Diaz-Mitoma, F. et al. "Oral Famciclovir for Suppression of Recurrent Genital Herpes." *Journal of the American Medical Association* 280(10)(1998):887.

Dietary Guidelines and Your Diet. Hyattsville, MD: USDA, 1992, No. HG–232, 1–11.

Dillingham, T. R. "Lumbar Supports for Prevention of Low Back Pain in the Workplace." *Journal of the American Medical Association* 279(22)(1998):1826.

Dimeo, F. et al. "Aerobic Exercise As Therapy for Cancer Fatigue." *Medicine and Science in Sports and Exercise* 30(4),(1998):475.

Disabella, V. & Sherman, C. "Exercise for Asthma Patients." *Physician and Sports Medicine* 26(6)(1998):75.

Dishman, R., and J. Sallis. "Determinants and Interventions for Physical Activity and Exercise." In C. Bouchard, et al., eds., *Physical Activity, Fitness, and Health.* Champaign, IL: Human Kinetics Publishers, 1994.

Dishman, R. K., ed. *Advances in Exercise Adherence.* Champaign, IL: Human Kinetics Publishers, 1994.

Dixon, A. E., et al. "Sudden Death in Sports Activities." *New England Journal of Medicine* 333(1995):1784.

"Drinking and Driving." *Alcohol Alert.* No. 31 PH362 January 1996. National Institute on Alcohol Abuse and Alcoholism.

Drinkwater, B. "Teach Osteoporosis Prevention Through Physical Activity." *ACSM's Health and Fitness* 2(2)(1998):12.

"Drug Abuse and Pregnancy." *NIDA Capsules.* Washington, DC: National Institute on Drug Abuse; U.S. Department of Health and Human Services, Public Health Service; Alcohol, Drug Abuse and Mental Health Administration, June 1989.

"Drug Ecstasy Could Cause Brain Damage." *Orange County Register,* Sept. 15, 1995.

Duda, M. "The Medical Risks and Benefits of Sauna, Steam Bath and Whirlpool Use." *Physician and Sportsmedicine* 15(1987):170.

Dunn, A. L. et al. "Comparison of Lifestyle and Structured Interventions to Increase Physical Activity and Cardiorespiratory Fitness." *Journal of the American Medical Association* 281(1999):327.

Dunn, A. L. et al. "Lifestyle Physical Activity Intervention." *American Journal of Preventive Medicine* 15(1998):398.

Durant, R. H., et al. "Use of Multiple Drugs Among Adolescents Who Use Anabolic Steroids." *New England Journal of Medicine* 328(1993):922.

Dye, C. *"Adam" & "Eve" & "Ecstasy": Facts about MDMA.* Tempe, AZ: D.I.N. Publications, 1988.

Dzewaltowski, D., et al. "Physical Activity Participation: Social Cognitive Theory Versus the Theories of Reasoned Action and Planned Behavior." *Journal of Sport and Exercise Psychology* 12(1990):388.

"Early Breast Cancer Trialists' Collaborative Group. Tamoxifen for Early Breast Cancer." *Lancet* 351(1998):1510.

Ebbens, W. P., Jensen, R. L. "Strength Training for Women." *Physician and Sports Medicine* 26(5)(1998):86.

Eddy, D. M., et al. "The Value of Mammography Screening in Women under 50 Years." *Journal of the American Medical Association* 259(1988):187.

Eisenberg, D. M. "Trends in Alternative Medicine in the US 1990–1997." *Journal of the American Medical Association* 280(18)(1998):1569.

Eisner, M. D. et al. "Bartenders' Respiratory Health After Establishment of Smoke-Free Bars and Taverns." *Journal of the American Medical Association* 280(22)(1998):1909.

Elkin, P. L. "Effects of Diet and Exercise on Cholesterol Levels." *New England Journal of Medicine* 339(21)(1998):552.

Engel, J. P. "Long Term Suppression of Genital Herpes." *Journal of the American Medical Association* 280(10)(1998):928.

Engels, H. J. et al. "An Empirical Evaluation of the Prediction of Maximal Heart Rate." *Research Quarterly for Exercise and Sport* 69(1)(1998):94.

Englehardt, M. et al. "Creatine Supplementation in Endurance Sports." *Medicine and Science in Sports and Exercise* 30(7),(1998):1123.

Erickson, S. M. & Sevier, T. L. "Osteoporosis in Active Women." *Physician and Sports Medicine* 25(11)(1997):61.

Etnier, J. L. et al. "The Influence of Physical Fitness and Exercise Upon Cognitive Functioning: A Meta Analysis." *The Journal of Sport and Exercise Psychology* 19(3)(1997):249.

Evans, W. J. "Exercise Training Guidelines for the Elderly." *Medicine and Science in Sports and Exercise* 31(1),(1999):12.

Farrel, S. W. et al. "Influences of Cardiorespiratory Fitness Levels and Other Predictors of Cardiovascular Disease Mortality in Men." *Medicine and Science in Sports and Exercise* 30(6)(1998):899.

Farzadegen, H. et al. "Sex Difference in HIV-1 Load and Progression of AIDS." *Lancet* 352(9139)(1998):1510.

Feigenbaum, M. S. and Pollock, M. L. "Strength Training: Rationale for Current Guidelines for Adult Fitness Programs." *Physician and Sports Medicine* 25(2)(1997):44.

Feignebaum, M. S. and Pollock, M. L. "Prescription of Resistance Training for Health and Disease." *Medicine and Science in Sports and Exercise* 31(1),(1999):38.

Ferenchick, G. S., et al. "Steroids and Cardiomyopathy: How Strong a Connection?" *Physician and Sportsmedicine* 19(1991):107–10.

Fessel, W. J., et al. "Early Treatment of HIV Infections." *New England Journal of Medicine* 333(1995):1782.

Field, R. "How Humans Sit." *The American Way* (April 15, 1988):28–29.

Fisher, H. R., et al. "Calculating Blood Alcohol Concentration (BAC) By Sex, Weight, Number of Drinks and Time." *Canadian Journal of Public Health* 78(5)(1987):300.

Fleck, S. J. "Cardiovascular Adaptations to Resistance Training." *Medicine and Science in Sports and Exercise* 20(1988):Supplement, 146.

Fletcher, G. F., et al. "American Heart Association Medical/Scientific Statement on Exercise." *Circulation* 86(1992):340.

Fogelholm, M. et al. "Assessment of Energy Expenditure in Overweight Women." *Medicine and Science in Sports and Exercise* 30(8),(1998):1191.

Fomby, E. W. and Mellon, M. B. "Identifying and Treating Myofascial Pain Syndrome." *The Physician and Sports Medicine.* 25(2)(1997):67.

Fontanarosa, P. B. "Alternative Medicine Meets Science." *Journal of the American Medical Association* 280(18)(1998):1618.

Food and Drug Administration. *Condoms and Sexually Transmitted Diseases.* Rockville, MD: U.S. Department of Health and Human Services, 1990.

"Foods, Drugs or Frauds?" *FDA Consumer,* May, 1985 (reprint).

Foy, S. F. et al. "7-Step Guide to Motivating Clients." *ACSM's Health and Fitness* 2(2)(1998):5.

Frankle, M., and D. Leffers. "Athletes on Anabolic-Androgenic Steroids: New Approach Diminishes Health Problems." *Physician and Sportsmedicine* 20(1992):75–87.

Franklin, B. "Exercise Training and Coronary Collateral Circulation." *Medicine and Science in Sport and Exercise* 23(1991):648.

Franklin, B. A. "A Common Misunderstanding About Heart Rate and Exercise." *ACSM's Health and Fitness* 2(1),(1998):18–19.

Franklin, B. A. "Homocysteine: A New Risk Factor for Heart Disease." *ACSM's Health and Fitness* 2(4)(1998):43.

Franklin, B. A. "Prevent Cardiac Events During Physical Activity." *ACSM's Health and Fitness* 2(2)(1998):8.

Franklin, B. A. "Pumping Iron: Rationale, Benefits, Safety, and Prescription." *ACSM's Health and Fitness Journal* 2(5)(1998):12.

Franks, B. D. "Individualized recommendations for physical activity." *President's Council on Physical Fitness and Sports Research Digest* 3(1)(1997):1.

Franks, B. D., et al. "Physical Activity Intensity: How Much Is Enough?" *ACSM's Health and Fitness* 1(6)(1997):14.

Freedman, A. M. "Philip Morris Draft Report May Help U.S. Case Against Tobacco." *Orange County Register,* Dec. 9, 1995.

Fuchs, C. S., et al. "Alcohol Consumption and Mortality Among Women." *New England Journal of Medicine* 332(1995):1245.

Fuchs, C. S. et al. "Dietary Fiber and Risk of Colorectal Cancer in Women." *New England Journal of Medicine* 340(4)(1999):169.

Gallup, G. "Leisure: Swimming, Fishing, Bicycling Are Top Sports Activities." *Gallup Report* 281(1989):28.

Garrick, J. G. and Schelkun, P. H. "Managing Ankle Sprains: Keys to Preserving Motion and Strains." *The Physician and Sports Medicine* 25(3)(1997):56.

Gaydos, C. A. "Chlamydia Trachomatis Infections in Female Military Recruits." *New England Journal of Medicine* 339(11)(1998):739.

George, J. D., Fellingham, G. W., & Fisher, A. G. "A Modified Version of the Rockport Fitness Walking Test for College Men and Women." *Research Quarterly for Exercise and Sport* 69(2)(1998):205.

Girdano, D. & Everly, G. *Controlling Stress and Tension: A Holistic Approach* (5th ed.). Englewood Cliffs, NJ: Prentice Hall, 1996.

Glantz, S. A., and W. W. Parmley. "Passive Smoking and Heart Disease: Mechanism and Risk." *Journal of the American Medical Association* 273(1995):1047.

Golding, L. A. "Engage Older Adults in Physical Activity." *ACSM's Health and Fitness* 2(2)(1998):24.

Golding, L. A. "Flexibility, Stretching, and Flexibility Testing." *ACSM's Health and Fitness* 1(1)(1997):17.

Goldman, L. K. & Glantz, S. A. "Evaluation of Antismoking Campaigns." *Journal of the American Medical Association* 279(10)(1998):772.

Golomb, L. M. et al. "Primary Dysmenorrhea and Physical Activity." *Medicine and Science in Sports and Exercise* 30(6)(1998):906.

Gorley, T. and Gordon, S. "An Examination of the Transtheoretical Model and Exercise Behavior in Older Adults." *Journal of Sport and Exercise Psychology* 17(1995):312.

Grady, D. "A Silent Killer Returns: Doctors Rethink Tactics to Lower Blood Pressure." *New York Times* July 14, 1998, F1.

Grahame, R., and J. M. Jenkins. "Joint Hypermobility—Asset or Liability." *Annals of Rheumatic Disease* 31(1972):109.

Grandal, N. A. et al. "Effects of Sodium Restriction on Blood Pressure and Other Factors." *Journal of the American Medical Association* 279(17)(1998):1383.

Graves, J. E., et al. "Physiological Responses to Walking with Hand Weights, Wrist Weights and Ankle Weights." *Medicine and Science in Sports and Exercise* 20(1988):265.

Greenberg, J. S. et al. "A Clinical Trial of Antioxidant Vitamins to Prevent Colorectal Adenoma." *The New England Journal of Medicine* 331(1994):141.

Grigg, W. "Quackery: It Costs More Than Money." *FDA Consumer* 22(1988):30.

Gulick, R. M. "HIV Treatment Strategies: Planning for the Long Term." *Journal of the American Medical Association* 279(12)(1998):957.

Gunby, P. "World No-Tobacco Day Targets Sports and the Arts." *Journal of the American Medical Association* 275(16)(1996):1220.

Haddock, B. L. et al. "Cardiorespiratory Fitness and Cardiovascular Disease Risk Factors in Postmenopausal Women." *Medicine and Science in Sports and Exercise* 30(6)(1998):1893.

Haennel, R., et al. "Effects of Hydraulic Circuit Training on Cardiovascular Function." *Medicine and Science in Sports and Exercise* 21(1989):605–11.

Hagg, R. S. et al. "Improved Survival Among HIV Infected Individuals Following Initiation of Antiretroviral." *Journal of the American Medical Association* 279(67)(1998):450.

Hallmark, M. A. et al. "Effects of Chromium and Resistive Training on Muscle Training Exercise on Strength and Body Composition." *Medicine and Science in Sports and Exercise* 28(61),(1998–6139):992.

Hardy, L., and D. Jones. "Dynamic Flexibility and Proprioceptive Neuromuscular Facilitation." *Research Quarterly for Exercise and Sport* 57(1986):150.

Harris, L. *Inside America.* New York: Vintage Books, 1987.

Haskell, W. L. "Physical Activity in the Prevention and Management of Coronary Heart Disease." *Physical Activity and Fitness Research Digest* 2(1995):1.

Haussenblas, H. A. et al. "Applications of the Theories of Reasoned Action and Planned Behaviors: A Meta Analysis." *The Journal of Sport and Exercise Psychology* 19(1997):36.

Hawley, J. A. "Fat Burning During Exercise: Can Ergogenics Change the Balance?" *Physician and Sports Medicine* 26(9)(1998):56.

"Herbal Roulette." *Consumers Report* 60(1995):689.

Hiatt, W., et al. "Benefits of Exercise Conditioning for Patients with Peripheral Arterial Disease." *Circulation* 81(1990):602.

Hirsch, M. S. et al. "Antiretroviral Drug Testing in Adults with HIV Infection." *Journal of the American Medical Association* 279(24)(1998):1984.

Hjelm, J. and Johnson, R. C. "Spiritual Health: An Annotated Bibliography" *Journal of Health Education* 27(1996), 248–252.

Hochhauser, M. and Rothenberger, J. *AIDS Education.* St. Louis: WCB/McGraw-Hill, 1996.

Hoeger, W. W. K., and D. R. Hopkins. "A Comparison of the Sit-and-Reach and the Modified Sit-and-Reach in the Measurement of Flexibility in Women." *Research Quarterly for Exercise and Sport* 31(June 1992):191–95.

Hopkins, D. R., and W. W. K. Hoeger. "A Comparison of the Sit-and-Reach Test and the Modified Sit-and-Reach Test in the Measurement of Flexibility for Males." *Journal of Applied Sport Science Research* 6(1992):7–10.

Howard, G. "Cigarette Smoking and Progression of Atherosclerosis." *Journal of the American Medical Association* 279(2)(1998):119.

Howley, E. T. and Franks, B. D. *Health Fitness Instructor's Handbook* (3rd ed.). Champaign, IL: Human Kinetics, 1997.

Hulley, S. et al. "Randomized Trial of Estrogen and Progestin for Secondary Prevention of CHD in Post Menopausal Women." *Journal of the American Medical Association* 280(7)(1998):605.

Inhofe, P. D., et al. "The Effects of Anabolic Steroid on Rat Tendon." *The American Journal of Sports Medicine* 23(1995):227.

Jackson, A. S., et al. "Generalized Equations for Predicting Body Density of Women." *Medicine and Science in Sports and Exercise* 12(1980):175.

Jacobson, B. "Effects of Amino Acids on Growth Hormone Release." *Physician and Sportsmedicine* 18(1990):63.

Jinot, J., and S. Bayard. "Respiratory Health Effects of Passive Smoking: EPA's Weight of Evidence Analysis." *Journal of Clinical Epidemiology* 47(1994):339.

Johnson, E. "Aquatic Exercise For Better Living on Land." *ACSM's Health and Fitness Journal* 2(3)(1998), 16.

Jonas, W. B. et al. "Alternative Medicine: Learning from the Past, Examining the Present, Advancing to the Future." *Journal of the American Medical Association* 280(18)(1998):1616.

Kahn, H. S. et al. "Increased Cancer Mortality Following a History of Non Melanoma Skin Cancer." *Journal of the American Medical Association* 280(10)(1998):910.

Kamb, M. L. et al. "Efficacy of Risk Reduction Counseling to Prevent HIV and STDs." *Journal of the American Medical Association* 280(13)(1998):1161.

Kamwendo, K., et al. "Neck and Shoulder Disorders in Medical Secretaries. Part I: Pain Prevalence and Risk Factors." *Scandinavian Journal of Rehabilitation Medicine* 23(1991):127–33.

Kamwendo, K., et al. "Neck and Shoulder Disorders in Medical Secretaries: Part II. Ergonomical Work Environment and Symptom Profile." *Scandinavian Journal of Rehabilitation Medicine* 23(1991):135–42.

Kanders, B., et al. "Interaction of Calcium Nutrition and Physical Activity on Bone Mass in Young Women." *Journal of Bone Mineral Research* 3(1988):145.

Kanter, M. "Free Radicals and Exercise: Effects of Nutritional Antioxidant Supplementation." *Exercise and Sport Sciences Reviews* 23(1995):375.

Karkowsky, N. "Exercise with Care—Fitness Is Not Risk Free." *FDA Consumer* 23(1989):25.

Katz, W. A. & Sherman, C. "Exercise for Osteoporosis." *Physician and Sports Medicine* 26(2)(1998):43.

Katz, W. A. & Sherman, C. "Osteoporosis: The Role of Exercise in Optimal Management." *Physician and Sports Medicine* 26(2)(1998):33.

Kavanaugh, T. "Does Exercise Improve Coronary Collateralization? A New Look at an Old Belief." *Physician and Sportsmedicine* 17(1989):96.

Keefe, C. "Body Miracles Aren't Found All Bottled Up." *Orange County Register,* April 2, 1995.

Kelleher, S. "R.S.I.: Treating Repetitive Motion Injuries is Fledgling Science." *Orange County Register,* March 1, 1995.

Kenyon, G. S. "Six Scales for Assessing Attitudes Toward Physical Activity." *Research Quarterly* 39(1968):566.

King, A. C., et al. "Determinants of Physical Activity and Interventions in Adults." *Medicine and Science in Sports and Exercise* 24(1992):S221 (Supplement).

Kisner, C., and L. A. Colby. *Therapeutic Exercise: Foundations and Techniques.* 2d ed. Philadelphia: F. A. Davis, Company, 1990.

Klein, K. K. "The Deep Squat as Utilized in Weight Training for Athletics and Its Effect on the Ligaments of the Knee." *Journal of Physical and Mental Rehabilitation* 15(1961):10.

Kleiner, S. "Fiber Facts." *Physician and Sportsmedicine* 18(1990):19.

Knudson, D. "Stretching: From Science to Practice." *Journal of Physical Education Recreation and Dance* 69(3)(1998):38.

Kobashigawa, J. A. et al. "A Controlled Trial of Exercise Rehabilitation After Heart Transplant." *New England Journal of Medicine* 340(4)(1999):272.

Koop, C. E. et al. "Reinventing American Tobacco Policy." *Journal of the American Medical Association* 279(7)(1998):550.

Koplan, J. P., et al. "The Risk of Exercise: A Public Health View of Injuries and Hazards." *Public Health Reports* 199(1985):189.

Kottke, F. J., et al. *Krusen's Handbook of Physical Medicine and Rehabilitation.* 4th ed. Philadelphia: W. B. Saunders Co., 1990.

Kraus, H., and W. Raab. *Hypokinetic Disease.* Springfield, IL: Charles C. Thomas, 1961.

Kreider, R. B., Fry, A. C., & O'Toole, M. L. *Overtraining in Sport.* Champaign, IL: Human Kinetics, 1998.

Kromhout, D. "Fish Consumption and Sudden Cardiac Death." *Journal of the American Medical Association* 279(1)(1998):65.

Kuipers, H., et al. "Influence of Anabolic Steroids on Body Composition, Blood Pressure, Lipid Profile and Liver Functions in Body Builders." *International Journal of Sports Medicine* 12(1991):413–18.

Kujala, U. M. et al. "Relationship of Leisure Time Physical Activity and Mortality." *Journal of the American Medical Association* 279(6)(1998):440.

Kuntzleman, C. T. and Wilkerson, R. "A Primer to Recommending Home Aerobic Equipment." *ACSM's Health and Fitness Journal* 1(6)(1997):24.

Kuritzky, L. and White, J. "Extend Yourself for Back Relief." *Physician and Sports Medicine* 25(1)(1998):65.

Kuritzky, L. and White, J. "Low Back Pain." *Physician and Sports Medicine* 25(1)(1998):56.

Kushi, L. H., et al. "Dietary Antioxidant Vitamins and Death from Coronary Heart Disease in Postmenopausal Women." *The New England Journal of Medicine* 334(1996):1156.

LaBree, M. "A Review of Anabolic Steroids: Uses and Effects." *Journal of Sports Medicine and Physical Fitness* 32(1991):618–26.

LaChance, P. F., and T. Hortobagyi. "Influence of Cadence on Muscular Performance During Push-ups and Pull-up Exercise." *Journal of Strength and Conditioning Research* 8(1994):76–79.

Lagakos, S. W. "Comparison of Immediate with Deferred Zidovudine Therapy for Asymptomatic HIV-infected Adults with CD4 Counts of 500 or More per Cubic Millimeter." *New England Journal of Medicine* 333(1995):1782.

Landers, D. "The Influence of Exercise on Mental Health." In Corbin, C. B. & Pangrazi, R. P. (ed.). *Towards a Better Understanding of Physical Fitness and Activity* Scottsdale, AZ: Holcomb-Hathaway, 1999, Chapter 16.

Laseter, J. T., and J. A. Russell. "Anabolic Steroid-Induced Tendon Pathology: A Review of the Literature." *Medicine and Science in Sports and Exercise* 23(1991):1–3.

Lauderman, S. H., and D. Burns. "Quantifying HIV." *Journal of the American Medical Association* 275(1996):640.

Layne, J. E. and Nelson, M. E. "The Effects of Progressive Resistance Training on Bone Density: A Review." *Medicine and Science in Sports and Exercise* 31(1)(1999):25.

Lazarus, R. S. "Theory-based Stress Measurement." *Psychological Inquiry* 1(1990), 3–13.

Leach, R. "The Impingement Syndrome." In B. Zarins, et al., eds., *Injuries to the Throwing Arm.* Philadelphia: W. B. Saunders Co., 1985.

Lee, C. D., Jackson, A. S., & Blair, S. N. "US Weight Guidelines: It Is Also Important to Consider Cardiorespiratory Fitness." *International Journal of Obesity* 22(supplement 2)(1998):S2.

Lee, I. "Exercise and Physical Health: Cancer and Immune Function." *Research Quarterly for Exercise and Sport* 66(1995):286.

Lee, I., et al. "Change in Body Weight and Longevity." *Journal of the American Medical Association* 268(1992):2045.

Lee, I., et al. "Physical Activity and Risk of Developing Colorectal Cancer Among College Alumni." *Journal of the National Cancer Institute* 83(1991):1324.

Lee, I., et al. "Time Trends in Physical Activity Among College Alumni 1962–1988." *American Journal of Epidemiology* 135(1992):915.

Lee, I., and R. S. Paffenbarger. "Do Physical Activity and Physical Fitness Avert Premature Mortality?" *Exercise and Sport Sciences Reviews* 24(1996):135.

Lemonick, M. D. "Are We Ready for Fat Free Fat?" *Time* 4(Jan. 22, 1996), 40.

Leutholtz, B. C. "Exercise Can Reduce Incidence and Severity of Hypertension." *ACSM's Health and Fitness* 2(5)(1998):36.

Levine, J. A. et al. "Role of Nonexercise Activity in Fat Burning in Humans." *Science* 283(5399)(1998):212.

Liemohn, W., et al. "Criterion Related Validity of the Sit and Reach Test." *Journal of Strength and Conditioning Research* 8(1994):91.

Liemohn, W. S., et al. "Unresolved Controversies in Back Management." *Journal of Orthopaedic and Sports Physical Therapy* 9(1988):239.

Lightsey, D. M. "Deceptive Tactics Used in Marketing Purported Ergogenic Aids." *National Strength and Conditioning Association Journal* 14:2(1992):26.

Lightsey, D., and J. Attaway. "Deceptive Tactics Used in Marketing Purported Ergogenic Aids." *National Strength and Conditioning Association Journal* 14(1992):26.

Little, D. R. *Easy Stress-Reducing Strategies.* North Hollywood, CA: D. R. Little and Health Fair Expo, 1992.

Little, J. C. "The Athlete's Neurosis—A Deprivation Crisis." In M. H. Sacks, and M. L. Sachs, *Psychology of Running.* Champaign, IL: Human Kinetics Publishers, 1981.

Lohman, T. G. Houtkooper, L. H., and Going, S. B. "Body Fat Measurement Goes Hi-Tech." *ACSM's Health and Fitness Journal* 1(1)(1998):?.

Lox, C. L. et al. "Exercise as an Intervention for Enhancing Subjective Well-Being in an HIV-1 Population." *Journal of Sport and Exercise Psychology* 17(4)(1995):345.

Loy, S. F. et al. "Easy Grip on Body Composition Measures." *ACSM's Health and Fitness* 2(5)(1998):16.

Lubell, A. "Potentially Dangerous Exercises: Are They Harmful to All?" *Physician and Sportsmedicine* 17(1989):187.

Lyman, S. A. et al. "Date Rape Drugs a Growing Concern." *Journal of Health Education* 29(5)(1998):271.

Maddi, S. R. and Khoshaba, D. M. "Hardiness and Mental Health." *Journal of Personality Assessment* 63(1994), 265–274.

Maddux, J. E. "Habit, Health, and Happiness." *Journal of Sport & Exercise Psychology* 19(1997):331.

Magill, R. A. *Motor Learning: Concepts and Applications.* 5th ed. Dubuque, IA: McGraw-Hill, 1998.

Malmivaara, A., et al. "The Treatment of Acute Low Back Pain—Bed Rest, Exercise or Ordinary Activity." *New England Journal of Medicine* 332(1995):351.

Marcus, B. H. "Exercise Behavior and Strategies for Intervention." *Research Quarterly for Exercise and Sport* 66(1995):319.

Marcus, B. H. et al. "Longitudinal Shifts in Employee's Stages and Processes of Exercise Behavior Change." *American Journal of Health Promotion* 10(1997):1105.

Markowitz, M. "A Preliminary Study of Ritonavir, an Inhibitor of HIV-1 Protease, to Treat HIV." *New England Journal of Medicine* 333(1995):1534.

Marrugat, J. et al. "Mortality Differences Between Men and Women Following First Myocardial Infarction." Journal of the American Medical Association 280(16)(1998):1405.

Martin D. R. "Athletic Shoes: Finding a Good Match." *The Physician and Sports Medicine* 25(9)(1997):138.

Martin, D. R. "How to Steer Patients Toward the Right Sport Shoe." *Physician and Sports Medicine* 25(9)(1997):138.

Massara G., and F. Scoppa. "Proprioceptive Muscle Stretching." ICHPER. SD 31(Winter 1994–95):38.

Mayer-Davis, E. J. et al. "Intensity and Amount of Physical Activity in Relation to Insulin Sensitivity." *Journal of the American Medical Association* 279(9)(1998):669.

Mayers, D. L. et al. "Drug-Resistant HIV-1: The Virus Strikes Back." *Journal of the American Medical Association* 279(24)(1998):2000.

McCulley, K. S. "Homocysteine, Folate, Vitamin B6 and Cardiovascular Disease." *Journal of the American Medical Association* 279(5)(1998):392.

McGinnis, J. M., and P. R. Lee. "Healthy People 2000 at Mid Decade." *Journal of the American Medical Association* 273(1995):1123.

McKenzie, R. *The Lumbar Spine: Mechanical Diagnosis and Therapy.* Upper Hutt, New Zealand: Spinal Publications, Ltd., 1981.

McMurray, R. G., et al. "Is Physical Activity or Aerobic Power More Influential on Reducing Cardiovascular Disease Risk Factors?" *Medicine and Science in Sports and Exercise* 30(10)(1998):1521.

"Methamphetamine Abuse on Rise." *Orange County Register,* Nov. 30, 1995.

Mitchell, T. L. & Gibbons, L. W. "Controlling Blood Lipids: A Practical Role for Diet and Exercise." *Physician and Sports Medicine* 26(10)(1998):41.

Monahan, T. "Perceived Exertion: An Old Exercise Tool Finds New Applications." *Physician and Sportsmedicine* 16(1988):174.

Morbidity and Mortality Weekly Reports. Published Weekly by the Centers for Disease Control and Prevention, Provides Updated Information on Health, Available on the WEB at *www.cdc.gov.epo/mmwr/mmwr.html.*

Morey, M. C. et al. "Physical and Functional Limitations in Community Dwelling Older Adults." *Medicine and Science in Sports and Exercise* 30(5),(1998):715.

Morgan, G. T. and McGlynn, G. H. *Cross-Training for Sports.* Champaign, IL: Human Kinetics, 1997.

Mosher, P., et. al, "Effects of 12 Weeks of Aerobic Circuit Training on Aerobic Capacity, Muscular Strength and Body Composition in College-Age Women." *Journal of Strength and Conditioning Research* 8(3):144–48.

Narod, S. A. et al. "Oral Contraception and the Risk of Ovarian Cancer." *New England Journal of Medicine* 339(7)(1998):424.

National Center for Health Statistics. *Health, United States, 1998: With Socioeconomic Statistics and Health Chartbook.* Hyattsville, MD: National Center for Health Statistics, 1998.

National Council for Reliable Health Information Newsletter. Published every other month it contains articles that give objective information about health products and food supplements. NCRHI, P. O. Box 1276, Loma Linda, CA 92354.

National Institutes of Health Developmental Panel. "Acupuncture." *Journal of the American Medical Association* 280(17)(1998):1518.

National Institutes of Health, National Heart Lung and Blood Institute. *Exercise and Your Heart.* Dallas, TX: American Heart Association, 1993.

National Institutes of Health. Interventions to Prevent HIV Risk Behaviors, *NIH Consensus Statement.* 15(2)(1997):1.

NCAF Newsletter The New Dietary Supplement Laws. *NCAF Newsletter* 17(1994):1.

NCAHF Asks FTC to Stop Antioxidant Supplement Advertising." *National Council Against Health Fraud Newsletter* 17(July–August 1994):1.

Neck Exercises for a Healthy Neck. Daly City, CA: Krames Communications, 1990.

Nelson, B. W. et al., "The Clinical Effects of Intensive, Specific Exercise on Chronic Low Back Pain: A Controlled Study of 895 Consecutive Patients with 1-Year Follow-up." *Orthopedics* 18(1995), 971–981.

Newton, F. "The Stressed Out Student—How Can We Help?" *On Campus* (1998).

Nieman, D. C. "Moderate Exercise Boosts the Immune System." *ACSM's Health and Fitness Journal* 1(5)(1997):19.

Norkin, C., and P. Levangie. *Joint Structure and Function: A Comprehensive Analysis.* Philadelphia: F. A. Davis, Co., 1983.

O'Connor, P. J., and S. D. Youngstedt. "Influence of Exercise on Human Sleep." *Exercise and Sport Sciences Reviews* 23(1995):105.

O'Grady, D. *Taking the Fear Out of Change.* Rainier, WA: Adams Publishing, 1995.

Oakley, G. P., and J. D. Erickson. "Vitamin A and Birth Defects: Continuing Caution is Needed." *New England Journal of Medicine* 333(1995):1414.

Oja, P. "Descriptive Epidemiology of Health-Related Physical Activity and Fitness." *Research Quarterly for Exercise and Sport* 66(1995):303.

Oliveria, S. A. et al. "The Association Between Cardiorespiratory Fitness and Prostate Cancer." *Medicine and Science in Sports and Exercise* 28(1),(1996):97.

Olson, M. S. and Williford, H. N. "Step Aerobics Fulfills Its Promise: High on Fitness, Low on Impact." *ACSM's Health and Fitness Journal* 2(2)(1997):2.

Omenn, G. S., et al. "Effects of Combination of Beta Carotine and Vitamin A on Lung Cancer and Cardiovascular Disease." *The New England Journal of Medicine* 334(1996):1150.

Ortal, M. & Sherman, C. "Exercise Against Depression." *Physician and Sports Medicine* 26(10)(1998):55.

Osness, W. H. "Exercise and the Older Adult." Reston, VA: AAHPERD, 1998.

Ossness, W. and Mulligan, L. "Physical Activity and Depression in Older Adults." *Journal of Physical Education Recreation and Dance* 69(9)(1998):16.

Otis, C. L., Drinkwater, B., Johnson, M., Loucks, A., & Wilmore, J. "ACSM Position Stand on the Female Athlete Triad." *Medicine and Science in Sports and Exercise* 29(5)(1997):i.

Otis, C. L. "Too Slim, Amenorrheic, Fracture Prone: The Female Athlete Triad." *ACSM's Health and Fitness Journal* 2(1)(1998):20.

Painter, K. "Drug Cuts AIDS Death Nearly in Half." *USA Today* October 8, 1998, 1A.

Parish, S., et al. "Cigarette Smoking, Tar Yield and Non-Fatal Myocardial Infarction." *British Medical Journal* 333(1995):471.

Parrott, A. C., et al. "Anabolic Steroid Use by Amateur Athletes: Effects upon Psychological Mood States." *Journal of Sports Medicine and Physical Fitness* (1994):292.

Payne, V. G. et al. "Resistance Training in Children and Youth: A Meta Analysis." *ACSM's Health and Fitness* 2(3)(1998):11.

Payne, W. A. & Hahn, D. B. *Understanding Your Health* (5th ed.) St. Louis: WCB/McGraw-Hill, 1998.

Perrine, J. J., and R. V. Edgerton. "Muscle Force-Velocity and Power Velocity Relationships under Isokinetic Loading." *Medicine and Science in Sports and Exercise* 10(1978):159.

Pescatello, L. S. and Murphy, D. "Lower Intensity Physical Activity is Advantageous for Fat Distribution and Blood Glucose Among Viscerally Obese Older Women." *Medicine and Science in Sports and Exercise* 30(9), (1998):1408.

Peterson, J. A., Bryant, C. X., and Franklin, B. A. "50 Nifty Ways to Reduce Fat in Your Diet." *Fitness Management* 14(11)(1998):40.

Peterson, J. "10 Ways to Avoid Heat-Related Conditions While Exercising." *ACSM's Health and Fitness Journal* 2(3)(1998):48.

Peterson, K. S. "Smoke and Marriage Don't Always Go Together." *USA Today* December 28, 1998, ID.

Petruzzello, S. J., et al. "A Meta-Analysis on the Anxiety-Reducing Effects of Acute and Chronic Exercise: Outcomes and Mechanisms." *Sports Medicine* 11(1991):143–82.

Physical Activity and Cardiovascular Health: NIH Consensus, *Online,* 1995 December 18–20; 13(3):1–13.

Pierce, J. P. et al. "Tobacco Industry Promotion of Cigarettes and Adolescent Smoking." *Journal of the American Medical Association* 279(7)(1998):511.

Pinger, R., Payne, W. A., Hahn, D. B., and Hahn, E. J. *Drugs: Issues for Today* (3rd ed.). St. Louis: WCB/McGraw-Hill, 1998.

Plowman, S. A. "Physical Fitness and Healthy Low Back Function." In Corbin, C. B. & Pangrazi, R. P. (ed.) *Towards a Better Understanding of Physical Fitness and Activity.* Scottsdale, AZ: Holcomb-Hathaway, 1999, Chapter 13.

Pollock, M. L., et al. "Measurement of Cardiorespiratory Fitness and Body Composition in the Clinical Setting." *Comprehensive Therapy* 6(1980):12.

Pollock, M. J. and Evans, W. J. "Resistance Training for Health and Disease." *Medicine and Science in Sports and Exercise* 31(1),(1999):10.

Pollock, M. L. and Vincent, K. R. "Resistance Training for Health." In Corbin, C. B. & Pangrazi, R. P. (ed.). *Towards a Better Understanding of Physical Fitness and Activity.* Scottsdale, AZ: Holcomb-Hathaway, 1999, Chapter 14.

Pope, H. G., et al. "Muscle Dysmorphia: An Underrecognized Form of Body Dysmorphic Disorder." *Psychosomatics* 38(6)(1997):548.

Potter, J. D. "Fiber and Colorectal Cancer: Where to Now?" *New England Journal of Medicine* 340(3)(1999):223.

Powell, K. E. et al. "Injury Rates from Walking, Gardening, Weightlifting, Outdoor Bicycling, and Aerobics." *Medicine and Science in Sports and Exercise* 30(8),(1998):1246.

Powers, S. K., and E. T. Howley. *Exercise Physiology.* 3rd ed. Dubuque, IA: Brown & Benchmark Publishers, 1997.

Pratt, M. "Benefits of Lifestyle Activity Vs. Structured Exercise." *Journal of the American Medical Association* 281(4)(1999):375.

Prendergast, M. L. "Substance Abuse Among College Students: A Review of Recent Literature." *Journal of College Health* 43(1994):99.

Prevost, M. C. et al. "Creatine Supplementation Enhances Intermittent Work Performance." *Research Quarterly for Exercise and Sport* 68(3)(1997):233.

Prochaska, J. O. and Markus, B. H. "The Trans-Theoretical Model: Applications to Exercise." In *Advances in Exercise Adherence,* Dishman, R. K. (ed.). Champaign, IL: Human Kinetics.

Questioning 40/40/30: A Guide to Understanding Sports Nutrition Advice. A 22-page booklet published jointly by the American College of Sport Medicine, The American Dietetics Association, The Women's Sports Foundation and the Cooper Institute for Aerobics Research, 1997.

Raisz, L. G. & Prestwood, K. M. "Estrogen and the Risk of Fracture—New Data—New Quest." *New England Journal of Medicine* 339(11)(1998):767.

Ransdell, L. B., Snow, H., & Ostlund, D. "Metabolic Syndrome X: Postmenopausal Women's Hidden Nemesis." *Journal of Women and Aging* 9(1)(1997):53.

Rapola, J. M., et al. "Effects of Vitamin E and Beta Carotine on the Indicence of Angina Pectoris: A Randomized Double Blind Controlled Trial." *Journal of the American Medical Association* 275(1996):693.

"Red Wine No 'Magic Bullet' for Heart Disease." *Health Digest* (July/August 1992):9.

Reeves, R. K., Laskowski, E. R., & Smith, J. "Weight Training Injuries: Part I." *Physician and Sport Medicine* 26(2)(1998):54.

Reeves, R. K., Laskowski, E. R., & Smith, J. "Weight Training Injuries: Part II." *Physician and Sports Medicine* 26(3)(1998):46.

Reibe, D. & Nigg, C. "Setting the State for Healthy Living." *ACSM's Health and Fitness* 2(3)(1998):11.

Reim, E. B. et al. "Folate and Vitamin B6 from Diet and Supplements in Relation to Risk of CHD Among Women." *Journal of the American Medical Association* 279(5)(1998):359.

Rejeski, W. J., et al. "Physical Activity and Health-Related Quality of Life." *Exercise and Sport Sciences Reviews* 24(1996):71.

Rexrode, K. M. et al. "Abdominal Adiposity and Coronary Heart Disease in Women." *Journal of the American Medical Association* 28(21)(1999):1843.

Roche, A. F., Hyemsfield, S. B., & Lohman, T. G. *Human Body Composition.* Champaign, IL: Human Kinetics, 1996.

Roitman, J. L. (ed.) *ACSM's Resource Manual for Guidelines for Exercise Testing and Prescription* (3rd ed.). Baltimore, MD: Williams & Wilkins, 1998.

Rosamond, W. D. et al. "Trends in the Incidence of Myocardial Infarction and the Mortality Due to CHD." *New England Journal of Medicine* 339(13)(1998):861.

Rosenberg, P. S. & Biggar, R. J. "Trends in HIV Incidence Among Young Adults in the US." *Journal of the American Medical Association* 279(23)(1998):1894.

Rosenfeld, I. "Acupuncture Goes Mainstream (Almost)." *Parade* August 16 (1998): 10.

Rosenfeld, I. "For A Good Nights Sleep." *Parade* October 25 (1998):8.

Rosenfeld, I. "What is Normal Cholesterol Anyway?" *Parade* July 12 (1998):4.

Ross, R. "Mechanisms of Disease: Atherosclerosis and Inflammatory Disease?" *Journal of the American Medical Association* 340(3)(1999):115.

Rubin, R. "Measuring Up is Tricky." *USA Today* June 10, 1998, D1.

Sallis, J. F. et al. "Environmental and Policy Intervention to Promote Physical Activity." *American Journal of Preventive Medicine* 15(1998):379.

Sallis, J. F. "Influences of Physical Activity on Children, Adolescents, and Adults or Determinants of Physical Activity." In Corbin, C. B. & Pangrazi, R. P. (ed.), *Towards a Better Understanding of Physical Fitness and Activity* Scottsfale, AZ: Holcomb-Hathaway, 1999, Chapter 4.

Sandor, R. P. "Heat Illness." *Physician and Sports Medicine* 25(6)(1997):35.

Saris, W. H. M. "Fit, Fat and Fat Free: The Metabolic Effects of Weight Control." *International Journal of Obesity* 22(Supplement 22)(1998):S15.

Schneider, K. S., et al. "Mission Impossible: Too Fat? Too Thin?" *People* 145(22)(1996):65.

Schtleben, T. R. et al. "Serum Lipoprotein Patterns in Long-Term Anabolic Steroid Users." *Research Quarterly for Exercise and Sport* 68(1)(1996):110.

Schwenk, T. L. "Psychoactive Drugs and Athletic Performance." *Physician and Sports Medicine* 25(1)(1997):32.

"Secondhand Smoke: Is it a Hazard?" *Consumer Reports* 60:1(1995):142.

Seligman, M. E. P. "Building Human Strength: Psychology's Forgotten Mission." *APA Monitor* 29(1)(1998):2.

Shangold, M. M. (1998). "Beyond the Exercise Prescription: Making Exercise as Way of Life." *Physician and Sports Medicine* 26(11)(1998):35.

Shelton, et al. "State Laws on Tobacco Control—United States, 1995." *Morbidity and Mortality Weekly Report* 44(1995), 1–7.

Shephard, R. J. "Readiness for Physical Activity." *Physical Activity and Fitness Research Digest* 1(1994):1.

Shephard, R. J. "Preparing for Physical Activity." In Corbin, C. B. & Pangrazi, R. P. (ed.), *Towards a Better Understanding of Physical Fitness and Activity.* Scottsdale, AZ: Holcomb-Hathway, 1999, Chapter 1.

Shephard, R. "Par-Q, Canadian Home Fitness Test and Exercise Screening Alternatives." *Sports Medicine* 5(1988):185.

Shephard, R. "Physical Activity, Health and Well-Being at Different Life Stages." *Research Quarterly for Exercise and Sport* 66(1995):298.

Shipple, B. "Relieving Low Back Pain With Exercise." *Physician and Sports Medicine* 25(8)(1997):51.

Shipple, B. "Treating Low Back Pain: Exercise Knowns and Unknowns." *Physician and Sports Medicine* 25(8)(1997):67.

Simons-Morton, D. G. et al. "Effects of Interventions in Health Care Settings on Physical Activity or Cardiovascular Fitness." *American Journal of Preventive Medicine* 15(1998):413.

Singh, A., et al. "Chronic Multivitamin-Mineral Supplementation Does Not Enhance Physical Performance." *Medicine and Science in Sports and Exercise* 24(1992):726.

Sjodin, A. M. et al. "The Influence of Physical Activity on BMR." *Medicine and Science in Sports and Exercise* 28(1),(1996):85.

Slavin, J. L., et al. "Amino Acid Supplements: Beneficial or Risky?" *Physician and Sportsmedicine* 16(1988):221.

Smith, A. D. "The Fit Woman in the 21st Century." *The Physician and Sports Medicine* 26(1998):23.

Smith, E. L., and S. L. Zook. "The Aging Process: Benefits of Regular Physical Activity." *Journal of Physical Education, Recreation and Dance* 57(1986):32.

Smith, G. D. et al. "Mortality Differences Between Black and White Men in the USA." *Lancet* 351(9107):934.

Smith, L. L., et al. "The Effects of Static and Ballistic Stretching on Delayed Onset Muscle Soreness and Creatine Kinase." *Research Quarterly for Exercise and Sport* 64(1993):103.

Smith-Warner, S. A. "Alcohol and Breast Cancer in Women." *Journal of the American Medical Association* 279:(7)(1998):535.

Sparling, P. B. et al. "Development of a Cadence Curl-up Test for College Students." *Research Quarterly for Exercise and Sport* 68(1)(1997):110.

Sparling, P. B. "Field Testing for Abdominal Muscular Fitness." *ACSM's Health and Fitness Journal* 1(5)(1997):30.

Stephanick, M. L. et al. "Effects of Diet and Exercise in Men and Postmenopausal Women with Low Levels of HDL Cholesterol and High Levels of LDL." *New England Journal of Medicine* 340(1)(1999):12.

Storms, W. W. and Joyner, D. M. "Update on Exercise-Induced Asthma." *The Physician and Sports Medicine* 25(3)(1997):45.

Studdert, D. M. "Medical Malpractice: Implications of Alternative Medicine." *Journal of the American Medical Association* 280(1998):1610.

Stuhr, R. M. "Strategies for Beating the Barriers to Exercise for Women." *ACSM's Health and Fitness Journal* 2(5)(1998):20.

Surgeon General's Office. *Surgeon General's Report on Physical Activity and Health.* Washington, DC: U.S. Government Printing Office, (1996).

Teegarden, D. et al. "Previous Physical Activity Relates to Bone Mineral Measures in Young Women." *Medicine and Science in Sports and Exercise* 28(1),(1996):105.

"Teenagers and AIDS." *Newsweek* (August 3, 1992):44.

Terbizan, D. J. & Strand, B. "How Much Exercise?" *Fitness Management* 14(9)(1998):32.

"The Antioxidant Scare." *National Council Against Health Fraud Newsletter* 17(May–June 1994):1.

"Thigh Cream Fails Test." *National Council Against Health Fraud Newsletter* 18(1995).

Thomas, D. Q. et al. "Nasal Strips and Mouthpieces Do Not Effect Power Output During Anaerobic Exercise." *Research Quarterly for Exercise and Sport* 69(2)(1998):201.

Thomis, M. A. I. et al. "Strength Training: Importance of Genetic Factors." *Medicine and Science in Sports and Exercise* 30(5),(1998):725.

Tofler, I. R., et al. "Physical and Emotional Problems of Elite Female Gymnasts." *New England Journal of Medicine* 335(4)(1998):281.

Turner, E. E. et al. "Psychological Benefits of Physical Activity Are Influenced by the Social Environment." *Journal of Sport and Exercise Psychology* 19(2)(1997):119.

University of California at Berkeley Wellness Letter, "The Breathtaking Promises of Melatonin." *University of California at Berkeley Wellness Letter* 12(1996):1.

University of California at Berkeley Wellness Letter, "Thin Thighs in a Bottle." *University of California at Berkeley Wellness Letter* 10(1994):1.

University of California at Berkeley Wellness Letter, "Weight, Fate, Set Point and Counterpoint." *University of California at Berkeley Wellness Letter* 11(1995):1.

U.S. Department of Agriculture and U.S. Department of Health and Human Services. *Nutrition and Your Health: Dietary Guidelines for Americans* (4th ed.). Washington, DC: U.S. Department of Agriculture and U.S. Department of Health and Human Services, 1995.

U.S. Department of Health and Human Services. *Alcohol and Health.* Seventh Special Report to the U.S. Congress from the Secretary of Health and Human Services. NIAAA, Rockville, MD: 1990.

U.S. Department of Health and Human Services. *Healthy People 2010 Objectives: Draft for Comment.* Washington, DC: U.S. Department of Health and Human Services, 1998.

U.S. Department of Health and Human Services. *Physical Activity and Health: A Report of the Surgeon General.* Atlanta, GA: U. S. Department of Health and Human Services, 1996.

Van Loan, M. D. "What Makes Good Bones: Factors Affecting Bone Health." *ACSM's Health and Fitness Journal,* 2(4)(1998):27.

Volek, J. S. "Creatine Supplementation and Its Possible Role in Improving Physical Performance." *ACSM's Health and Fitness Journal* 1(4)(1997):23.

Volski, R. V., et al. "Lower Spine Screening in the Shooting Sports." *Physician and Sportsmedicine* 14(1986):101.

von Poppel, H. "Lumbar Supports and Education for Prevention of Low Back Pain in Industry." *Journal of the American Medical Association* 279(27)(1998):1789.

Vuori, I. "Exercise and Physical Health: Musculoskeletal Health and Functional Capacities." *Research Quarterly for Exercise and Sport* 66(1995):276.

Walker, L. S. et al. "Chromium Picolinate Effects On Body Composition and Muscular Performance in Wrestlers." *Medicine and Science in Sports and Exercise* 30(12),(1998):1730.

Wallace, J. P. "Exercise Can Reduce High Blood Pressure." *ACSM's Health and Fitness* 2(1)(1998):29.

Wallman, H. "Low Back Pain: Is It Really All Behind You? An Excellent 7-Step Abdominal Strengthening Program." *ACSM's Health and Fitness* 2(5)(1998):30.

Wardlaw, G. M., Insel, P. M., and Seyler, M. F. *Contemporary Nutrition* (2nd ed.). St. Louis: Mosby, 1994.

Wechsler, H. et al. "Increased Level of Cigarettes Use Among College Students: A Cause for National Concern." *Journal of the American Medical Association* 280(19)(1998):1673.

Weibe, D. J. "Hardiness and Stress Moderation: A Test of Proposed Mechanisms." *Journal of Personality and Social Psychology* 60(1991), 89–99.

Weinhouse, S., et al. "American Cancer Society Guidelines on Diet, Nutrition and Cancer." *CA- A Cancer Journal for Clinicians* 41(1991): 334.

Weinstock, C. P. "The Grazing of America: A Guide to Healthy Snacking." *FDA Consumer* 23(1989):8.

Weisfuse, I. B. "Gonorrhea Control and Antimicrobial Resistance." *Lancet* 352(9107)(1998):928.

Weitman, A., and B. Stamford. "Is Excessive Sweating Healthy?" *Physician and Sportsmedicine* 11(1983):195.

Wells, K. B., et al. "The Functioning and Well-Being of Depressed Patients." *Journal of the American Medical Association* 262(1989):914.

Wenger, N. K. and Drinkwater, B. L. (eds.) "Series of seven articles on Exercise and Heart Disease In Women." *Medicine and Science in Sports and Exercise* 28(1),(1996):3.

"We're Sticking by Our Beta-Carotene." *University of California at Berkeley Wellness Letter* 10(July 1994):1.

Wescott, W. L. *Strength Fitness: Physiological Principles and Training Techniques.* 4th ed. Dubuque, IA. Brown & Benchmark, 1995.

Wescott, W. L. and Baechle, T. R. *Strength Training for Seniors.* Champaign, IL: Human Kinetics, 1999.

Wescott, W. L. "How Long? How Often?" *Fitness Management* 14(7)(1998):48.

Whitehead, J. R. "Physical Activity and Intrinsic Motivation." In Corbin, C. B. & Pangrazi, R. P. (ed.). *Towards a Better Understanding of Physical Fitness and Activity.* Scottsdale, AZ: Holcomb-Hathaway, 1999, Chapter 5.

Willett, W. C. "Weight, Weight Change and CHD." *Journal of the American Medical Association* 273(1995):461.

Williams, M. H. *Nutrition for Sport and Fitness* 4th ed. St. Louis: WCB/McGraw-Hill, 1995.

Williams, M. "Nutrition Ergenics and Sport Performance." In Corbin, C. B. & Pangrazi, R. P. (ed.), *Towards a Better Understanding of Physical Fitness and Activity.* Scottsdale, AZ: Holcomb-Hathaway, 1999, Chapter 22.

Williams, P. C. *Low Back and Neck Pain: Causes and Conservative Treatment.* Springfield, IL: Charles C. Thomas, 1974.

Williams, R. & Williams, V. *Anger Kills: 17 Strategies for Controlling Hostility that Can Harm You.* New York: Times Books/Random House, 1994.

Williford, H. N., et al. "Is Low-Impact Aerobic Dance an Effective Cardiovascular Workout?" *Physician and Sportsmedicine* 17(1989):95.

Wilmore, J. H. & Costill, D. L. *Physiology of Sport and Exercise (2nd ed.).* Champaign, IL: Human Kinetics, 1999.

Wilmore, J. H. "Exercise, Obesity and Weight Control." In Corbin, C. B. & Pangrazi, R. P. (ed.). *Towards a Better Understanding of Physical Fitness and Activity.* Scottsdale, AZ: Holcomb-Hathaway, 1999, Chapter 16.

Wilt, T. J. *"Saw Palmetto Extracts for Treatment of Benign Prostatic Hyperplasia."* Journal of the American Medical Association 280(18)(1998):1604.

Winkley, M. A. et al. "Ethnic and Socioeconomic Differences in Cardiovascular Disease Risk Factors." *Journal of the American Medical Association* 280(4)(1998):356.

Wynder, E. L., et al. "High Fiber Intake: Indicators of a Healthy Lifestyle." Journal of the American Medical Association 275(1996):486.

Yesalis, C. E. & Cowart, V. S. *The Steroids Game.* Champaign, IL: Human Kinetics, 1998.

Young, J. C. "Exercise and Type II Diabetes." *ACSM's Health and Fitness* 2(3)(1998):24.

Youngstedt, S. D. "Does Exercise Truly Enhance Sleep?" *Physician and Sports Medicine* 25(10)(1997):72.

Zamula, E. "Back Talk: Advice for Suffering Spines." FDA Consumer 23(1989):28.

Zeni, A. I., et al. "Energy Expenditure With Indoor Machines." Journal of the American Medical Association 275(1996):1424.

Credits

Photos

Concept 1
CO1: © James Kay/Adstock Photos, p. 7 top left: © Charles B. Corbin, p. 7 top right: © Vic Bider/Photo Edit, p. 7 bottom right: © Bonnie Kamin/Photo Edit, p. 7 middle left: © David Young Wolff/Photo Edit, p. 7 bottom left, p. 8 top left: © David R. Frazier Photolibrary, p. 8 top middle: © Vic Bider/Photo Edit, p. 8 top right: Kevin Syms/David R. Frazier Photolibrary, p. 8 bottom left: Corel, p. 8 bottom middle: © Scott Stallard/The Image Bank, p. 8 bottom right: © David R. Frazier Photolibrary, p. 10: © David Frazier Photolibrary, p. 13: © Tony Freeman/Photo Edit

Concept 2
CO2: © Mark Ahn, p. 24: © Bob Daemmrich/Stock Boston, p. 28: © Tom McCarthy/Photo Edit

Concept 3
CO3: © Charles B. Corbin, p. 43: Charles B. Corbin

Concept 4
CO4: © Kevin Syms/David R. Frazier Photolibrary, p. 53: © David Young Wolff/Photo Edit.

Concept 5
CO5: © Richard Price/FPG, p. 62: © David Young Wolff/Photo Edit, p. 65: © David Madison, p. 69: © Tony Freeman/Photo Edit

Concept 6
CO6: © David Young Wolff/Photo Edit, p. 86: © Charles B. Corbin

Concept 7
CO7: ©Esbin Anderson/The Image Works, p. 97: © Randy Taylor/Leo de Wys, Inc., p. 99 left: © David Frazier Photolibrary, p. 99 right: Myrleen Ferguson/Photo Edit.

Concept 8
CO8: © Tefe Rakle/The Image Bank, p. 113 left: © Charles B. Corbin, p. 113 right: © Mark Ahn, p. 125 © Charles B. Corbin

Concept 9
CO9: © Corel, p. 132: © Keri Weatherly/Corbis, p. 136: © Tony Freeman/Photo Edit, p. 137 © Mark Ahn, p. 140: © Ken Akers/First Image West

Concept 10
CO10: © David Stocklein/Ad Stock, p. 147: © Corel

Concept 11
CO11: © Mark Ahn, p. 171: © Sue Benett/Ad Stock, p. 175 © Mark Ahn, p. 178: © Mark Ahn, p. 186: © David Stocklein/ Ad Stock, p. 198: © Charles B. Corbin

Concept 12
CO12: © Mark Ahn, p. 210: © Charles B. Corbin

Concept 13
CO13: James W. Kay/Ad Stock, p. 233 © Mark Ahn

Concept 14
CO14: Corel, p. 251, 253: Corel, p. 255: David R. Frazier Photolibrary, p. 258 Corel

Concept 15
CO15: © Charles B. Corbin, p. 277 © Charles B. Corbin, p. 278: © David R. Laurie, p. 281: © Bob Daemmrich/Stock Boston

Concept 16
CO16: © Novastock/Photo Edit, p. 312 Corel, p. 314: © John Coletti/Stock Boston, p. 318 Corel, p. 319 Joanne Scott/Greg Kidd, p. 322 © David R. Frazier Photolibrary

Concept 17
CO17: © Mark Ahn, p. 336: © Mark Ahn, p. 337: © Cindy Charles/Photo Edit

Concept 18
CO18: © Brian Bailey/Tony Stone Images, p. 350: © Spencer Grant/Photo Edit, p. 352: Roswell Angier/Stock Boston

Concept 19
CO19: © David Stocklein/Ad Stock, p. 366: © Gary A. Conner/Photo Edit, p. 367: © Michael Newman/Photo Edit

Concept 20
CO20: © Gary Buss/FPG, p. 388: © Dennis McDonald/Photo Edit

Concept 21
CO21: © Corel, p. 398: © Stacy Pick/Stock Boston

Concept 22
CO22: © Mike Howell/Leo de Wys, Inc., p. 414: © Richard Hutchings/Photo Edit, p. 415: Courtesy of Partnership for a Drug Free America

Concept 23
CO23: © David Frazier Photolibrary, p. 425: © David Frazier Photo Library, p . 426: CDC-Atlanta, GA.

Concept 24
CO24: © David Frazier Photolibrary, p. 435: © Larry Mulvehill/Photo Researchers, Inc., p. 438 © James A. Prince/Photo Researchers, Inc.

Concept 25
CO25: © David R. Laurie, p. 447: © Charles B. Corbin, p. 449: © B. Bachmann/Image Works, p. 451, 452: © Mark Ahn

Concept 26
CO26: © Myrleen Furgeson/Photo Edit, p. 466: David R. Frazier Photolibrary.

Index

Laboratory Worksheets